Exercise Physiology

**Theory and Application
to Fitness and Performance**

Exercise Physiology

Theory and Application
to Fitness and Performance

Scott K. Powers
University of Florida

Edward T. Howley
University of Tennessee—Knoxville

 Wm. C. Brown Publishers

Book Team

Editor *Chris Rogers*
Developmental Editor *Sue Pulvermacher-Alt*
Production Editor *David Welsh*
Art Editor *Janice M. Roerig*
Photo Editor *Michelle Oberhoffer*
Permissions Editor *Vicki Krug*
Visuals Processor *Joseph P. O'Connell*

 Wm. C. Brown Publishers

President *G. Franklin Lewis*
Vice President, Publisher *George Wm. Bergquist*
Vice President, Publisher *Thomas E. Doran*
Vice President, Operations and Production *Beverly Kolz*
National Sales Manager *Virginia S. Moffat*
Advertising Manager *Ann M. Knepper*
Marketing Manager *Kathy Law Laube*
Production Editorial Manager *Colleen A. Yonda*
Production Editorial Manager *Julie A. Kennedy*
Publishing Services Manager *Karen J. Slaght*
Manager of Visuals and Design *Faye M. Schilling*

The credits section for this book begins on page C-1, and is considered an extension of the copyright page.

Library of Congress Catalog Card Number: 89–45909

ISBN 0–697–00502–X

Printed in the United States of America by Wm. C. Brown Publishers, 2460 Kerper Boulevard, Dubuque, IA 52001

10 9 8 7 6 5 4 3 2

Brief Contents

Contents

Preface

*T*his book is intended for physical educators, coaches, physical therapists, and exercise specialists interested in exercise physiology, sports performance, adult fitness, or cardiopulmonary rehabilitation. The general aim of this text is to provide the student with an up-to-date understanding of the physiology of exercise. In addition, the book contains extensive practical applications, including work tests to evaluate cardiorespiratory fitness, and information on training for improvements in health-related fitness and performance.

This volume is intended for use in a one-semester, upper-level undergraduate or beginning graduate exercise physiology course. Clearly, the text contains more material than can be covered during a typical fifteen-week semester. This is by design. The book was written to be comprehensive in order to afford instructors a large degree of freedom to select the material that they consider most important for the makeup of their class.

Given the nature and complexity of the material, some exercise physiology texts fall short by being too abbreviated and poorly illustrated, while others are too detailed or too advanced. We have therefore attempted to write a textbook that is well illustrated and contains current information with sufficient detail for the interested student of exercise physiology. Features that make this book unique are described briefly in the following sections.

Contents and Organization

All topics in exercise physiology addressed within this text are presented in a contemporary fashion with up-to-date references provided. The text is divided into three sections: (1) Physiology of Exercise, (2) Physiology of Health and Fitness, and (3) Physiology of Performance. Section one (Physiology of Exercise) contains 13 chapters that provide the necessary background for the beginning student of exercise physiology to understand the role of the major organ systems of the body in maintaining homeostasis during exercise. Indeed, a major theme in section one of the book is that almost all organ systems of the body work to help maintain a relatively stable internal environment during exercise. Included in section one are chapters covering an overview of biological control systems, bioenergetics, exercise metabolism, endocrine function during exercise, techniques for measurement of work, power, and energy expenditure, neuromuscular function during exercise, cardiopulmonary responses to exercise, acid-base regulation during exercise, temperature regulation, and the effects of endurance training on various organ systems.

The chapters in the first section provide an up-to-date presentation of exercise physiology without consideration as to how that information is applied to fitness or performance. The purpose of the second and third sections of the text is to address these concerns. These last two sections distinguish between exercise programs that are appropriate for attainment of health-related fitness goals versus those needed to realize world-class or individual maximal performance goals. Section two of the text (Physiology of Health and Fitness) contains five chapters dealing with health-related fitness: (1) factors that limit health and fitness, (2) work tests used to evaluate cardiorespiratory fitness, (3) training methods for fitness, (4) exercise concerns for special populations, and (5) body composition and nutritional concerns for health.

Section three of the text includes seven chapters dealing with the physiology of performance: (1) factors affecting performance, (2) work tests to evaluate performance, (3) training techniques for improvement of performance, (4) training concerns for special populations, (5) nutrition, body composition, and performance, (6) environmental influences on performance, and (7) ergogenic aids. A unique aspect of sections two and three of the book is the inclusion of two chapters on exercise training for special populations. These chapters include discussions of exercise for women, asthmatics, diabetics, and the elderly.

Writing Style

The concepts in this text are presented in a simple and straightforward style. Illustrations and examples are commonly used to clarify or further explain a concept. Technical terms are defined as they are presented and are also organized in a glossary at the end of the book.

Pedagogical Aids

As an aid to help students study and learn the material within *Exercise Physiology,* the following pedagogical devices are included in the text:

1. Each chapter begins with a list of learning objectives.
2. A detailed outline of the topics to be discussed (with page references) is contained at the start of each chapter.
3. Key terms to be learned are listed at the front of each chapter.
4. Key terms are highlighted and defined in the text.
5. Most chapters include special or practical applications that are contained within a "box" format.
6. An outlined summary is found at the end of each chapter.
7. A list of study questions is included at the end of each chapter.
8. A suggested reading list and an up-to-date reference list is found at the completion of most chapters.
9. Supplementary appendices are included.
10. A glossary of terms is provided at the end of the book.

Ancillary Material

The following materials are available from Wm. C. Brown Publishers to supplement the use of this textbook in the teaching of exercise physiology:

1. *Instructor's Manual* by Scott K. Powers and Edward T. Howley. The Instructor's Manual provides a chapter-by-chapter overview of key concepts to be stressed by the instructor as well as a multiple choice test bank. The Instructor's Manual also provides suggestions for laboratory exercises and is free to adopters.
2. *Exercise Physiology Transparency Set.* Thirty-one transparency acetates are offered free to adopters of this text.

Acknowledgments

A text like *Exercise Physiology* is not the effort of two authors, but represents the contributions of hundreds of scientists throughout the world. While it is not possible to acknowledge every contributor to this work, we would like to recognize the following scientists who have greatly influenced our thinking, careers, and lives in general: Drs. Bruno Balke, Ralph Beadle, Ronald Byrd, Jerome Dempsey, Stephen Dodd, H. V. Forster, B. D. Franks, Steven Horvath, Henry Montoye, Francis Nagle, and Hugh G. Welch. Additional thanks is due to the following scholars who reviewed earlier drafts of this volume and offered comments for improvement that we trust they will recognize:

Phillip A. Bishop
University of Alabama

William Floyd
University of Wisconsin–LaCrosse

Robert Grueninger
Eastern Montana College

Craig G. Johnson
St. Mary's College

James H. Johnson
Smith College

Martin W. Johnson
Mayville State University

Francis J. Nagle
University of Wisconsin–Madison

Roberta L. Pohlman
Wright State University

Phil Watts
Northern Michigan University

Finally, we wish to offer thanks to our editors, Chris Rogers, Sue Pulvermacher-Alt, and David Welsh of Wm. C. Brown Publishers for their excellent support and cooperation during the writing of this work.

Scott K. Powers   Gainesville, Florida
Edward T. Howley   Knoxville, Tennessee

Dedicated to Lou and Ann
for their love, patience,
and support

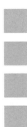

Section 1

Physiology of Exercise

1 Physiology of Exercise in the U.S.—Its Past, Its Future

Objectives

By studying this chapter, you should be able to do the following:

1. Name the three Nobel Prize winners whose research work involved muscle or muscular exercise.
2. Describe the role of the Harvard Fatigue Laboratory in the history of exercise physiology in the United States.
3. Describe factors influencing physical fitness in the United States over the past century.

Outline

*D*oes one have to have a "genetic gift" of speed to be a world-class runner, or is it all due to training? What happens to your heart rate when you take a fitness test that increases in intensity each minute? What changes occur in your muscles as a result of an endurance training program that allows you to run at faster speeds over longer distances? The answer to these and other questions are provided throughout this text. However, we go beyond simple statements of fact to try and show how information about physiology of exercise is applied to the prevention of and rehabilitation from coronary heart disease, the performances of elite athletes, and the ability of a person to work in adverse environments such as high altitudes. The recent acceptance of terms such as *sports physiology, sports nutrition,* and *sports medicine* is evidence of the growth of interest in the application of physiology of exercise to real-world problems. Before we take you on this journey, a brief look at our past is needed to understand where we are and where we are going.

European Heritage

A good starting place to discuss the history of exercise physiology in the United States is in Europe. Three scientists, A. V. Hill of Britain, August Krogh of Denmark, and Otto Meyerhof of Germany, received Nobel Prizes for research on muscle or muscular exercise (4). Hill, who is well known for his work on O_2 debt, introduced the term "maximal oxygen intake" in 1924 as a description of the upper limit of performance. We will discuss both of these topics in detail in later chapters. Meyerhof is recognized for his work in the metabolism of glucose, which can lead to the production of lactic acid, a factor long implicated in fatigue. While Krogh received his Nobel Prize for his research on capillary circulation, he is also known for designing a considerable amount of instrumentation used in exercise physiology research: a precise gas analyzer to measure CO_2 within 0.001%, and a precision balance to weigh human subjects within a few grams (8) are but two examples. The August Krogh Institute in Denmark contains some of the most prominent exercise physiology laboratories in the world.

There are several other European scientists who must be mentioned, not only because of their contributions to the physiology of exercise, but also because their names are commonly used in a discussion of exercise physiology. J. S. Haldane did some of the original work on the role of CO_2 in the control of breathing. Haldane also developed the respiratory gas analyzer that bears his name (8). C. G. Douglas did pioneering work with Haldane in the role of O_2 and lactic acid in the control of breathing during exercise, including some work conducted at various altitudes. The canvas-and-rubber gas collection bag used for many years in exercise physiology laboratories around the world carries Douglas' name. A contemporary of Douglas, who did the classic work on how O_2 binds to hemoglobin, was Christian Bohr of Denmark. The "shift" in the oxygen–hemoglobin dissociation curve due to the addition of CO_2 bears his name. It was in Bohr's lab that Krogh got his start on a career studying respiration and exercise in humans (8).

Harvard Fatigue Laboratory

A focal point in the history of exercise physiology in the United States is found in the Harvard Fatigue Laboratory. Professor L. J. Henderson organized the laboratory within the Business School to conduct

Table 1.1 Active research areas in the Harvard Fatigue Laboratory

Metabolism
   Maximal oxygen uptake
   Oxygen debt
   Carbohydrate and fat metabolism during long-
      term work
Environmental physiology
   Altitude
   Dry and moist heat
   Cold
Clinical physiology
   Gout
   Schizophrenia
   Diabetes
Aging
   Basal metabolic rate
   Maximal oxygen uptake
   Maximal heart rate
Blood
   Acid-base balance
   O_2 saturation: role of PO_2, PCO_2, and carbon
      monoxide
Nutrition
   Nutritional assessment techniques
   Vitamins
   Foods
Physical fitness
   Harvard step test

physiological research on industrial hazards. Dr. David Bruce Dill was the research director from the time the laboratory opened in 1927 until it closed in 1947 (11). Table 1.1 shows that the laboratory conducted research in numerous areas, in the laboratory and in the field, and the results of those early studies have been supported by recent investigations. Dill's classic text, *Life, Heat, and Altitude* (7), is recommended reading for any student of exercise and environmental physiology. Much of the careful and precise work of the laboratory was conducted using the now-classic Haldane analyzer for respiratory gas analysis and the van Slyke apparatus for blood-gas analysis. The advent of computer-controlled equipment in the 1980s has made data collection easier, but has not improved on the accuracy of measurement.

The Harvard Fatigue Laboratory attracted doctoral students as well as scientists from other countries. Many of the alumni from the laboratory are recognized in their own right for excellence in research in the physiology of exercise. Two doctoral students, Steven Horvath and Sid Robinson, went on to distinguished careers at the Institute of Environmental Stress in Santa Barbara, and at Indiana University, respectively. Foreign "Fellows" included E. Asmussen, E. H. Christensen, M. Nielsen, and the Nobel Prize-winner August Krogh from Denmark. These scientists brought new ideas and technology to the lab, participated in laboratory and field studies with the other staff members, and published some of the most important work in the physiology of exercise between 1930–1980. Rudolpho Margaria, from Italy, went on to extend his classic work on oxygen debt, and describe the energetics of locomotion. Peter F. Scholander, from Norway, gave us his chemical gas analyzer that is now the primary method of calibrating tank gas used to standardize electronic gas analyzers (11). (See figure 1.1.)

In summary, under the leadership of Dr. D. B. Dill, The Harvard Fatigue Laboratory became a model for research investigations into exercise and environmental physiology, especially as it relates to humans. When the laboratory closed and the staff dispersed, the ideas, techniques and approaches to scientific inquiry were distributed throughout the world, and with them, Dill's influence in the area of environmental and exercise physiology. Dr. Dill continued his research outside Boulder City, Nevada into the 1980s. He died at the age of 93 in 1986.

Physical Fitness

Physical fitness is a popular topic today and its popularity has been a major factor in motivating college students to pursue careers in physical education, physiology of exercise, health education, nutrition, physical therapy, and medicine. In 1980 the Public Health Service listed "physical fitness and exercise" as one of fifteen areas of concern related to improving the country's overall health (22). While this might appear to be an unprecedented event, similar interests and concerns

Figure 1.1 Comparison of old and new technology used to measure oxygen consumption and carbon dioxide production during exercise. (*Top:* The Carnegie Institute of Washington, D.C.; *Bottom:* Quinton Instrument Co.)

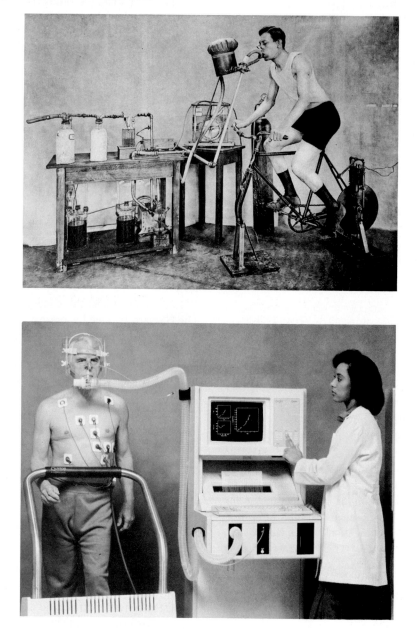

about physical fitness existed in this country over 100 years ago. Between the Civil War and WWI physical education was primarily concerned with the development and maintenance of fitness, and many of the leaders in physical education were trained in medicine (5, p. 5). For example, Dr. Dudley Sargent, hired by Harvard University in 1879, set up a physical training program with individual exercise prescriptions to improve an individual's structure and function to achieve "that prime physical condition called fitness—fitness for work, fitness for play, fitness for anything a man may be called upon to do" (25, p. 297).

While Sargent was clearly ahead of his time in promoting health-related fitness, a primary force driving this country's interest in physical fitness was war. Concerns about health and fitness were raised during WWI and WWII when large numbers of draftees failed the induction exams due to mental and physical defects (10, p. 407). These concerns influenced the type of physical education programs in the schools during these years, making them resemble pre-military training programs (27, p. 484).

The present interest in physical activity and health was stimulated in the early 1950s by two major findings: (a) autopsies of young soldiers killed during the Korean War showed significant coronary artery disease to be already developed and (b) Hans Kraus showed that American children performed poorly on a minimal muscular fitness test compared to European children (27, p. 516). Due to the latter finding, President Eisenhower initiated a conference in 1955 that resulted in the formation of the President's Council on Youth Fitness. The American Association for Health, Physical Education, and Recreation (AAHPER) supported these activities and in 1957 developed the AAHPER Youth Fitness Test with national norms to be used in physical education programs throughout the country. Before he was inaugurated, President Kennedy expressed his concerns about the nation's fitness in an article published in *Sports Illustrated,* called "The Soft American" (15).

For the physical vigor of our citizens is one of America's most precious resources. If we waste and neglect this resource, if we allow it to dwindle and grow soft, then we will destroy much of our ability to meet the great and vital challenges which confront our people. We will be unable to realize our full potential as a nation.

During Kennedy's term the council's name was changed to the President's Council on Physical Fitness, to highlight the concern for fitness. The council experienced another name change in the Nixon administration to the current President's Council on Physical Fitness and Sports, which supports fitness, not only in the school, but also in business and industry. Items in the Youth Fitness Test were changed over the years and in 1980 the AAHPER published a separate *Health-Related Physical Fitness Test Manual* (1) to distinguish between "performance testing" (e.g., fifty-yard dash) and "fitness testing" (e.g., skinfold thickness). This health-related test battery is consistent with the direction of lifetime fitness programs, being concerned with obesity, cardiorespiratory fitness, and low-back function. Unfortunately, this new health-related fitness test has not been as readily accepted by physical education professionals as one might have expected.

Paralleling this interest in the physical fitness of youth was the rising concern about the death rate from coronary heart disease in the middle-aged American male population. Epidemiological studies of the health status of a population underscored the fact that degenerative diseases related to poor health habits (e.g., high fat diet, smoking, inactivity) were responsible for more deaths than the classic infectious and contagious diseases. In 1966 a major symposium highlighted the need for more research in the area of physical activity and health (23). In the 1970s there was an increase in the use of exercise tests to diagnose heart disease and to aid in the prescription of exercise programs to improve cardiovascular health. Large corporations developed "executive" fitness programs to improve the health status of that high-risk group. While most Americans are now familiar with such programs and some students of exercise physiology seek careers in "Corporate Fitness," such programs are not new. The following photos, taken from the 1923 edition of McKensie's *Exercise in Education and Medicine* (18),

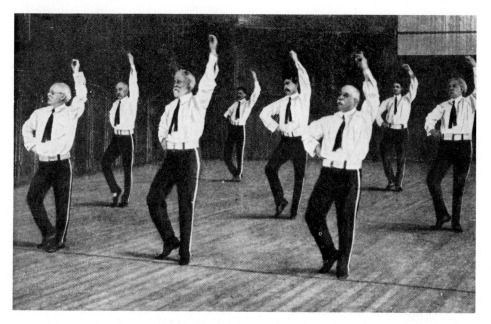

show a group of businessmen in costume doing dance exercises (figure 1.2), and fitness facilities on the roof of a large inner-city department store (figure 1.3). In short, the idea that regular physical activity is an important part of a healthy life-style has been "rediscovered."

Science in Physical Education

Undergraduate academic preparation in physical education has changed over the past two decades to represent the scientific knowledge base that is needed to deal with the issues related to fitness, performance, and skill acquisition. There has been an increase in the number of physical education programs requiring undergraduates to take one year of calculus, chemistry, and physics, and courses in organic chemistry, biochemistry, anatomy, physiology, and nutrition. In many colleges and universities, there is now little difference between the first two years of requirements in a prephysical therapy or pre-medical track and the physical education track associated with fitness and exercise physiology. The differences among these tracks relate to the "application" courses that follow: kinesiology, physiology of exercise, fitness assessment, exercise prescription, exercise leadership, etc., belonging to the latter track. However, it must again be pointed out that this new trend is but another example of a rediscovery of old roots rather than a revolutionary change. Kroll describes two four-year professional physical education programs in the 1890s, one at Stanford and the other at Harvard, that were the forerunners of today's programs (16, pp. 51–64). They included the detailed scientific work and application courses with clear prerequisites cited. Finally, considerable time was allotted for laboratory work. No doubt Lagrange's 1890 text, *Physiology of Bodily Exercise* (17), served as an important reference source for these students. The expectations and goals of those programs were more or less identical to the current exercise physiology undergraduate tracks. In fact, one of the aims of the Harvard program was to allow a student to pursue the study of medicine after completing two years of study (16, p. 61).

Figure 1.3 Roof of the John Wanamaker store, Philadelphia, showing running track, basketball, and tennis courts.

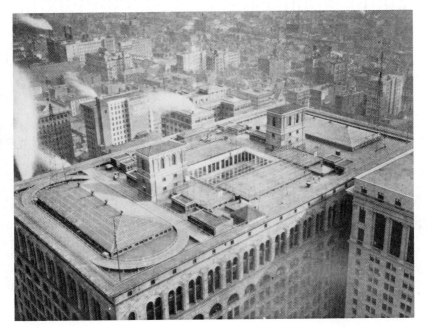

Graduate Study and Research in the Physiology of Exercise

While the Harvard Fatigue Laboratory was closing in 1947, the country was on the verge of a tremendous expansion in the number of universities offering graduate study and research opportunities in exercise physiology. In a 1950 survey, only sixteen colleges or universities had research laboratories in departments of physical education (12). By 1966, 151 institutions had research facilities, fifty-eight of them in exercise physiology (27, p. 526). This expansion was due to the availability of more scientists trained in the research methodology of exercise physiology, the increased number of students attending college due to the GI Bill and student loans, and the increase in federal dollars to improve the research capabilities of universities.

"The scholar's work will be multiplied many fold through the contribution of his students." This quote, taken from Montoye and Washburn (21) expresses a view that has helped attract researchers and scholars to universities. Evidence to support this quote was presented in the form of genealogical charts of contributors to the *Research Quarterly* (20). These charts showed the tremendous influence a few people had through their students in the expansion of research in physical education. Probably the best example of this is Thomas K. Cureton, Jr. of the University of Illinois, a central figure in the training of productive researchers in exercise physiology and fitness. The Illinois Research Laboratory dates from 1944 (16, pp. 177–83) and it focused attention on the physiology of fitness. The *Proceedings* of a symposium honoring Cureton in 1969 listed the sixty-eight Ph.D. students who completed their work under his direction (9). While Cureton's scholarly record includes hundreds of research articles and dozens of books dealing with physical fitness, the publications of his students in the areas of epidemiology, fitness, cardiac rehabilitation, and exercise physiology represent the "multiplying effect" that students have on a scholar's productivity.

An example of a major university program that can trace its lineage to the Harvard Fatigue Laboratory is found at Pennsylvania State University. Dr. Ancel Keys, a staff member at the Harvard Fatigue Laboratory, brought Henry Longstreet Taylor back to the Laboratory for Physiological Hygiene at the University of Minnesota, where he received his Ph.D. in 1941. Taylor subsequently advised the research work of Elsworth R. Buskirk, who designed and directs the Laboratory for Human Performance Research (Noll Laboratory) at Pennsylvania State University. Noll Laboratory continues in the tradition of the Harvard Fatigue Laboratory with a comprehensive research program of laboratory and field research into basic exercise, environmental, and industrial research questions (3). However, it is clear that excellent research in exercise and environmental physiology is conducted in laboratories other than those that have a tie to the Harvard Fatigue Lab. Laboratories are found in physical education departments, physiology departments in medical schools, clinical medicine programs at hospitals, and in independent facilities like the Cooper Clinic. The proliferation and specialization of research involving exercise is discussed in the next section.

Professional Societies and Research Journals

The expansion of interest in exercise physiology and its application to fitness and rehabilitation resulted in an increase in the number of professional societies where scientists and clinicians could present their work. Prior to 1950 the two major societies concerned with physiology of exercise and its application were the American Physiological Society (APS) and the American Alliance of Health, Physical Education, and Recreation (AAHPER). The need to bring together physicians, physical educators, and physiologists interested in physical activity and health into one professional society resulted in the incorporation of the American College of Sports Medicine (ACSM) in 1955. The ACSM now has more than 11,000 members with regional chapters throughout the country, each holding its own annual meeting to present research, sponsor symposia and promote sports medicine. Since 1980 there has been an increase in the

numbers of professional societies to meet the needs of practitioners involved in fitness (e.g., Association for Fitness in Business) and cardiopulmonary rehabilitation (e.g., American Association of Cardiovascular and Pulmonary Rehabilitation).

The growth of research journals has paralleled the increased number of professional societies. During the time of the Harvard Fatigue Laboratory much of the research was published in the following journals: *Journal of Biological Chemistry, American Journal of Physiology, Arbeitsphysiologie* (European Journal of Occupational and Applied Physiology), *Journal of Clinical Investigation, Journal of Aviation Medicine, Journal of Nutrition,* and *Journal of Physiology.* In 1948 the American Physiological Society published the *Journal of Applied Physiology* to bring together the research work in exercise and environmental physiology. In 1969 the American College of Sports Medicine published the research journal *Medicine and Science in Sports* to support the growing productivity of its members. In the past ten years the *International Journal of Sports Medicine, Sports Medicine,* and *Journal of Cardiopulmonary Rehabilitation* have been introduced to report and review research.

One of the clear consequences of this increase in research activity is the degree to which scientists are having to specialize in order to be competitive for research grants and to manage the research literature. Laboratories may focus on neuromuscular physiology, cardiac rehabilitation, or the influence of exercise on bone structure. Graduate students are having to specialize earlier in their careers as researchers, and undergraduates must investigate graduate programs very carefully to make sure they meet their career goals (13).

This specialization in research has generated comments about the need to emphasize "basic" research examining the mechanisms underlying a physiological issue rather than "applied" research, which might describe responses of persons to exercise, environmental, or nutritional factors. It would appear that both types of research are needed and, to some extent, such a separation is arbitrary. For example, one scientist might study the interaction of exercise intensity and diet on muscle hypertrophy, another may characterize the changes in muscle cell size and contractile protein, a

Box 1.1 Bruno Balke

Given the introduction to this chapter, it should be no surprise that some scientists who have had an impact on the present state of exercise physiology, fitness, and cardiac rehabilitation in the United States received their training in Europe. Dr. Bruno Balke received his training in medicine and physical education in Germany, and was invited to this country by Dr. Ulrich Luft in 1950. During the 1950s he did research on high-altitude tolerance and high-speed flight for the Civil Aeromedical Research Institute and the United States Air Force. His research on work capacity testing on the treadmill led to the development of the exercise test protocols that bear his name. In addition, his distance-run field test to evaluate cardiovascular fitness (maximal aerobic power) was modified by Ken Cooper for use in the well-known *Aerobics* book (6).

Balke was active in the early days of the American College of Sports Medicine (ACSM), serving as its president in 1966. He was a prime mover in the development of the ACSM certifications for exercise leaders of fitness and cardiac rehabilitation programs (see later discussion) and was actively involved in the teaching and practical examinations associated with those certification workshops.

Balke left government service in 1963 to create the Biodynamics Laboratory at The University of Wisconsin, Madison. Francis J. Nagle followed in 1964, and both had joint appointments with the physical education and physiology departments. Balke's quantitative approach to human physiological questions, especially as they related to fitness and performance, set the standard for other graduate exercise physiology programs. Balke enjoyed teaching others how to do things and viewed as his greatest accomplishment the graduation of the Ph.D. students from his lab who would now teach others (14). As of 1987, fifty-two Ph.D. students were graduated from the Biodynamics Program (19). This is another example of how a scholar's work is multiplied by his or her students.

---

third might study changes in the energetics of muscle contraction relative to cytoplasmic enzyme activities, and a fourth might study gene expression needed to synthesize that contractile protein. Where does "applied" research begin and "basic" research end? In the introduction to his text on *Human Circulation* (24), Loring Rowell quoted T. H. Huxley, which bears on this issue.

I often wish that this phrase "applied science," had never been invented. For it suggests that there is a sort of scientific knowledge of direct practical use, which can be studied apart from another sort of scientific knowledge, which is of no practical utility, and which is termed "pure science." But there is no more complete fallacy than this. What people call applied science is nothing but the application of pure science to particular classes of problems. It consists of deductions from those principles, established by reasoning and observation, which constitute pure science. No one can safely make these deductions until he has a firm grasp of the principles; and he can obtain that grasp only by personal experience of the operations of observation and of reasoning on which they are found. (Huxley, 1948)

It is clear that we are moving along a continuum from the role of exercise in the prevention of disease in whole populations (epidemiology) to the domain of a cell biologist. We hope that all forms of inquiry are supported by fellow scientists such that present theories related to exercise physiology are continually questioned and modified. Lastly, we completely agree with the sentiments expressed in a quote ascribed to Arthur B. Otis: "Physiology is a good way to make a living and still have fun." (26)

Translation of Exercise Physiology to the Consumer

Some of the practical implications of the "fitness boom" include an increase in the number of "health spas" offering fitness or weight-control programs, and an explosion in the number of diet and exercise books selling easy ways to shed pounds and inches. It is clear that there has been and continues to be a need to provide correct information to the consumer about the "facts" related to exercise and weight control, and to provide some guidelines about the qualities to look for in an instructor associated with health and fitness programs. Most readers are familiar with the videotapes and books based on fitness programs of movie stars and are also aware that some of what is offered may not be very sound. Fortunately, there are a number of well-known scientists and scholars in the area of exercise physiology and fitness who are now writing "popular" books related to fitness issues.

Concern over the qualifications of fitness instructors has been addressed by professional societies that offer "certification programs" for those interested in a career in fitness programming. The American College of Sports Medicine (ACSM) provided a leadership role in this area by initiating certification programs in 1975 for those involved in cardiac rehabilitation programs. These certifications include that of the Preventive and Rehabilitation Program Director, Preventive and Rehabilitation Exercise Specialist, and the Exercise Test Technologist. Later, in response to the needs of those fitness personnel who conduct exercise programs for the apparently healthy individual, the ACSM developed the following certification programs: Exercise Leader/Aerobics, Health/Fitness Instructor, and Health/Fitness Director. These certification programs are based on sets of behavioral objectives describing what the candidate must know. The exams are recognized nationwide by those involved in fitness programs as imparting a high standard of professional achievement (2).

Colleges and universities have also responded to this need by the consumer to have qualified personnel direct exercise and weight-control programs. Many physical education departments offer undergraduate and graduate courses to train students for a career in fitness and cardiac rehabilitation programs, or for advanced graduate study leading to a career in research and teaching at the university level. The growth in these programs occurred at the same time that there was a glut in the job market for physical education positions in the public schools. The colleges and universities had simply overproduced physical education teachers at a time when teaching positions were decreasing. One can only hope that as more and more colleges and universities develop these undergraduate fitness tracks that the quality of the graduate will be maintained and the market will not be saturated. On the other hand, the increase in the number of well-educated people who can provide quality programming for the apparently healthy individual might be properly timed for the expected teacher shortage in the school systems in the 1990s.

Summary

1. Three physiologists, A. V. Hill, August Krogh, and Otto Meyerhof received the Nobel Prize for work related to muscle or to muscular exercise.

2. The Harvard Fatigue Laboratory is a focal point in the development of exercise physiology in the United States. Dr. D. B. Dill directed the laboratory from its opening in 1927 until its closing in 1947. The body of research in exercise and environmental physiology produced by that laboratory forms the basis of much of what we know today.

3. Fitness has been an issue in this country from the latter part of the 19th century until the present. The presence of war has exerted a strong influence on fitness programs in the public schools. Recent interest in fitness is related to the growing concern over the high death rates from disease processes due to preventable factors, like diet, exercise, and smoking. The government and professional organizations have responded to this need by educating the public about these problems. Schools are now using health-related fitness tests such as the skinfold estimation of body

fatness, rather than the more traditional performance tests, to evaluate a child's physical fitness.

4. Colleges and universities have responded to this interest in fitness by including a thorough preparation in the sciences in undergraduate physical education programs. Undergraduates can now take advanced study in exercise physiology, fitness, and cardiac rehabilitation at numerous universities. This expansion of graduate study has resulted in an increase in the number of research studies and scholarly journals that publish them. In addition, there has been an increase in the number of professional societies to meet the needs of these individuals.

5. In order to meet the needs of the consumer for correct information and programs about physical activity and health, university and college physical education departments have developed new areas of study in exercise physiology and fitness. Organizations like the American College of Sports Medicine have developed certification programs to establish a standard of knowledge and skill to be achieved for those who lead health-related exercise programs.

Study Questions

1. Name the three Nobel Prize winners whose research involved muscle or muscular exercise.
2. Who directed the Harvard Fatigue Laboratory?
3. What were some of the forces driving the fitness movement in the first half of the 20th century?
4. Compared to the first half of the 20th century, what factors or events in the latter half triggered a renewed interest and concern about physical fitness?
5. Identify three professional organizations and four research journals that support the work of those in exercise physiology, fitness, and cardiac rehabilitation.

Suggested Readings

Cannon, W. B. 1965. *The Way of an Investigator.* New York: Hafner.
Hill, A. V. 1966. *Trails and Trials in Physiology.* Baltimore: The Williams & Wilkins Company.

References

1. American Alliance for Health, Physical Education, Recreation and Dance. 1980. *Lifetime Health Related Physical Fitness: Test Manual.* Reston, Va.: American Alliance for Health, Physical Education, Recreation and Dance.
2. American College of Sports Medicine. 1986. *Guidelines for Exercise Testing and Prescription,* 3d ed. Philadelphia: Lea & Febiger.
3. Buskirk, E. R. 1987. Personal communication based on "Our extended family: Graduates from the Noll Lab for Human Performance Research." Noll Laboratory, Pennsylvania State University, University Park, Pa. 16802
4. Chapman, C. B., and J. H. Mitchell. 1965. The physiology of exercise. *Scientific American* 212:88–96.
5. Clarke, H. H., and D. H. Clarke. 1978. *Developmental and Adapted Physical Education.* Englewood Cliffs, N.J.: Prentice-Hall, Inc.
6. Cooper, K. H. 1968. *Aerobics.* New York: Bantam Books.
7. Dill, D. B. 1938. *Life, Heat, and Altitude.* Cambridge, Mass.: Harvard University Press.
8. Fenn, W. O., and H. Rahn, eds. 1964. *Handbook of Physiology: Respiration,* Volume 1. American Physiological Society, Washington, D.C.
9. Franks, B. Don. 1969. *Exercise and Fitness 1969.* Chicago, Ill.: The Athletic Institute.
10. Hackensmith, C. W. 1966. *History of Physical Education.* New York: Harper & Row, Publishers.
11. Horvath, S. M., and E. C. Horvath. 1973. *The Harvard Fatigue Laboratory: Its History and Contributions.* Englewood Cliffs, N.J.: Prentice-Hall, Inc.
12. Hunsicker, P. A. 1950. A survey of laboratory facilities in college physical education departments. *Research Quarterly* 21:420–23.

13. Ianuzzo, D., and R. S. Hutton. 1987. A prospectus for graduate students in muscle physiology and biochemistry. *Sports Medicine Bulletin* 22:17–18, The American College of Sports Medicine, Indianapolis.

14. Jackson, M. A. 1977. Bruno Balke welcomes—and creates—avalanches. *Physician and Sportsmedicine* 7:93–98.

15. Kennedy, J. F. 1960. The Soft American. *Sports Illustrated* 13:14–17.

16. Kroll, W. P. 1971. *Perspectives in Physical Education.* New York: Academic Press.

17. Lagrange, F. 1890. *Physiology of Bodily Exercise.* New York: D. Appleton and Company.

18. McKenzie, R. T. 1923. *Exercise in Education and Medicine.* Philadelphia: W.B. Saunders Company.

19. Montoye, H. J. 1987. Personal communication based on The University of Wisconsin Alumni Class Roster. Department of Physical Education and Dance, The University of Wisconsin, Madison.

20. Montoye, H. J., and R. Washburn. 1980. Research quarterly contributors: An academic genealogy. *Research Quarterly for Exercise and Sport* 51:261–66.

21. Montoye, H. J., and R. Washburn. 1980. Genealogy of scholarship among academy members. *The Academy Papers,* Washington, D.C.: AAHPERD 13:94–101.

22. Powell, K. E., and R. S. Paffenbarger. 1985. Workshop on epidemiologic and public health aspects of physical activity and exercise: A summary. *Public Health Reports* 100:118–26.

23. Proceedings of the International Symposium on Physical Activity and Cardiovascular Health. 1967. *Canadian Medical Association Journal* 96:695–915.

24. Rowell, L. B. 1986. *Human Circulation: Regulation During Physical Stress.* New York: Oxford University Press.

25. Sargent, D. A. 1906. *Physical Education.* Boston: Ginn and Co.

26. Stainsby, W. N. 1987. Part two: "For what is a man profited?" *Sports Medicine Bulletin* 22:15. The American College of Sports Medicine, Indianapolis.

27. Van Dalen, D. B., and B. L. Bennett. 1971. *A World History of Physical Education: Cultural, Philosophical, Comparative,* 2d ed. Englewood Cliffs, N.J.: Prentice-Hall, Inc.

2 Control of the Internal Environment

Objectives

*B*y studying this chapter, you should be able to do the following:
1. Define the terms homeostasis and steady state.
2. Diagram and discuss a biological control system.
3. Give an example of a biological control system.
4. Explain the term *negative feedback*.
5. Define what is meant by the gain of a control system.

Outline

Key Terms

biological control system
effector
gain
homeostasis
integrating center
negative feedback
receptor
steady state

If you had a body temperature of 100° F while sitting at rest, you would know that something is wrong. As children we learned that normal body temperature is 98.6° F and that values above or below normal signify a problem. How does the body manage to maintain core temperature within a narrow range? Further, how is it that during exercise, when the body is producing great amounts of heat, that we generally do not experience overheating problems? What keeps body temperature fairly normal?

Over a hundred years ago the French physiologist Claude Bernard observed that the "melieu interior" (internal environment) of the body remained remarkably constant despite a changing external environment. The fact that the body manages to maintain a relatively constant internal environment in spite of various stressors such as exercise, heat, cold, or fasting is not an accident but the result of many complex control systems. Control mechanisms that are responsible for maintenance of a stable internal environment constitute a major chapter in exercise physiology, and it is helpful to examine their function in light of simple control theory. Therefore, the purpose of this chapter is to introduce the concept of "control systems" and to discuss how the body maintains a rather constant internal environment during periods of stress.

Homeostasis: Dynamic Constancy

The term **homeostasis** was coined by Walter Cannon in 1932 and is defined as the maintenance of a constant or unchanging internal environment. A similar term, **steady state,** is often used by exercise physiologists to denote a steady physiological environment. Although the terms steady state and homeostasis are often used interchangeably, homeostasis generally refers to a relatively constant internal environment during unstressed conditions resulting from many compensating regulatory responses (1, 10, 11). In contrast, a steady state does not necessarily mean that the internal environment is completely normal, but simply that it is unchanging. In other words, a balance has been achieved between the demands placed on the body and the body's response to those demands. An example that is useful in distinguishing between these two terms is the case of body temperature during exercise. Figure 2.1 illustrates the changes in body core temperature during sixty minutes of constant-load submaximal exercise in a thermoneutral environment (i.e., low humidity and low temperature). Note that core temperature reaches a new and steady level within forty minutes after commencement of exercise. This plateau of core temperature represents a steady state since temperature is constant; however, this constant temperature is above the normal resting body temperature and thus does not represent a true homeostatic condition. Therefore, the term homeostasis is generally reserved for describing normal resting conditions, and the term steady state is often applied to exercise where the physiological variable in question is unchanging but may not equal the "true" resting value.

Although the concept of homeostasis means that the internal environment is unchanging, this does not mean that the internal environment remains absolutely constant. In fact, most physiological variables vary around some "set" value and thus homeostasis represents a rather dynamic constancy. An example of this dynamic constancy is the carbon dioxide concentration (called tension or pressure) in arterial blood. Figure

Figure 2.1 Changes in body core temperature during sixty minutes of submaximal exercise in a thermoneutral environment. Note that body temperature reaches a plateau by thirty-five to forty-five minutes of exercise.

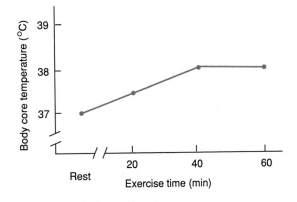

Figure 2.2 Changes in arterial CO_2 tension across time during normal breathing. Notice that although the arterial CO_2 tension oscillates across time, the mean CO_2 tension remains unchanged.

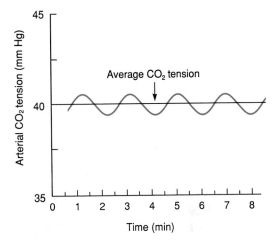

2.2 shows the change in CO_2 pressure in arterial blood across time. Note the oscillatory change in arterial CO_2 pressure, but the mean (average) CO_2 pressure remains around 40 mm Hg. The reason such an oscillation occurs in physiological variables is probably related to the "feedback" nature of biological control systems, which will be discussed later in the chapter (7, 9, 15).

Control Systems of the Body

The body has literally hundreds of different control systems, and the overall goal of most is to regulate some physiological variable at or near a constant value (6, 10, 16). The most intricate of these control systems resides inside the cell itself and acts to regulate cellular activities such as protein breakdown and synthesis, energy production, and maintenance of the appropriate amounts of stored nutrients. Almost all organ systems of the body work to help maintain homeostasis. For example, the lungs (pulmonary system) and heart (circulatory system) work together to replenish oxygen and to remove carbon dioxide from the extracellular fluid. The fact that the cardiopulmonary system is usually able to maintain normal levels of oxygen and carbon dioxide even during periods of strenuous exercise is not an accident but the end result of a good control system.

Nature of the Control Systems

To develop a better understanding of how the body maintains a stable internal environment, let's begin with an analogy of a simple nonbiological control system such as a thermostat-regulated heating and cooling system in a home. Suppose the thermostat is set at 20° C. Any change in room temperature away from the 20° C "set point" results in the appropriate response by either the furnace or the air conditioner to return the room temperature back to 20° C. If the room temperature rises above the set point, the thermostat signals the air conditioner to start, which returns the room temperature to 20° C. In contrast, a decrease in temperature below the set point results in the thermostat signaling the heating system to begin operation (figure 2.3). In both cases the response by the heating or cooling systems was to correct the condition, low or high temperature, that initially turned it on.

A **biological control system** can be defined as a series of interconnected components that serve to maintain a physical or chemical parameter of the body constant (10, 17). The general components of a biological control system are: (1) receptor, (2) integrating center, and

Figure 2.3 A thermostat-controlled heating/cooling system. An increase in temperature above the "set point" signals the air conditioner to turn on. In contrast, a decrease in room temperature below the set point results in turning on the furnace. This system illustrates a nonbiological control system.

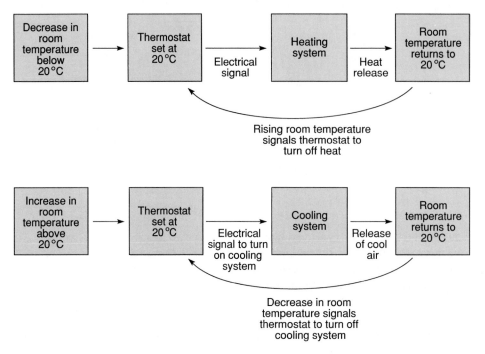

(3) effector. Figure 2.4 represents the schema of such a control system. The signal to begin the operation of a control system is the stimulus (i.e., some detectable change in the environment), such as temperature, blood pressure, etc. The stimulus excites a **receptor** (component capable of detecting change of the variable in question), which sends a message to the **integrating center,** which can be thought of as a control box. The integrating center assesses the strength of the stimulus and sends an appropriate output message to a component known as the **effector,** which is concerned with correcting the disturbance by responding in a manner that changes the internal environment back to normal. The return of the internal environment towards normal results in a decrease in the original stimulus that triggered the initial control system's response. This type of feedback is termed negative feedback and is discussed in detail in the next section.

Negative Feedback

Most control systems of the body operate via **negative feedback** (2, 7). An example of negative feedback can be seen in the respiratory system's regulation of the CO_2 concentration in extracellular fluid. In this case, an increase in extracellular CO_2 above normal levels triggers a receptor, which sends information to the respiratory control center (intregrating center) to increase breathing. The effector in this example is the respiratory muscles. This increase in breathing will lower extracellular CO_2 concentrations back to normal, thus reestablishing homeostasis. The reason that this type of feedback is termed negative is that the response of the control system is negative (opposite) to the stimulus.

Figure 2.4 Schematic of the components that comprise a biological control system. The process begins with a change in the internal environment (stimulus), which excites a receptor to send information about the change to an integrating control center. The integrating center makes an assessment of the amount of response needed to correct the disturbance and sends the appropriate message to the effector. The effector is responsible for correcting the disturbance and thus the stimulus is removed.

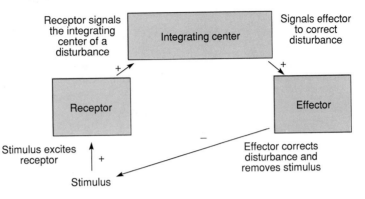

Gain of a Control System

The precision with which a control system maintains homeostasis is termed the gain of the system. **Gain** can be thought of as the amount of amplification of the system. A control system with a large gain is more capable of correcting alterations in homeostasis than a system with a low gain. The gain of a negative feedback control system is defined as the ratio of the amount of correction needed to maintain homeostasis to the amount of the abnormality that exists after correction by the system (7):

$$\text{Gain} = \frac{\text{Amount of correction needed}}{\text{Amount of abnormality that exists after correction}}$$

Consider the following example of the feedback gain of the temperature control system during exposure to cold. Suppose a person dressed in shorts leaves a comfortable room (i.e., 22° C) and enters a cold room (i.e., 0° C) for a twenty-minute stay. Upon entering the cold room the person's body temperature is 37° C, but after twenty minutes it had decreased to 36° C. During cold exposure various control systems automatically decrease skin blood flow to minimize heat loss, and initiate shivering to increase heat production, which prevents body temperature from decreasing drastically. The feedback gain of this control system can be calculated as follows:

$$\text{Feedback gain} = \frac{22° \text{ C} - 0° \text{ C}}{37° \text{ C} - 36° \text{ C}} = \frac{22}{1} = 22$$

A high feedback gain of twenty-two means that for each degree change in body temperature that occurs during this type of cold exposure, there would be twenty-two times greater change in temperature if it were not for the control system! It is not surprising that the temperature control system has a high gain given the importance of maintaining a reasonably constant body temperature.

Examples of Homeostatic Control

As an aid to better understand biological control systems, consider a few examples of homeostatic control.

Regulation of Arterial Blood Pressure

An excellent illustration of homeostatic control that uses negative feedback is the "baroreceptor system," which is responsible for the regulation of blood pressure. The baroreceptors are pressure-sensitive receptors located in the carotid arteries and the arch of the aorta. When arterial pressure increases above normal levels, these baroreceptors are stimulated and nerve

Figure 2.5 Example of negative feedback mechanism to lower blood pressure. A similar mechanism helps to increase blood pressure if it decreases below normal.

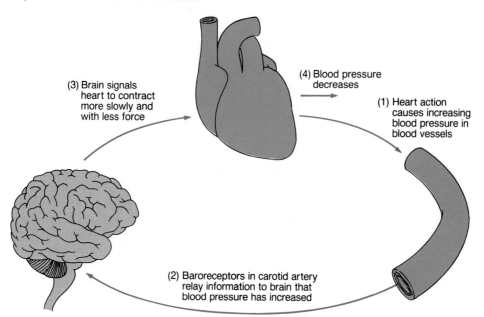

(3) Brain signals heart to contract more slowly and with less force

(4) Blood pressure decreases

(1) Heart action causes increasing blood pressure in blood vessels

(2) Baroreceptors in carotid artery relay information to brain that blood pressure has increased

impulses are transmitted to the cardiovascular control center in the medulla of the brain. In turn, the cardiovascular control center decreases the number of impulses transmitted to the heart, which lowers the amount of blood pumped by the heart and arterial pressure returns to normal (figure 2.5). In contrast, a reduction in arterial pressure reduces the number of impulses transmitted from the baroreceptors to the brain, which causes the cardiovascular control center to increase the number of impulses transmitted to the heart to produce an increase in blood pressure (7).

Regulation of Blood Glucose

Homeostasis is also a function of the endocrine system (chapter 5). The body contains eight major endocrine glands, which synthesize and secrete blood-borne chemical substances called hormones. Hormones are transported via the circulatory system throughout the body as an aid to regulate circulatory and metabolic functions (2, 8). For instance, the hormone insulin regulates cellular uptake and the metabolism of glucose and is therefore important in the regulation of the blood glucose concentration. After a large carbohydrate meal, blood levels of glucose increase above normal. This rise in blood glucose signals the pancreas to release insulin, which then acts to lower blood glucose by increasing cellular uptake. Likewise, a low blood glucose level results in decreased insulin release, which serves to reduce glucose uptake (figure 2.6).

Exercise: A Test of Homeostatic Control

Muscular exercise can be considered a dramatic test of the body's homeostatic control systems since exercise has the potential to disrupt many homeostatic variables. For example, during heavy exercise skeletal muscle produces large amounts of lactic acid, which causes an increase in intracellular and extracellular acidity (4, 12, 13, 18). This increase in acidity represents a serious challenge to the body's acid-base control system (3, 5) (chapter 11). Additionally, heavy exercise results in large increases in muscle O_2 requirements and large amounts of CO_2 are produced. These changes must be countered by increases in breathing (pulmonary ventilation) and blood flow to

Figure 2.6 Illustration of the regulation of blood glucose concentration. Changes in blood glucose concentration from the normal range regulate insulin secretion. Insulin, in turn, acts to regulate blood glucose levels (completing the negative feedback loop) and to maintain homeostasis. In this system the Islets of Langerhans in the pancreas are both the sensors and the effector organs. They sense the change in blood glucose from normal and release insulin appropriately.

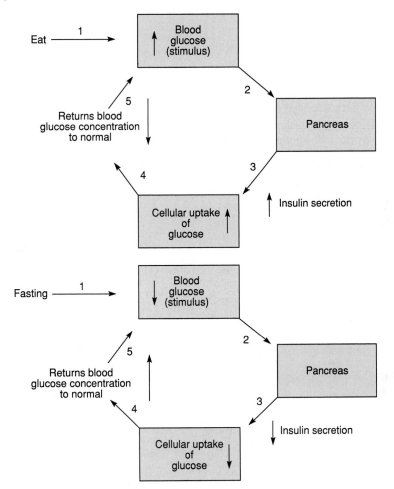

increase O_2 delivery to the exercising muscle and remove metabolically produced CO_2. Further, during heavy exercise the working muscles produce large amounts of heat that must be removed to prevent overheating. The body's control systems must respond rapidly to prevent drastic alterations in the internal environment.

In a strict sense, the body rarely maintains true homeostasis while performing intense exercise or during prolonged exercise in a hot/humid environment. Heavy exercise or prolonged work results in disturbances in the internal environment that are generally too great for even the highest gain control systems to overcome and thus a steady state is not possible. Specific details concerning individual control systems (i.e., circulatory, respiratory, etc.), which affect the internal environment during exercise, are discussed in chapters 4–12.

Summary

1. Homeostasis is defined as the maintenance of a constant or unchanging internal environment. The body's hundreds of control systems function to maintain homeostasis. A biological control system is composed of a receptor, an integrating center, and an effector. Most control systems act by way of negative feedback.

2. The degree with which a control system maintains homeostasis is termed the gain of the system. Gain can be defined mathematically as the following ratio:

$$\text{Gain} = \frac{\text{Amount of correction needed}}{\text{Amount of abnormality that exists after correction}}$$

3. Exercise represents a test of the body's ability to maintain homeostasis. In general, the body's many control systems are capable of maintaining a steady state during most types of submaximal exercise in a cool environment. However, intense exercise or prolonged work in a hostile environment (i.e., high temperature/humidity) may exceed the ability of a control system to maintain a steady state.

Study Questions

1. Define the term homeostasis. How does the term homeostasis differ from the term steady state?
2. Cite an example of a biological homeostatic control system.
3. Draw a simple diagram that demonstrates the relationships between the components of a biological control system.
4. Briefly, explain the role of the receptor, the integrating center, and the effector organ in a biological control system.
5. Explain the term negative feedback. Give a biological example of negative feedback.
6. Discuss the concept of gain associated with a biological control system.

Suggested Readings

Guyton, Arthur. 1986. *Textbook of Medical Physiology.* Philadelphia: Saunders Company.

Jones, R. 1973. *Principles of Biological Regulation: An Introduction to Feedback Systems.* New York: Academic Press.

Toates, F. 1975. *Control Theory in Biology and Experimental Psychology.* London: Hutchinson Education Ltd.

References

1. Adolph, E. 1968. *Origins of Physiological Regulations.* New York: Academic Press.
2. Asterita, M. 1985. *Physiology of Stress.* New York: Human Sciences Press.
3. Brooks, G., and T. Fahey. 1984. *Exercise Physiology: Human Bioenergetics and its Applications.* New York: John Wiley & Sons.
4. Edwards, R. H. T. 1983. "Biochemical Bases of Fatigue in Exercise Performance: Catastrophe Theory of Muscular Fatigue." In *Biochemistry of Exercise.* Champaign, Ill.: Human Kinetics Publishers.
5. Fox, S. 1984. *Human Physiology.* Dubuque, Ia.: Wm. C. Brown.
6. Frisancho, A. 1979. *Human Adaptation.* St. Louis. C. V. Mosby.
7. Guyton, Arthur. 1986. *Textbook of Medical Physiology.* Philadelphia: W. B. Saunders Company.
8. Hole, J. 1984. *Human Anatomy and Physiology.* Dubuque, Ia.: Wm. C. Brown.
9. Iyengar, S. 1984. *Computer Modeling of Complex Biological Systems.* Boca Raton, Fla.: CRC Press.
10. Jones, R. 1973. *Principles of Biological Regulation: An Introduction to Feedback Systems.* New York: Academic Press.
11. Mason, E. 1983. *Human Physiology.* Reading, Mass.: Benjamin Cummings.
12. Poortmans, J. 1983. "The Intracellular Environment in Peripheral Fatigue." In *Biochemistry of Exercise.* Champaign, Ill.: Human Kinetics Publishers.
13. Sahlin, K. 1983. "Effects of Acidosis on Energy Metabolism and Force Generation in Skeletal Muscle." In *Biochemistry of Exercise.* Champaign, Ill.: Human Kinetics Publishers.

14. Schmidt-Nielson, K. 1983. *Animal Physiology: Adaptation and Environment.* London: Cambridge University Press.

15. Spain, J. 1982. *Basic Microcomputer Models in Biology.* London: Addison-Wesley Publishing Company.

16. Toates, F. 1975. *Control Theory in Biology and Experimental Psychology.* London: Hutchinson Education Ltd.

17. Vander, S., J. Sherman, and D. Luciano. 1985. *Human Physiology.* New York: McGraw-Hill.

18. Vollestad, N., and O. Sejersted. 1988. Biochemical correlates of fatigue. *European Journal of Applied Physiology* 57:336–37.

3 *Bioenergetics*

Objectives

*B*y studying this chapter, you should be able to do the following:
1. Discuss the function of the cell membrane, nucleus, and mitochondria.
2. Define the following terms: (1) endergonic reactions, (2) exergonic reactions, (3) coupled reactions, (4) first and second law of thermodynamics, and (5) bioenergetics.
3. Describe the role of enzymes as catalysts in cellular chemical reactions.
4. List and discuss the nutrients that are used as fuels during exercise.
5. Identify the high-energy phosphates.
6. Discuss the biochemical pathways involved in anaerobic ATP production.
7. Discuss the aerobic production of ATP.
8. Describe the general scheme used to regulate metabolic pathways involved in bioenergetics.
9. Discuss the interaction between aerobic and anaerobic ATP production during exercise.
10. Identify the enzymes that are considered rate limiting in glycolysis and the Krebs cycle.

Outline

Key Terms

adenosine diphosphate (ADP)
adenosine triphosphate (ATP)
aerobic
anaerobic
ATPase
ATP–CP system
bioenergetics
cell membrane
coupled reactions
creatine phosphate (CP)
cytoplasm
electron transport chain
endergonic reactions
energy of activation
enzymes
exergonic reactions
FAD
glucose
glycogen
glycogenolysis
glycolysis

inorganic
inorganic phosphate (Pi)
isocitrate dehydrogenase
Krebs cycle
lactic acid
mitochondrion
NAD
nucleus
organic
oxidative phosphorylation
phosphofructokinase

All cells possess the capability to convert foodstuffs (i.e., fats, proteins, carbohydrates) into a biologically useable form of energy. This process is termed **bioenergetics** and is of major interest to sports physiologists and physical educators. In order to run, jump, or swim, skeletal muscle cells must be able to continuously extract energy from food nutrients. In fact, the inability to transform energy contained in foodstuffs into useable biological energy would limit performance in endurance activities. The explanation for this is simple. In order to continue to contract, muscle cells must have a continuous source of energy. When energy is not readily available, muscular contraction is not possible and thus work must stop. Therefore, given the importance of cellular energy production during exercise, it is critical that the student of exercise physiology develop a thorough understanding of bioenergetics. It is the purpose of this chapter to introduce both general and specific concepts associated with bioenergetics.

Cell Structure

Cells were discovered in the 17th century by the English scientist Robert Hook. Advancements in the microscope over the past 300 years have led to improvements in our understanding of cell structure and function. In order to understand bioenergetics, it is important to have some appreciation for the structure of the cell. Four elements (an element is a basic chemical substance) compose over 95% of the human body. These most common elements are oxygen (65%), carbon (18%), hydrogen (10%), and nitrogen (3%) (12, 28). Additional elements found in rather small amounts in the body include sodium, iron, zinc, potassium, and

calcium. These various elements are linked together by chemical bonds to form molecules or compounds. Compounds that contain carbon are called **organic** compounds while those that do not contain carbon are termed **inorganic.** For example, water (H_2O) lacks carbon and is thus inorganic. In contrast, proteins, fats, and carbohydrates contain carbon and are organic compounds.

As the basic functional unit of the body, the cell is a highly organized factory capable of synthesizing the large number of compounds necessary for normal cellular function. Figure 3.1 illustrates the structure of a typical cell. Note that all cells are not alike nor do they perform the exact same functions. The hypothetical cell pictured in figure 3.1 simply illustrates parts of cells that are contained in most cell types found in the body. In general, cell structure can be divided into three major parts:

1. **Cell membrane.** The cell membrane is a semipermeable barrier that separates the cell from the extracellular environment. The two most important functions of the cell membrane are to enclose the components of the cell and to regulate the passage of various types of substances in and out of the cell (12, 18).

2. **Nucleus.** The nucleus is a large, round body within the cell that contains the cellular genetic components (genes). The nucleus functions to regulate protein synthesis, which determines cell composition and controls cellular activity.

3. **Cytoplasm** (called sarcoplasm in muscle cells). This is the fluid portion of the cell between the nucleus and the cell membrane. Contained

Figure 3.1 A typical cell and its major organelles.

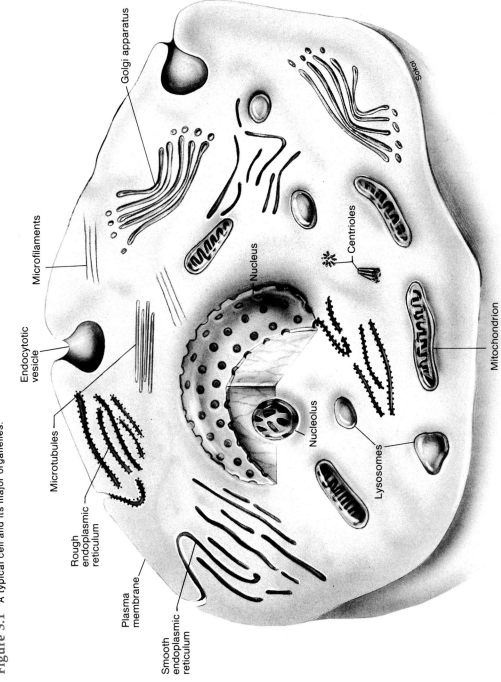

Golgi apparatus

Sokol

Microfilaments

Centrioles

Nucleus

Endocytotic vesicle

Mitochondrion

Microtubules

Nucleolus

Rough endoplasmic reticulum

Lysosomes

Plasma membrane

Smooth endoplasmic reticulum

within the cytoplasm are various organelles (minute structures) that are concerned with specific cellular functions. One such organelle, the **mitochondrion** is often called the powerhouse of the cell and is involved in the oxidative conversion of foodstuffs into useable cellular energy.

Biological Energy Transformation

In a broad sense, bioenergetics refers to the flow of energy in living systems. Cells must maintain a highly ordered structure in order to perform life-sustaining functions using energy obtained from their environment. The following discussion focuses upon those physical laws that govern bioenergetics.

Thermodynamics

The energy flow in living systems obeys the first and second laws of thermodynamics. According to the first law of thermodynamics, energy cannot be created nor destroyed, but can be changed from one form to another (2, 26). This law is sometimes called the "law of conservation of energy" and is familar to most of us. The second law of thermodynamics asserts that as a result of energy transformations, the universe and its components (i.e., living systems) have increased amounts of disorder (called entropy) (12, 24). Only energy that is in an organized state (called free energy) can be used to perform useful work. This means that entropy increases as a result of every energy transformation in the cell, and, as a result, the amount of free energy decreases. Therefore, according to the second law of thermodynamics, systems tend to go from a state of higher free energy to one of lower free energy (12).

Cellular Chemical Reactions

Energy transfer in the body occurs via the releasing of energy trapped within chemical bonds of various molecules. Chemical bonds that contain relatively large amounts of potential energy are often referred to as "high energy bonds." As mentioned previously, bioenergetics is concerned with the transfer of energy from foodstuffs into a biologically useable form. This energy transfer in the cell occurs as a result of a series of chemical reactions. Many of these reactions require that energy be added to the reactants (**endergonic reactions**) before the reaction will "go." However, since energy is added to the reaction, the products contain more free energy than the original reactants.

Reactions that give off energy as a result of the chemical process are known as **exergonic reactions.** Figure 3.2 illustrates that the amount of energy released via exergonic reactions is the same whether the energy is released in one single reaction or many small, controlled steps that usually occur in cells.

Coupled Reactions

Many of the chemical reactions that occur within the cell are called **coupled reactions.** Coupled reactions are reactions that are linked together, with the liberation of free energy in one reaction being used to "drive" a second reaction. Figure 3.3 illustrates this point. In this example, energy released by an exergonic reaction is being used to drive an energy-requiring reaction (endergonic reaction) in the cell. This is like two meshed gears in which the turning of one (energy releasing, exergonic gear) causes the movement of the second (endergonic gear). In other words, energy-liberating reactions are "coupled" to energy-requiring reactions.

Enzymes

The speed of chemical reactions that occur in the body is regulated by catalysts called **enzymes.** Enzymes are proteins that play a major role in the regulation of metabolic pathways in the cell. Enzymes do not cause a reaction to occur, but simply regulate the rate or speed at which the reaction takes place. Further, the enzyme does not change the nature of the reaction nor its final result.

Chemical reactions occur when the reactants have sufficient energy to proceed. The energy required to initiate chemical reactions is called the **energy of activation** (5, 28). Enzymes work as catalysts by lowering the energy of activation. The end result is to increase the rate at which these reactions take place. Figure 3.4 illustrates this concept. Note that the energy of activation is greater in the noncatalyzed reaction on the left when compared to the enzyme-catalyzed reaction pictured in the right. By reducing the energy of

Figure 3.2 The breakdown of glucose into carbon dioxide and water via cellular oxidation results in a release of energy. Reactions that result in a release of free energy are termed exergonic.

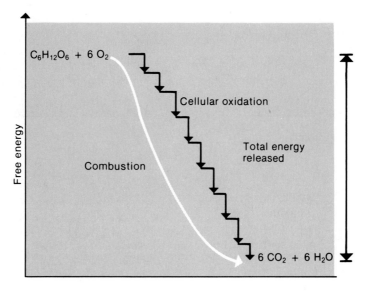

Figure 3.3 Model showing the coupling of exergonic and endergonic reactions. Note that the energy given off by the exergonic reaction (driveshaft) powers the endergonic reactions (smaller gear).

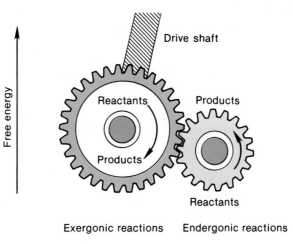

Figure 3.4 Enzymes catalyze reactions by lowering the energy of activation. That is, the energy required to start the reaction is reduced. Note the difference in the energy of activation in the catalyzed reaction versus the noncatalyzed reaction.

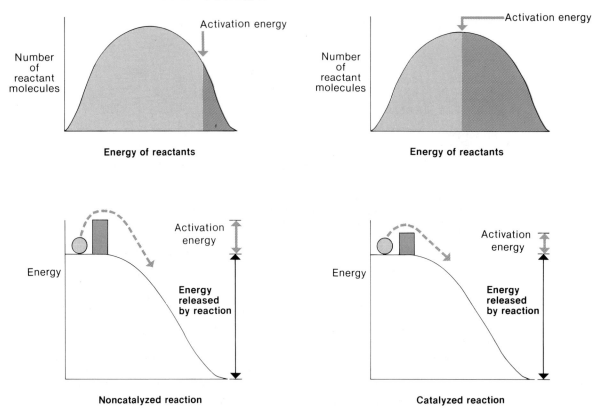

activation, enzymes increase the number of molecules that have sufficient energy to participate in the reaction and thus the reaction speed increases.

The ability of enzymes to lower the energy of activation results from unique structural characteristics. In general, enzymes are rather large protein molecules with a three-dimensional shape. Each type of enzyme has characteristic ridges and grooves. The pockets that are formed from the ridges or grooves located on the enzyme are called active sites. These active sites are important since it is the unique shape of the active site that causes a specific enzyme to adhere to a particular reactant molecule (called a substrate). The concept of how enzymes fit with a particular substrate molecule is analogous to the idea of a lock and key (figure 3.5).

The shape of the enzyme's active site is specific for the shape of a particular substrate, which allows the two molecules (enzyme + substrate) to form a complex known as the enzyme-substrate complex. After formation of the enzyme-substrate complex, the energy of activation needed for the reaction to occur is lowered and the reaction is more easily brought to completion. This is followed by the dissociation of the enzyme and the product.

Although there is a standardized naming system for enzymes, most textbooks use common names that generally reflect the job category of the enzyme and the reaction it catalyzes. Almost all enzyme names end with the suffix "ase." For example, kinases are a group of enzymes that add phosphate groups to the sub-

Figure 3.5 Lock-and-key model of enzyme action. See text for details.

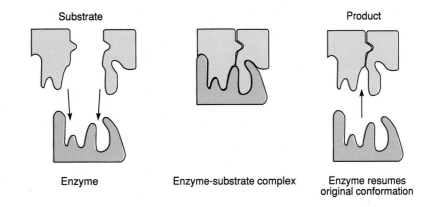

Substrate   Product

Enzyme   Enzyme-substrate complex   Enzyme resumes
                                                  original conformation

Box 3.1 Factors that Alter Enzyme Activity

The activity of an enzyme, as measured by the rate at which its substrates are converted into products, is influenced by a variety of factors. Two of the more important factors include the temperature and pH (pH is a measure of acidity) of the solution.

Individual enzymes have an optimum temperature at which they are most active. In general, a small rise in body temperature increases the activity of most enzymes. This is useful during exercise since muscular work results in an increase in body temperature. The resulting elevation in enzyme activity would enhance bioenergetics (ATP production) by speeding up the rate of reactions involved in the production of biologically useful energy. In contrast, a decrease in temperature or a large increase in temperature results in a decrease in enzyme activity.

The pH of body fluids has a profound effect on enzyme activity. The relationship between pH and enzyme activity is similar to the temperature/enzyme activity relationship; that is, individual enzymes have a pH optimum. If the pH is altered from the optimum, the enzyme activity is reduced. This has important implications during exercise. For example, during intense exercise the concentration of lactic acid increases in body fluids. Lactic acid is a relatively strong acid and results in a decrease in the pH of body fluids away from the optimum pH of most enzymes involved in bioenergetics. The end result is a decreased ability to provide a biologically useful form of energy for muscular contraction. In fact, extreme acidity is an important limiting factor in various types of intense exercise. This will be discussed in detail in chapter 19.

strates with which they react. Further, dehydrogenases are enzymes that remove hydrogens from their substrates. An example of a specific enzyme whose name contains both the substrate and job category is lactate dehydrogenase (found in skeletal muscle, heart, and liver). This enzyme catalyzes the conversion of lactic acid to pyruvic acid and vice versa, with the direction dependent on the relative concentrations of the reactants on either side of the arrow:

$$\text{Lactate dehydrogenase}$$
$$\text{Lactic acid} \longleftrightarrow \text{Pyruvic acid}$$
$$+ \qquad\qquad\qquad +$$
$$\text{NAD} \qquad\qquad \text{NADH} + \text{H}^+$$

Fuels for Exercise

The body uses carbohydrate, fat, and protein nutrients consumed daily to provide the necessary energy to maintain cellular activities both at rest and during exercise. During exercise, the primary nutrients used for energy are fats and carbohydrates, with protein contributing less than 5%–15% of the total energy used (5, 9, 13, 14, 21).

Carbohydrates
Carbohydrates are composed of atoms of carbon, hydrogen, and oxygen. Stored carbohydrates provide the body with a rapidly available form of energy, with one gram of carbohydrate yielding approximately 4 kcal of energy (23). Plants synthesize carbohydrates from the interaction of CO_2, water, and solar energy in a process called photosynthesis. Carbohydrates exist in three forms (22, 28): (1) monosaccharides, (2) disaccharides, and (3) polysaccharides. Monosaccharides are simple sugars such as glucose and fructose. **Glucose** is familar to most of us and is often referred to as "blood sugar." It is found in foods or can be formed in the digestive tract as a result of cleavage of more complex carbohydrates. Fructose is contained in fruits or honey and is considered to be the sweetest of the simple carbohydrates (22, 23).

Disaccharides are composed of the combination of two monosaccharides. For example, table sugar is called sucrose and is composed of glucose and fructose. Maltose, also a disaccharide, is composed of two glucose molecules. Sucrose is considered to be the most common dietary disaccharide in the United States and constitutes approximately 25% of the total caloric intake of most Americans (22). It occurs naturally in many carbohydrates such as cane sugar, beets, honey, and maple syrup.

Polysaccharides are complex carbohydrates that contain three or more monosaccharides. Polysaccharides may be rather small molecules (i.e., three monosaccharides) or relatively large molecules containing hundreds of monosaccharides. In general, polysaccharides are classified as either plant or animal polysaccharides. The two most common forms of plant polysaccharides are cellulose and starch. Humans lack the digestive enzymes necessary to digest cellulose and thus cellulose forms fiber in the diet and is discarded as waste in the fecal material. On the other hand, starch, found in corn, grains, beans, potatoes, and peas, is easily digested by humans and is an important source of carbohydrates in the American diet (22). After ingestion, starch is broken down to form monosaccharides and may be used as energy immediately by cells or stored in another form within cells for future energy needs.

Glycogen is the term used for the polysaccharide stored in animal tissue. It is synthesized within cells by linking glucose molecules together. Glycogen molecules are generally large and may consist of hundreds to thousands of glucose molecules. Cells store glycogen as a means of supplying carbohydrates as an energy source. For example, during exercise, individual muscle cells break down glycogen into glucose (this process is called **glycogenolysis**) and use the glucose as a source of energy for contraction. On the other hand, glycogenolysis also occurs in the liver with the free glucose being released into the bloodstream and transported to tissues throughout the body.

Total glycogen stores in the body are relatively small and can be depleted within a few hours as a result of prolonged exercise. Therefore, glycogen synthesis is an ongoing process within cells. Diets low in carbohydrates tend to hamper glycogen synthesis, while high-carbohydrate diets enhance glycogen synthesis (chapter 23).

Fats
Although fats contain the same chemical elements as carbohydrates, the ratio of carbon to oxygen in fats is much greater than that found in carbohydrates. Stored body fat is an ideal fuel for prolonged exercise since fat molecules contain large quantities of energy per unit of weight. One gram of fat contains about 9 kcal of energy, which is over twice the energy content of either carbohydrates or protein (23, 30, 31). Fats are insoluble in water and can be found in both plants and animals. In general, fats are classified in three general groups (22): (1) simple fats, (2) compound fats, and (3) derived fats. Simple or neutral fats are common in

the body and consist primarily of triglycerides. Triglycerides are composed of three molecules of free fatty acids and one molecule of glycerol (not a fat but a type of alcohol). Triglycerides constitute the most common storage form of fat in the body and in times of need can be broken down into their component parts and both the glycerol and free fatty acids can be used as energy substrates.

Compound fats are ...   ation with
                                          e not used
                                          rcise (25,
                                          compound
                                          lipids are
                                          re synthe-
                                          biological
                                          structural
                                          nsulating
                                          er impor-
                                          Lipopro-
                                          transport
                                          ot water-
                                          he blood,
                                          ible mol-

                                          "derived
                                          rgy sub-
                                          d briefly
                                          arer un-
                                          s. These
                                          r simple
                                          d fat is
                                          nt of all
                                          ery cell
                                          n foods.
                                          choles-
                                          rmones
                                          5). Al-
                                          l func-

..., high blood cholesterol levels have been implicated in the development of coronary artery disease (33) (chapter 18).

Proteins

Proteins are composed of many tiny subunits called amino acids. At least twenty different types of amino acids are needed by the body to form various tissues, enzymes, blood proteins, etc. Nine amino acids, called essential amino acids, cannot be synthesized by the body and therefore must be consumed in foods. Proteins are formed by linking amino acids together by chemical bonds called peptide bonds. As a potential fuel source, proteins contain approximately 4 kcal per gram (23). In order for proteins to be used as substrates for the formation of high-energy compounds, they must be broken down into their constituent amino acids. Proteins may contribute fuel for exercise in two ways. First, the amino acid alanine can be converted in the liver to glycogen. Liver glycogen can be degraded into glucose and transported to working skeletal muscle via the circulation. Second, many amino acids (i.e., isoleucine, alanine, leucine, valine, etc.) can be converted into metabolic intermediates (i.e., compounds that may directly participate in bioenergetics) in muscle cells and directly contribute as fuel in the bioenergetic pathways (7, 30, 31).

High-Energy Phosphates

The immediate source of energy for muscular contraction is the high-energy phosphate compound, **adenosine triphosphate (ATP)**. Although ATP is not the only energy-carrying molecule in the cell, it is the most important one, and without sufficient amounts of ATP most cells quickly die.

The structure of ATP consists of three main parts: (1) an adenine portion, (2) a ribose portion, and (3) three phosphates linked together (figure 3.6). The formation of ATP occurs by combining **adenosine diphosphate (ADP)** and **inorganic phosphate (Pi)** and requires a rather large amount of energy. Some of this energy is stored in the chemical bond joining ADP and Pi. Accordingly, this bond is called a high-energy bond. When the enzyme **ATPase** breaks this bond, energy is released and this energy can be used to do work (i.e., muscular contraction):

$$\text{ATP} \xrightarrow{\text{ATPase}} \text{ADP} + \text{Pi} + \text{energy}$$

Figure 3.6 Top portion of figure demonstrates the structural formation of adenosine triphosphate (ATP). Lower portion of the figure depicts the breakdown of ATP with the resultant release of energy.

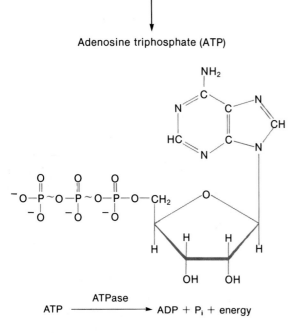

Adenosine diphosphate (ADP)

+

Inorganic phosphate (P_i)

Adenosine triphosphate (ATP)

$$ATP \xrightarrow{\text{ATPase}} ADP + P_i + \text{energy}$$

ATP is often called the universal energy donor and serves to couple the energy released from the breakdown of foodstuffs into a useable form of energy required by the diverse energy-requiring processes in cells. For example, figure 3.7 presents a model depicting ATP as the universal energy donor in the cell. The cell uses exergonic reactions (breakdown of foodstuffs) to form ATP via endergonic reactions. This newly formed ATP can then be used to drive the energy-requiring processes in the cell. Therefore, energy-liberating reactions are linked to energy-requiring reactions like two meshed gears.

Bioenergetics

Muscle cells store limited amounts of ATP. Therefore, because muscular exercise requires a constant supply of ATP to provide the needed energy for contraction, metabolic pathways must exist in the cell with the capability to produce ATP rapidly. Indeed, muscle cells can produce ATP by any one or a combination of three metabolic pathways: (1) by **creatine phosphate (CP)** formation of ATP, (2) formation of ATP via the degradation of glucose or glycogen (called glycolysis), and (3) oxidative formation of ATP. Formation of ATP via the CP pathway or glycolysis does not involve the use of O_2 and is called an **anaerobic** (without O_2) pathway. Oxidative formation of ATP by the use of O_2 is termed **aerobic** metabolism. A detailed discussion of the operation of the three metabolic pathways involved in the formation of ATP during exercise follows.

Anaerobic ATP Production
The simplest and consequently the most rapid method of producing ATP involves the donation of a phosphate group and its bond energy from CP to ADP to form ATP (3, 16, 34):

$$CP + ADP \xrightarrow[\text{Creatine kinase}]{} ATP + C$$

The reaction is catalyzed by the enzyme creatine kinase. As rapidly as ATP is broken down to ADP + Pi at the onset of exercise, ATP is reformed via the CP reaction. However, muscle cells store only small amounts of CP and thus the total amount of ATP that can be formed via this reaction is limited. The combination of stored ATP and CP is called the **ATP-CP system** or the "phosphagen system" and provides energy for muscular contraction at the onset of exercise and during short-term high-intensity exercise (i.e., one to five seconds). CP reformation requires ATP and occurs only during recovery from exercise (6, 10).

The importance of the ATP-CP system in athletics can be appreciated by considering short-term intense exercise such as sprinting 50 meters, high jumping, performing a rapid weight-lifting move, or a football player racing 10 yards downfield. All of these activities require only a few seconds to complete and thus

Figure 3.7 Model of ATP serving as the universal energy donor that drives the energy needs of the cell. On the left, the energy released from the breakdown of foodstuffs is used to form ATP. On the right, the energy released from the breakdown of ATP is used to "drive" the energy needs of the cell.

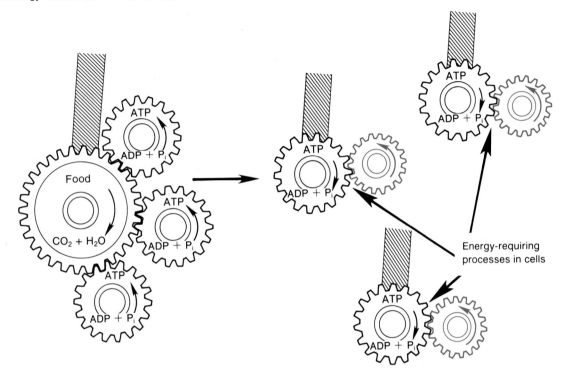

need a rapid supply of ATP. The ATP-CP system provides a simple one-reaction method of producing ATP for these types of activities.

A second metabolic pathway capable of producing ATP rapidly without the involvement of O_2 is termed **glycolysis.** Glycolysis involves the breakdown of glucose or glycogen to form two molecules of pyruvic acid or lactic acid (figure 3.8). Simply stated, glycolysis is an anaerobic pathway used to transfer bond energy from glucose to rejoin Pi to ADP. This process involves nine enzymatically catalyzed steps and occurs in the sarcoplasm of the muscle cell. In short, glycolysis produces a net gain of two molecules of ATP and two molecules of pyruvic or lactic acid per glucose molecule.

Let's consider glycolysis in more detail. First, although the end result of glycolysis is energy producing (exergonic), glycolysis must be "primed" by the addition of ATP at two points at the beginning of the

pathway (figure 3.8). The purpose of the ATP priming is to add phosphate groups (called phosphorylation) to glucose and to fructose-6-phosphate. Note that if glycolysis begins with glycogen as the substrate, the addition of only one ATP is required (glycogen does not require phosphorylation by ATP, but is phosphorylated by inorganic phosphate instead). Further, figure 3.8 points out that two molecules of ATP are produced at each of two separate reactions near the end of the glycolytic pathway; thus, the net gain of glycolysis is two ATP if glucose is the substrate and three ATP if glycogen is the substrate.

Hydrogens are frequently removed from nutrient substrates in bioenergetic pathways and are transported by "carrier molecules." Two biologically important carrier molecules are **nicotinamide adenine dinucleotide (NAD)** and **flavin adenine dinucleotide (FAD).** Both NAD and FAD transport hydrogens

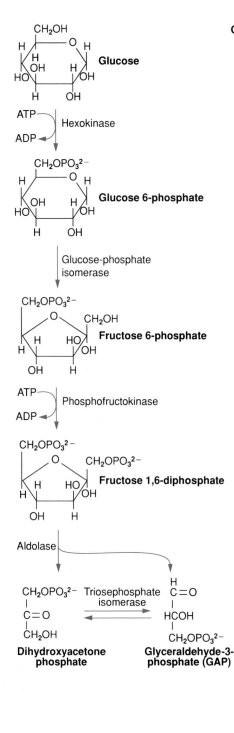

Figure 3.8 Step-by-step reactions of the breakdown of glucose to form pyruvate or lactic acid. This metabolic pathway is called glycolysis.

Box 3.2 The Concept of Oxidation-Reduction Reactions

When a molecule accepts electrons from an electron donor it is said to become reduced; when a molecule gives up electrons the molecule has undergone a process called oxidation. Oxidation-reduction reactions are always coupled. In other words, a molecule cannot be reduced unless another molecule is oxidized first. The molecule that gives up the electrons is called a reducing agent, while the molecule that accepts the electrons is referred to as an oxidizing agent.

Oxidation does not mean oxygen is involved in this process. The term oxidation is derived from the fact that oxygen has the tendency to accept electrons. Hence, oxygen is a strong

oxidizing agent. Cells make use of this fact by using oxygen as the final electron acceptor in the electron transport chain.

Two molecules that play an important role as oxidizing agents in cellular bioenergetics are nicotinamide adenine dinucleotide (NAD) and flavin adenine dinucleotide (FAD). Each NAD and FAD molecule can accept two electrons (see text for specific details). An example of these reactions are as follows:

$$FAD + 2H \longrightarrow FADH + H$$
$$\text{and}$$
$$NAD + 2H \longrightarrow NADH + H$$

and their associated energy to be used for later generation of ATP in the mitochondrion via aerobic processes. In order for the chemical reactions in glycolysis to proceed, two hydrogens must be removed from glyceraldehyde 3-phosphate, which then forms 1, 3-diphosphoglycerate. The hydrogen acceptor in this reaction is NAD (figure 3.8). Here NAD accepts one of the hydrogens while the remaining hydrogen is free in solution. Upon accepting the hydrogen, NAD is converted to its reduced form, NADH (see Box 3.2). Adequate amounts of NAD must be available to accept the hydrogen atoms that must be removed from glyceraldehyde 3-phosphate if glycolysis is to continue (1, 8, 20). How is NAD reformed from NADH? There are two ways that the cell restores NAD from NADH. First, if sufficient oxygen (O_2) is available, the hydrogens from NADH can be "shuttled" into the mitochondria of the cell and can contribute to the aerobic production of ATP. Second, if O_2 is not available to accept the hydrogens in the mitochondria, pyruvic acid can accept the hydrogens to form **lactic acid** (figure 3.9). The enzyme that catalyzes this reaction is lactate dehydrogenase (LDH), with the end result being the formation of lactic acid and the reformation of NAD. Therefore, the reason for lactic acid formation is the "recycling" of NAD (i.e., NADH → NAD) so that glycolysis can continue.

In summary, glycolysis is the breakdown of glucose or glycogen into pyruvic acid or lactic acid with the net production of two or three ATP depending on whether the pathway began with glucose or glycogen, respectively. Figure 3.10 summarizes glycolysis in a simple flowchart. Note that glucose is a six-carbon molecule and that pyruvic acid and lactic acid are three-carbon molecules. Thus, this explains the production of two molecules of pyruvic acid and lactic acid from one molecule of glucose. Since O_2 is not directly involved in glycolysis the pathway is considered anaerobic. However, in the presence of O_2 in the mitochondria, pyruvate can participate in the aerobic production of ATP. Thus, in addition to being an anaerobic pathway capable of producing ATP without O_2, glycolysis can be considered the first step in the aerobic degradation of carbohydrates. This will be discussed in detail in the next section.

Aerobic ATP Production

Aerobic production of ATP occurs inside the mitochondria and involves the interaction of two cooperating metabolic pathways: (1) Krebs cycle and (2) electron transport chain. The primary function of the **Krebs cycle** is to complete the oxidation (hydrogen removal) of carbohydrates, fats, or proteins and to use

Figure 3.9 The addition of two hydrogen atoms to pyruvic acid forms lactic acid and NAD, which can be used again in glycolysis. The reaction is catalyzed by the enzyme lactate dehydrogenase (LDH).

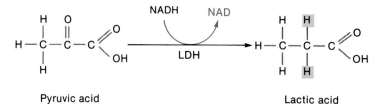

Pyruvic acid　　　　　　　　　　　　　　　Lactic acid

NAD and FAD as hydrogen (energy) carriers. The importance of hydrogen removal is that hydrogens (by virtue of the electrons that they possess) contain potential energy. This energy can be used in the electron transport chain to combine ADP + Pi to reform ATP. Oxygen is the final hydrogen acceptor at the end of the electron transport chain and water is formed (i.e., $H_2 + O \rightarrow H_2O$). The process of aerobic production of ATP is termed **oxidative phosphorylation.**

Krebs Cycle

The Krebs cycle is named after the biochemist Hans Krebs, whose pioneering research has increased our understanding of this rather complex pathway. Entry into the Krebs cycle requires preparation of a two-carbon molecule, acetyl Co-A. Acetyl Co-A can be formed from the breakdown of either carbohydrates, fats, or proteins. For the moment let's focus on the formation of acetyl Co-A from pyruvate (pyruvate can be formed from both carbohydrates and proteins). Figure 3.11 depicts the cyclic nature of the reactions involved in the Krebs cycle. Note that pyruvate (three-carbon molecule) is broken down to form acetyl Co-A (two-carbon molecule) and the remaining carbon is given off as CO_2. Next, acetyl Co-A combines with oxaloacetic acid (four-carbon molecule) to form citric acid (six carbons). What follows is a series of six reactions to regenerate oxaloacetic acid and two molecules of CO_2, and the pathway begins all over again.

For every molecule of glucose entering glycolysis two molecules of pyruvate are formed, and in the presence of O_2, are converted to two molecules of acetyl Co-A. This means that each molecule of glucose results in two turns of the Krebs cycle. With this in mind let's examine the Krebs cycle in more detail. Remember that the primary function of the Krebs cycle is to remove hydrogens and the energy associated with those hydrogens from various substrates involved in the cycle. Figure 3.12 illustrates that during each turn of the Krebs cycle three molecules of NADH and one molecule of FADH are formed. For every pair of electrons passed through the electron transport chain from NADH to oxygen, enough energy is available to form three molecules of ATP (30, 32). For every FADH molecule that is formed, enough energy is available to produce two molecules of ATP. Thus, in terms of ATP production, FADH is not as energy rich as NADH.

In addition to the production of NADH and FADH, the Krebs cycle results in direct formation of an energy-rich compound, guanosine triphosphate (GTP) (30) (figure 3.12). GTP is a high-energy compound that can transfer its terminal phosphate group to form ATP. The direct formation of GTP in the Krebs cycle is called substrate-level phosphorylation and accounts for only a small amount of the total energy conversion in the Krebs cycle since most of the Krebs cycle energy yield (i.e., NADH and FADH) is taken to the electron transport chain to form ATP.

Up to this point we have focused on the role that carbohydrates play in producing acetyl Co-A to enter the Krebs cycle. How do fats and proteins undergo aerobic metabolism? The answer can be found in figure 3.13. Note that fats (triglycerides) are broken down to form fatty acids and glycerol. These fatty acids

Figure 3.10 A simple summary of the anaerobic metabolism of glucose via glycolysis. Note that the end result of the anaerobic breakdown of one molecule of glucose is two molecules of lactate.

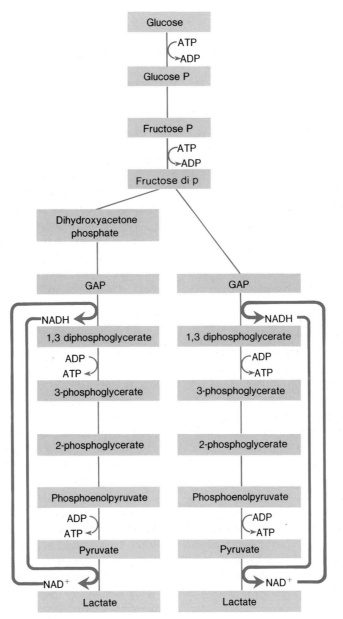

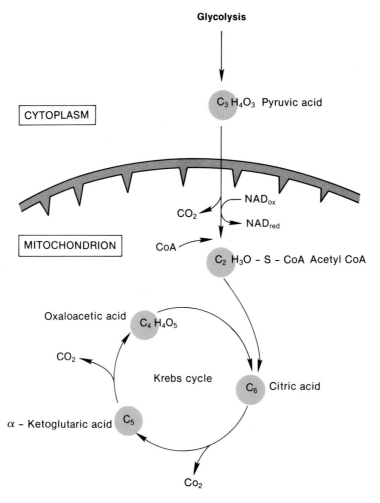

Glycolysis

CYTOPLASM

$C_3 H_4 O_3$ Pyruvic acid

NAD_{ox}

CO_2

NAD_{red}

MITOCHONDRION

CoA

$C_2 H_3 O - S - CoA$ Acetyl CoA

Oxaloacetic acid $C_4 H_4 O_5$

CO_2

Krebs cycle

C_6 Citric acid

α – Ketoglutaric acid C_5

CO_2

can then undergo a series of reactions to form acetyl Co-A (called beta oxidation) and thus enter the Krebs cycle (30, 31). Although glycerol can be converted into an intermediate of glycolysis, it is unlikely that this occurs to a great extent in skeletal muscle and thus glycerol is not an important fuel during exercise (13, 17).

As mentioned previously, protein is not considered a major fuel source during exercise since it contributes less than 5%–15% of the fuel utilized during exercise (9, 13, 21). Proteins can enter bioenergetic pathways in a variety of places. However, the first step is the breakdown of the protein into its amino acid subunits. What happens next depends on which amino acid is involved. For example, some amino acids can be converted to glucose or pyruvic acid, some to acetyl Co-A, and still others to Krebs-cycle intermediates. The role of proteins in bioenergetics is summarized in figure 3.13.

In summary, the Krebs-cycle completes the oxidation of carbohydrates, fats, or proteins and supplies electrons to be passed through the electron transport

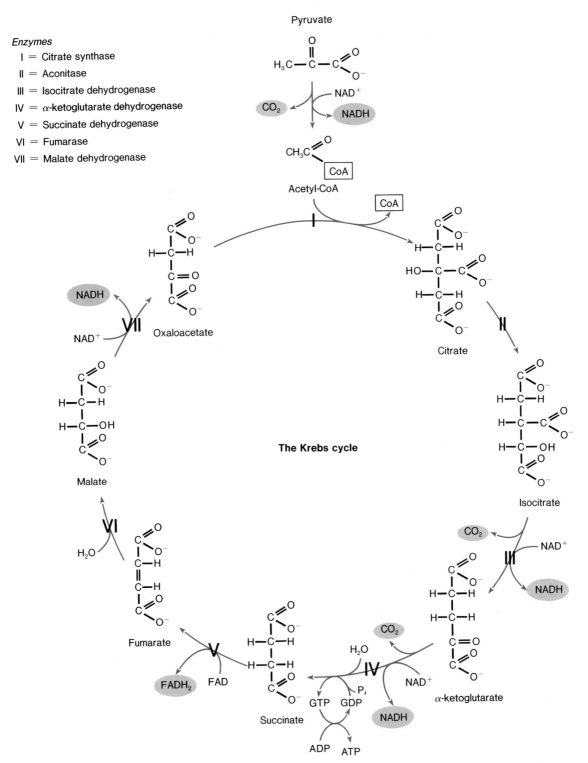

Enzymes

I = Citrate synthase
II = Aconitase
III = Isocitrate dehydrogenase
IV = α-ketoglutarate dehydrogenase
V = Succinate dehydrogenase
VI = Fumarase
VII = Malate dehydrogenase

Pyruvate

Acetyl-CoA

The Krebs cycle

Oxaloacetate

Citrate

Isocitrate

Malate

α-ketoglutarate

Fumarate

Succinate

Figure 3.12 The molecular structures of the compounds involved in the Krebs cycle. Note the formation of three molecules of NADH and one molecule of FADH per turn of the cycle.

Figure 3.13 The relationship between the metabolism of proteins, carbohydrates, and fats. The overall interaction between the metabolic breakdown of these three foodstuffs is often referred to as the metabolic pool.

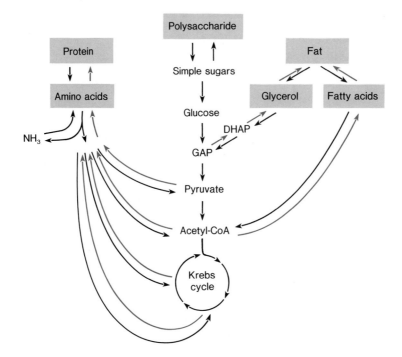

chain to provide the energy for the aerobic production of ATP. Enzymes catalyzing Krebs-cycle reactions are located inside the mitochondria.

Electron Transport Chain

Oxidative phosphorylation or the aerobic production of ATP occurs in the mitochondria. The pathway responsible for this process is called the **electron transport chain** or respiratory chain. Aerobic production of ATP is possible due to a mechanism that uses the potential energy available in reduced hydrogen carriers such as NADH and FADH to rephosphorylate ADP to ATP. The reduced hydrogen carriers do not directly react with oxygen. Instead, electrons containing the bond energy of the hydrogen atoms are passed down a series of electron carriers known as cytochromes. During this passage of electrons down the cytochrome

pathway enough "bond" energy is released to rephosphorylate ADP to form ATP at three different sites (29) (figure 3.14).

The hydrogen carriers that bring the electrons to the electron transport chain come from a variety of sources. Recall that two NADH are formed per glucose molecule that is degraded via glycolysis (figure 3.8). These NADH are outside the mitochondria and their hydrogens must be transported across the mitochondrial membrane by special "shuttle" mechanisms. However, the bulk of the electrons that enter the electron transport chain comes from those NADH and FADH formed as a result of Krebs-cycle oxidations.

Figure 3.14 outlines the pathway for electrons entering the electron transport chain. Simply stated, pairs of electrons from NADH or FADH are passed down

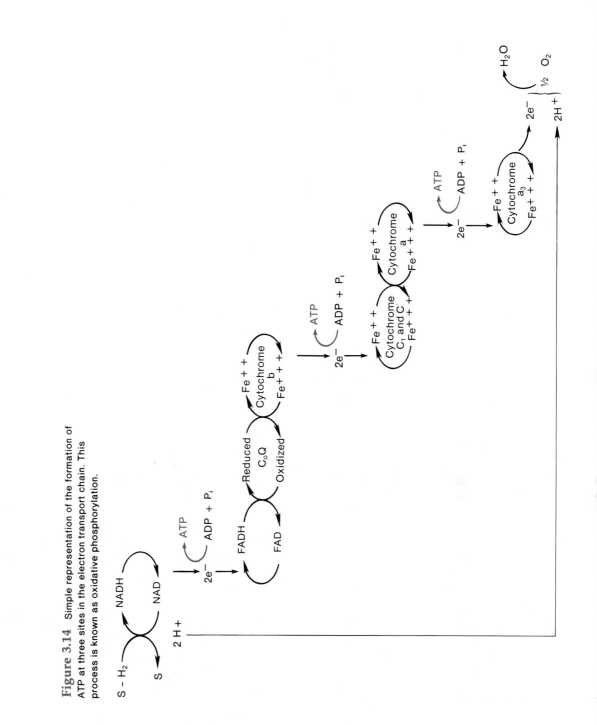

Figure 3.14 Simple representation of the formation of ATP at three sites in the electron transport chain. This process is known as oxidative phosphorylation.

Table 3.1 Aerobic ATP talley from the breakdown of one molecule of glucose

Metabolic Process	High-Energy Products	ATP from Oxidative Phosphorylation	ATP Subtotal
Glycolysis	2 ATP	—	2 (total if anaerobic)
	2 NADH	6	8 (if aerobic)
Pyruvic acid to acetyl CoA	2 NADH	6	14
Krebs cycle	2 GTP	—	16
	6 NADH	18	34
	2 FADH	4	38
		Grand total:	38 ATP

a series of compounds that undergo oxidation and reduction, with ATP synthesis occurring at three places along the way. Notice that FADH enters the cytochrome pathway at a point just below the entry level for NADH (figure 3.14). This is important because the level of FADH entry bypasses one of the sites of ATP formation and thus each molecule of FADH that enters the electron transport chain has enough energy to form only two ATP. In contrast, NADH entry into the electron transport chain results in the formation of three ATP. At the end of the electron transport chain oxygen accepts the electrons that are passed along, and combines with hydrogen to form water. If O_2 is not available to accept those electrons, oxidative phosphorylation is not possible and ATP formation in the cell must occur via anaerobic metabolism.

Aerobic ATP Talley

It is now possible to compute the overall ATP production as a result of the aerobic breakdown of glucose or glycogen. Let's begin by counting the total energy yield of glycolysis. Recall that the net ATP production of glycolysis was two ATP per glucose molecule. Further, when O_2 is present in the mitochondria, two NADH produced by glycolysis can then be shuttled into the mitochondria with the energy used to synthesize an additional six ATP (table 3.1). Thus, glycolysis can produce two ATP directly via substrate-level phosphorylation and an additional six ATP by the energy contained in the two molecules of NADH.

How many ATP are produced as a result of the oxidation-reduction activities of the Krebs cycle? Table 3.1 shows that two NADH are formed when pyruvic acid is converted to acetyl CoA, yielding 6 ATP. Note that two GTP (similar to ATP) are produced via substrate-level phosphorylation and that a total of six NADH and two FADH are produced. Hence, the NADH/ATP total is twenty-four (eight NADH × three ATP per NADH = twenty-four ATP), with four ATP for the two FADH. Therefore, the total ATP yield for the aerobic degradation of glucose is thirty-eight ATP. The aerobic ATP yield for glycogen breakdown is thirty-nine ATP since the net glycolytic production of ATP by glycogen is one ATP more than that of glucose.

How efficient is oxidative phosphorylation as a system of converting energy from foodstuffs into biologically useable energy? This can be calculated by computing the ratio of the energy contained in the ATP molecules produced via aerobic respiration divided by the total potential energy contained in the glucose. For example, a mole (a mole is one gram molecular weight) of ATP, when broken down, has an energy yield of 7.3 kcal. The potential energy released from the oxidation of a mole of glucose is 686 kcal. Thus, an efficiency figure for aerobic respiration can be computed as follows (19):

Efficiency of respiration =

$$\frac{38 \text{ moles ATP/mole glucose} \times 7.3 \text{ kcal/mole ATP}}{686 \text{ kcal/mole glucose}}$$

$$\times 100 = 40\%$$

Therefore, the efficiency of aerobic respiration is approximately 40% with the remaining 60% of free energy of glucose oxidation being released as heat.

Control of Bioenergetics

The biochemical pathways that result in the production of ATP are regulated by very precise control systems. Each of these pathways contain a number of reactions that are catalyzed by specific enzymes. In general, if ample substrate is available, an increase in the number of enzymes present results in an increased rate of chemical reactions. Therefore, regulation of one or more enzymes in a biochemical pathway would provide a means of controlling the rate of that particular pathway. Indeed, metabolism is regulated by control of enzymatic activity. Most metabolic pathways have one enzyme that is considered "rate limiting." This rate-limiting enzyme determines the speed of the particular metabolic pathway involved.

How does a rate-limiting enzyme work to control the speed of reactions? First, as a rule, rate-limiting enzymes are found early in a metabolic pathway. This position is important since products of the pathway might accumulate if the rate-limiting enzyme was located near the end of a pathway. Second, the activity of rate-limiting enzymes is regulated by modulators. Modulators are substances that increase or decrease enzyme activity. In the control of energy metabolism, ATP is the classic example of an inhibitor, while ADP and Pi are examples of substances that stimulate enzymatic activity (4). The fact that large amounts of cellular ATP would inhibit the metabolic production of ATP is logical since large amounts of ATP would indicate that ATP usage in the cell is low. An example of this type of negative feedback is illustrated in figure 3.15. In contrast, an increase in cell levels of ADP and Pi (low ATP) would indicate that ATP utilization is high. Therefore, it makes sense that ADP and Pi should stimulate the production of ATP to meet the increased energy need.

Control of ATP-CP System

Creatine phosphate breakdown is regulated by creatine kinase activity. Creatine kinase is activated when sarcoplasmic concentrations of ADP increase, and is inhibited by high levels of ATP. At the onset of exercise, ATP is split into ADP $+$ Pi to provide energy for muscular contraction. This immediate increase in ADP concentrations stimulates creatine kinase activity to trigger the breakdown of CP to resynthesize ATP. If exercise is continued, glycolysis and finally aerobic metabolism begin to produce adequate ATP to meet the muscles' energy needs. The increase in ATP concentration, coupled with a reduction in ADP concentration, inhibits creatine kinase activity (table 3.2). Regulation of the ATP-CP system is an example of a "negative feedback" control system which was introduced in chapter 2.

Control of Glycolysis

Although several factors serve to control glycolysis, the most important rate-limiting enzyme in glycolysis is **phosphofructokinase (PFK)**. Note that PFK is located near the beginning of glycolysis (figure 3.8). Table 3.2 lists known modulators of PFK. When exercise begins, ADP/Pi levels rise and enhance PFK activity, which serves to increase the rate of glycolysis. In contrast, at rest when cellular ATP levels are high, PFK activity is inhibited and glycolytic activity is slowed. Further, high cellular levels of free fatty acids or citrate (produced via Krebs cycle) also inhibit PFK activity. Similar to the control of the ATP-CP system, regulation of PFK activity operates via negative feedback.

Another important regulating enzyme in glycolysis is phosphorylase, which is responsible for degrading glycogen to glucose. This reaction provides the glycolytic pathway with the necessary glucose at the origin of the pathway. At the beginning of exercise, calcium (Ca^{++}) is released from the sarcoplasmic reticulum in muscle. This rise in sarcoplasmic Ca^{++} concentration indirectly activates phosphorylase which immediately begins to break down glycogen to glucose for entry into glycolysis. Additionally, phosphorylase activity may be stimulated by high levels of the hormone, epinephrine.

Figure 3.15 An example of a "rate-limiting" enzyme in a simple metabolic pathway. Here, a buildup of the product serves to inhibit the rate-limiting enzyme, which in turn slows down the reactions involved in the pathway.

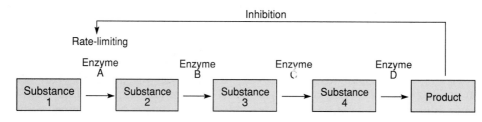

Table 3.2 *Factors known to affect the activity of rate-limiting enzymes of metabolic pathways involved in bioenergetics*

Pathway	Rate-Limiting Enzyme	Stimulators	Inhibitors
ATP-PC system	Creatine kinase	ADP	ATP
Glycolysis	Phosphofructokinase	ADP, Pi, pH↑	ATP, CP, citrate, FFA, pH↓
Glycolysis	Phosphorylase	Ca^{++}, cyclic AMP	ATP
Krebs cycle	Isocitrate dehydrogenase	ADP, Pi	ATP
Electron transport chain	Cytochrome oxidase	ADP, Pi	ATP

Epinephrine, released at a faster rate during heavy exercise, results in the formation of the compound, cyclic AMP (chapter 5). It is cyclic AMP, not epinephrine, that directly activates phosphorylase. Thus, the influence of epinephrine on phosphorylase is indirect.

Control of Krebs Cycle/Electron Transport Chain

The Krebs cycle, like glycolysis, is subject to enzymatic regulation. The rate-limiting enzyme here is **isocitrate dehydrogenase.** Isocitrate dehydrgenase, like PFK, is inhibited by ATP and stimulated by increasing levels of ADP/Pi (30, 31).

Finally, it is not surprising that the electron transport chain is also regulated by the amount of ATP and ADP/Pi present (4, 31). When exercise begins, ATP levels decline and ADP/Pi levels increase and the electron transport chain is stimulated to begin aerobic production of ATP. When exercise stops, cellular levels

of ATP increase and ADP/Pi concentrations decline and thus the electron transport activity is reduced when normal levels of ATP, ADP, and Pi are reached.

Interaction between Aerobic/Anaerobic ATP Production

It is important to emphasize the interaction of anaerobic and aerobic metabolic pathways in the production of ATP during exercise. Although it is common to hear someone speak of aerobic versus anaerobic exercise, in reality the energy to perform most types of exercise comes from a combination of anaerobic/aerobic sources (5, 16, 22, 25). This point is illustrated in table 3.3. Notice that the contribution of anaerobic ATP production is greater in short-term high-intensity activities, while aerobic metabolism predominates in longer activities. For example, approximately 90% of the energy to perform a 100-meter dash would come

Table 3.3 *Contribution of aerobic/anaerobic production of ATP during maximal exercise as a function of the duration of the event*

| | Duration of Maximal Exercise | | | | | | | | |
| | Seconds | | | Minutes | | | | | |
	10	30	60	2	4	10	30	60	120
Percent aerobic	10	20	30	40	65	85	95	98	99
Percent anaerobic	90	80	70	60	35	15	5	2	1

Data from references 5 and 25.

from anaerobic sources, with most of the energy coming via the ATP-CP system. Similarly, energy to run 400 meters (i.e., 55 seconds) would be largely anaerobic (70%–75%). However, ATP and CP stores are limited and thus glycolysis must supply much of the ATP during this type of an event.

On the other end of the energy spectrum, events like the marathon (i.e., 26.2-mile race) rely on aerobic production of ATP for the bulk of the needed energy. Where does the energy come from in events of moderate length (i.e., two to thirty minutes)? Table 3.3 provides an estimation of the percentage anaerobic/aerobic yield in events over a wide range of durations. Although these estimates are based on laboratory measurements of running or exercising on a cycle ergometer, they can be related to other athletic events that require intense effort by comparing the length of time spent in the activity.

In summary, the shorter the activity, the greater the contribution of anaerobic energy production; conversely, the longer the activity, the greater the contribution of aerobic energy production. A more detailed discussion of the metabolic responses to various types of exercise is contained in chapter 4.

Summary

1. In general, cell structure can be divided into three major parts: (1) cell membrane, (2) nucleus, and (3) cytoplasm (called sarcoplasm in muscle).

2. Bioenergetics refers to the energy flow in living systems. All chemical reactions that occur in cells obey the laws of thermodynamics. The speed of cellular chemical reactions is regulated by enzymes that serve as catalysts for these reactions.

3. The body uses carbohydrate, fat, and protein nutrients consumed daily to provide the necessary energy to maintain cellular activities both at rest and during exercise. During exercise, the primary nutrients used for energy are fats and carbohydrates, with protein contributing less than 5% of the total energy used.

4. The immediate source of energy for muscular contraction is the high-energy phosphate, ATP. ATP is degraded via the enzyme ATPase as follows:

$$ATP \xrightarrow{\text{ATPase}} ADP + Pi + energy$$

5. Formation of ATP without the use of O_2 is termed anaerobic metabolism. In contrast, production of ATP using O_2 as the final electron acceptor is referred to as aerobic metabolism.

6. The ATP-CP system and "anaerobic glycolysis" are two metabolic pathways that are capable of producing ATP without O_2. Oxidative phosphorylation or aerobic ATP

production occurs in the mitochondria as a result of a complex interaction between the Krebs cycle and the electron transport chain.

7. The aerobic metabolism of one molecule of glucose results in the production of thirty-eight ATP molecules, whereas the aerobic ATP yield for glycogen breakdown is thirty-nine ATP. The overall efficiency of aerobic respiration is approximately 40%, with the remaining 60% of free energy of glucose oxidation being released as heat.

8. Metabolism is regulated by enzymatic activity. An enzyme that regulates a metabolic pathway is termed the "rate-limiting" enzyme. The rate-limiting enzyme for glycolysis is phosphofructokinase, while the controlling enzyme for the Krebs cycle is isocitrate dehydrogenase. In general, cellular levels of ATP and ADP/Pi regulate the rate of metabolic pathways involved in the production of ATP. High levels of ATP inhibit further ATP production while low levels of ATP and high levels of ADP/Pi stimulate ATP production.

9. Energy to perform exercise comes from an interaction of anaerobic and aerobic pathways. In general, the shorter the activity (high intensity), the greater the contribution of anaerobic energy production. In contrast, long-term activities (low to moderate intensity) utilize ATP that comes primarily from aerobic sources.

Study Questions

1. List and briefly discuss the function of the three major components of cell structure.
2. Briefly explain the first and second laws of thermodynamics.
3. Define the following terms: (1) bioenergetics, (2) endergonic reactions, (3) exergonic reactions, (4) organic reactions, and (5) coupled reactions.
4. Discuss the role of enzymes as catalysts. What is meant by the expression "energy of activation"?
5. Briefly, identify the common forms of carbohydrates, proteins, and fats. What role does each play as an energy source during exercise?
6. Define the terms glycogen, glycogenolysis, and glycolysis.
7. What are high-energy phosphates? Explain the statement that "ATP is the universal energy donor."
8. Define the terms aerobic and anaerobic.
9. Briefly discuss the function of glycolysis in bioenergetics. What role does NAD play in glycolysis?
10. Discuss the operation of the Krebs cycle and the electron transport chain in the aerobic production ATP. What is the function of NAD and FAD in these pathways?
11. What is the efficiency of the aerobic degradation of glucose?
12. How is bioenergetics controlled? What are rate-limiting enzymes and how do they operate?
13. What enzyme regulates glycolysis? Krebs cycle?
14. Briefly, discuss the interaction of anaerobic versus aerobic ATP production during exercise.

Suggested Readings

Brazy, P., and L. Mandel. 1986. Does availability of inorganic phosphate regulate cellular oxidative metabolism? *News in Physiological Sciences* 1:100–2.

Cerretelli, P., D. Rennie, and D. Pendergast. 1980. Kinetics of metabolic transients during exercise. *International Journal of Sports Medicine* 55:171–80.

Davies, J., and B. Littlewood. 1979. *Elementary Biochemistry.* Englewood Cliffs, N.J.: Prentice-Hall, Inc.

Holloszy, J. 1982. Muscle metabolism during exercise. *Archives of Physical and Rehabilitation Medicine* 63:231–34.

Jequier, E., and J. Flatt. 1986. Recent advances in human bioenergetics. *News in Physiological Sciences* 1:112–14.

References

1. Armstrong, R. 1979. "Biochemistry: Energy Liberation and Use." In (R. Strauss, ed.) *Sports Medicine and Physiology*. Philadelphia: W. B. Saunders Company.
2. Bennett, C. 1967. *College Physics*. New York: Barnes and Noble.
3. Bessman, S., and C. Carpender. 1985. The creatine phosphate shuttle. *Annual Review of Biochemistry* 54:831–62.
4. Brazy, P., and L. Mandel. 1986. Does availability of inorganic phosphate regulate cellular oxidative metabolism? *News in Physiological Sciences* 1:100–2.
5. Brooks, G., and T. Fahey. 1984. *Exercise Physiology: Human Bioenergetics and its Applications*. New York: John Wiley & Sons.
6. Cerretelli, P., D. Rennie, and D. Pendergast. 1980. Kinetics of metabolic transients during exercise. *International Journal of Sports Medicine* 55:171–80.
7. Davies, J., and B. Littlewood. 1979. *Elementary Biochemistry*. Englewood Cliffs, N.J.: Prentice-Hall, Inc.
8. De Zwaan, A., and G. Thillard. 1985. "Low and High Power Output Modes of Anaerobic Metabolism: Invertebrate and Vertebrate Categories." In (R. Giles, ed.) *Circulation, Respiration, and Metabolism*, 166–92. Berlin: Springer-Verlag.
9. Dolny, D., and P. Lemon. 1988. Effect of ambient temperature on protein breakdown during prolonged exercise. *Journal of Applied Physiology* 64:550–55.
10. di Prampero, P., U. Boutellier, and P. Pietsch. 1983. Oxygen deficit and stores at the onset of muscular exercise in humans. *Journal of Applied Physiology* 55:146–53.
11. Fox, S. 1984. *Human Physiology*. Dubuque, Ia.: Wm. C. Brown.
12. Giese, A. 1979. *Cell Physiology*. Philadelphia: W. B. Saunders Company.
13. Gollnick, P. 1985. Metabolism of substrates: Energy substrate metabolism during exercise and as modified by training. *Federation Proceedings* 44:353–56.
14. Gollnick, P. et al. 1985. Differences in metabolic potential of skeletal muscle fibers and their significance for metabolic control. *Journal of Experimental Biology* 115:191–95.
15. Hole, J. 1984. *Human Anatomy and Physiology*. Dubuque, Ia.: Wm. C. Brown.
16. Holloszy, J. 1982. Muscle metabolism during exercise. *Archives of Physical and Rehabilitation Medicine* 63:231–34.
17. Holloszy, J., and E. Coyle. 1984. Adaptations of skeletal muscle to endurance exercise and their metabolic consequences. *Journal of Applied Physiology* 56:831–38.
18. Jain, M. 1972. *The Biomolecular Lipid Membrane: A System*. New York: Reinhold Company.
19. Jequier, E., and J. Flatt. 1986. Recent advances in human bioenergetics. *News in Physiological Sciences* 1:112–14.
20. Johnson, L. 1983. *Biology*. Dubuque, Ia.: Wm. C. Brown.
21. Lemon, P., and J. Mullin. 1980. Effect of initial muscle glycogen levels on protein catabolism during exercise. *Journal of Applied Physiology* 48:624–29.
22. McArdle, W., F. Katch, and V. Katch. 1986. *Exercise Physiology*. Philadelphia. Lea & Febiger.
23. McMurray, W. 1977. *Essentials of Human Metabolism*. New York: Harper & Row.
24. Miller, F. 1977. *College Physics*. New York: Harcourt Brace Jovanovich.
25. Mole, P. 1983. "Exercise Metabolism." In *Exercise Medicine: Physiological Principles and Clinical Application*. New York: Academic Press.
26. Nave, C., and B. Nave. 1975. *Physics of the Health Sciences*. Philadelphia: W. B. Saunders Company.
27. Newsholme, E. 1979. The control of fuel utilization by muscle during exercise and starvation. *Diabetes* 28 (Suppl.):1–7.
28. Sears, C., and C. Stanitski. 1976. *Chemistry for the Health-Related Sciences*. Englewood Cliffs, N.J.: Prentice-Hall, Inc.
29. Senior, A. 1988. ATP synthesis by oxidative phosphorylation. *Physiological Reviews* 68:177–216.
30. Stryer, L. 1981. *Biochemistry*. San Francisco: W. H. Freeman.
31. Suttie, J. 1977. *Introduction to Biochemistry*. New York: Holt, Rinehart & Winston.
32. Weibel, E. 1984. *The Pathway for Oxygen*. London: Harvard University Press.
33. West, J. 1985. *Best's and Taylor's Physiological Basis of Medical Practice*. Baltimore: Williams and Wilkins.
34. Whipp, B., and M. Mahler. 1980. Dynamics of pulmonary gas exchange during exercise. In (J. West, ed.) *Pulmonary Gas Exchange, Volume 2*. New York: Academic Press.

4 Exercise Metabolism

Objectives

*B*y studying this chapter, you should be able to do the following:

1. Discuss the relationship between exercise intensity/duration and the bioenergetic pathways that are most responsible for production of ATP during various types of exercise.
2. Define the term oxygen deficit.
3. Define the term lactate threshold.
4. Discuss several possible explanations for the sudden rise in blood-lactate concentration during incremental exercise.
5. List the factors that regulate fuel selection during different types of exercise.
6. Explain why fat metabolism is dependent on carbohydrate metabolism.
7. Define the term oxygen debt.
8. Give the physiological explanation for the observation that the O_2 debt is greater following intense exercise when compared to the O_2 debt following light exercise.

Outline

Key Terms

anaerobic threshold
EPOC
free fatty acid (FFA)
gluconeogenesis
lactate threshold
lipase
lipolysis
oxygen debt
oxygen deficit
respiratory exchange ratio (R)

Exercise poses a serious challenge to the bioenergetic pathways in the working muscle. For example, during heavy exercise the body's total energy expenditure may increase fifteen to twenty-five times above rest. Most of this increase in energy production is used to provide ATP for contracting skeletal muscles, which may increase their energy utilization 200 times over that of rest (1). Therefore, it is apparent that skeletal muscles have a great capacity to produce and use large quantities of ATP during exercise. This chapter will describe the metabolic responses to various types of exercise, the selection of fuels used to produce ATP, a general scheme showing how exercise metabolism is regulated, and finally, the metabolic response during recovery from exercise.

Metabolic Responses to Exercise

The point was made in chapter 3 that short-term high-intensity exercise lasting less than ten seconds utilizes primarily anaerobic metabolic pathways to produce ATP. In contrast, an event like the marathon makes primary use of aerobic ATP production to provide the needed ATP for work. However, events lasting longer than ten to twenty seconds and less than ten minutes generally produce the needed ATP for muscular contraction via a combination of both anaerobic/aerobic pathways. In fact, most sports use a combination of anaerobic/aerobic pathways for production of the needed ATP for muscular contraction. The next four sections consider which bioenergetic pathways are involved in energy production in specific types of exercise.

Rest-to-Exercise Transitions

Suppose an individual steps onto a treadmill belt that is moving at 6 mph. Within one step the muscles must increase their rate of ATP production from that required for standing to that required for running at 6 mph. If not, the individual would exit off the back of the treadmill. What metabolic changes must occur in skeletal muscle at the beginning of exercise to provide the necessary energy to continue movement? In the transition from rest to light or moderate exercise, oxygen consumption ($\dot{V}O_2$) increases rapidly and reaches a steady state within one to four minutes (6, 13, 50) (figure 4.1). The fact that $\dot{V}O_2$ does not increase instantaneously to a steady state value suggests that anaerobic energy sources contribute to the overall production of ATP at the beginning of exercise. Indeed, there is much evidence to suggest that at the onset of exercise the ATP-CP system is the first active bioenergetic pathway followed by glycolysis and, finally, aerobic energy production (2, 12, 22, 36, 45, 53). However, after a steady state is reached, the body's ATP requirement is met via aerobic metabolism. The major point to be emphasized concerning the bioenergetics of rest-to-work transitions is that several energy systems are involved. In other words, the energy needed for exercise is not provided by simply turning on or turning off various bioenergetic pathways, but rather is provided by a mixture of several metabolic systems operating with considerable overlap.

The term **oxygen deficit** applies to the lag in oxygen uptake at the beginning of exercise. Specifically, the oxygen deficit is defined as the difference between oxygen uptake in the first few minutes of exercise and an equal time period after steady state has been obtained (6). This is represented as the shaded area in

Figure 4.1 The time course of oxygen uptake ($\dot{V}O_2$) in the transition from rest to submaximal exercise.

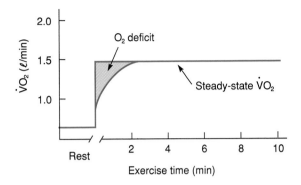

Figure 4.2 Differences in the time course of oxygen uptake during the transition from rest to submaximal exercise between trained and untrained subjects. Note that the time to reach steady-state is slower in untrained subjects when compared to the trained. See text for details.

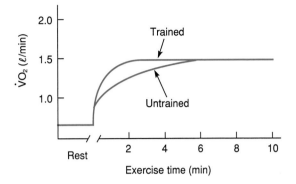

the left-hand portion of figure 4.1. Note that the time to reach steady state is shorter in trained individuals when compared to untrained subjects (32, 50) (figure 4.2). This difference in the time course of oxygen uptake at the onset of exercise between trained and untrained subjects results in the trained subjects having a lower oxygen deficit when compared to the untrained. What is the explanation for this difference? It seems likely that the trained subjects have a better-developed aerobic bioenergetic capacity resulting from either cardiovascular or muscular adaptations induced by endurance training (17, 32, 50, 51). Practically speaking, this means that aerobic ATP production is active earlier at the beginning of exercise and results in less production of lactic acid in the trained individual when compared to the untrained. Chapter 13 provides a detailed analysis of this adaptation to training.

Short-Term Intense Exercise
The energy to perform short-term exercise of high intensity comes primarily from anaerobic metabolic pathways. Whether the ATP production is dominated by the ATP-CP system or glycolysis depends primarily on the length of the activity (1, 2, 36, 40). For example, the energy to run a 50-meter dash, or complete a single play in a football game comes principally from the ATP-CP system. In contrast, the energy to complete the 400-meter dash (i.e., 55 seconds) comes from a combination of the ATP-CP system, glycolysis,

and aerobic metabolism, with glycolysis producing most of the ATP. In general, the ATP-CP system can supply almost all the needed ATP for work for events lasting one to five seconds; intense exercise lasting longer than five to six seconds begins to utilize the ATP-producing capability of glycolysis. It should be emphasized that the transition from the ATP-CP system to an increased dependence upon glycolysis during exercise is not an abrupt change but rather a gradual shift from one pathway to another.

Events lasting longer than forty-five seconds use a combination of all three energy systems (i.e., ATP-CP, glycolysis, aerobic system). This point was emphasized in table 3.3 in chapter 3. In general, intense exercise lasting approximately sixty seconds utilizes 70%/30% (anaerobic/aerobic) energy production, while events lasting two minutes utilize anaerobic and aerobic bioenergetic pathways almost equally to supply the needed ATP (see table 3.3).

Prolonged Exercise
The energy to perform long-term exercise (i.e., > ten minutes) comes primarily from aerobic metabolism. A steady state oxygen uptake can generally be maintained during submaximal exercise of moderate duration. However, two exceptions to this rule exist. First, prolonged exercise in a hot/humid environment results in a "drift" upward of oxgyen uptake; therefore,

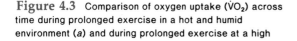

Figure 4.3 Comparison of oxygen uptake ($\dot{V}O_2$) across time during prolonged exercise in a hot and humid environment (*a*) and during prolonged exercise at a high relative work rate ($>$ 70% $\dot{V}O_2$ max) (*b*). Note that in both conditions there is a steady "drift" upward in $\dot{V}O_2$. See text for description.

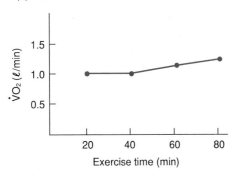

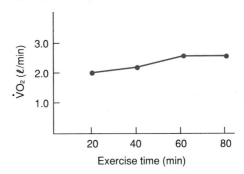

a steady state is not maintained in this type of exercise (47). Second, continuous exercise at a high relative work rate (i.e., $>$ 70% $\dot{V}O_2$ max) results in a slow rise in oxygen uptake across time (28) (figure 4.3). In each of these two types of exercise, the drift upward in $\dot{V}O_2$ is probably due principally to the effects of increasing body temperature and to a lesser degree to rising blood levels of the hormones epinephrine and norepinephrine (11, 24, 25, 28, 39). Both of these variables tend to increase the metabolic rate resulting in increased oxygen uptake across time.

Incremental Exercise

The maximal capacity to transport and utilize oxygen during exercise ($\dot{V}O_2$ max) is considered by many exercise scientists to be the most valid measurement of cardiovascular fitness. Indeed, incremental or graded exercise tests are often employed by physicians to examine patients for possible heart disease and by physical educators to determine a subject's cardiovascular fitness. These tests are usually conducted on a treadmill or a cycle ergometer. However, an arm crank ergometer can be employed for testing paraplegics or athletes whose sport involves arm work (e.g., swimmers, rowers, etc.). The test generally begins with the subject performing a brief warm-up followed by an increase in the work rate every one to three minutes until the subject cannot maintain the desired power output.

This increase in work rate can be achieved on the treadmill by increasing either the speed of the treadmill or the incline. On the cycle or arm ergometer, the increase in power output is obtained by increasing the resistance against the flywheel.

Figure 4.4 illustrates the change in oxygen uptake during a typical incremental exercise test on a cycle ergometer. Oxygen uptake increases as a linear function of the work rate until $\dot{V}O_2$ max is reached. When $\dot{V}O_2$ max is reached, an increase in power output does not result in an increase in oxygen uptake; thus, $\dot{V}O_2$ max represents a "physiological ceiling" for the ability of the oxygen transport system to deliver O_2 to contracting muscles.

Lactate Threshold

It is generally believed that most of the ATP production used to provide energy for muscular contraction during the early stages of an incremental exercise test comes from aerobic sources (48, 54). However, as the exercise intensity increases, blood levels of lactic acid begin to rise in an exponential fashion (figure 4.5). This appears in untrained subjects around 50%–60% of $\dot{V}O_2$ max, while it occurs at higher work rates in trained subjects (i.e., 65%–80% $\dot{V}O_2$ max). Although much controversy exists, many investigators believe that this sudden rise in lactic acid during incremental exercise represents a point of increasing reliance on anaerobic

Figure 4.4 Changes in oxygen uptake ($\dot{V}O_2$) during an incremental exercise test. The observed plateau in $\dot{V}O_2$ represents $\dot{V}O_2$ max.

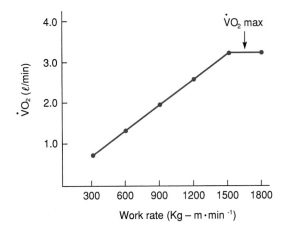

metabolism (i.e., glycolysis) (15, 57–61). The most common term used to depict the point of a systematic rise in blood lactic acid during exercise is the **anaerobic threshold** (10, 14, 34, 38, 43, 49, 58, 59, 64). However, arguments over terminology exist and this lactic acid inflection point has also been called the **lactate threshold** and the "onset of blood lactate accumulation (OBLA)" by some investigators (21, 30). To avoid confusion, we will refer to the sudden rise in blood lactic acid during incremental exercise as the lactate threshold.

The basic argument against the term "anaerobic threshold" centers around the question of whether the rise in blood lactic acid during incremental exercise is due to a lack of oxygen in the working muscle or perhaps other reasons. Historically, rising blood lactic acid levels have been considered an indication of increased anaerobic metabolism within the contracting muscle due to low levels of O_2 in the individual muscle cells (58, 59). However, whether the end product of glycolysis is pyruvic or lactic acid depends on a variety of factors. First, if the rate of glycolysis is rapid, then NADH production may exceed the transport capacity of the shuttle mechanisms that move hydrogens from the sarcoplasm into the mitochondria (55, 56, 63).

Also, blood levels of epinephrine and norepinephrine begin to rise at 50%–65% of $\dot{V}O_2$ max during incremental exercise and have been shown to stimulate the glycolytic rate, and therefore increase the rate of NADH production (56). Failure of the shuttle system to keep up with the rate of NADH production by glycolysis would result in pyruvic acid accepting some "unshuttled" hydrogens, and the formation of lactic acid could occur independent of whether the muscle cell had sufficient oxygen for aerobic ATP production (figure 4.6).

A second explanation for the formation of lactic acid in exercising muscle is related to the enzyme that catalyzes the conversion of pyruvate to lactic acid. The enzyme responsible for this reaction is lactate dehydrogenase (LDH) and exists in several forms. Recall that the reaction is as follows:

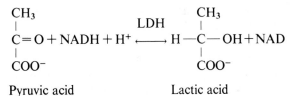

Pyruvic acid   Lactic acid

This reaction is reversible in that lactic acid can be converted back to pyruvic acid under the appropriate conditions. Human skeletal muscle is generally classified into three different fiber types (chapter 8). Briefly, two of these fiber types are labeled as being either "fast twitch" or "slow twitch." As the names imply, fast-twitch fibers are recruited during intense rapid exercise, while slow-twitch fibers are used primarily during low-intensity activity. Fast-twitch fibers contain a form of LDH, which favors the conversion of pyruvic acid to lactic acid (35, 54). In contrast, slow-twitch fibers contain an LDH form that promotes the conversion of lactic acid to pyruvic acid. Therefore, lactic acid formation might occur in fast-twitch fibers during exercise simply because of the type of LDH present. Thus, lactic acid production would again be independent of oxygen availability in the muscle cell. Early in an incremental exercise test it is likely that slow-twitch fibers are first called into action. However,

Figure 4.5 Changes in blood lactic acid concentrations during incremental exercise. The sudden rise in lactate is known as the lactate threshold.

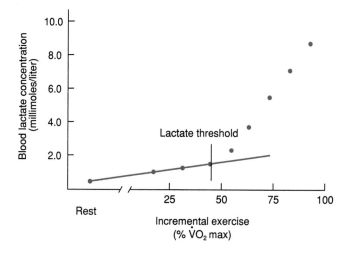

as the work rate rises the need to recruit more and more fast-twitch fibers increases. Therefore, the involvement of more fast-twitch fibers may result in increased lactic acid production and thus be responsible for the lactate threshold.

A final explanation for the lactate threshold may be related to the rate of removal of lactic acid from the blood during incremental exercise. When a researcher removes a blood sample from an exercising subject the concentration of lactic acid in that sample is the difference between the amount of lactic acid entry into the blood and the rate of lactic acid removal from the blood. At any given time during exercise, some muscles are producing and releasing lactic acid into the blood, and some tissues (i.e., liver, skeletal muscles, heart, etc.) are removing lactic acid. Therefore, the concentration of lactic acid in the blood at any given time can be expressed mathematically in the following way:

$$\text{Blood lactic acid concentration} = \text{lactic acid entry into the blood} - \text{blood lactic acid removal}$$

Thus a rise in the blood lactic acid concentration can occur due to either an increase in lactic acid production or a decrease in lactic acid removal. Recent evidence suggests that the rise in blood lactic acid levels in animals during incremental exercise may be due to both an increase in lactic acid production and a decrease in the rate of lactic acid removal (9, 20). See chapter 13 for a discussion of how endurance training affects lactic acid production.

In summary, controversy exists over both the terminology and the mechanism to explain the sudden rise in blood lactic acid concentrations during incremental exercise. It seems possible that any one or combination of the above explanations (including lack of O_2) might provide an explanation for the lactate threshold. Figure 4.7 contains a summary of possible mechanisms to explain the lactate threshold. The search for definitive evidence to explain the mechanism(s) altering the blood lactate concentration during incremental exercise will continue for years to come.

Figure 4.6 Failure of the mitochondrial "hydrogen shuttle" system to keep pace with the rate of glycolytic production of NADH + H⁺ results in the conversion of pyruvic acid to lactic acid.

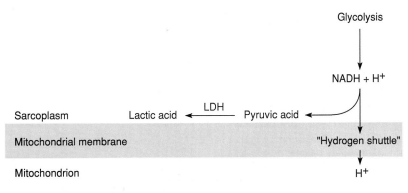

Figure 4.7 Possible mechanisms to explain the lactate threshold during incremental exercise. See text for details.

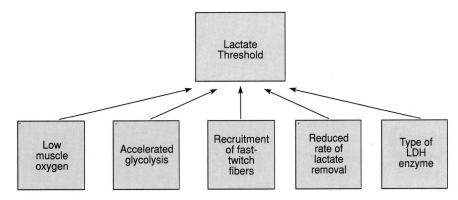

Practical Use of the Lactate Threshold

Regardless of the physiological mechanism to explain the lactate threshold, the point of exponential rise in lactic acid during graded exercise has important implications for predicting sports performance and perhaps in planning training programs for endurance athletes. For example, several studies have demonstrated that the lactate threshold used in combination with other physiological measurements (i.e., $\dot{V}O_2$ max, etc.) is a useful predictor of success in distance running (23, 44). Further, the lactate threshold might serve as a guideline for coaches and athletes in planning the level of exercise intensity needed to optimize training results. This will be discussed in more detail in chapters 16 and 21.

Estimation of Fuel Utilization during Exercise

A noninvasive technique that is commonly used to estimate the percent contribution of carbohydrate or fat to energy metabolism during exercise is the ratio of carbon dioxide output ($\dot{V}CO_2$) to the volume of oxygen consumed ($\dot{V}O_2$). This ratio ($\dot{V}CO_2/\dot{V}O_2$) is called the **respiratory exchange ratio (R)**. During steady state conditions the $\dot{V}CO_2/\dot{V}O_2$ ratio is often termed the respiratory quotient (RQ). For simplicity, we will refer to the $\dot{V}CO_2/\dot{V}O_2$ ratio as the respiratory exchange ratio (R). How can the R be used to estimate whether fat or carbohydrate is being used as a fuel? The answer is related to the fact that fat and carbohydrate differ in the amount of O_2 used and CO_2 produced during oxidation. When using R as a predictor of fuel utilization during exercise, the role that protein contributes to ATP production during exercise is ignored. This is reasonable since protein generally plays a small role as a substrate during physical activity. Therefore, the R during exercise is often termed a "nonprotein R."

Let's consider the R for fat first. When fat is oxidized, O_2 combines with carbon to form CO_2 and joins with hydrogen to form water. The chemical relationship is as follows:

Fat (palmitic acid) $C_{16}H_{32}O_2$
Oxidation: $C_{16}H_{32}O_2 + 23\ O_2 \rightarrow 16\ CO_2 + 16\ H_2O$
Therefore the $R = 16\ CO_2 \div 23\ O_2 = 0.70$

In order for R to be used as an estimate of substrate utilization during exercise, the subject must have reached a steady state. This is important because only during steady state exercise is the $\dot{V}CO_2$ and $\dot{V}O_2$ reflective of O_2 and CO_2 exchange in the tissues. For example, if a person is hyperventilating (i.e., breathing too much for a particular metabolic rate), excessive CO_2 loss could bias the ratio of $\dot{V}CO_2$ to $\dot{V}O_2$ and invalidate the use of R to estimate which fuel is being consumed.

Carbohydrate oxidation also results in a predictable ratio of the volume of oxygen consumed to the amount of CO_2 produced. The oxidation of carbohydrate results in an R of 1.0:

Table 4.1 *Percentage of fat and carbohydrate metabolized as determined by a nonprotein respiratory exchange ratio (R)*

R	% Fat	% Carbohydrate
0.70	100	0
0.75	83	17
0.80	67	33
0.85	50	50
0.90	33	67
0.95	17	83
1.00	0	100

Glucose $= C_6H_{12}O_6$
Oxidation: $C_6H_{12}O_6 + 6\ O_2 \rightarrow 6\ CO_2 + 6\ H_2O$
$R = \dot{V}CO_2 \div \dot{V}O_2 = 6\ CO_2 \div 6\ O_2 = 1$

Fat oxidation requires more O_2 than does carbohydrate oxidation. This is due to the fact that carbohydrate contains more O_2 than does fat (56).

It is unlikely that either fat or carbohydrate would be the singular substrate used during most types of submaximal exercise. Therefore, the exercise R would likely be somewhere between 1.0 and 0.70. Table 4.1 lists a range of R values and the percentage of fat or carbohydrate metabolism they represent. Note that a nonprotein R of 0.85 represents a condition where fat and carbohydrate contribute equally as energy substrates. Further, notice that the higher the R, the greater the role of carbohydrate as an energy source, and the lower the R, the greater the contribution of fat.

Factors Governing Fuel Selection

Proteins play only a minor role as a substrate during exercise, with fat and carbohydrate serving as the major sources of energy during activity in the healthy individual consuming a balanced diet. In general, carbohydrates are used as the primary fuel during high-intensity exercise (26, 27). Further, carbohydrates

Figure 4.8 Shift from carbohydrate metabolism toward fat metabolism during prolonged exercise.

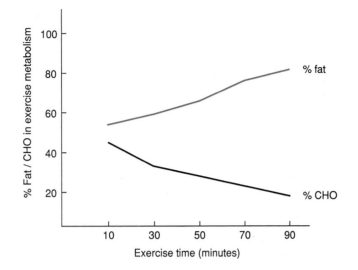

serve as the major substrate at the onset of low-to-moderate-intensity exercise. However, during prolonged work (i.e., > thirty minutes) there is gradual shift from carbohydrate metabolism toward an increasing reliance on fat as a substrate (46). Figure 4.8 demonstrates this point. Whether fat or carbohydrate is the primary substrate during work is determined largely by the availability of the fuel to the individual muscle cell and those factors that regulate glycolysis, the Krebs cycle, and the electron transport chain.

Regulation of Protein Metabolism
In the 1960s and early 1970s, protein was believed to contribute less than 2% of the fuel utilized during exercise. However, recent evidence suggests that the total contribution of protein to the fuel supply during exercise may reach 5%–15% depending on exercise duration (5, 12, 41, 42, 62). The role that protein plays as a substrate during exercise is principally dependent on body carbohydrate stores and the availability of branch-chained amino acids and the amino acid alanine (4). Skeletal muscle can directly metabolize certain types of amino acids (i.e., valine, leucine, isoleucine) to produce ATP (refer to figure 3.13 for a review). In

the liver, alanine can be converted to glucose and returned via the blood to skeletal muscle to be utilized as a substrate.

Any factor that increases the amino acid pool (amount of available amino acids) in the liver or in skeletal muscle can theoretically enhance protein metabolism. One such factor is prolonged exercise (i.e., > 120 minutes). Dohm and associates (18, 19) have demonstrated that enzymes capable of degrading muscle proteins (proteases) are activated following long-term exercise. The mechanism to explain activation of these proteases during prolonged exercise is not currently known. However, the practical aspect of this finding is that during the course of prolonged exercise, proteases become active and amino acids are liberated from their parent proteins. This rise in the amino acid pool results in an increased use of amino acids as fuel for exercise.

Regulation of Carbohydrate Metabolism
Most of the carbohydrate used as a substrate during exercise comes from glycogen stores in muscle, with the remaining portion coming from blood glucose (26, 37). Glycogen or glucose enters the bioenergetic process via glycolysis; therefore, any factor that stimulates glycolysis increases carbohydrate metabolism.

Figure 4.9 Illustration of the effect of an increase of ADP + P$_i$ on glycolysis. Note that a lack of O$_2$ results in (−) inhibition of the electron transport chain and ultimately an enhanced (+) rate of glycolysis.

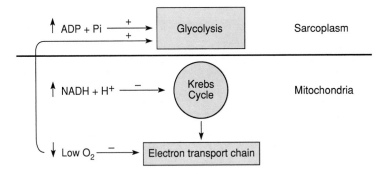

Several variables contribute to the regulation of carbohydrate metabolism during exercise. First, when oxygen is not available in muscle cells, the activity of the Krebs cycle and electron transport chain is halted. Thus, the only source of ATP production during this situation is the ATP-CP system and glycolysis. Under these anaerobic conditions there is an accumulation of NADH and ADP + Pi. The increase in NADH and therefore a reduction in NAD inhibits the Krebs cycle, and the increase in ADP + P$_i$ stimulates glycolysis (figure 4.9).

Several hormones play a role in the regulation of carbohydrate metabolism. We will mention only two here since details of hormonal activity during exercise are discussed in chapter 5. Briefly, the hormone epinephrine, which is released during periods of high stress or heavy exercise, stimulates glycolysis and thus promotes carbohydrate metabolism (56). Further, the hormone insulin increases glycolysis by aiding in the uptake of glucose into the cell and increasing the formation of fat, which reduces the availability of free fatty acids as a substrate.

Regulation of Fat Metabolism

When an individual consumes more energy (i.e., food) than he or she expends, this additional energy is stored in the form of fat. A gain of 3,500 kcal of energy results in the storage of one pound of fat. Most fat is stored in the form of triglycerides in adipocytes (fat cells), but some is stored in muscle cells as well. The major factor that determines the role of fat as a substrate during exercise is its availability to the muscle cell. In order to be metabolized, triglycerides must be broken down by a process called **lipolysis** into **free fatty acids** (FFA) (three molecules) and glycerol (one molecule). When triglycerides are split, FFA can then be converted into Acetyl CoA and enter the Krebs cycle.

Similar to carbohydrate metabolism, fat metabolism is regulated by those variables that regulate lipolysis. What factors regulate lipolysis? Triglycerides are broken down into FFA and glycerol by enzymes called **lipases.** These lipases are generally inactive until stimulated by the hormones epinephrine, norepinephrine, and glucagon. For example, during prolonged exercise, blood levels of epinephrine rise, which increases lipase activity and thus promotes lipolysis. This increase in lipolysis results in an increase in blood and muscle levels of FFA and promotes fat metabolism. In general, lipolysis is a rather slow process and an increase in fat metabolism occurs only after several minutes of exercise. This point is illustrated in figure 4.8 by the slow increase in fat metabolism across time during prolonged submaximal exercise.

The mobilization of FFA into the blood is inhibited by the hormone insulin and high blood levels of lactic acid. Insulin inhibits lipolysis by direct inhibition of lipase activity. Normally, blood insulin levels decline during prolonged exercise (chapter 5). However, if a

Box 4.1 Regulation of Glycogen Breakdown during Exercise

Much of the carbohydrate broken down via glycolysis during exercise comes from intramuscular glycogen stores. Glycogen storage in muscle is dependent on the availability of glucose and the activity of the enzyme glycogen snythetase. Breakdown of glycogen (glycogenolysis) into individual glucose molecules is dependent on the enzyme phosphorylase. In nonworking muscle, phosphorylase is generally found in an inactive form and thus must be "activated" before glycogen breakdown can occur. This activation of phosphorylase is regulated by two mechanisms. The mechanism that best explains the activation of phosphorylase at the beginning of exercise is linked to a substance called "calmodulin." Calmodulin is found in muscle and is activated at the onset of exercise by the release of calcium from the sarcoplasmic reticulum (chapter 8). Active calmodulin then activates phosphorylase, which promotes glycogenolysis (see chapter 5 for details of calmodulin activity).

The second system that may activate phosphorylase during exercise is controlled by the hormone epinephrine. Epinephrine binds to a receptor on the cell membrane, which results in the formation of "cyclic AMP," which then activates phosphorylase (chapter 5 contains additional information on cyclic AMP). This mechanism is probably operative during prolonged exercise, but is too slow to explain the immediate glycogenolysis at the onset of muscular contraction.

---

high-carbohydrate meal or drink is consumed immediately prior to exercise, blood glucose levels rise and more insulin is released from the pancreas. This elevation in blood insulin results in diminished lipolysis and a reduction in fat metabolism.

Exercise above the lactate threshold results in elevated blood levels of lactic acid, which promotes the recombination of FFA and glycerol to form triglycerides. The end result of this process is a reduction in the availability of FFA as a substrate. The lack of fat as a substrate for working muscles under these conditions dictates that carbohydrate will be the primary fuel.

Interaction of Fat/Carbohydrate Metabolism

During short-term exercise it is unlikely that muscle stores of glycogen or blood glucose levels would be depleted. However, during prolonged exercise (e.g., > 120 minutes) muscle stores of glycogen and blood glucose levels can reach very low levels (2, 12, 26). This depletion of available carbohydrate reduces the rate of glycolysis. This affects fat metabolism in the following manner. Pyruvic acid (produced via glycolysis) is in equilibrium with oxaloacetic acid (an intermediate in the Krebs cycle) (56). When the rate of glycolysis is greatly reduced due to the unavailability of substrate, pyruvic acid levels in the sarcoplasm begin to decline. The fall is followed by a conversion of oxaloacetic acid to pyruvic acid:

$$\text{Pyruvic acid} \xleftarrow[\text{Pyruvate carboxylase}]{\hspace{3cm}} \text{Oxaloacetic acid}$$

As a result, oxaloacetic acid levels decrease in the mitochondria and slow the rate of the Krebs cycle, which is limited by the availability of oxaloacetic acid. This results in a diminished rate of ATP production via fat metabolism since fat can only be metabolized via Krebs-cycle oxidation. Hence, when carbohydrate stores are depleted in muscle, the rate at which fat is metabolized is reduced. Therefore, "fats burn in the flame of carbohydrates" (56). The role that glycogen depletion may play in limiting performance during prolonged exercise is discussed in chapter 19.

Recovery from Exercise: Metabolic Responses

Metabolism remains elevated for several minutes immediately following exercise. The magnitude and duration of this elevated metabolism is influenced by the

Figure 4.10 Oxygen deficit and debt during light/moderate exercise (*a*) and during heavy exercise (*b*).

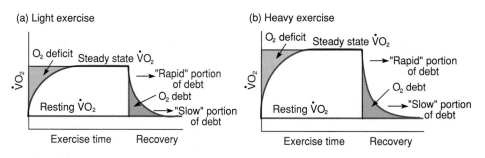

(a) Light exercise

O_2 deficit   Steady state $\dot{V}O_2$

→ "Rapid" portion of debt

$\dot{V}O_2$

O_2 debt

Resting $\dot{V}O_2$

→ "Slow" portion of debt

Exercise time   Recovery

(b) Heavy exercise

O_2 deficit   Steady state $\dot{V}O_2$

→ "Rapid" portion of debt

$\dot{V}O_2$

O_2 debt

Resting $\dot{V}O_2$

→ "Slow" portion of debt

Exercise time   Recovery

intensity of the exercise (3, 34). This point is illustrated in figure 4.10. Note that oxygen uptake is greater and remains elevated for a longer time period following high-intensity exercise when compared to exercise of light-to-moderate intensity. The reason(s) for this observation will be discussed shortly.

Historically, the term **oxygen debt** has been applied to mean the excess oxygen uptake above rest following exercise. The prominent British physiologist A. V. Hill (33) first used the term O_2 debt and reasoned that the excess oxygen consumed (above rest) following exercise was repayment for the O_2 deficit incurred at the onset of exercise. Evidence collected in the 1920s and 1930s by Hill and other researchers in Europe suggested that the oxygen debt could be divided into two portions: the rapid portion immediately following exercise (i.e., approximately two to three minutes post exercise) and the slow portion, which persisted for greater than thirty minutes after exercise. The rapid portion is represented by the steep decline in oxygen uptake following exercise, and the slow portion is represented by the slow decline in $\dot{V}O_2$ across time following exercise (figure 4.10). The rationale for the two divisions of the O_2 debt was based on the belief that the rapid portion of the O_2 debt represented the oxygen that was required to resynthesize stored ATP and CP and replace tissue stores of O_2 ($\sim$ 20% of the O_2 debt), while the slow portion of the debt was due to the oxidative conversion of lactic acid to glycogen in the liver ($\sim$ 80% of the O_2 debt).

In contrast to the historical view, recent evidence has shown that only about 20% of the oxygen debt is used to convert the lactic acid produced during exercise to glycogen (the process of glycogen synthesis from noncarbohydrate sources is called **gluconeogenesis**) (7, 8). Therefore, the notion that the "slow" portion of the O_2 debt is due entirely to oxidative conversion of lactic acid to glycogen does not appear to be accurate. Several investigators have argued that the term oxygen debt be eliminated from the literature because the elevated oxygen consumption following exercise does not appear to be entirely due to the "borrowing" of oxygen from the body's oxygen stores (7, 8, 12, 24). In recent years several replacement terms have been suggested. One such term is **EPOC,** which stands for "excess post exercise oxygen consumption" (12, 24).

If the EPOC is not exclusively used to convert lactic acid to glycogen, why does oxygen consumption remain elevated post exercise? Several possibilities exist. First, at least part of the O_2 consumed immediately following exercise is used to restore CP in muscle and O_2 stores in blood and tissues (6, 24). Restoration of both CP and oxygen stores in muscle is completed within two to three minutes of recovery (29). This is consistent with the classic view of the fast portion of the oxygen debt. Further, heart rate and breathing remain elevated above resting levels for several minutes following exercise; therefore, both of these activities require additional O_2 above resting levels. Other factors that may result in the EPOC are an elevated body

Box 4.2 Removal of Lactic Acid Following Exercise

What happens to the lactic acid that is formed during exercise? Classical theory proposed that the majority of the post-exercise lactate was converted into glycogen by the "Cori cycle" in the liver and resulted in an elevated post-exercise oxygen uptake (i.e., O_2 debt). However, recent evidence suggests that this is not the case and that lactate is mainly oxidized after exercise (7, 8). That is, lactate is converted to pyruvate and used as a substrate by the heart, skeletal muscle, etc. It is estimated that approximately 70% of the lactate produced during exercise is oxidized, while 20% is converted to glycogen and the remaining 10% is converted to amino acids.

Figure 4.11 demonstrates the time course of lactic acid removal from the blood following strenuous exercise. Note that lactate removal is more rapid if continuous light exercise is performed as compared to a resting recovery. The explanation for these findings is linked to the fact that light exercise enhances oxidation of lactate by the working muscle (16, 31). It is estimated that the optimum intensity of recovery exercise to promote blood lactate removal is around 30%–40% of $\dot{V}O_2$ max (16). Higher exercise intensities would likely result in an increased muscle production of lactic acid and therefore hinder removal.

Figure 4.11 Blood lactate removal following strenuous exercise. Note that lactic acid can be removed more rapidly from the blood during recovery if the subject engages in continuous light exercise.

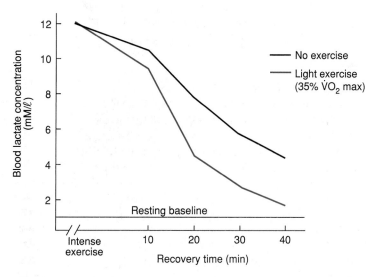

Figure 4.12 A summary of factors that might contribute to "excess post exercise oxygen consumption." See text for details.

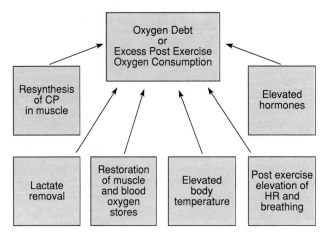

temperature and specific circulating hormones. Increases in body temperature result in an increased metabolic rate (called the Q_{10} effect) (11, 28, 47). Further, it has been argued that high levels of epinephrine or norepinephrine result in increased oxygen consumption after exercise (25). However, both of these hormones are rapidly removed from the blood following exercise and therefore may not exist long enough to have a significant impact on the EPOC.

Earlier it was mentioned that the EPOC was greater following high-intensity exercise when compared to the EPOC following light-to-moderate work. The explanation for this observation is related, in part, to the differences between the two exercise intensities in the amount of body heat gained, the amount of CP depleted, and the blood levels of epinephrine and norephinephrine. First, assuming similar ambient conditions (i.e., room temperature/relative humidity) and equal exercise time, high-intensity exercise will result in greater body heat gain than light exercise. Secondly, depletion of CP is dependent on exercise intensity. Since high-intensity exercise would utilize more CP, additional oxygen would be required during recovery for resynthesis. Finally, intense exercise results in greater

blood concentrations of epinephrine and norepinephrine when compared to light work. All of these factors may contribute to the EPOC being greater following intense exercise when compared to light exercise. Figure 4.12 contains a summary of factors thought to contribute to the "excess post exercise oxygen consumption."

Summary

1. In the transition from rest to light or moderate exercise, oxygen uptake increases rapidly, reaching a steady state within one to four minutes. The failure of oxygen uptake to increase instantly at the beginning of exercise suggests that anaerobic pathways contribute to the overall production of ATP early in exercise. However, after a steady state is reached, the body's ATP requirement is met via aerobic metabolism.

2. During high-intensity short-term exercise (i.e., two to twenty seconds), the muscle's ATP production is dominated by the ATP-CP system. Intense exercise lasting more than

twenty seconds relies more on anaerobic glycolysis to produce much of the needed ATP. Finally, high-intensity events lasting longer than forty-five seconds use a combination of the ATP-CP system, glycolysis, and the aerobic system to produce the needed ATP for muscular contraction.

3. The energy to perform prolonged exercise (i.e., > ten minutes) comes primarily from aerobic metabolism.

4. Oxygen uptake increases in a linear fashion during incremental exercise until $\dot{V}O_2$ max is reached. The point at which blood lactate rises systematically during graded exercise is termed the lactate threshold or anaerobic threshold. The lactate threshold has practical uses such as in performance prediction and as a marker of training intensity.

5. Regulation of fuel selection during exercise is under complex control. In general, carbohydrates are used as the major fuel source early in exercise and during high-intensity work. However, during prolonged exercise there is a gradual shift from carbohydrate metabolism toward fat metabolism.

6. One of the experimental techniques used to study the role of fat or carbohydrate as a substrate during exercise is measurement of the respiratory exchange ratio (R) ($\dot{V}CO_2 \div \dot{V}O_2$) during steady state exercise.

7. The term *oxygen debt* is defined as the O_2 consumption above rest following exercise. The O_2 debt consists of several parts. First, some of the O_2 debt is used to resynthesize stored CP in the muscle and replace O_2 stores in both muscle and blood. Other factors that contribute to the "slow" portion of the O_2 debt include an elevated body temperature, O_2 required to convert lactate to glycogen (gluconeogenesis), and elevated blood levels of epinephrine and norepinephrine.

Study Questions

1. Identify the predominant energy systems used to produce ATP during the following types of exercise:
   a. short-term intense exercise (i.e., < ten seconds duration).
   b. 400-meter dash
   c. twenty-kilometer race (i.e., 12.4 miles)

2. Graph the change in oxygen uptake during the transition from rest to steady state submaximal exercise. Label the oxygen deficit. Where does the ATP come from during the transition period from rest to steady state?

3. Graph the change in oxygen uptake and blood lactate concentration during incremental exercise. Label the point on the graph that might be considered the lactate threshold or lactate inflection point.

4. Discuss several possible reasons why blood lactate begins to rise rapidly during incremental exercise.

5. Briefly, explain how the respiratory exchange ratio is used to estimate which substrate is being utilized during exercise. What is meant by the term "nonprotein R"?

6. List two factors that play a role in the regulation of carbohydrate metabolism during exercise.

7. List those variables that regulate fat metabolism during exercise.

8. Define the following terms: (a) triglyceride, (b) lipolysis, and (c) lipases.

9. Graph the change in oxygen uptake during recovery from exercise. Label the oxygen debt.

10. How does modern theory of EPOC differ from the classical oxygen debt theory proposed by A. V. Hill?

Suggested Readings

Armstrong, R. 1979. Biochemistry: Energy liberation and use. In (R. Strauss, ed.) *Sports Medicine and Physiology.* Philadelphia: W. B. Saunders Company.

Brooks, G., and T. Fahey. 1984. *Exercise Physiology: Human Bioenergetics and Its Applications.* New York: John Wiley & Sons.

Gollnick, P. 1985. Metabolism of substrates: Energy substrate metabolism during exercise and as modified by training. *Federation Proceedings* 44:353–56.

Holloszy, J. 1982. Muscle metabolism during exercise. *Archives of Physical and Rehabilitation Medicine* 63:231–34.

Lemon, P. 1987. Protein and exercise: Update 1987. *Medicine and Science in Sports and Exercise* 19 (Suppl.):S179–S190.

References

1. Armstrong, R. 1979. Biochemistry: Energy liberation and use. In (R. Strauss, ed.) *Sports Medicine and Physiology.* Philadelphia: W. B. Saunders Company.

2. Astrand, P., and K. Rodahl. 1986. *Textbook of Work Physiology.* New York: McGraw-Hill.

3. Barnard, R., and M. Foss. 1969. Oxygen debt: Effect of beta adrenergic blockade on the lactacid and alactacid components. *Journal of Applied Physiology* 27:813–16.

4. Bates, P. et al. 1980. Exercise and protein turnover in the rat. *Journal of Physiology* (London) 303:41P.

5. Berg, A., and J. Keul. 1980. Serum alanine during long-lasting exercise. *International Journal of Sports Medicine* 1:199–202.

6. Boutellier, U. et al. 1984. Aftereffects of chronic hypoxia on $\dot{V}O_2$ kinetics and on O_2 deficit and debt. *European Journal of Applied Physiology* 53:87–91.

7. Brooks, G. 1985. "Lactate: Glycolytic End Product and Oxidative Substrate during Sustained Exercise in Mammals—the Lactate Shuttle." In (R. Giles, ed.) *Circulation, Respiration, and Metabolism.* Berlin: Springer-Verlag.

8. Brooks, G. 1986. The lactate shuttle during exercise and recovery. *Medicine and Science in Sports and Exercise* 18:360–68.

9. Brooks, G. 1986. Lactate production under fully aerobic conditions: The lactate shuttle during rest and exercise. *Federation Proceedings* 45:2924–29.

10. Brooks, G. 1985. Anaerobic threshold: Review of the concept and directions for future research. *Medicine and Science in Sports and Exercise* 17:22–23.

11. Brooks, G. et al. 1971. Temperature, skeletal muscle, mitochondrial functions, and oxygen debt. *American Journal of Physiology* 220:1,053–59.

12. Brooks, G., and T. Fahey. 1984. *Exercise Physiology: Human Bioenergetics and Its Applications.* New York: John Wiley & Sons.

13. Cerretelli, P. et al. 1977. Oxygen uptake transients at the onset and offset of arm and leg work. *Respiration Physiology* 30:81–97.

14. Davis, J. et al. 1976. Anaerobic threshold and maximal aerobic power for three modes of exercise. *Journal of Applied Physiology* 41:544–50.

15. Davis, J. 1985. Anaerobic threshold: Review of the concept and directions for future research. *Medicine and Science in Sports and Exercise* 17:6–18.

16. Dodd, S. et al. 1984. Blood lactate disappearance at various intensities of recovery exercise. *Journal of Applied Physiology* 57:1462–65.

17. Dodd, S. et al. 1988. Effects of beta-blockade on ventilation and gas exchange during the rest-to-work transition. *Aviation, Space, and Environmental Medicine* 59:255–58.

18. Dohm, G. et al. 1978. Changes in tissue protein levels as a result of endurance exercise. *Life Sciences* 23:845–50.

19. Dohm, G. et al. 1981. Influence of exercise on free amino acid concentrations in rat tissues. *Journal of Applied Physiology* 50:41–44.

20. Donovan, C., and G. Brooks. 1983. Endurance training affects lactate clearance, not lactate production. *American Journal of Physiology* 244:E83–E92.

21. England, P. et al. 1985. The effect of acute thermal dehydration on blood lactate accumulation during incremental exercise. *Journal of Sports Sciences* 2:105–11.

22. Essen, B., and L. Kaijser. 1978. Regulation of glycolysis in intermittent exercise in man. *Journal of Physiology* 281:499–511.

23. Farrell, P. et al. 1979. Plasma lactate accumulation and distance running performance. *Medicine and Science in Sports* 11:338–44.

24. Gaesser, G., and G. Brooks. 1984. Metabolic bases of excess post-exercise oxygen consumption: A review. *Medicine and Science in Sports and Exercise* 16:29–43.

25. Gladden, B., W. Stainsby, and B. MacIntosh. 1982. Norepinephrine increases canine muscle $\dot{V}O_2$ during recovery. *Medicine and Science in Sports and Exercise* 14:471–76.

26. Gollnick, P. 1985. Metabolism of substrates: Energy substrate metabolism during exercise and as modified by training. *Federation Proceedings* 44:353–56.

27. Gollnick, P., W. Bayly, and D. Hodgson. 1986. Exercise intensity, training, diet, and lactate concentration in muscle and blood. *Medicine and Science in Sports and Exercise* 18:334–40.

28. Hagberg, J., J. Mullin, and F. Nagle. 1978. Oxygen consumption during constant load exercise. *Journal of Applied Physiology* 45:381–84.

29. Harris, R. et al. 1976. The time course of phosphocreatine resynthesis during recovery of the quadriceps muscle in man. *Pflugers Archives* 367:137–42.

30. Heck, H., and A. Mader. 1985. Justification of the 4-mmol/l lactate threshold. *International Journal of Sports Medicine* 6:117–30.

31. Hermanson, L., and I. Stensvold. 1972. Production and removal of lactate during exercise in man. *Acta Physiologica Scandinavica* 86:191–201.

32. Hickson, R., H. Bomze, and J. Holloszy. 1978. Faster adjustment of O_2 uptake to the energy requirement of exercise in the trained state. *Journal of Applied Physiology* 44:877–81.

33. Hill, A. 1914. The oxidative removal of lactic acid. *Journal of Physiology* (London) 48:x–xi.

34. Hollman, W. 1985. Historical remarks on the development of the aerobic-anaerobic threshold up to 1966. *International Journal of Sports Medicine* 6:109–16.

35. Holloszy, J. 1982. Muscle metabolism during exercise. *Archives of Physical and Rehabilitation Medicine* 63:231–34.

36. Hultman, E. 1973. Energy metabolism in human muscle. *Journal of Physiology* (London) 231:56.

37. Hultman, E., and H. Sjoholm. 1983. Substrate availability. In *Biochemistry of Exercise*, eds. H. Knuttgen, J. Vogel, and J. R. Poortmans. Champaign, Ill.:Human Kinetics Publishers.

38. Jones, N., and R. Ehrsam. 1982. The anaerobic threshold. *Exercise and Sports Science Review* 10:49–83.

39. Kalis, J. et al. 1988. Effects of beta blockade on the drift in O_2 consumption during prolonged exercise. *Journal of Applied Physiology* 64:753–58.

40. Knuttgen, H., and B. Saltin. 1972. Muscle metabolites and oxygen uptake in short-term submaximal exercise in man. *Journal of Applied Physiology* 32:690–94.

41. Lemon, P., and F. Mullin. 1980. Effect of initial glycogen levels on protein metabolism during exercise. 48:624–29.

42. Lemon, P., and R. Nagle. 1980. Effects of exercise on protein and amino acid metabolism. *Medicine and Science in Sports and Exercise* 13:141–49.

43. Mader, A., and H. Heck. 1986. A theory of the metabolic origin of the anaerobic threshold. *International Journal of Sports Medicine* 7:45–65.

44. Marti, B., T. Abelin, and H. Howald. 1987. A modified fixed blood lactate threshold for estimating running speed for joggers in 16-Km races. *Scandavian Journal of Sports Sciences* 9:41–45.

45. Medbo, J. et al. 1988. Anaerobic capacity determined maximal accumulated O_2 deficit. *Journal of Applied Physiology* 64:50–60.

46. Powers, S., W. Riley, and E. Howley. 1980. A comparison of fat metabolism in trained men and women during prolonged aerobic work. *Research Quarterly for Exercise and Sport* 52:427–31.

47. Powers, S., E. Howley, and R. Cox. 1982. Ventilatory and metabolic reactions to heat stress during prolonged exercise. *Journal of Sports Medicine and Physical Fitness* 22:32–36.

48. Powers, S. et al. 1983. Effects of caffeine ingestion on metabolism and performance during graded exercise. *European Journal of Applied Physiology* 560:301–7.

49. Powers, S., S. Dodd, and R. Garner. 1984. Precision of ventilatory and gas exchange alterations as a predictor of the anaerobic threshold. *European Journal of Applied Physiology* 52:173–77.

50. Powers, S. Dodd, and R. Beadle. 1985. Oxygen uptake kinetics in trained athletes differing in $\dot{V}O_2$ max. *European Journal of Applied Physiology* 39:407–15.

51. Powers, S. et al. 1987. Oxygen deficit-debt relationships in ponies during submaximal treadmill exercise. *Respiratory Physiology* 70:251–63.

52. Refsum, H., L. Gjessing, and S. Stromme. 1978. Changes in plasma amino acid distribution and urine amino acid excretion during prolonged heavy exercise. *Scandinavian Journal of Clinical and Laboratory Investigation* 39:407–13.

53. Riley, W., S. Powers, and H. Welch. 1981. The effect of two levels of muscular work on urinary creatinine excretion. *Research Quarterly for Exercise and Sport* 52:339–47.

54. Skinner, J., and T. McLellan. 1980. The transition from aerobic to anaerobic exercise. *Research Quarterly* 51:234–48.

55. Stainsby, W. 1986. Biochemical and physiological bases for lactate production. *Medicine and Science in Sports and Exercise* 18:341–43.

56. Stryer, L. 1981. *Biochemistry.* San Francisco: W. H. Freeman.

57. Wasserman, K. 1986. Anaerobiosis, lactate, and gas exchange during exercise: The issues. *Federation Proceedings* 45:2904–9.

58. Wasserman, K., and M. McIlroy. 1964. Detecting the threshold of anaerobic metabolism. *American Journal of Cardiology* 14:844–52.

59. Wasserman, K. et al. 1973. Anaerobic threshold and respiratory gas exchange during exercise. *Journal of Applied Physiology* 35:236–43.

60. Wasserman, K., B. Whipp, and J. Davis. 1981. Respiratory physiology of exercise: Metabolism, gas exchange, and ventilatory control. In (J. Widdicombe, ed.) *International Review of Physiology, Respiratory Physiology III.* Baltimore: University Park Press.

61. Wasserman, K., W. Beaver, and B. Whipp. 1986. Mechanisms and pattern of blood lactate increase during exercise in man. *Medicine and Science in Sports and Exercise* 18:344–52.

62. White, T., and G. Brooks. 1981. (C^{14}) Glucose, alanine, and leucine oxidation in rats at rest and two intensities of running. *Journal of Physiology* 240:R147–R152.

63. Wilson, D. et al. 1977. Effect of oxygen tension on cellular energetics. *American Journal of Physiology* 233:C135–C140.

64. Yoshida, T. 1986. Effect of dietary modifications on the anaerobic threshold. *Sports Medicine* 3:4–9.

5 Hormonal Responses to Exercise

Objectives

By studying this chapter, you should be able to do the following:

1. Describe the concept of hormone-receptor interaction.
2. Identify the four factors influencing the concentration of a hormone in the blood.
3. Describe the mechanism by which steroid hormones act on cells.
4. Describe the "second messenger" hypothesis of hormone action using the adenylate cyclase-cyclic AMP and Ca^{++}-calmodulin examples.
5. Describe the role of the hypothalamus-releasing factors in the control of hormone secretion from the anterior pituitary gland.
6. Describe the relationship of the hypothalamus to the secretion of hormones from the posterior pituitary gland.
7. Identify the site of release, stimulus for release, and the predominant action of the following hormones: epinephrine, norepinephrine, glucagon, insulin, cortisol, aldosterone, thyroxine, growth hormone, estrogen, and testosterone.
8. Discuss the use of testosterone (an anabolic steroid) and growth hormone on muscle growth and their potential side effects.
9. Contrast the role of plasma catecholamines with intracellular factors in the mobilization of muscle glycogen during exercise.
10. Graphically describe the changes in the following hormones during graded and prolonged exercise and discuss how those changes influence the four mechanisms used to maintain the blood glucose concentration: insulin, glucagon, cortisol, growth hormone, epinephrine, and norepinephrine.
11. Describe the interaction of changing hormone and substrate levels in the blood on the mobilization of free fatty acids from adipose tissue.

Outline

Key Terms

acromegaly
adenylate cyclase
adrenal cortex
adrenocorticotrophic hormone (ACTH)
aldosterone
alpha glycerol phosphate
alpha receptors
anabolic steroid
androgenic steroid
androgens
angiotensin I and II
anterior pituitary
antidiuretic hormone (ADH)
beta receptors
calcitonin
calmodulin
catecholamines
cortisol
cyclic AMP
diabetes mellitus
endocrine gland
endorphin
epinephrine (E)
estrogens
follicle-stimulating hormone (FSH)
General Adaptation Syndrome (GAS)
glucagon
glucocorticoids

growth hormone (GH)
hormone
hypothalamic somatostatin
hypothalamus
insulin
luteinizing hormone (LH)
mineralocorticoids
neuroendocrinology
norepinephrine (NE)
pancreas
phosphodiesterase
pituitary gland
posterior pituitary gland
prolactin
receptor
releasing hormone
renin
second messengers
sex steroids
somatomedins
somatostatin
steroids
testosterone
thyroid gland
thyroid-stimulating hormone (TSH)
thyroxine
triiodothyronine

As presented in the last chapter, the fuels for muscular exercise include muscle glycogen and fat, plasma glucose and free fatty acids, and to a lesser extent, amino acids. These fuels must be provided for activities as diverse as the 100-meter dash and the 26-mile, 385-yard marathon, or fatigue will occur. What controls the delivery of fuel? What stimulates the adipose tissue to release more FFA? How is the liver made aware of the need to replace the glucose that is being removed from the blood by exercising muscles? If glucose is not replaced, a hypoglycemic (low-blood-glucose condition) will occur. Hypoglycemia is a topic of crucial importance in a discussion of exercise as a challenge to homeostasis. Blood glucose is the primary fuel for the central nervous system (CNS), and without optimal CNS function during exercise, the chance of fatigue and even risk of serious injury are increased. While blood glucose was used as an example, it is clear that sodium, calcium, potassium, and water concentrations, as well as blood pressure and pH levels also should be maintained within tight limits during exercise. It should be no surprise then that there are a variety of automatic control systems maintaining these variables within these limits. Chapter 2 presented an overview of automatic control systems that maintain homeostasis. This chapter will expand on that by providing information on **neuroendocrinology,** a branch of physiology dedicated to the systematic study of control systems. The first part of the chapter will present a brief introduction to each hormone, indicate the factor controlling its secretion, and discuss its role in homeostasis. Following that, we will discuss how hormones control the delivery of carbohydrates and fats during exercise.

Neuroendocrinology

The two major homeostatic systems involved in the control and regulation of various functions (cardiovascular, renal, metabolic, etc.) are the nervous and endocrine systems. Both are structured to sense information, organize an appropriate response, and then deliver the message to the proper organ or tissue. Often, the two systems work together to maintain homeostasis, and the term "neuroendocrine response" is reflective of that interdependence. The two systems differ in the way the message is delivered: the endocrine system releases hormones into the blood to circulate to tissues, while nerves use neurotransmitters to relay messages from one nerve to the other, or from a nerve to a tissue.

Endocrine glands release **hormones** (chemical messengers) directly into the blood, which carries the hormone to a tissue to exert an effect. It is the binding of the hormone to a specific protein **receptor** that allows the hormone to exert its effect. In that way the hormone can circulate to all tissues while affecting only a few—those with the specific receptor. Hormones can be divided into several classes based on chemical makeup: amino acid derivatives, peptides/protein, and **steroids.** The chemical structure influences the way in which the hormone is transported in the blood and the manner in which it exerts its effect on the tissue. For example, while steroid hormones' lipid-like structure requires that they be transported bound to plasma protein (to "dissolve" in the plasma), that same structure allows them to diffuse through cell membranes to exert their effects. This will be discussed in detail in a later section. Hormones exist in very small quantities in the blood and are measured in microgram, nanogram (10^{-9} g), and picogram (10^{-12} g) amounts.

Clearly, the quantity of hormone needed to bring about an effect is small and it wasn't until the 1950s that analytical techniques were improved to the point of monitoring these low plasma concentrations.

Blood Hormone Concentration

The effect a hormone exerts on a tissue is directly related to the concentration of the hormone in the plasma and the number of active receptors to which it can bind. The hormone concentration in the plasma is dependent on (1) the rate of secretion of the hormone from the endocrine gland, (2) the rate of metabolism or excretion of the hormone, (3) for some hormones, the quantity of transport protein in the plasma, and (4) changes in the plasma volume.

Control of Hormone Secretion

The rate at which a hormone is released from an endocrine gland is dependent on the magnitude of the input and whether it is stimulatory or inhibitory in nature. The input in every case is a chemical one, be it an ion (e.g., Ca^{++}) or substrate (e.g., glucose) in the plasma, a neurotransmitter such as acetylcholine or norepinephrine, or another hormone. Most endocrine glands are under the direct influence of more than one type of input, which may either reinforce or interfere with each other's effect. An example of this interaction is found in the control of insulin release from the pancreas. Figure 5.1 shows that the pancreas, which produces insulin, responds to changes in plasma glucose and amino acids, norepinephrine released from sympathetic neurons, as well as circulating epinephrine, parasympathetic neurons, which release acetylcholine, and a variety of hormones. An elevation of plasma glucose and amino acids increase insulin secretion ($+$), while an increase in sympathetic nervous system activity (epinephrine and norepinephrine) decrease ($-$) insulin secretion. It is this magnitude of inhibitory versus exitatory input that determines whether there will be an increase or decrease in the secretion of insulin (85).

Metabolism and Excretion of Hormones

The concentration of a hormone in the plasma is also influenced by the rate at which it is metabolized (inactivated) and/or excreted. Inactivation can take place

at or near the receptor, or in the liver, the major site for hormone metabolism. In addition, the kidneys can metabolize a variety of hormones, or excrete them in their free (active) form. In fact, the rate of excretion of a hormone in the urine has been used as an indicator of its rate of secretion during exercise (6, 19, 46). Since blood flow to the kidneys and liver decreases during exercise, the rate at which hormones are inactivated or excreted decreases. This results in an elevation of the plasma level of the hormone over and above that due to higher rates of secretion.

Transport Protein

The concentration of some hormones is influenced by the quantity of transport protein in the plasma. Steroid hormones and thyroxine are transported bound to plasma proteins. In order for a hormone to exert its effect on a cell it must be "free" to interact with the receptor, and not "bound" to the transport protein. The amount of free hormone is dependent on the quantity of transport protein, and the capacity and affinity of the protein to bind the hormone molecules. (Capacity refers to the maximal quantity of hormone that can be bound to the transport protein, and affinity refers to the tendency of the transport protein to bind to the hormone.) An increase in the quantity, capacity, or affinity of transport protein would reduce the amount of free hormone, and its effect on tissue (27, 60). For example, high levels of estrogen achieved during pregnancy increase the quantity of thyroxine's transport protein, causing a reduction in free thyroxine. The thyroid gland produces more thyroxine to correct this problem.

Plasma Volume

Changes in plasma volume will change the hormone concentration independent of changes in the rate of secretion or inactivation of the hormone. During exercise, plasma volume decreases due to the movement of water out of the cardiovascular system. This causes an increase in the concentration of hormones in the plasma.

In summary, the plasma hormone concentration determines the magnitude of the effect at the tissue level. The hormone concentration can be changed by

Figure 5.1 The secretion of a hormone can be modified by a number of factors, some exerting a positive influence and others, a negative influence.

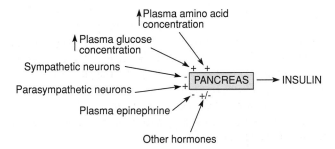

altering the rate of secretion or inactivation of the hormone, the quantity of transport protein, or the plasma volume. Given the influence of these four factors on the plasma hormone concentration, one must be careful in drawing conclusions about endocrine gland activity when viewing changes in the hormone concentration in plasma (8).

Mechanism of Hormone Action

Hormones are carried by the circulation to all tissues, but affect only certain tissues. Tissues responsive to specific hormones have specific protein receptors capable of binding those hormones. These protein receptors should not be viewed as static fixtures associated with cells, but like any cellular structures, are subject to change. Receptor number may decrease when exposed to a chronically elevated level of a hormone (down-regulation), resulting in a diminished response for the same hormone concentration. The opposite case, chronic exposure to a low concentration of a hormone, may lead to an increase in receptor number (up-regulation), with the tissue becoming very responsive to the available hormone. Since there is a finite number of receptors on or in a cell, a situation can arise in which the concentration of a hormone is so high that all receptors are bound to the hormone. This is called saturation, and any additional increase in the plasma hormone concentration will have no additional effect (25). Further, since the receptors are specific to a hormone, any chemical similar in "shape" will compete for the limited receptor sites. A major way in which

endocrine function is studied is to use chemicals (drugs) to block receptors and observe the consequences.

The initial event in a hormone's effect on a cell is its binding to a specific receptor. It is the hormone-receptor interaction that triggers events, and varying the concentration of the hormone, the number of receptors on the cell, or the affinity of the receptor for the hormone will all influence the magnitude of the effect on the cell. Mechanisms by which hormones modify cellular activity include (1) the alteration of membrane transport mechanisms, (2) stimulation of DNA in the nucleus to initiate the synthesis of a specific protein, and (3) the activation of special proteins in the cells by "second messengers."

Membrane Transport

After binding to a receptor on a membrane, the major effect of some hormones is to activate carrier molecules in the membrane to increase the movement of substrates or ions from outside to inside the cell. The facilitated diffusion of glucose and the active transport of amino acids are examples of this effect due to the action of insulin.

Stimulation of DNA in the Nucleus

Due to their lipid-like nature, steroid hormones easily diffuse through cell membranes where they become bound to a protein receptor in the cytoplasm of the cell. Figure 5.2 shows that the steroid-receptor complex enters the nucleus and binds to a specific protein linked to DNA, which contains the instruction codes

Figure 5.2 The mechanism by which steroid hormones act on target cells. The steroid hormone, represented by the triangle with the letter "H," binds to a cytoplasmic receptor to be transported to the nucleus where it stimulates DNA to bring about a change in cellular activity.

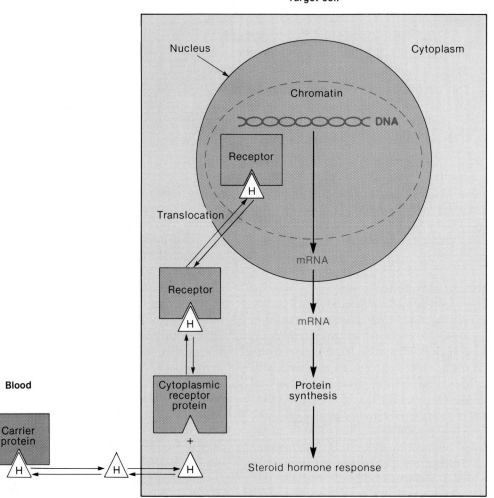

for protein synthesis. This initiates the steps leading to the synthesis of a specific messenger RNA (mRNA) that carries the codes from the nucleus to the cytoplasm where the specific protein is synthesized. While thyroid hormones are not steroid hormones, they act in a similar manner. These processes—the activation of DNA and the synthesis of specific protein—take time to turn on (making the hormones involved "slow acting" hormones), but their effects are longer lasting than those generated by "second messengers" (36).

Second Messengers

Many hormones, because of their size or highly charged structure, cannot easily cross cell membranes. These hormones exert their effect by binding to a receptor on the membrane surface, where they either activate

Figure 5.3 The cyclic AMP "second messenger" mechanism by which hormones act on target cells.

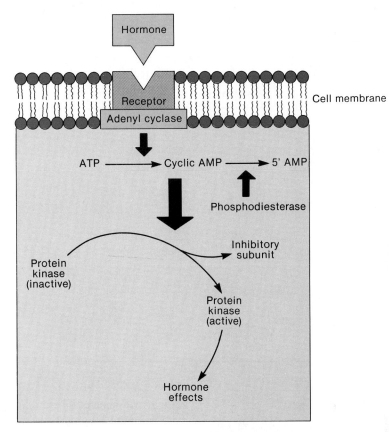

a membrane-bound enzyme, **adenylate cyclase,** or modify an ion channel that either increases or decreases Ca^{++} influx into the cell. If the hormone-receptor interaction activates adenylate cyclase, then **cyclic AMP** (cyclic 3′, 5′-adenosine monophosphate) is formed from ATP (see figure 5.3). In turn, cyclic AMP activates inactive protein kinases, which directly alter cellular activity. The cyclic AMP is inactivated by **phosphodiesterase,** which converts cyclic AMP to 5′AMP. Factors that interfere with phosphodiesterase activity, such as caffeine, would increase the effect of the hormone by allowing cyclic AMP to exert its effect for a longer period of time. For example, caffeine exerts this effect on adipose tissue causing free fatty acids to be mobilized at a faster rate (see chapter 24).

If the hormone-receptor interaction activates a Ca^{++} ion channel, then Ca^{++} enters the cell, binds to and activates a protein called **calmodulin,** which can influence enzyme activity, as could cyclic AMP (see figure 5.4). Intracellular Ca^{++} can also be elevated when an organelle such as the sarcoplasmic reticulum of muscle cells releases Ca^{++} during exercise. Cyclic AMP and Ca^{++} are viewed as **second messengers** in the events following the hormone's binding to a receptor on the cell membrane. These two second messengers should not be viewed as being independent of each other because changes in one can affect the action of the other.

Figure 5.4 The Ca^{++}-calmodulin "second messenger" mechanism by which hormones act on target cells.

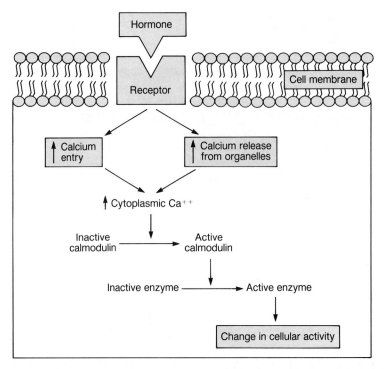

Hormones: Regulation and Action

This section will present the major endocrine glands, their hormones, the effect the hormones have on tissues, and how the concentration of each hormone is regulated. This information is essential in order to discuss the role of the neuroendocrine system in the adaptation to exercise.

Hypothalamus and the Pituitary Gland

The **pituitary gland** is located at the base of the brain, attached to the **hypothalamus.** The gland has two lobes, the anterior lobe (adenohypophysis), which is a true endocrine gland, and the posterior lobe (neurohypophysis), which is neural tissue extending from the hypothalamus. Both lobes are under the direct control of the hypothalamus. In the case of the **anterior pituitary,** hormone release is controlled by chemicals (**releasing hormones** or factors) that originate in neurons located in the hypothalamus. These releasing hormones stimulate or inhibit the release of specific hormones from the anterior pituitary. The posterior pituitary gland receives its hormones from special neurons originating in the hypothalamus. The hormones move down the axon to blood vessels in the posterior hypothalamus where they are discharged into the general circulation.

Anterior Pituitary Gland

The anterior pituitary hormones include **adrenocorticotrophic hormone (ACTH), follicle-stimulating hormone (FSH), luteinizing hormone (LH), thyroid-stimulating hormone (TSH), growth hormone (GH),** and **prolactin.** Figure 5.5 shows each hormone and its target tissue. While prolactin directly stimulates the breast to produce milk, the majority of the hormones secreted from the anterior pituitary control the release of other hormones. TSH controls the rate of thyroid hormone formation and secretion from the thyroid

Figure 5.5 Summary of the hormones released from the anterior pituitary gland, and their target tissues.

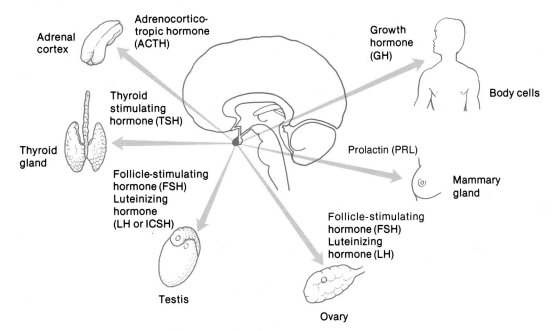

gland; ACTH stimulates the production and secretion of cortisol in the adrenal cortex; LH stimulates the production of testosterone in the testes and estrogen in the ovary; and finally, GH stimulates the release of **somatomedins** from the liver. However, as we will see, growth hormone exerts important effects on protein, fat, and carbohydrate metabolism.

Growth Hormone. Growth hormone (GH) is secreted from the anterior pituitary gland and exerts profound effects on the growth of all tissues. GH stimulates tissue uptake of amino acids and the synthesis of new protein, and long-bone growth. In addition, GH opposes the action of insulin to reduce the use of plasma glucose, increases the synthesis of new glucose in the liver (gluconeogenesis), and increases the mobilization of fatty acids from adipose tissue to spare plasma glucose. Given these characteristics, it should be no surprise that GH increases with exercise to help maintain the plasma glucose concentration (this will be covered in detail in a later section). Some of these effects are due to the direct effect of GH on tissues, while others are due to somatomedins, which are growth factors released from the liver in response to GH. Growth hormone, because of its role in protein synthesis, is being used by some athletes to enhance muscle mass. There are problems with this approach to better performance through chemistry (see Box 5.1).

Growth hormone secretion is controlled by releasing hormones secreted from the hypothalamus. Growth hormone releasing hormone (GHRH) stimulates GH release from the anterior pituitary, while another factor, **hypothalamic somatostatin,** inhibits it. The GH and somatomedin levels in blood exert a negative feedback effect on the continued secretion of GH. As shown in figure 5.6, additional input to the hypothalamus that can influence the secretion of GH includes exercise, stress (broadly defined), a low plasma-glucose concentration, and sleep (85).

Box 5.1 Growth Hormone and Performance

An excess of growth hormone (GH) during childhood is tied to gigantism, while an inadequate secretion causes dwarfism. The latter condition requires the administration of GH (along with other growth-promoting hormones) during the growing years if the child is to regain his or her position on the normal growth chart. GH needed for this was originally obtained by extracting it from pituitary glands obtained from cadavers—an expensive and time-consuming proposition. Due to the success of genetic engineering, human GH is now available in large quantities.

If an excess of GH occurs during adulthood, a condition called *acromegaly* occurs. The additional GH during adulthood does not affect growth in height since the epiphyseal growth plates at the ends of the long bones have closed. Unfortunately, the excess GH causes permanent deformities as seen in a thickening of the bones in the face, hands, and feet. Until recently, the usual cause of acromegaly was a tumor in the anterior pituitary gland that resulted in an excess secretion of GH. That is no longer

the case. In an unfortunate drive to reap the muscle-growth-stimulating effects of GH, body builders and strength trainers are injecting the now readily available human GH, along with other hormones (see Box 5.3). Evidence exists showing that GH increases protein synthesis in muscle; however, it is connective tissue protein, collagen, that is increased more than contractile protein. Consistent with these observations, strength gains do not parallel gains in muscle size (66). Like all hormones that have multiple effects, you can't have one without the other. It is not an uncommon observation to see young adults, male and female, in weight training and body building facilities with permanent deformities on the face and hands associated with the development of **acromegaly.** Chronic use of GH may lead to diabetes, muscle disease, and shortened life span (66, 93). Concern is so great that some are recommending that growth hormone be reclassified as a "controlled substance" to reduce its availability (15, 83).

Posterior Pituitary Gland

The **posterior pituitary gland** releases two hormones, oxytocin and **antidiuretic hormone (ADH),** which is also called vasopressin. Oxytocin is a powerful stimulator of smooth muscle, especially at the time of childbirth, and is also involved in the milk "let down" response needed for the release of milk from the breast. The baby's sucking of the nipple during breast feeding initiates a reflex through the hypothalamus to release oxytocin.

Antidiuretic Hormone. Antidiuretic hormone (ADH) does what its name implies: it reduces water loss from the body. ADH favors the reabsorption of water from the kidney tubules back into the capillaries to maintain body fluid. There are two major stimuli that result in an increased secretion of ADH: (1) high

plasma osmolality (a low water concentration) that can be caused by excessive sweating without water replacement, and (2) a low plasma volume, which can be due to either the loss of blood, or inadequate fluid replacement. There are osmoreceptors in the hypothalamus that sense the water concentration in the interstitial fluid. When the plasma has a high concentration of particles (low water concentration) the osmoreceptors shrink, and a neural reflex to the hypothalamus stimulates ADH release, which causes a reduction in water loss at the kidney. If the osmolality of the plasma is normal, but the volume of plasma is low, stretch receptors in the left atrium initiate a reflex leading to ADH release to attempt to maintain body fluid. During exercise plasma volume decreases and osmolality increases, and for exercise intensities

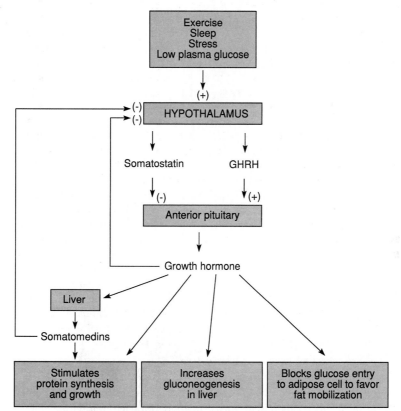

in excess of 60% of $\dot{V}O_2$ max, ADH secretion is increased as shown in figure 5.7 (13). This favors the conservation of water to maintain plasma volume (87).

Thyroid Gland

The **thyroid gland** is stimulated by TSH to synthesize two iodine-containing hormones: **triiodothyronine (T_3)** and **thyroxine (T_4)**. T_3 contains three iodine atoms and T_4 contains four. TSH is also the primary stimulus for release of T_3 and T_4 into the circulation where they are bound to plasma proteins. Remember, it is the "free" hormone concentration that is important in bringing about an effect on tissue.

Thyroxine

Thyroid hormones are central in establishing the overall metabolic rate, (i.e., a hypothyroid (Low T_3) individual would be characterized as being lethargic, and hypokinetic). It is this effect of the hormone that has been linked to weight-control problems; however, only a small percentage of obese individuals are hypothyroid. T_3 and T_4 act as permissive hormones in that they permit other hormones to exert their full effect. There is a relatively long latent period between the time T_3 and T_4 are elevated, and when their effects are observed. The latent period is six to twelve hours for T_3 and two to three days for T_4. However, once initiated, their effects are long lasting (36). The control of T_3

Figure 5.7 Percent change in the plasma antidiuretic hormone (ADH) concentration with increasing exercise intensity.

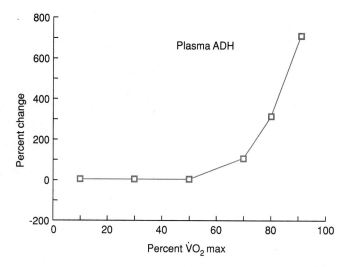

and T_4 secretion is another example of the negative feedback mechanism introduced in chapter 2. As the plasma concentrations of T_3 and T_4 increase, they inhibit the release of TSH-releasing hormone from the hypothalamus as well as TSH itself. This self-regulating system insures the necessary level of T_3 and T_4 for the maintenance of a normal metabolic rate. During exercise the "free" hormone concentration increases due to changes in the binding characteristic of the transport protein and the hormones are taken up at a faster rate by tissues. In order to counter the higher rate of removal of T_3 and T_4, TSH secretion increases and causes an increased secretion of these hormones from the thyroid gland (84).

Calcitonin

The thyroid gland also secretes **calcitonin,** which is involved in a minor way in the regulation of plasma calcium (Ca^{++}), a crucial ion for normal muscle and nerve function. Control of this hormone is by another negative feedback mechanism. As the plasma Ca^{++} concentration increases, calcitonin release is increased. Calcitonin blocks the release of Ca^{++} from bone to lower the plasma Ca^{++} concentration. As the Ca^{++} concentration is decreased, the rate of calcitonin secretion is reduced.

Parathyroid Gland

Parathyroid hormone is the primary hormone involved in plasma Ca^{++} regulation. The parathyroid gland releases parathyroid hormone in response to a low plasma Ca^{++} concentration. The hormone stimulates bone to release Ca^{++} into the plasma, and simultaneously increases the renal absorption of Ca^{++}; both raise the plasma Ca^{++} level. Parathyroid hormone also stimulates the kidney to convert a form of Vitamin D into a hormone that increases the absorption of Ca^{++} from the gastrointestinal tract. Exercise increases the concentration of parathyroid hormone in the plasma (62, 63).

Adrenal Gland

The adrenal gland is really two different glands, one secreting steroid hormones (**adrenal cortex**) and one secreting the **catecholamines, epinephrine (E)** and **norepinephrine (NE)** (adrenal medulla).

Adrenal Medulla

The adrenal medulla is part of the sympathetic nervous system and 80% of its hormonal secretion is epinephrine, which affects receptors in the cardiovascular and respiratory systems, gastrointestinal (GI) tract, liver, endocrine glands, muscle, and adipose tissue. E and NE are involved in the maintenance of blood pressure and the plasma glucose concentration. Their role in the cardiovascular system is discussed in chapter 9 and their involvement in the mobilization of substrate for exercise is discussed in a later section. E and NE also respond to strong emotional stimuli, and are the bases of Cannon's "fight or flight" hypothesis of how the body responds to challenges from the environment (10). Cannon's view was that the activation of the sympathetic nervous system prepared you to either confront a danger, or flee from it. Expressions such as "The adrenalin must really be pumping now" would be a rough translation of this hypothesis.

E and NE bind to adrenergic (from adrenaline, the European name for epinephrine) receptors on target tissues. The receptors are divided into two major classes: **alpha** (α) and **beta** (β), with subgroups (α_1 and α_2; β_1 and β_2). The response generated in the target tissue, both size and direction, is dependent on the receptor type and whether E or NE is involved. Epinephrine can bind to both alpha and beta receptors equally, while NE is primarily a stimulator of alpha receptors, and only a weak stimulator of beta receptors. Table 5.1 summarizes the effects E and NE have on a variety of tissues relative to the type of adrenergic receptor involved (25). The values in table 5.1 indicate which catecholamine, E or NE, has a greater effect on alpha and beta receptors in different tissues.

Adrenal Cortex

The adrenal cortex secretes a variety of steroid hormones having rather distinct physiological functions. The hormones can be grouped into three different categories: (1) **mineralocorticoids** (aldosterone), involved in the maintenance of the Na^+ and K^+ concentrations in plasma, (2) **glucocorticoids** (cortisol), involved in plasma glucose regulation, and (3) **sex steroids (androgens** and **estrogens**), which support prepubescent growth, with androgens being associated with post-pubescent sex drive in women. The chemical precursor common to all of these steroid hormones is cholesterol, and while the final active hormones possess minor structural differences, their physiological functions differ greatly.

Aldosterone. **Aldosterone** (mineralocorticoid) is an important regulator of Na^+ reabsorption and K^+ secretion at the kidney. Aldosterone is directly involved in Na^+/H_2O balance and, consequently, plasma volume and blood pressure (chapter 9). There are two levels of control over aldosterone secretion. The release of aldosterone from the adrenal cortex is controlled directly by the plasma K^+ concentration. An increase in K^+ concentration increases aldosterone secretion, which stimulates the kidney's active transport mechanism to secrete K^+ ions. This control system uses the negative feedback loop we have already seen. Aldosterone secretion is also controlled by another more complicated mechanism. Figure 5.8 shows that a decrease in plasma volume, a fall in blood pressure at the kidney, or an increase in sympathetic nerve activity to the kidney stimulates special cells in the kidney to secrete an enzyme called **renin.** Renin enters the plasma and converts angiotensinogen to **angiotensin I,** which is, in turn, converted to **angiotensin II** by a "converting enzyme" in the lung. Angiotensin II stimulates aldosterone release, which increases Na^+ reabsorption. The stimuli for aldosterone and ADH secretion are also the signals that stimulate thirst, a necessary ingredient to restore body fluid volume. During light exercise there is little or no change in plasma renin activity or aldosterone (62); however, when a heat load is imposed during light exercise, both renin and aldosterone secretion are increased (27). When exercise intensity approaches 50% $\dot{V}O_2$ max (figure 5.9) renin, angiotensin, and aldosterone increase in parallel showing the linkage within this homeostatic system (67, 84).

Cortisol. The primary glucocorticoid secreted by the adrenal cortex is **cortisol.** Cortisol contributes to the maintenance of plasma glucose during long-term fasting and exercise by a variety of mechanisms: (1) promotes the breakdown of tissue protein (by inhibiting protein synthesis) to form amino acids, which are then used by the liver to form new glucose (gluconeogenesis); (2) stimulates the mobilization of free

Table 5.1 *Adrenergic receptors (alpha or beta) found in various organ systems. The effects of epinephrine (E) and norepinephrine (NE) on these receptors is rated on a three-point scale (1 = greatest effect).*

Organ (or Organ System)	Receptor	Response	Relative Order of Catecholamine Potency	
			NE*	E*
Heart	Beta	Increased heart rate; increased contractility; increased conduction velocity	3	2
Blood vessels	Alpha	Constriction	2	1
	Beta†	Dilatation	3	2
Bronchi	Beta	Relaxation	3	2
Intestine				
Muscle	Alpha, beta	Inhibition	2	1
Sphincters	Alpha	Contraction	2	1
Bladder				
Detrusor muscle	Beta	Relaxation	3	2
Trigone muscle of sphincter	Alpha	Contraction	2	1
Uterus	Alpha, beta	Variable§	2	1
Eye				
Radial muscle	Alpha	Contraction	2	1
Ciliary muscle	Beta	Relaxation	3	2

*NE = norepinephrine; E = epinephrine
†Only demonstrated in skeletal muscle and visceral muscle vessels.
†Probably not active in intestine.
§Response is dependent upon stage of menstrual cycle and pregnancy.
Source: Reproduced with permission from Carrier, O., Jr.: Pharmacology of the Peripheral Autonomic Nervous System. Copyright © 1972 by Year Book Medical Publishers, Inc., Chicago.

fatty acids from adipose tissue; (3) stimulates liver enzymes involved in the metabolic pathway leading to glucose synthesis, and (4) blocks the entry of glucose into tissues, forcing those tissues to use more fatty acids as fuel (36, 85).

Cortisol secretion is controlled in the same manner as thyroxine. The hypothalamus secretes cortico-trophic-releasing hormone (CRH), which causes the anterior pituitary gland to secrete more ACTH into the general circulation. ACTH binds to receptors on the adrenal cortex and increases cortisol secretion. As the cortisol level increases, CRH and ACTH are inhibited in another negative feedback system. However, the hypothalamus, like any brain center, receives neural input from other areas of the brain. This input can influence the secretion of hypothalamic-releasing hormones beyond the level seen in a negative feedback system. Over fifty years ago Hans Selye observed that a wide variety of stressful events such as burns, bone breaks, and heavy exercise led to predictable increases in ACTH and cortisol; he called this response the **General Adaptation Syndrome (GAS).** A key point in this

Figure 5.8 Summary of how the renin-angiotensin-aldosterone system functions to maintain salt and water balance and blood pressure.

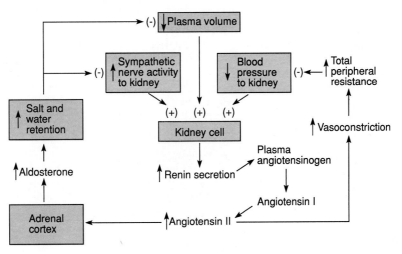

Figure 5.9 Parallel increases in renin activity, angiotensin II, and aldosterone with increasing intensities of exercise. Data are expressed as the percent change from resting values.

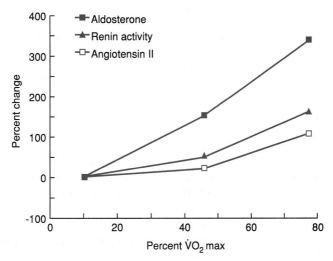

Figure 5.10 Control of cortisol secretion, showing the balance of positive and negative input to the hypothalamus, and cortisol's influence on metabolism.

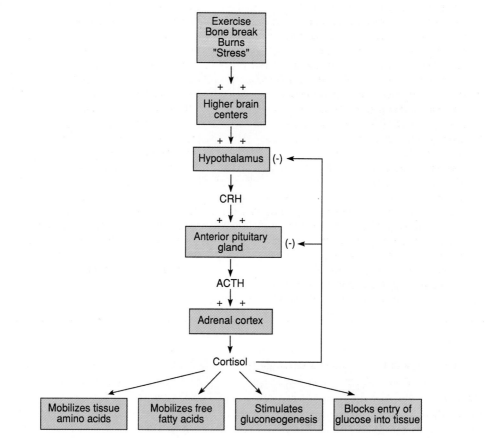

pattern was the release of ACTH and cortisol to aid in the adaptation. His GAS had three stages: (1) **the alarm reaction,** involving cortisol secretion, (2) **stage of resistance,** where repairs are made, and (3) **stage of exhaustion,** in which repairs are not adequate, and sickness or death results (77). A summary of cortisol's actions and its regulation is presented in figure 5.10. The usefulness of the GAS is seen in times of "stress" caused by tissue damage. The cortisol stimulates the breakdown of tissue protein to form amino acids, which can then be used at the site of the tissue damage for repair.

Pancreas

The **pancreas** is both an exocrine and endocrine gland. The exocrine secretions include digestive enzymes and bicarbonate, which are secreted into ducts leading to the small intestine. The hormones, released from special groups of cells in the islets of Langerhans, include **insulin, glucagon,** and **somatostatin.**

Insulin

Insulin is secreted from beta cells of the islets of Langerhans. Insulin is the most important hormone during the absorptive state (when nutrients are entering the

Box 5.2 Endorphins and Exercise

The reader may be familiar with the expression "runner's high" as a description of the good feeling some individuals experience during long-distance runs. This experience has been linked to **endorphins,** endogenous morphine-like substances, which interact with opiate receptors in the brain areas involved in the transmission of information about pain. β-endorphin is formed in the anterior pituitary from β-lipotrophin, which is itself generated during the formation of adrenocorticotrophic hormone (ACTH) (85). Given the close relationship between these substances and ACTH, which is the cornerstone of Selye's General Adaptation Syndrome, investigators became interested in how plasma levels of β-lipotrophin and β-endorphin would respond to exercise stress. Studies conducted in the early 1980s found that exercise caused parallel changes in plasma ACTH and β-endorphin (26). A summary of research up through 1984 supported this observation in that all studies showed an elevation in β-lipotrophin/β-endorphin with exercise in men (22) and women (68). As chemical techniques improved to separate β-endorphin from β-lipotrophin, other studies were conducted. In one study in which subjects exercised at 60% $\dot{V}O_2$ max for one hour, no changes in β-endorphin were reported (58). Along with this finding, other investigators found no changes in β-endorphin during a graded exercise test to exhaustion (32). These results do not mean that these morphine-like substances are not involved in the acute and long-term adaptations to exercise. The plasma levels may simply not reflect the influence of these substances on neuroendocrine function in the brain (35, 39). Consistent with this cautious interpretation of the results, Morgan (69) emphasizes the need to explore alternative hypotheses in studying the effect of exercise on mood changes.

blood from the small intestine). Insulin stimulates tissues to take up and store nutrient molecules as glycogen, proteins, and fats. Insulin's best-known role is in the facilitated diffusion of glucose across cell membranes. A lack of insulin causes an accumulation of glucose in the plasma since the tissues cannot take it up. The plasma glucose concentration can become so high that reabsorption mechanisms in the kidney are overwhelmed and glucose is lost to the urine, taking large volumes of water with it. This condition is called **diabetes mellitus.**

As mentioned earlier in this chapter, insulin secretion is influenced by a wide variety of factors: plasma glucose concentration, plasma amino acid concentration, sympathetic and parasympathetic nerve stimulation, and various hormones. The rate of secretion of insulin is dependent on the level of excitatory and inhibitory input to the beta cells of the pancreas (see figure 5.1). The blood glucose concentration is a major source of input that is part of a simple negative feedback loop: as plasma glucose concentration increases (following a meal), the beta cells directly monitor this increase and secrete additional insulin to enhance tissue uptake of glucose. This increased uptake lowers the plasma glucose concentration, and insulin secretion is reduced.

Glucagon

Glucagon, secreted by the alpha cells in the islets of Langerhans, exerts an effect opposite that of insulin. Glucagon secretion increases in response to a low-plasma glucose concentration, which is monitored by the alpha cells. Glucagon stimulates both the mobilization of glucose from liver stores (glycogenolysis) and free fatty acids from adipose tissue (to spare blood glucose as a fuel). Lastly, along with cortisol, glucagon stimulates gluconeogenesis in the liver. Glucagon secretion is also influenced by factors other than the glucose concentration, notably, the sympathetic nervous

Figure 5.11 Control of testosterone secretion and sperm production by hypothalamus and anterior pituitary.

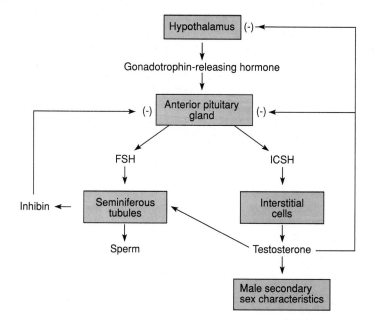

Testosterone

Testosterone is secreted by the interstitial cells of the testes and is controlled by interstitial cell stimulating hormone (ICSH—also known as LH), produced in the anterior pituitary. LH is, in turn, controlled by a releasing hormone secreted by the hypothalamus. Sperm production from the seminiferous tubules of the testes requires follicle-stimulating hormone (FSH) from the anterior pituitary and testosterone. Figure 5.11 shows testosterone secretion to be controlled by a negative feedback loop involving the anterior pituitary gland and the hypothalamus. Sperm production is controlled, in part, in another negative feedback loop involving the hormone inhibin.

Testosterone is both an **anabolic** and **androgenic** steroid in that it stimulates protein synthesis and is responsible for the characteristic changes in boys at adolescence that lead to the high muscle mass/fat mass ratio. Plasma testosterone increases by 10%–30% during prolonged submaximal work (86) and during

system. A complete description of the role of insulin and glucagon in the maintenance of blood glucose during exercise is presented later in this chapter.

Somatostatin

Pancreatic somatostatin is secreted by the delta cells of the islets of Langerhans. Pancreatic somatostatin secretion is increased during the absorptive state and modifies the activity of the GI tract to control the rate of entry of nutrient molecules into the circulation. It may also be involved in the regulation of insulin secretion.

Testes and Ovaries

Testosterone and **estrogen** are the primary sex steroids secreted by the testis and ovary, respectively. These hormones are not only important in establishing and maintaining reproductive function, they determine the secondary sex characteristics associated with masculinity and femininity.

Figure 5.12 Role of estrogen in the development of female secondary sex characteristics and maturation of the ovum.

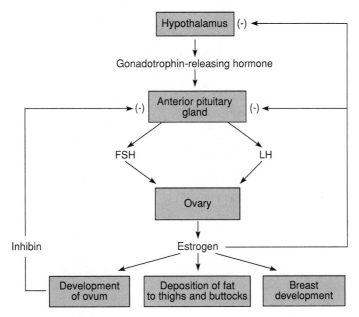

graded exercise taken to near-maximum (90) or maximum levels (16). Some feel that these small changes are due to a reduction in plasma volume (90), or to a decrease in the rate of inactivation and removal of testosterone (84). However, others have concluded on the basis of a parallel increase in the LH concentration, that the increase in plasma testosterone is due to an increased rate of production (16). While the testosterone response to exercise is small, there is evidence that it increases over the course of a long-term training program (24). Most readers probably recognize testosterone or one of its synthetic analogs as one of the most abused drugs in the drive to increase muscle mass and performance. Such use is not without its problems (see Box 5.3).

Estrogen

Estrogen is really a group of hormones that exerts similar physiological effects. These hormones include estradiole, estrone, and estriol. Estrogen stimulates breast development, female fat deposition, and other secondary sex characteristics (see figure 5.12). During the early part of the menstrual cycle called the **follicular phase,** LH stimulates the production of androgens in the follicle, which are subsequently converted to estrogens under the influence of FSH. Following ovulation, the **luteal phase** of the menstrual cycle begins, and both estrogens and progesterone are produced by the corpus luteum, a secretory structure occupying the space where the ovum was located (85). Figure 5.13 shows the changes in these hormones during a normal menstrual cycle. How does exercise affect these hormones?

In one study (55) the plasma levels of LH, FSH, estradiole, and progesterone were measured at rest and at three different work rates during both the follicular and luteal phases of the menstrual cycle. The patterns of response of these hormones during graded exercise were very similar in the two phases of the menstrual cycle (55). Figure 5.14 (page 90) shows only small changes in progesterone and estradiole with increasing

Box 5.3 Anabolic Steroids and Performance

Testosterone, as both an anabolic and androgenic steroid, causes size changes as well as male secondary sexual characteristics, respectively. Due to these combined effects scientists developed steroids to maximize the anabolic effects and minimize the androgenic effects. These synthetic steroids were developed to promote tissue growth in patients who had experienced atrophy as a result of prolonged bed rest. It was not long before the thought occurred that these anabolic steroids might be helpful in developing muscle mass and strength in athletes.

Numerous studies were conducted to determine whether or not these steroids would bring about the desired changes, with about an even split in the results (5, 92, 93). In these studies the scientists used the recommended therapeutic dosage, as required by committees approving research with human subjects. Unfortunately, the "results" of many personal studies conducted in various gyms and weight training facilities throughout the world disagreed with these scientific results. It is generally accepted that anabolic steroids can enhance muscle mass and strength (92, 93). Why the disagreement in results between the controlled scientific studies and these latter "studies"? In the weight room it is not uncommon for a person looking for greater "strength through chemistry" to take 10 to 100 times the recommended dosage. In effect, it was impossible to compare the results of the controlled scientific studies with those done in the gym.

By the mid 1980s, the steroid problem had reached a level that prompted both professional and college teams to institute testing of athletes to control drug use. Olympic and Pan American athletes were also tested to disqualify those who used the steroid. The problem escalated when athletes started to take pure testosterone rather than the anabolic steroid. Part of the reason for the switch was to reduce the chance of detection when drug testing was conducted, and part was related to the availability of testosterone. The loss of the gold medal by Canadian sprinter Ben Johnson in the 1988 Olympic Games indicates that testing has caught up with those willing to break the rules.

Like the GH example presented in Box 5.1, the use of testosterone or synthetic anabolic steroids can bring about undersirable effects. Adverse reactions to chronic anabolic steroid use in males include a decrease in testicular function, including a reduction in sperm production to zero (2, 4). Due to the similarity in its chemical structure and the means by which sex steroids are synthesized in the body, an excess of testosterone in males can result in plasma estrogen levels similar to that seen in women; breast development can result (3). Females taking anabolic steroids experience an increase in male secondary sex characteristics (including deepening of voice and beard growth), clitoral enlargement, and a disruption in menstrual function. Further, anabolic steroid abuse is linked to two disease processes: (1) an increase in the risk of coronary artery disease (CHD) due to a decrease in serum high-density lipoprotein cholesterol (38, 56, 61, 88), and (2) an increase in liver cancer (92, 93).

intensities of work. Given that LH and FSH changed little or not at all during the luteal phase, the elevation in progesterone and estrogen were believed to be due to changes in plasma volume and to a decreased rate of removal rather than an increased rate of secretion (8, 84). Another study (7) found little or no difference in the metabolic response to exercise between the two phases of the menstrual cycle. However, subjects who fasted responded differently than those who did not. This indicated that nutritional status must be maintained in both phases of the menstrual cycle to correctly judge the influence of each phase on the

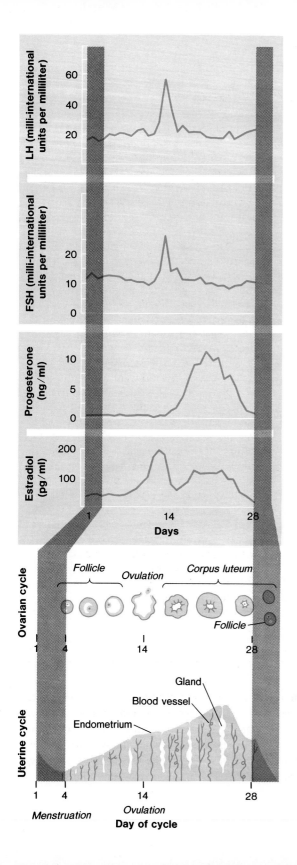

Figure 5.13 Changes in the plasma concentrations of LH, FSH, estradiol, and progesterone during a normal menstrual cycle.

Figure 5.14 Percent change (from resting values) in the plasma FSH, LH, progesterone, and estradiole concentrations during graded exercise in the follicle and luteal phases of the menstrual cycle.

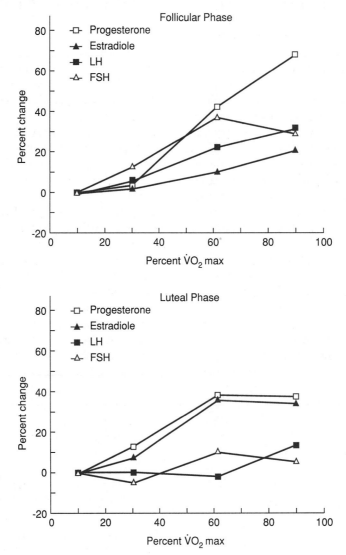

physiological responses to exercise. This suggestion received strong support from recent experiments in which women exercised at 63% $\dot{V}O_2$ max for ninety minutes after twenty-four hours on a carbohydrate-poor diet. The subjects experienced hypoglycemia in the luteal phase, but not in the follicular phase of the cycle during the exercise test (59). Interested readers are referred to Eston's review (20) of research on the menstrual cycle and athletic performance.

While the changes in estrogen and progesterone during an acute exercise bout are small, concern is being raised about the effect of chronic heavy exercise on the menstrual cycle of distance runners, gymnasts, and ballet dancers. For example, it has been shown that 29% of endurance athletes have primary (delay of menarche until age sixteen) or secondary (absence of menstruation in women who have had normal menstrual cycles) amenorrhea (89). Special attention is now being directed at the issue of secondary amenorrhea (64). Athletic amenorrhea is associated with chronically low estradiole levels, which can have a deleterious effect on bone mineral content. Osteoporosis, usually associated with the elderly (see chapter 17), is now being reported in athletes with amenorrhea (8).

Table 5.2 contains a summary of the information on each of the endocrine glands, their secretion(s), actions, controlling factors, the stimuli that elicit a response, and the effect of exercise on the hormonal response. This would be a good place to stop and review before proceeding to the discussion of the hormonal control of muscle glycogen mobilization, and the maintenance of the plasma glucose concentration during exercise.

Hormonal Control of Substrate Mobilization during Exercise

The type of substrate and the rate at which it is utilized during exercise depends to a large extent on the intensity and duration of the exercise. While diet and the training state of the person are important, and will be considered in chapters 21 and 23, the factors of intensity and duration of exercise ordinarily have prominence. Because of this, our discussion of the hormonal control of substrate mobilization during exercise will be divided into two parts. The first part will deal with control of muscle glycogen utilization, and the second part with the control of blood-glucose mobilization from the liver and free fatty acids (FFA) from adipose tissue.

Muscle-Glycogen Utilization

At the onset of most types of exercise and for the entire duration of very strenuous exercise, muscle glycogen is the primary carbohydrate fuel for muscular work (76). The intensity of exercise, which is inversely related to exercise duration, determines the rate at which muscle glycogen is used as a fuel. Figure 5.15 shows a family of lines, the slopes of which define rates of glycogen utilization (76). The heavier the exercise, the faster glycogen is broken down. This process of glycogen breakdown, glycogenolysis, is initiated by second messengers, which activate protein kinases in the muscle cell, as described in figures 5.3 and 5.4. Plasma epinephrine, a powerful stimulator of cyclic AMP formation when bound to β receptors on a cell, was believed to be primarily responsible for glycogenolysis. The data in figure 5.16 showing the changes in plasma E and NE, with increasing intensities of exercise (70), is consistent with this view: as the intensity of exercise increased, plasma E and NE increased, increasing the rate of glycogen degradation. However, there is more to this story.

In order to test the hypothesis that glycogenolysis in muscle was controlled by circulating E and NE during exercise, investigators had subjects take propranolol, a drug that blocks beta adrenergic receptors on the muscle cell membrane. Subjects worked for two minutes at an intensity of exercise that caused the muscle glycogen to be depleted to half its initial value and the muscle lactate concentration to be elevated tenfold. Surprisingly, the propranolol had no effect on the rate of glycogen depletion or lactate formation (40). Other experiments have also shown that propranolol has little effect on slowing the rate of glycogen breakdown during exercise (54). How could this be?

As mentioned in chapter 3, enzymatic reactions in a cell are under the control of both intracellular and extracellular factors. In the aforementioned example

Table 5.2 Summary of endocrine glands, their hormones, their action, factors controlling their secretion, stimuli that elicit a response, and the effect of exercise

Endocrine Gland	Hormone	Action	Controlling Factors	Stimuli	Exercise Effect
Anterior pituitary	Growth hormone (GH)	Increases growth, FFA mobilization, and gluconeogenesis; decreases glucose uptake	Hypothalamic GH-releasing hormone; hypothalamic somatostatin	Exercise; "stress"; Low blood glucose	↑
	Thyroid-stimulating hormone (TSH)	Increases T_3 and T_4 production and secretion	Hypothalamic TSH-releasing hormone	Low plasma T_3 and T_4	↑
	Adrenocorticotrophic hormone (ACTH)	Increases cortisol synthesis and secretion	Hypothalamic ACTH-releasing hormone	"Stress"; bone breaks; heavy exercise; burns, etc.	?
	Gonadotrophins: Follicle-stimulating hormone (FSH); luteinizing hormone (LH)	Female: estrogen and progesterone production and ovum development Male: testosterone production and sperm development	Hypothalamic gonadotrophic-releasing hormone. Females: plasma estrogen and progesterone. Males: plasma testosterone	Cyclic or intermittent firing of neurons in the hypothalamus	Small or no change
	Prolactin	Increases breast milk production	Prolactin-inhibiting hormone (dopamine)	Sucking of nipple	?
	Endorphins	Blocks pain by acting on opiate receptors in brain	ACTH-releasing hormone ???	"Stress"	Mixed
Posterior pituitary	Antidiuretic hormone (ADH) (vasopressin)	Decreases water loss at kidney; peripheral resistance	Hypothalamic neurons	Plasma volume; plasma osmolarity	↑

	Hormone	Action	Control	Stimulus	
	Oxytocin	Decreases uterine contractions; milk "let down"	Hypothalamic neurons	Uterine receptors; sucking of nipple	?
Thyroid	Triiodothyronine (T₃); thyroxine (T₄)	Increases metabolic rate, mobilization of fuels, growth	TSH; plasma T₃ and T₄	Low T₃ and T₄	↑ "Free" T₃ and T₄
	Calcitonin	Decreases plasma calcium	Plasma calcium	Elevated plasma calcium	?
Parathyroid	Parathyroid hormone	Increases plasma calcium	Plasma calcium	Low plasma calcium	
Adrenal cortex	Cortisol	Increases gluconeogenesis, free fatty acid mobilization and protein synthesis; decreases glucose utilization	ACTH	See ACTH, above	↑ Heavy exercise; ↓ light exercise
	Aldosterone	Increases potassium secretion and sodium reabsorption at kidney	Plasma potassium concentration and renin-angiotensin system	Low blood pressure and plasma volume; elevated plasma potassium and sympathetic activity to kidney	←
Adrenal medulla	Epinephrine (80%); norepinephrine	Increases glycogenolysis, FFA mobilization, heart rate, stroke volume, and peripheral resistance	Output of baroreceptors; glucose receptor in hypothalamus; brain and spinal centers	Low blood pressure, and blood glucose; too much "stress"; emotion	←
Pancreas	Insulin	Increases glucose, amino acid and FFA uptake into tissues	Plasma glucose and amino acid concentrations; autonomic nervous system	Elevated plasma glucose and amino acid concentrations; elevated epinephrine and norepinephrine	→

Table 5.2 *Continued*

Endocrine Gland	Hormone	Action	Controlling Factors	Stimuli	Exercise Effect
	Glucagon	Increases glucose and FFA mobilization; gluconeogenesis	Plasma glucose and amino acid concentrations; autonomic nervous system	Low plasma glucose and amino acid concentrations; elevated epinephrine and norepinephrine	←
Testes	Testosterone	Protein synthesis; secondary sex characteristics; sex drive; sperm production	FSH and LH (ICSH)	Increased FSH and LH	Small ↑
Ovaries	Estrogen	Fat deposition; secondary sex characteristics; ovum development	FSH and LH	Increased FSH and LH	Small ↑

Figure 5.15 Glycogen depletion in the quadriceps muscle during bicycle exercise of increasing exercise intensities.

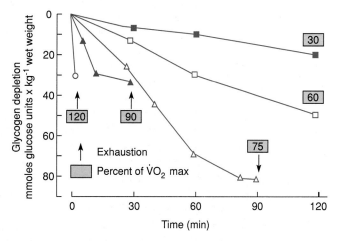

Figure 5.16 Percent change (from resting values) in the plasma epinephrine and norepinephrine concentrations with graded exercise.

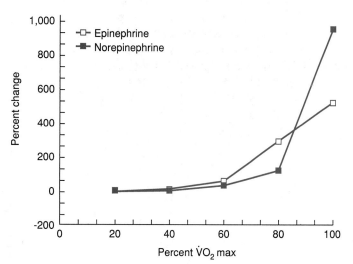

Figure 5.17 The breakdown of muscle glycogen, glycogenolysis, can be initiated by either the Ca^{++}-calmodulin mechanism or the cyclic AMP mechanism. When a drug blocks the β-receptor, glycogenolysis can still occur.

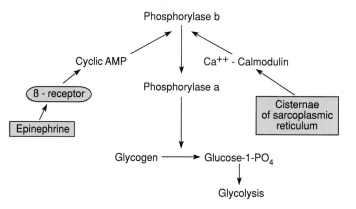

with propranolol, plasma E may not have been able to activate adenylate cyclase to form the cyclic AMP needed to activate the protein kinases to initiate glycogen breakdown. However, when a muscle cell is stimulated to contract, Ca^{++}, which is stored in the cisternae of the sacoplasmic reticulum, floods the cell. Some Ca^{++} ions are used to initiate contractile events (chapter 8), but other Ca^{++} ions bind to calmodulin, which, in turn, activates the protein kinases needed for glycogenolysis (see figure 5.4). In this case, the increased intracellular Ca^{++} (rather than cAMP) is the initial event stimulating muscle glycogen breakdown. Recent experiments in which the increased secretion of catecholamines was blocked during exercise confirmed the propranolol experiments, showing that an intact sympathoadrenal system was not necessary to initiate glycogenolysis in skeletal muscle (11).

Observations of glycogen depletion patterns support this view. Individuals who do heavy exercise with one leg will cause elevations in plasma E and NE, which circulate to all muscle cells. The muscle glycogen, however, is depleted only from the exercised leg (49), suggesting that intracellular factors (e.g., Ca^{++}) are more responsible for these events. Further, in experiments in which individuals engaged in intermittent intense exercise interspersed with a rest period (interval work), the glycogen was depleted faster from fast-twitch fibers (18, 19, 33). The plasma E and NE concentrations should be the same outside both fast- and slow-twitch muscle fibers, but the glycogen was depleted at a faster rate from the fibers used in the activity. This is only reasonable since a "resting" muscle fiber should not be using glycogen at a high rate. This discussion does not mean that E cannot or does not cause glycogenolysis (12, 94), and there is ample evidence to show that a surge of E will in fact cause that to occur (52, 79, 80, 81). Figure 5.17 summarizes these events.

Blood Glucose Homeostasis during Exercise

As mentioned in the introduction, a focal point of hormonal control systems is the maintenance of the plasma glucose concentration during times of inadequate carbohydrate intake (fasting/starvation) and accelerated glucose removal from the circulation (exercise). In both cases body energy stores are used to meet the challenge, and the hormonal response to these two different situations, exercise and starvation, is quite similar.

The plasma glucose concentration is maintained through four different processes: (1) mobilization of glucose from liver glycogen stores, (2) mobilization of plasma FFA from adipose tissue to spare plasma glucose, (3) synthesis of new glucose (gluconeogenesis) from amino acids and glycerol, and (4) blocking of glucose entry into cells to force a substitution of FFA as fuel. The overall aim of these four processes is to provide fuel for work while maintaining the plasma glucose concentration.

While the hormones will be presented separately, keep in mind that each of the above processes is controlled by more than one hormone, and all four processes are involved in the adaptation to exercise. Some hormones act in a "permissive" way, or are "slow acting," while others are "fast acting" controllers of substrate mobilization. For this reason, this discussion of the hormonal control of plasma glucose will be divided into two sections, one dealing with permissive and slow-acting hormones, and the other dealing with fast-acting hormones.

Permissive and Slow-Acting Hormones

Thyroxine, cortisol, and growth hormone are involved in the regulation of carbohydrate, fat, and protein metabolism. These hormones are discussed in this section because they act to either facilitate the actions of other hormones, or respond to stimuli in a slow manner. Remember, that to act in a permissive manner the hormone concentration doesn't have to change. However, as you will see, there are certain stressful situations in which permissive hormones can achieve such elevated plasma concentrations that they act directly to influence carbohydrate and fat metabolism rather than to simply facilitate the actions of other hormones.

Thyroxine. The discussion of substrate mobilization during exercise must include thyroxine, a hormone whose concentration doesn't change dramatically when one goes from the resting to the exercise state. As mentioned earlier, the thyroid hormones T_3 and T_4 are important in establishing the overall metabolic rate, and in allowing other hormones to exert their full effect (permissive hormone). Thyroxine accomplishes this latter function by influencing either the number of receptors on the surface of a cell (for other hormones to interact with), or the affinity of the receptor for the hormone. For example, without thyroxine, epinephrine has little effect on the mobilization of free fatty acids from adipose tissue. During exercise there is an increase in "free" thyroxine due to changes in the binding characteristics of the transport protein (84). T_3 and T_4 are removed from the plasma by tissues during exercise at a greater rate than at rest. In turn, TSH secretion from the anterior pituitary is increased to stimulate the secretion of T_3 and T_4 from the thyroid gland to maintain the plasma level (30). A low thyroxine (hypothyroid) state would interfere with the ability of other hormones to mobilize fuel for exercise (71, 84).

Cortisol. The primary glucocorticoid in humans is cortisol, and as figure 5.18 shows, it stimulates FFA mobilization from adipose tissue, mobilizes tissue protein to yield amino acids for glucose synthesis in the liver (gluconeogenesis), and decreases the rate of glucose utilization by cells (36). There are problems, however, when one tries to describe the cortisol response to exercise. Given the GAS of Selye, events other than exercise can influence the cortisol response. Figure 5.19 shows how a naive subject might view a treadmill test on first exposure. The wires, noise, and blood sampling could all influence the level of arousal of the subject and result in a cortisol response not tied to a need to mobilize additional substrate. Results supporting such a proposition were reported in the following study (74). Twelve subjects walked on a treadmill at five times their resting metabolic rate (5 METs) for thirty minutes, and blood samples were taken for cortisol analysis. Ten of the twelve subjects showed a decrease in cortisol due to the exercise, while the other two, who were anxious, had an increase. Clearly, the perception of the subject can influence the cortisol response to mild exercise.

As the exercise intensity increases, one might expect the cortisol secretion to increase. This is true, but only within certain limits. Bonen (6) showed the importance of exercise duration as a factor influencing the cortisol response when the urinary excretion of cortisol was not changed by exercise at 76% $\dot{V}O_2$ max for ten minutes, but was increased about two-fold when the duration was extended to thirty minutes. Davies and Few (17) extended our understanding of the cortisol response to exercise when they studied subjects who worked for one-hour durations with the intensity

Figure 5.18 Role of cortisol in the maintenance of plasma glucose.

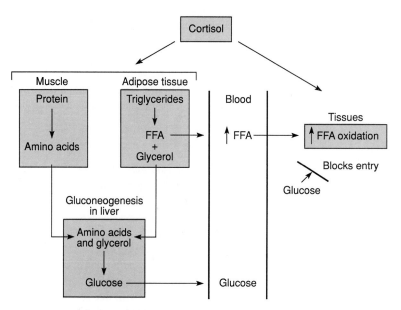

Figure 5.19 The perception of the subject can influence the hormonal response to exercise. (© George Moudry)

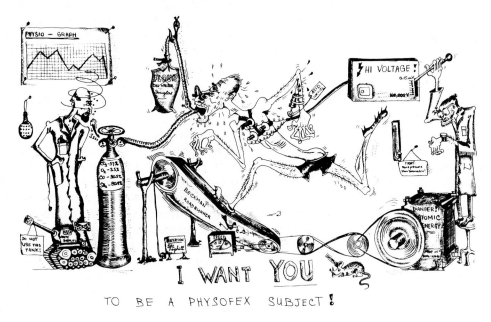

Figure 5.20 Percent change (from resting values) in the plasma cortisol concentration with increasing exercise intensity.

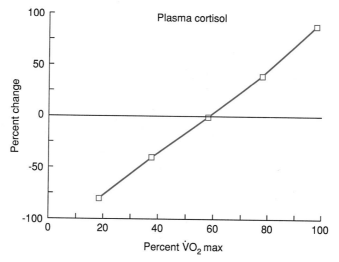

varying from 40%–80% $\dot{V}O_2$ max. Exercise at 40% $\dot{V}O_2$ max resulted in a decrease in plasma cortisol over time, while the response was reversed for exercise at 80% $\dot{V}O_2$ max. Figure 5.20 shows the plasma cortisol concentration measured at sixty minutes into each of the above exercise tests plotted against % $\dot{V}O_2$ max. When the exercise intensity exceeded 60% $\dot{V}O_2$ max, the cortisol concentration increased; below that, the cortisol concentration decreased. What caused these changes? Using radioactive cortisol, they found that during light exercise the cortisol was removed faster than the adrenal cortex could secrete it, and during intense exercise the increase in plasma cortisol was due to a higher rate of secretion that could more than match the rate of removal, which had doubled.

What is interesting is that for low-intensity, long-duration exercise where the effects of cortisol would go a long way in helping to maintain the plasma glucose concentration, the concentration of cortisol does not change very much. Even if it did, the effects on metabolism would not be immediately noticeable. The direct effect of cortisol is mediated through the stimulation of DNA, resulting in mRNA formation which, in turn, leads to protein synthesis, a slow process. In essence, cortisol, like thyroxine, exerts primarily a permissive effect on substrate mobilization during acute exercise, allowing other fast-acting hormones to deal with glucose and FFA mobilization. Given that athletic competitions (triathlon, ultra marathon, most team sports) can result in tissue damage, the reason for changes in the plasma cortisol concentration might be other than the need to mobilize fuel for exercising muscles. In these situations cortisol's role in dealing with inflammation and tissue repair would come to the forefront.

Growth Hormone. Growth hormone is a major factor in the synthesis of tissue protein, acting either directly, or through the enhanced secretion of somatomedins from the liver. However, GH can also influence fat and carbohydrate metabolism. Figure 5.21 shows that growth hormone supports the action of cortisol, mentioned earlier: it decreases glucose uptake by tissue, increases FFA mobilization, and enhances gluconeogenesis in the liver. The net effect is to preserve the plasma glucose concentration.

Describing the plasma GH response to exercise is as difficult as describing cortisol's response to exercise since GH can also be altered by a wide variety of

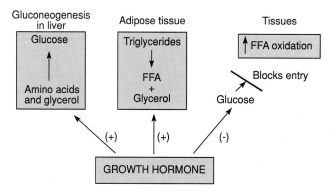

Figure 5.21 Role of plasma growth hormone in the maintenance of plasma glucose.

stresses: physical, chemical, and psychological (14, 34, 82). Given that, the comments mentioned earlier about cortisol should be kept in mind. Figure 5.22a shows plasma GH to increase with increasing intensities of exercise, achieving values twenty-five times resting at maximal work (82). Figure 5.22b shows the plasma GH concentration to increase over time in exercise requiring 60% $\dot{V}O_2$ max that is carried out for sixty minutes (9). What is interesting, compared to other hormonal responses, is that the trained runners had a higher response compared to a group of nonrunners (see later discussion). Values were about five to six times resting by sixty minutes. In summary, GH, a hormone primarily concerned with protein synthesis, can achieve plasma concentrations during exercise where it exerts a direct but "slow-acting" effect on carbohydrate and fat metabolism.

Fast-Acting Hormones

In contrast to the aforementioned "permissive" and slow-acting hormones, there are very-fast-responding hormones whose actions quickly return the plasma glucose to normal. Again, while each will be presented separately, they collectively behave in a predictable way during exercise to maintain the plasma glucose concentration.

Epinephrine and Norepinephrine. Epinephrine and norepinephrine have already been discussed relative to muscle glycogen mobilization. However, as figure 5.23 shows, they are also involved in the mobilization of glucose from the liver, FFA from adipose tissue, and may interfere with the uptake of glucose by tissues (75). While the plasma NE can increase ten- to twenty-fold during exercise and can achieve a plasma concentration that can exert a physiological effect (78), the primary means by which NE acts is when released from sympathetic neurons onto the surface of the tissue under consideration. The plasma level of NE is usually taken as an index of overall sympathetic nerve activity. Epinephrine, released from the adrenal medulla, is viewed as the primary catecholamine in the mobilization of glucose from liver. Figure 5.24 shows plasma E and NE to increase linearly with duration of exercise (48, 72). These changes, of course, are related to cardiovascular adjustments to exercise, as well as to the mobilization of fuel. These responses favor the mobilization of glucose and FFA to maintain the plasma glucose concentration. While it is sometimes difficult to separate the effect of E from NE, E seems to be more responsive to changes in the plasma glucose concentration. A low plasma glucose concentration stimulates a receptor in the hypothalamus to increase E secretion while having only a modest effect on plasma NE. In contrast, when the blood pressure

Figure 5.22 (*a*) Percent change (from resting values) in the plasma growth hormone concentration with increasing exercise intensity. (*b*) Percent change (from resting values) in the plasma growth hormone concentration during exercise at 60% $\dot{V}O_2$ max for runners and nonrunners (controls).

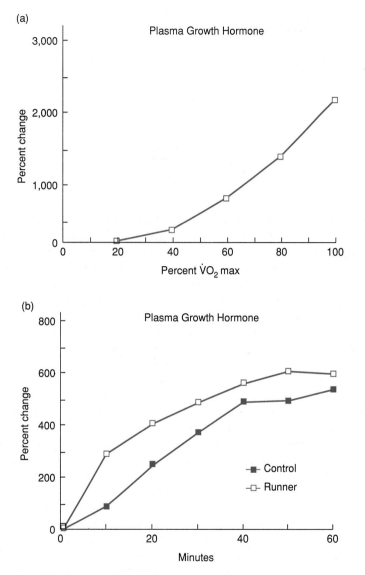

Figure 5.23 Role of catecholamines in substrate mobilization.

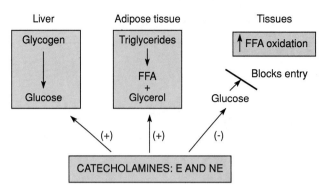

Figure 5.24 Percent change (from resting values) in the plasma epinephrine and norepinephrine concentrations during exercise at ~60% $\dot{V}O_2$ max.

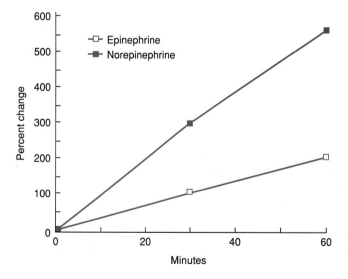

is challenged as during an increased heat load, the primary catecholamine involved is norepinephrine (72). Epinephrine binds to beta receptors on the liver and stimulates the breakdown of liver glycogen to form glucose for release into the plasma. If these receptors are blocked with propranolol, a beta receptor blocking drug, the plasma glucose concentration is more difficult to maintain during exercise. In addition, since the propranolol binds beta receptors on adipose tissue, less

FFA are released and the muscles have to rely more on muscle glycogen as the fuel (29).

Figure 5.25 shows that endurance training causes a very rapid decrease in the plasma E and NE responses to a fixed exercise bout. Within three weeks the concentration of both catecholamines is clearly depressed (91). In spite of this the mobilization of glucose from the liver and FFA from adipose tissue continues, indicating the complexity of the control

Figure 5.25 Changes in plasma epinephrine and norepinephrine with endurance training.

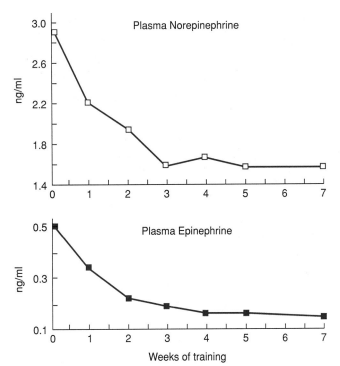

over the mobilization of fuel (see later discussion on hormone/substrate interaction). However, during a very stressful event a trained individual has a greater capacity to secrete E than an untrained individual (57). This suggests that physical training, which stimulates the symphathetic nervous system on a regular basis, increases the capacity of the adrenal medulla to respond to extreme challenges.

Insulin and Glucagon. These two hormones will be discussed together since they respond to the same stimuli, but exert opposite actions in the mobilization of liver glucose and adipose tissue FFA. Figure 5.26 shows insulin to be the primary hormone involved in the uptake and storage of glucose and FFA, and glucagon to cause the mobilization of those fuels from storage, as well as increase gluconeogenesis.

Given that insulin is directly involved in the uptake of glucose into tissue, and that glucose uptake by muscle can increase seven- to twenty-fold during exercise (23), what should happen to the insulin concentration during exercise? While it is surprising to many, Figure 5.27a shows that the insulin concentration actually decreases during exercise of increasing intensity (28, 41, 73). This of course is an appropriate response. If exercise were associated with an increase in insulin, the plasma glucose would be taken up into all tissues (including adipose tissue) at a faster rate, leading to an immediate hypoglycemia. The lower insulin concentration during exercise favors the mobilization of glucose from the liver and FFA from adipose tissue, both of which are necessary to maintain the plasma glucose concentration. Figure 5.27b shows that plasma insulin decreases during moderate-intensity, long-term exercise (37). It should be pointed out that following

Figure 5.26 Effect of insulin and glucagon on glucose and fatty-acid uptake and mobilization.

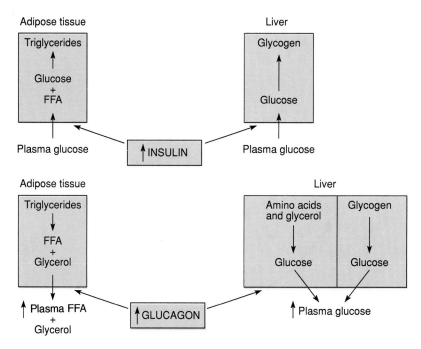

an endurance training program the plasma insulin concentration does not decrease to the same degree during exercise. One reason for the smaller change in plasma insulin is related to the training state of the individual, while another is simply related to the fact that the person performed exercise a day or two before the experiment. Acute (a single bout) and chronic exercise have been shown to increase the sensitivity of insulin receptors such that less insulin is needed to have the same effect on the uptake of glucose into tissue (43, 51).

With plasma insulin decreasing with long-term exercise, it should be no surprise that the plasma glucagon concentration is increasing (37). This increase in plasma glucagon, shown in figure 5.28, favors the mobilization of FFA from adipose tissue and glucose from the liver, as well as an increase in gluconeogenesis. Overall, the reciprocal responses of insulin and glucagon favor the maintenance of the plasma glucose concentration at a time when the muscle is using

plasma glucose at a high rate. Figure 5.28 also shows that following an endurance training program the glucagon response to a fixed exercise task is diminished to the point that there is no increase during exercise. In effect, endurance training allows the plasma glucose concentration to be maintained with little or no change in insulin and glucagon. The increased ability of a trained person to use fat as a fuel is consistent with this reduction in the glucagon response to submaximal exercise in that less liver glycogen is required to maintain the plasma glucose concentration.

These findings raise several questions. If the plasma glucose concentration is relatively constant during exercise, and the plasma glucose concentration is a primary stimulus for insulin and glucagon secretion, what caused the insulin secretion to decrease and glucagon secretion to increase? The answer lies in the multiple levels of control over hormonal secretion mentioned earlier. There is no question that changes in the plasma glucose concentration provide an important level of

Figure 5.27 (*a*) Percent change (from resting values) in the plasma insulin concentration with increasing intensities of exercise. (*b*) Percent change (from resting values) in the plasma insulin concentration during prolonged exercise at 60% $\dot{V}O_2$ max showing the effect of endurance training on that response.

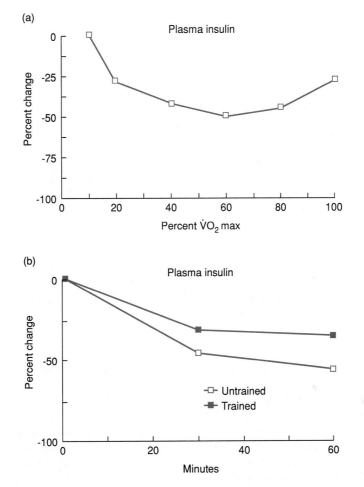

control over the secretion of glucagon and insulin (29). However, when the plasma glucose concentration is relatively constant, the sympathetic nervous system can modify the secretion of insulin and glucagon. Figure 5.29 shows that E and NE stimulate alpha-adrenergic receptors on the beta cells of the pancreas to decrease insulin secretion during exercise when the plasma glucose concentration is normal. Figure 5.29 also shows that E and NE stimulate beta receptors on the alpha cells of the pancreas to increase glucagon secretion when the plasma glucose concentration is normal.

These effects have been confirmed through the use of adrenergic receptor blocking drugs. When phentolamine, an alpha blocker, is given, insulin secretion increases with exercise. When propranolol is given, the glucagon concentration remains the same or decreases with exercise (65). Figure 5.30 summarizes the effect the sympathetic nervous system has on the mobilization of fuel for muscular work. Endurance training decreases the sympathetic nervous system response to a fixed exercise bout, resulting in less stimulation of adrenergic receptors on the pancreas.

Figure 5.28 Percent change (from resting values) in the plasma glucagon concentration during prolonged exercise at 60% V̇O₂ max showing the effect of endurance training on that response.

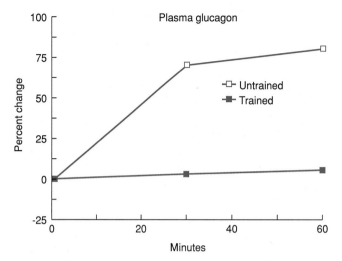

Figure 5.29 Effect of epinephrine and norepinephrine on insulin and glucagon secretion from the pancreas during exercise.

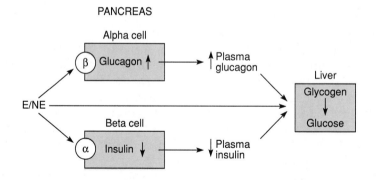

Figure 5.30 Effect of increased sympathetic nervous system activity on free-fatty-acid and glucose mobilization during submaximal exercise.

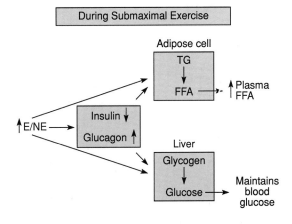

The observation that plasma insulin decreases with prolonged submaximal exercise raises another question. How can exercising muscle take up glucose seven to twenty times faster than at rest if the insulin concentration is decreasing? The answer, interestingly, relates to the high intramuscular Ca^{++} concentration that exists during exercise. The Ca^{++} concentration can influence the carrier molecule involved in the transport of glucose into the cell to enhance glucose uptake into the muscle (45). In this way, plasma insulin can decrease to facilitate the mobilization of FFA and glucose without affecting glucose entry into muscle.

In summary, figures 5.31a and 5.31b show the changes in the above hormones (except for thyroxine). The decrease in insulin and the increase in all the other hormones favor the mobilization of glucose from the liver, FFA from adipose tissue, gluconeogenesis in the liver, while inhibiting the uptake of glucose. These combined actions maintain homeostasis relative to the plasma glucose concentration so that the central nervous system can have the fuel it needs.

Hormone-Substrate Interaction

In the examples mentioned above, insulin and glucagon responded as they did during exercise with a normal plasma glucose concentration due to the influence of the sympathetic nervous system. It must be mentioned that if there were a sudden change in the plasma glucose concentration during exercise, these hormones would respond to that change. For example, if the ingestion of glucose during exercise causes an elevation of plasma glucose, the plasma concentration of insulin would increase. This hormonal change would reduce FFA mobilization and force the muscle to use additional muscle glycogen (1).

During intense exercise plasma glucagon, GH, cortisol, epinephrine and NE are elevated and insulin is decreased. These hormonal changes favor the mobilization of FFA from adipose tissue that would spare carbohydrate and help maintain the plasma glucose concentration. If that is the case, why is the respiratory exchange ratio (R) increasing with increasing intensities of exercise? The answer lies, in part, to the elevation of lactate that occurs at this same time.

Figure 5.31 (*a*) Summary of the hormonal responses to exercise of increasing intensity. (*b*) Summary of the hormonal responses to moderate exercise of long duration.

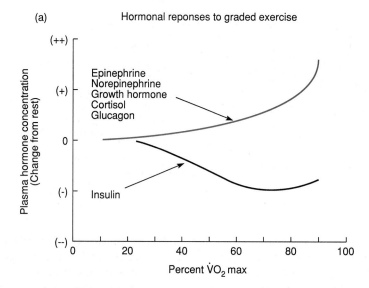

(a)   Hormonal reponses to graded exercise

Plasma hormone concentration (Change from rest)

(++)

(+)   Epinephrine
        Norepinephrine
        Growth hormone
        Cortisol
        Glucagon

0

(-)   Insulin

(--)

0   20   40   60   80   100

Percent $\dot{V}O_2$ max

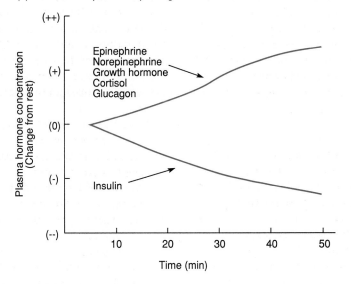

(b) Hormonal responses to prolonged exercise

Plasma hormone concentration (Change from rest)

(++)

(+)   Epinephrine
        Norepinephrine
        Growth hormone
        Cortisol
        Glucagon

(0)

(-)   Insulin

(--)

10   20   30   40   50

Time (min)

Figure 5.32 Effect of lactic acid on the mobilization of free fatty acids from the adipose cell.

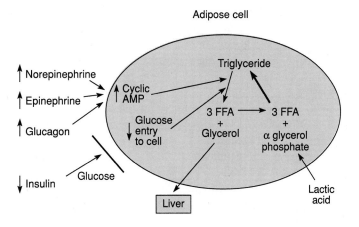

Figure 5.32 shows that while the hormones previously mentioned are stimulating the adipose cell to degrade TG to FFA and glycerol, the lactate enters the cell, is converted to **alpha glycerol phosphate,** and reverses the process (50). The result is that FFA are not released from the adipose cell, the plasma FFA level falls, and the muscle must use more carbohydrate as a fuel (higher R). One of the effects of endurance training is to decrease the lactate concentration at any fixed work rate. Such an adpatation would reduce the inhibition of this mobilization of FFA from adipose tissue.

Summary

1. Endocrine glands release hormones directly into the blood to alter the activity of tissues possessing receptors that can bind with the hormone. The effect a hormone exerts on a tissue is directly related to the concentration of the hormone and the number of active receptors on the tissue.

2. Hormone concentration is determined by the rate of secretion of the hormone from the endocrine gland, the rate of inactivation or excretion of the hormone, the quantity of transport protein in the plasma (for some hormones), and the changes in plasma volume.

3. The mechanisms by which hormones modify cellular activity include the alteration of membrane transport mechanisms, stimulation of DNA in the nucleus to initiate protein synthesis, and activation of special proteins in the cell by "second messengers."

4. Adenylate cyclase is activated by a variety of hormones to form cyclic AMP, which activates protein kinases in the cell. Elevations in intracellular Ca^{++} can activate calmodulin, which, in turn, activates protein kinases in the cell.

5. The hypothalamus controls the activity of both the anterior pituitary and posterior pituitary glands. Releasing hormones from the hypothalamus control the secretion of most hormones from the anterior pituitary. The posterior pituitary hormones are synthesized in the hypothalamus and move down neurons to be released.

6. Growth hormone (GH) increases protein synthesis, gluconeogenesis, and free fatty acid mobilization, and decreases glucose entry to tissue. GH increases with increasing exercise intensity. Because of its association with protein synthesis, it has become one of the most abused drugs in athletics.

7. Antidiuretic hormone (ADH) (vasopressin) increases the reabsorption of water at the kidney. Plasma ADH increases with increasing exercise intensity.

8. The thyroid gland secretes T_3 and T_4, which influence the metabolic rate, growth, and the action of other hormones. During exercise there is an increase in the concentration of "free" T_3 and T_4 due to changes in the binding characteristics of the plasma proteins transporting these hormones. TSH secretion increases with strenuous exercise to counter the higher rate of removal of T_3 and T_4, maintaining the plasma concentration of these hormones.

9. Calcitonin and parathyroid hormone are involved in the regulation of plasma calcium. Parathyroid hormone increases with exercise.

10. The adrenal medulla secretes the catecholamines epinephrine (E) and norepinephrine (NE). E is the adrenal medulla's primary secretion (80%), while NE is primarily secreted from the adrenergic neurons of the sympathetic nervous system. These hormones are involved in the regulation of metabolism (FFA and glucose mobilization) and blood pressure. In addition, E is involved in the mobilization of muscle glycogen. Both E and NE increase with exercise when the intensity exceeds 50% $\dot{V}O_2$ max. Endurance training causes a marked reduction in the E and NE responses to a fixed-exercise bout.

11. The adrenal cortex secretes aldosterone (mineralocorticoid), cortisol (glucocorticoid), and estrogens and androgens (sex steroids). Aldosterone regulates Na^+ and K^+ balance. Aldosterone secretion increases with strenuous exercise, driven by the renin-angiotensin system. Cortisol increases gluconeogenesis, free fatty acid mobilization, and decreases protein synthesis and glucose uptake by tissue. Work loads requiring more than 60% $\dot{V}O_2$ max cause an increase in plasma cortisol. Cortisol also responds to many types of "stress," and forms the basis of Selye's General Adaptation Syndrome (GAS).

12. The pancreas secretes insulin, glucagon, and somatostatin. Insulin is the primary hormone of the absorptive state when nutrients are entering the blood from the GI tract. Insulin promotes the uptake and storage of glucose, amino acids, and fatty acids. During exercise plasma insulin decreases to facilitate the mobilization of glucose from the liver and fatty acids from adipose tissue. Glucagon's actions are opposite those of insulin. Plasma glucagon increases with exercise causing a mobilization of FFA and glucose, and stimulating gluconeogenesis in the liver. Training causes the changes in plasma insulin and glucagon during exercise to be less dramatic.

13. Testosterone, secreted from the testes in response to FSH and ICSH (LH), is involved in protein synthesis, the appearance of secondary sex characteristics, and sperm production. Testosterone increases 10%–30% during exercise, with portions of the increase due to reductions in plasma volume, decreases in the rate of removal, and increases in the rate of secretion from the testes. Testosterone and its synthetic analogs (anabolic steroids) are some of the most abused drugs in athletics. There is no question that muscle size and strength are increased with large doses of these drugs. There is also no question that sperm production, testes size, and HDL cholesterol decrease while taking the drug.

14. Estrogen, secreted by the ovary in response to FSH and LH stimulation, is involved in fat deposition, the appearance of secondary sex characteristics, and ovum development. Estrogen increases slightly with exercise, with the increase explained primarily by a decreased rate of removal and a decrease in plasma volume. Chronic heavy exercise is associated with amenorrhea and low-plasma estrogens, which can lead to osteoporosis.

15. Muscle glycogen mobilization is increased by E stimulation of cyclic AMP formation, and the pattern of the E response to exercise is consistent with the high rates of glycolysis in heavy exercise. However, the fact that β-adrenergic blockade does not diminish this response in heavy exercise suggests that the Ca^{++}-calmodulin activation of glycogen breakdown is an important mechanism.

16. Plasma glucose is maintained during exercise by increasing liver glucose mobilization, using more plasma FFA, increasing gluconeogenesis, and decreasing glucose uptake by tissues. The decrease in plasma insulin, and the increase in plasma E, NE, GH, glucagon, and cortisol during exercise control these factors to maintain the glucose concentration.

17. Glucose is taken up seven to twenty times faster during exercise than at rest—even with the decrease in plasma insulin. The increase in intracellular Ca^{++} associated with exercise seems to increase the membrane transport of glucose.

18. The plasma FFA concentration decreases during heavy exercise even though the adipose cell is stimulated by a variety of hormones to increase triglyceride breakdown to FFA and glycerol. The high levels of lactate during heavy exercise seem to interfere with this process. The lactate is converted to alpha glycerol phosphate and used in the resynthesis of triglycerides.

Study Questions

1. Draw and label a diagram of a negative feedback mechanism for hormonal control using cortisol as an example.
2. List the factors that can influence the blood concentration of a hormone.
3. Discuss the use of testosterone and growth hormone as aids to increase muscle size and strength, and potential long-term consequences.
4. Identify the four mechanisms involved in maintaining the blood glucose concentration.
5. Draw a summary graph of the changes in the following hormones with exercise of increasing intensity or duration: epinephrine, norepinephrine, cortisol, growth hormone, insulin, and glucagon.
6. Briefly explain how glucose can be taken into the muscle at a high rate during exercise when plasma insulin is decreasing.
7. Explain how free fatty acid mobilization from the adipose cell decreases during maximal work in spite of the cell being stimulated by all the hormones.
8. Discuss the effect of glucose ingestion on the mobilization of free fatty acids during exercise.

Suggested Readings

Brooks, G., and T. Fahey. 1984. *Exercise Physiology: Human Bioenergetics and Its Applications.* New York: John Wiley and Sons.

Fox, E. L., and D. K. Mathews. 1981. *The Physiological Basis of Physical Education and Athletics,* 3d ed. Philadelphia: W. B. Saunders Company.

Lamb, D. R. 1984. *Physiology of Exercise: Responses and Adaptations,* 2d ed. New York: Macmillan Publishing Company.

McArdle, W. D., F. I. Katch, and V. L. Katch. 1986. *Exercise Physiology: Energy, Nutrition, and Human Performance,* 2d ed. Philadelphia: Lea & Febiger.

References

1. Ahlborg, G., and P. Felig. 1976. Influence of glucose ingestion on fuel-hormone response during prolonged exercise. *Journal of Applied Physiology* 41:683–88.
2. Alen, M., and K. Hakkinen. 1985. Physical health and fitness of an elite bodybuilder during 1 year of self-administration of testosterone and anabolic steroids: a case study. *International Journal of Sports Medicine* 6:24–29.
3. Alen, M., M. Reinila, and R. Vihko. 1985. Response of serum hormones to androgen administration in power athletes. *Medicine and Science in Sports and Exercise* 17:354–59.

4. Alen, M., and J. Suominen. 1984. Effect of androgenic and anabolic steroids on spermatogenesis in power athletes. *International Journal of Sports Medicine* 5:189–92.

5. American College of Sports Medicine. 1984. The use of anabolic-androgenic steroids in sports. In *Position Stands and Opinion Statements*. Indianapolis: The American College of Sports Medicine.

6. Bonen, A. 1976. Effects of exercise on excretion rates of urinary free cortisol. *Journal of Applied Physiology* 40:155–58.

7. Bonen, A. et al. 1983. Effects of menstrual cycle on metabolic responses to exercise. *Journal of Applied Physiology: Respiratory Environmental and Exercise Physiology* 55:1506–13.

8. Bunt, J. C. 1986. Hormonal alterations due to exercise. *Sports Medicine* 3:331–45.

9. Bunt, J. C. et al. 1986. Sex and training differences in human growth hormone levels during prolonged exercise. *Journal of Applied Physiology* 61:1796–1801.

10. Cannon, W. B. 1953. *Bodily Changes in Pain, Hunger, Fear and Rage,* 2d ed. Boston: Charles T. Branford Company.

11. Cartier, L., and P. D. Gollnick. 1985. Sympathoadrenal system and activation of glycogenolysis during muscular exercise. *Journal of Applied Physiology* 58:1122–27.

12. Christensen, N. J., and H. Galbo. 1983. Sympathetic nervous activity during exercise. *Annual Review of Physiology* 45:139–53.

13. Convertino, V. A., L. C. Keil, and J. E. Greenleaf. 1983. Plasma volume, renin and vasopressin responses to graded exercise after training. *Journal of Applied Physiology: Respiratory Environmental and Exercise Physiology* 54:508–14.

14. Copinschi, G. et al. 1967. Effect of various blood-sampling procedures on serum levels of immunoreactive human growth hormone. *Metabolism: Clinical and Experimental* 16:402–9.

15. Cowart, V. S. 1988. Human growth hormone: the latest ergogenic aid. *The Physician and Sportsmedicine* 16(3):175–85.

16. Cumming, D. C. et al. 1986. Reproductive hormone increases in response to acute exercise in men. *Medicine and Science in Sports and Exercise* 18:369–73.

17. Davies, C. T. M., and J. D. Few. 1973. Effects of exercise on adrenocorticol function. *Journal of Applied Physiology* 35:887–91.

18. Edgerton, V. R. et al. 1975. Glycogen depletion in specific types of human skeletal muscle fibers in intermittent and continuous exercise. In *Metabolic Adaptation to Prolonged Physical Exercise,* ed. by H. Howald and J. R. Poortmans, 402–15. Verlag Basel, Switzerland: Birkhauser.

19. Essen, B. 1978. Glycogen depletion of different fibre types in human skeletal muscle during intermittent and continuous exercise. *Acta Physiologica Scandinavica* 103:446–55.

20. Eston, R. G. 1984. The regular menstrual cycle and athletic performance. *Sports Medicine* 1:431–45.

21. Euler, U. S. von. 1969. Sympatho-adrenal activity and physical exercise. In *Biochemistry of Exercise, Medicine and Sport* 3, ed. J. R. Poortmans, 170–81. New York: Karger, Basal.

22. Farrell, P. A. 1985. Exercise and endorphins—male responses. *Medicine and Science in Sports and Exercise* 17:89–93.

23. Felig, P., and J. Wahren. 1975. Fuel homeostasis in exercise. *The New England Journal of Medicine* 293:1078–84.

24. Fellmann, N. et al. 1985. Effects of endurance training on the androgenic response to exercise in man. *International Journal of Sports Medicine* 6:215–19.

25. Fox, S. I. 1984. *Human Physiology.* Dubuque, Ia: Wm. C. Brown.

26. Fraioli, F. et al. 1980. Physical exercise stimulates marked concomitant release of β-endorphin and adrenocorticotropic hormone (ACTH) in peripheral blood in man. *Experientia* 36:987–89.

27. Francesconi, R. P., M. Sawka, and K. B. Pandolf. 1983. Hypohydration and heat acclimatization: plasma renin and aldosterone during exercise. *Journal of Applied Physiology: Respiratory Environmental and Exercise Physiology* 55:1790–94.

28. Galbo, H., J. J. Holst, and N. J. Christensen. 1975. Glucagon and plasma catecholamine responses to graded and prolonged exercise in man. *Journal of Applied Physiology* 38:70–76.

29. Galbo, H. et al. 1976. Glucagon and plasma catecholamines during beta-receptor blockade in exercising man. *Journal of Applied Physiology* 40:855–63.

30. Galbo, H. et al. 1977. Thyroid and testicular hormone responses to graded and prolonged exercise in man. *European Journal of Applied Physiology* 36:101–6.

31. Ganong, W. F. 1979. *Review of Medical Physiology.* Los Altos, Calif.: Lange Medical Publications.
32. Goldfarb, A. H. et al. 1987. Serum β-endorphin levels during a graded exercise test to exhaustion. *Medicine and Science in Sports and Exercise* 19:78–82.
33. Gollnick, P. D. et al. 1975. Glycogen depletion patterns in human skeletal muscle fibers after varying types and intensities of exercise. In *Metabolic Adaptation to Prolonged Physical Exercise,* ed. H. Howald and J. R. Poortmans, 416–21. Verlag Basel, Switzerland: Birkhauser.
34. Greenwood, F. C., and J. Landon. 1966. Growth hormone secretion in response to stress in man. *Nature* 210:540–41.
35. Grossman, A., and J. R. Sutton. 1985. Endorphins: What are they? How are they measured? What is their role in exercise? *Medicine and Science in Sports and Exercise* 17:74–81.
36. Guyton, A. C. 1986. *Textbook of Medical Physiology,* 7th ed. Philadelphia: W. B. Saunders Company.
37. Gyntelberg, F. et al. 1977. Effect of training on the response of plasma glucagon to exercise. *Journal of Applied Physiology: Respiratory, Environmental and Exercise Physiology* 43:302–5.
38. Hakkinen, K., and M. Alen. 1986. Physiological performance, serum hormone, enzyme and lipids of an elite power athlete during training with and without androgens and during prolonged detraining. *Journal of Sports Medicine* 26:92–100.
39. Harber, V. J., and J. R. Sutton. 1984. Endorphins and exercise. *Sports Medicine* 1:154–71.
40. Harris, R. C., J. Bergstrom, and E. Hultman. 1971. The effect of propranolol on glycogen metabolism during exercise. In *Muscle Metabolism during Exercise,* (B. Pernow and B. Saltin, ed.) 301–5. New York: Plenum Press.
41. Hartley, L. H. et al. 1972. Multiple hormonal responses to graded exercise in relation to physical training. *Journal of Applied Physiology* 33:602–6.
42. ———. 1972. Multiple hormonal responses to prolonged exercise in relation to physical training. *Journal of Applied Physiology* 33:607–10.
43. Heath, G. W. et al. 1983. Effect of exercise and lack of exercise on glucose tolerance and insulin sensitivity. *Journal of Applied Physiology: Respiratory, Environmental and Exercise Physiology* 55:512–17.
44. Hole, J. W. 1978. *Human Anatomy and Physiology.* Dubuque, Ia: Wm. C. Brown.
45. Holloszy, J. O., and H. T. Narahara. 1967. Enhanced permeability of sugar associated with muscle contraction: studies of the role of Ca^{++}. *Journal of General Physiology* 50:551–62.
46. Howley, E. T. 1976. The effect of different intensities of exercise on the excretion of epinephrine and norepinephrine. *Medicine and Science in Sports* 8:219–22.
47. ———. 1980. The excretion of catecholamines as an index of exercise stress. In *Exercise in Health and Disease,* ed. F. J. Nagle and H. J. Montoye, 171–83. Springfield, Ill: Charles C. Thomas.
48. Howley, E. T. et al.1983. Effect of hyperoxia on metabolic and catecholamine responses to prolonged exercise. *Journal of Applied Physiology: Respiratory, Environmental and Exercise Physiology* 54:54–63.
49. Hultman, E. 1967. Physiological role of muscle glycogen in man with special reference to exercise. In *Circulation Research* XX and XXI, ed. C. B. Chapman, 1–99 and 1–114. New York: The American Heart Association.
50. Issekutz, B., and H. Miller. 1962. Plasma free fatty acids during exercise and the effect of lactic acid. *Proceedings of the Society of Experimental Biology and Medicine* 110:237–39.
51. Ivy, J. L. et al. 1983. Exercise training and glucose uptake by skeletal muscle in rats. *Journal of Applied Physiology: Respiratory, Environmental and Exercise Physiology* 55:1393–96.
52. Jasson, E., P. Hjemdahl, and L. Kaijser. 1986. Epinephrine-induced changes in carbohydrate metabolism during exercise in male subjects. *Journal of Applied Physiology* 60:1466–70.
53. Johnson, L. G. 1983. *Biology.* Dubuque, Ia: Wm. C. Brown.
54. Juhlin-Dannfelt, A. C. et al. 1982. Effects of β-adrenergic receptor blockade on glycolysis during exercise. *Journal of Applied Physiology: Respiratory, Environmental and Exercise Physiology* 53:549–54.
55. Jurkowski, J. E. et al. 1978. Ovarian hormonal responses to exercise. *Journal of Applied Physiology: Respiratory, Environmental and Exercise Physiology* 44:109–14.

56. Kantor, M. A. et al. 1985. Androgens reduce HDL_2-cholesterol and increase hepatic triglyceride lipase activity. *Medicine and Science in Sports and Exercise* 17:462–65.

57. Kjaer, M., and H. Galbo. 1988. Effects of physical training on the capacity to secrete epinephrine. *Journal of Applied Physiology* 64:11–16.

58. Langenfeld, M. E., L. S. Hart, and P. C. Kao. 1987. Plasma β-endorphin responses to one-hour bicycling and running at 60% max. *Medicine and Science in Sports and Exercise* 19:83–86.

59. Lavoie, J. M. et al. 1987. Menstrual cycle phase dissociation of blood glucose homeostasis during exercise. *Journal of Applied Physiology* 62:1084–89.

60. Laycock, J. F., and P. H. Wise. 1983. *Essential Endocrinology.* New York: Oxford University Press.

61. Leeds, E. M. et al. 1986. Effects of jumping exercise and anabolic steroids on total and lipoprotein cholesterol concentrations in male and female rats. *Medicine and Science in Sports and Exercise* 18:663–67.

62. Ljunghall, S. et al. 1986. Prolonged low-intensity exercise raises the serum parathyroid hormone levels. *Clinical Endocrinology.* 25:535–42.

63. Ljunghall, S. et al. 1988. Increase in serum parathyroid hormone levels after prolonged exercise. *Medicine and Science in Sports and Exercise* 20:122–25.

64. Loucks, A. B., and S. M. Horvath. 1985. Athletic amenorrhea: a review. *Medicine and Science in Sports and Exercise* 17:56–72.

65. Luyckx, A. S., and P. J. Lefebvre. 1974. Mechanisms involved in the exercise-induced increase in glucagon secretion in rats. *Diabetes* 23:81–93.

66. Macintyre, J. G. 1987. Growth hormone and athletes. *Sports Medicine* 4:129–42.

67. Maher, J. T. et al. 1975. Aldosterone dynamics during graded exercise at sea level and high altitude. *Journal of Applied Physiology* 39:18–22.

68. McArthur, J. W. 1985. Endorphins and exercise in females: Possible connection with reproductive dysfunction. *Medicine and Science in Sports and Exercise* 17:82–88.

69. Morgan, W. P. 1985. Affective beneficence of vigorous physical activity. *Medicine and Science in Sports and Exercise* 17:94–100.

70. Painter, P. C., E. T. Howley, and J. N. Liles. 1982. Changes in plasma cAMP and catecholamines in men subjected to the same relative amount of physical work stress. *Aviation, Space, and Environmental Medicine* 53:683–86.

71. Paul, P. 1971. Uptake and oxidation of substrates in the intact animal during exercise. In *Muscle Metabolism during Exercise,* ed. B. Pernow and B. Saltin, 225–48. New York: Plenum Press.

72. Powers, S. K., E. T. Howley, and R. H. Cox. 1982. A differential catecholamine response during prolonged exercise and passive heating. *Medicine and Science in Sports and Exercise* 14:435–39.

73. Pruett, E. D. R. 1970. Glucose and insulin during prolonged work stress in men living on different diets. *Journal of Applied Physiology* 28:199–208.

74. Raymond, L. W., J. Sode, and J. R. Tucci. 1972. Adrenocorticotrophic response to non-exhaustive muscular exercise. *Acta Endocrinologica* 70:73–80.

75. Rizza, R. et al. 1979. Differential effects of epinephrine on glucose production and disposal in man. *American Journal of Physiology* 237:E356–E362.

76. Saltin, B., and J. Karlsson. 1971. Muscle glycogen utilization during work of different intensities. In *Muscle Metabolism During Exercise,* ed. B. Pernow and B. Saltin, 289–99. New York: Plenum Press.

77. Selye, H. 1976. *The Stress of Life.* New York: McGraw-Hill Book Company.

78. Silverberg, A. B. et al. 1978. Norepinephrine: hormone and neurotransmitter in man. *American Journal of Physiology* 234:E252–E256.

79. Spriet, L. L., J. M. Ren, and E. Hultman. 1988. Epinephrine infusion enhances muscle glycogenolysis during prolonged electrical stimulation. *Journal of Applied Physiology* 64:1439–44.

80. Stainsby, W. N., C. Sumners, and G. M. Andrew. 1984. Plasma catecholamines and their effect on blood lactate and muscle lactate output. *Journal of Applied Physiology* 57:321–25.

81. Stainsby, W. N., C. Sumners, and P. D. Eitzman. 1985. Effects of catecholamines on lactic acid output during progressive working contractions. *Journal of Applied Physiology* 59:1809–14.

82. Sutton, J., and L. Lazarus. 1976. Growth hormone in exercise: Comparison of physiological and pharmacological stimuli. *Journal of Applied Physiology* 41:523–27.

83. Taylor, W. M. 1988. Synthetic human growth hormone: a call for federal control. *The Physician and Sportsmedicine.* 16(3):189–92.

84. Terjung, R. 1979. Endocrine response to exercise. In (R. S. Hutton and D. I. Miller, ed.) *Exercise and Sport Science Reviews, Volume 7,* 153–79. New York: Macmillan Publishing Company.

85. Vander, A. J., J. H. Sherman, and D. S. Luciano. 1985. *Human Physiology: The Mechanisms of Body Function,* 4th ed. New York: McGraw-Hill Book Company.

86. Vogel, R. B. et al. 1985. Increase of free and total testosterone during submaximal exercise in normal males. *Medicine and Science in Sports and Exercise* 17:119—23.

87. Wade, C. E. 1984. Response, regulation, and actions of vasopressin during exercise: a review. *Medicine and Science in Sports and Exercise* 16:506–11.

88. Webb, O. L., P. M. Laskarzewski, and C. J. Glueck. 1984. Severe depression of high-density lipoprotein cholesterol levels in weight lifters and body builders by self-administered exogenous testosterone and anabolic-androgenic steroids. *Metabolism* 33:971–75.

89. Weicker, H. et al. 1984. Changes in sexual hormones with female top athletes. *International Journal of Sports Medicine* 5:200–2.

90. Wilkerson, J. E., S. M. Horvath, and B. Gutin. 1980. Plasma testosterone during treadmill exercise. *Journal of Applied Physiology: Respiratory, Environmental and Exercise Physiology* 49:249–53.

91. Winder, W. W. et al. 1978. Time course of sympathoadrenal adaptation to endurance exercise training in man. *Journal of Applied Physiology: Respiratory, Environmental and Exercise Physiology* 45:370–74.

92. Wright, J. E. 1980. Anabolic steroids and athletics. In (R. S. Hutton and D. I. Miller, ed.) *Exercise and Sports Sciences Reviews, Volume 8,* 149–202. New York: Macmillan Publishing Company.

93. Wright, J. E. 1982. *Anabolic Steroids and Sports,* Vol. II. New York: Sports Science Consultants.

94. Yakovlev, N. N., and A. A. Viru. 1985. Adrenergic regulation of adaptation to muscular activity. *International Journal of Sports Medicine* 6:255–65.

6 Measurement of Work, Power, and Energy Expenditure

Objectives

*B*y studying this chapter, you should be able to do the following:
1. Define the terms work, power, energy, and gross efficiency.
2. Give a brief explanation of the procedure used to calculate work performed during: (a) cycle ergometer exercise and (b) treadmill exercise.
3. Describe the concept behind the measurement of energy expenditure using: (a) direct calorimetry and (b) indirect calorimetry.
4. Discuss the procedure to estimate the energy expenditure during horizontal treadmill walking and running.
5. Define the following terms: (1) kilogram-meter, (b) relative $\dot{V}O_2$, (c) MET, and (d) open-circuit spirometry.
6. Describe the procedure used to calculate gross efficiency during steady state exercise.

Outline

Key Terms

absolute $\dot{V}O_2$
cycle ergometer
direct calorimetry
ergometer
ergometry
gross efficiency
indirect calorimetry
kilogram-meter
kilocalorie (kcal)
MET
open-circuit spirometry
percent grade
power
relative $\dot{V}O_2$
work

Measurement of energy expenditure and power output has many applications in exercise science. For example, adequate knowledge of the energy requirements of physical activities (i.e., running) is important to a coach in planning a training and dietary program for athletes. This same information can be used by a fitness specialist to prescribe exercise for adults entering a fitness program. Therefore, an understanding of human energy expenditure, how it is measured, and its practical significance is critical for the coach, physical educator, fitness specialist, or exercise physiologist. It is the purpose of this chapter to discuss those concepts necessary for understanding the measurement of human work output and the associated energy expenditure.

Work and Power Defined

Work

Work is defined by the physicist as the product of force times distance:

$$\text{Work} = \text{Force} \times \text{distance}$$

If you lift a 5 kilogram (kg) weight (1 kg = 2.2 pounds) upward over the vertical distance of 2 meters (m), the work performed would be:

$$\text{Work} = 5 \text{ kp} \times 2 \text{ m}$$
$$= 10 \text{ kpm}$$

Here the force exerted by the 5-kg weight is 5 kiloponds (kp), and the distance traveled is 2 meters, with the resulting amount of work performed being expressed in kilopond-meters (kpm). The explanation for the shift from kg to kp in the example just given is that kg is a measure of mass, not force. That is, one

kp is the force acting upon the mass of 1 kg at the normal acceleration of gravity. Note that there are a number of units that can be used to express both work and energy expenditure. Table 6.1 contains a list of terms that are in common use today.

It is often difficult to compute how much work is performed during sporting events. For instance, a shot-putter performs work since the shot has mass and is moved vertically; however, the exact amount of vertical displacement of the shot is difficult to measure without sophisticated photographic equipment, and thus computation of work performed is not a simple problem. In contrast, a weight lifter performing a clean and jerk is lifting a known amount of weight over a fixed vertical distance, making calculation of work quite easy.

Power

Power is the term used to describe how much work is accomplished per unit of time. This can be written as:

$$\text{Power} = \text{Work} \div \text{time}$$

The concept of power is important since it describes the rate at which work is being performed (work rate). It is the work rate or power output that describes the intensity of exercise. Given enough time, any healthy adult could perform a total work output of 2,000 kpm during a twenty-four-hour period. However, only a few highly trained athletes could perform this amount of work in sixty seconds (s). Calculation of power output using this example can be done as follows:

$$\text{Power} = 2,000 \text{ kpm} \div 60 \text{ s}$$
$$= 33.33 \text{ kpm} \cdot \text{s}^{-1}$$

Table 6.2 contains a list of ways that power can be expressed.

Table 6.1 Units used to express the amount of work performed or energy expended

Term	Abbreviation	Conversion Table
Kilogram-meter	kg-m	1 kg-m = 9.81 joules 1 kg-m = 7.23 ft-lbs 1 kg-m = 9.81 × 10 ergs 1 kg-m = 2.34 × 10^{-3} kcal
Kilopond-meter	kpm	1 kpm = 1 kg-m
Kilocalorie	kcal	1 kcal = 4,186 joules 1 kcal = 426.8 kpm 1 kcal = 3,087 ft-lbs
Joule*	J	1 J = 2.38 × 10^{-4} kcal 1 J = 0.737 ft-lbs 1 J = 0.101 kg-m
Foot-pounds	ft-lbs	1 ft-lb = 0.1383 kg-m

*The joule is the basic unit adopted by the System International (called SI unit) for expression of energy expenditure or work.

Table 6.2 Terms and units used to express power

Term	Abbreviation	Conversion Table
Watt*	W	1 W = 0.001 kilowatt 1 W = 1 J · s^{-1} 1 W = 6.12 kpm · min^{-1}
Horsepower	hp	1 hp = 745.1 W 1 hp = 745.7 J · s^{-1} 1 hp = 10.69 kcal · min^{-1}
Kilopond-meter · min^{-1}	kpm · min^{-1}	1 kpm · min^{-1} = 0.163 W

*The watt is the basic unit adopted by the System International (called SI units) for expression of power.

Measurement of Work and Power

Bench Step

The term **ergometry** pertains to the measurement of work output. The word **ergometer** refers to the apparatus or device used to measure a specific type of work. One of the earliest ergometers employed to measure work capacity in humans was the bench step. This ergometer is still in use today and simply involves the subject stepping up and down on a bench at a specified rate. Calculation of the work performed during bench stepping is very easy. Suppose a 70-kg man steps up and down a 50-centimeter (0.5 meter) bench for ten minutes at a rate of thirty steps per minute. The amount of work performed during this ten-minute task can be computed as follows:

Force = 70 kp (i.e., body weight = 70 kg)
Distance = 0.5 m · $step^{-1}$ × 30 steps · min^{-1}
$\qquad$ × 10 min = 150 m
Therefore, total work performed = 70 kp × 150 m
$\qquad\qquad\qquad\qquad\qquad$ = 10,500 kpm

The power output can be calculated as:

Power = 10,500 kpm ÷ 10 min
$\qquad$ = 1,050 kpm · min^{-1}

Cycle Ergometer

One of the most popular ergometers in use today is the **cycle ergometer.** This type of ergometer is a stationary exercise bicycle that permits accurate measurement of the amount of work performed. The most common type of cycle ergometer is the Monark® friction-braked cycle, which incorporates a belt wrapped around the wheel (called a flywheel). The belt can be loosened or tightened to provide a change in resistance. Distance traveled can be determined by computing the distance covered per revolution of the flywheel times the number of revolutions. Consider the following example for computation of work and power using the cycle ergometer. Calculate work given:

Duration of exercise = 10 min
Resistance against flywheel = 1.5 kp
Distance traveled per revolution = 6 m
Total revolutions = 600 (10 min $\times$ 60 rev $\cdot$ min^{-1})
Hence, total work = 1.5 kp $\times$ (6 m $\cdot$ rev^{-1}
$\times$ 600 rev)
= 5,400 kpm

Calculation of the power output in the above example is computed by dividing the total work performed by time:

$$Power = 5,400 \text{ kpm} \div 10 \text{ min}$$
$$= 540 \text{ kpm} \cdot \text{min}^{-1}$$

Treadmill

Calculation of the work performed while a subject runs or walks on a treadmill is not generally possible when the treadmill is horizontal. Although running horizontally on a treadmill requires energy, the vertical displacement of the body's center of gravity is not easily measured. Therefore, measurement of work performed during horizontal walking or running is complicated. However, quantifiable work is being performed when walking or running up a slope, and calculation of the amount of work done is a simple task.

Table 6.3 Determination of percent grade from angles of incline

Degrees	Sine	Percent Grade
1	0.0175	1.75
2	0.0349	3.49
3	0.0523	5.23
4	0.0698	6.98
5	0.0872	8.72
6	0.1045	10.45
7	0.1219	12.19
8	0.1392	13.92
9	0.1564	15.64
10	0.1736	17.36

The incline of the treadmill is expressed in units called "percent grade." **Percent grade** is defined as the amount of vertical rise per 100 units of belt travel. For instance, a subject walking on a treadmill at a 10% grade travels ten meters vertically for every 100 meters of the belt travel. Percent grade is calculated by multiplying the sine of the treadmill angle times 100. Examples of this calculation are presented in table 6.3. In practice, the treadmill angle (expressed in degrees) can be determined by simple trigometric computations, or by using a measurement device called an inclinometer (7,15).

To calculate the work output during treadmill exercise, you must know both the subject's body weight and the distance traveled vertically. Vertical travel can be computed by multiplying the distance the belt traveled times the percent grade. This can be written as:

$$\text{Vertical displacement} = \% \text{ grade} \times D$$

where percent grade is expressed as a fraction and the value of D is calculated by multiplying the treadmill speed (m $\cdot$ min^{-1}) times the total minutes of exercise

Figure 6.1 Determination of the "percent grade" on an inclined treadmill. Theta (Θ) represents the angle of inclination. Percent grade is computed as the sine of angle Θ × 100.

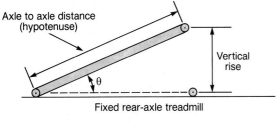

Grade = Sine θ = Rise ÷ Hypotenuse

(figure 6.1). Consider the following sample calculation of work output during treadmill exercise. Calculate work given:

Subject's body weight = 70 kg (i.e., force = 70 kp)
Treadmill speed = 200 m · min⁻¹
Treadmill angle = 7.5 % grade
$$(7.5\% \div 100 = 0.075 \text{ as fractional grade})$$
Exercise time = 10 min
Total vertical distance traveled = 200 m · min⁻¹
$$\times 0.075 \times 10 \text{ min}$$
$$= 150 \text{ m}$$
Therefore, total work performed = 70 kp × 150 m
$$= 10{,}500 \text{ kpm}$$

Measurement of Energy Expenditure

Measurement of an individual's energy expenditure at rest or during a particular activity has many practical applications. One direct application applies to exercise-assisted weight loss programs. Clearly, knowledge of the energy cost of walking, running, or swimming at various speeds is useful to individuals who use these modes of exercise as an aid in weight loss. Further, an industrial engineer might measure the energy cost of various tasks around a job site and use this information to assist in making the appropriate

job assignments to workers (12, 24). In this regard, the engineer might recommend that the supervisor assign those jobs that demand large energy requirements to workers that are physically fit and possess high work capacities. In general, there are two techniques employed in the measurement of human energy expenditure: (1) direct calorimetry and (2) indirect calorimetry.

Direct Calorimetry

When the body uses energy to do work, heat is liberated. This production of heat by cells occurs via both cellular respiration (bioenergetics) and cell work. The general process can be drawn schematically as (3, 25):

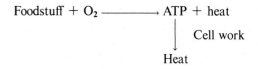

The process of cellular respiration was discussed in detail in chapter 3. Note that the rate of heat production in an animal is directly proportional to the metabolic rate. Therefore, measuring heat production (calorimetry) by an animal gives a direct measurement of metabolic rate.

One unit commonly employed to measure heat is the calorie. A calorie is defined as the amount of heat required to raise the temperature of one gram of water by one degree Celsius. Since the calorie is very small, the term **kilocalorie (kcal)** is generally used to express energy expenditure and the energy value of foods. One kcal is equal to 1,000 calories. The process of measuring an animal's metabolic rate via measurement of heat production is called **direct calorimetry,** and has been used by scientists since the 18th century. This technique involves placement of the animal in a tight chamber (called a calorimeter), which is insulated from the environment (usually by a jacket of water surrounding the chamber), and allowance is made for free exchange of O_2 and CO_2 from the chamber (figure 6.2). The animal's body heat raises the temperature of the water circulating around the chamber. Therefore, by measuring the volume of water flowing through the chamber per minute and the amount of temperature

Figure 6.2 Diagram of a simple calorimeter used to measure metabolic rate via measurement of production of body heat. This method of determining metabolic rate is called direct calorimetry.

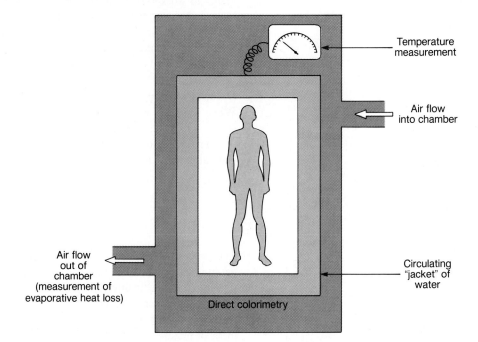

change of the water per unit of time, the amount of heat production can be computed. In addition, heat is lost from the animal by evaporation of water from the skin and respiratory passages. This heat loss can be measured and added back to the total heat picked up by the water to yield an estimate of the rate of energy utilization by the animal (15).

Indirect Calorimetry

Although direct calorimetry is considered to be a precise technique for measurement of metabolic rate, construction of a chamber that is large enough for humans is expensive. Also, use of direct calorimetry to measure metabolic rate during exercise is complicated since the ergometer used may produce heat. Fortunately, another procedure can be used to measure

metabolic rate. This technique is termed **indirect calorimetry** because it does not involve the direct measurement of heat production. The principle of indirect calorimetry can be explained by the following relationship:

$$\text{Foodstuffs} + O_2 \longrightarrow \text{Heat} + CO_2 + H_2O$$
$$\text{(Indirect calorimetry)} \qquad \text{(Direct calorimetry)}$$

Since a direct relationship exists between O_2 consumed and the amount of heat produced in the body, measurement of O_2 consumption provides an estimate of metabolic rate (2, 3, 10). In order to convert the amount of O_2 consumed into heat equivalents, it is necessary to know the type of nutrient (i.e., carbohydrate, fat, or protein) that was metabolized. The energy liberated when fat is the only foodstuff metabolized is

Figure 6.3 Modern open-circuit spirometry utilizing electronic gas analyzers and computer technology.

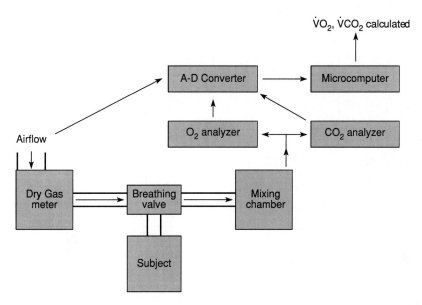

4.7 kcal $\cdot$ l O_2^{-1}, while the energy released when only carbohydrates are used is 5.05 kcal $\cdot$ l O_2^{-1}. Although it is not exact, the caloric expenditure of exercise is often estimated to be approximately 5 kcal per liter of O_2 consumed. Therefore, a person exercising at an oxygen consumption of 2.0 l $\cdot$ min^{-1} would expend approximately 10 kcal of energy per minute (2 l O_2 $\cdot$ min^{-1} $\times$ 5 kcal $\cdot$ l O_2^{-1} = 10 kcal $\cdot$ min^{-1}).

The most common technique used to measure oxygen consumption today is termed **open-circuit spirometry.** Modern-day open-circuit spirometry employs computer technology and is shown diagrammatically in figure 6.3 (21). The volume of air inspired is measured via a gasometer or similar device with the expired gas channeled to a small mixing chamber to be analyzed for O_2 and CO_2 content by electronic gas analyzers. Information concerning the volume of air inspired and the fraction of O_2 and CO_2 in the expired gas is sent to a digital computer by way of a device called an analog-to-digital converter (converts a voltage signal to a digital signal). The computer is programmed to perform the necessary calculations of

$\dot{V}O_2$ (volume of O_2 consumed per min) and the volume of carbon dioxide produced ($\dot{V}CO_2$). In short, $\dot{V}O_2$ is calculated in the following way:

$$\dot{V}O_2 =$$
[volume of O_2 inspired] $-$ [volume of O_2 expired]

See appendix A for details of $\dot{V}O_2$ and $\dot{V}CO_2$ calculations.

Estimation of Energy Expenditure

Researchers studying the oxygen cost (O_2 cost = $\dot{V}O_2$ at steady state) of exercise have demonstrated that it is possible to estimate the energy expended during physical activity with reasonable precision (6, 8, 14, 20). Walking and running are examples of two activities that have been studied in detail. The O_2 requirements of walking and running graphed as a function of speed are presented in figure 6.4. Note that the relationship between the relative O_2 requirement (ml $\cdot$ kg^{-1} $\cdot$ min^{-1}) and walking/running speed is a straight line (1). The fact that this relationship is linear over

Figure 6.4 The relationship between speed and $\dot{V}O_2$ cost is linear for both walking and running. Note that $\times$ equals the walking/running speed in meters $\cdot$ min^{-1}.

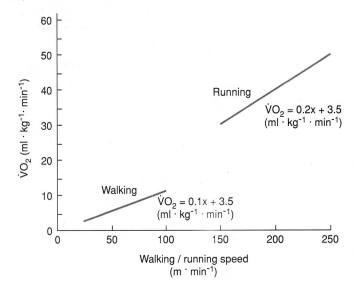

a wide range of speeds is convenient and makes the calculation of the O_2 cost (or energy cost) very easy (see Box 6.1 and Box 6.2 for examples). Estimation of the energy expenditure of other types of activities is more complex than for running or walking. For example, estimation of energy expenditure during tennis is dependent on whether the match is singles or doubles, and is also influenced by the participants' skill level. Nonetheless, a gross estimate of the energy expended during a tennis match is possible. Appendix B contains a list of activities and their estimated energy costs.

The need to express the energy cost of exercise in simple units has led to the development of the term MET. One **MET** is defined as a metabolic equivalent (2). It is equal to resting $\dot{V}O_2$, which is approximately 3.5 ml $\cdot$ kg^{-1} $\cdot$ min^{-1}. Thus, the energy cost of exercise can be described in multiples of resting $\dot{V}O_2$ (i.e., METs), which will simplify the quantification of exercise energy requirement. A physical activity requiring a 10-MET energy expenditure represents a $\dot{V}O_2$ of 35 ml $\cdot$ kg^{-1} $\cdot$ min^{-1} (10 METs $\times$ 3.5 ml $\cdot$ kg^{-1} $\cdot$ min^{-1} per MET = 35 ml $\cdot$ kg^{-1} $\cdot$ min^{-1}). The **absolute $\dot{V}O_2$** requirement of an activity requiring 10 METs can be calculated by multiplying the individual's body weight times the $\dot{V}O_2$ (ml $\cdot$ kg^{-1} $\cdot$ min^{-1}). Therefore, the $\dot{V}O_2$ requirement for a 60-kg individual performing a 10-MET activity would be:

$$\dot{V}O_2 \text{ (ml} \cdot \text{min}^{-1}) = 35 \text{ ml} \cdot \text{kg}^{-1} \cdot \text{min}^{-1} \times 60 \text{ kg}$$
$$= 2,100 \text{ ml} \cdot \text{min}^{-1}$$

Calculation of Exercise Efficiency

Exercise physiologists have long searched for ways to mathematically describe the efficiency of human movement. Although disagreement exists as to the most valid technique of calculating efficiency, the economy of exercise is most often described by the term **gross efficiency** (5, 9, 20, 27, 28). Gross efficiency is defined as the mathematical ratio of work output divided by the energy expended:

$$\% \text{ gross efficiency} = \frac{\text{Work output}}{\text{Energy expended}} \times 100$$

Box 6.1 Estimation of the O_2 Requirement of Treadmill Walking

The O_2 requirement of horizontal treadmill walking can be estimated with reasonable accuracy for speeds between 50 and 100 m · min^{-1} using the following formula (2, 15):

$$\dot{V}O_2 (ml · kg^{-1} · min^{-1}) = 0.1\ ml · kg^{-1} · min^{-1}/(m · min^{-1}) \times speed\ (m · min^{-1})$$
$$+ 3.5\ ml · kg^{-1} · min^{-1} (resting\ \dot{V}O_2)$$

This equation tells us that the O_2 requirement of walking increases as a linear function of walking speed. The slope of the line is 0.1 and the Y intercept is 3.5 ml · kg^{-1} · min^{-1} (resting $\dot{V}O_2$). The O_2 cost of grade walking is:

$$\dot{V}O_2 (ml · kg^{-1} · min^{-1}) = 1.8\ ml · kg^{-1} · min^{-1} \times [speed\ (m · min^{-1}) \times \%\ grade\ (expressed\ as\ a\ fraction)]$$

The total O_2 requirement of graded treadmill walking is the sum of the horizontal O_2 cost and the vertical O_2 cost. For example, the O_2 cost of walking at 80 m · min^{-1} at 5% grade would be:

$$Horizontal\ O_2\ cost = 0.1\ ml · kg^{-1} · min^{-1} \times 80\ m · min^{-1} + 3.5\ ml · kg^{-1} · min^{-1}$$
$$= 11.5\ ml · kg^{-1} · min^{-1}$$
$$Vertical\ O_2\ cost = 1.8\ ml · kg^{-1} · min^{-1} \times (0.05 \times 80) = 7.2\ ml · kg^{-1} · min^{-1}$$

Hence, the total O_2 requirement of walking would amount to:

$$11.5\ ml · kg^{-1} · min^{-1} + 7.2\ ml · kg^{-1} · min^{-1} = 18.7\ ml · kg^{-1} · min^{-1}$$

This O_2 requirement can be expressed in METs by dividing the measured (or estimated) $\dot{V}O_2$ (ml · kg^{-1} · min^{-1}) by 3.5 ml · kg^{-1} · min^{-1} per MET:

$$18.7\ ml · kg^{-1} · min^{-1} \div 3.5\ ml · kg^{-1} · min^{-1}\ per\ MET = 5.3\ METs$$

Formulas are taken from reference 1.

Box 6.2 Estimation of the O_2 Requirement of Treadmill Running

The O_2 requirements of horizontal treadmill running for speeds greater than 134 m · min^{-1} can be estimated in a similar manner to the procedure used to estimate the O_2 requirement for treadmill walking. It is also possible to estimate the O_2 requirement for running up a grade. This calculation is done in two parts:

1. First, the O_2 cost of the horizontal component is calculated using the following formula:

$$\dot{V}O_2 (ml · kg^{-1} · min^{-1}) = 0.2\ ml · kg^{-1} · min^{-1}/m · min^{-1} \times speed\ (m · min^{-1}) + 3.5\ ml · kg^{-1} · min^{-1}$$
$$(resting\ \dot{V}O_2)$$

2. Second, the O_2 requirement of the vertical component is computed using the relationship that running 1 m/min vertically requires 0.9 ml · kg^{-1} · min^{-1}. The vertical velocity is computed by multiplying running speed times the fractional grade. Therefore, the formula to estimate the O_2 cost of vertical treadmill work while running is as follows:

$$\dot{V}O_2 (ml · kg^{-1} · min^{-1}) = 0.9\ ml · kg^{-1}\ per\ m · min^{-1} \times vertical\ velocity\ (m · min^{-1})$$

Formulas are taken from reference 1.

No machine is 100% efficient since some energy is lost due to friction of the moving parts. Likewise, the human machine is not 100% efficient because energy is lost as heat. It is estimated that the gasoline automobile engine operates with a gross efficiency of approximately 20%–25%. Similarly, gross efficiency for humans exercising on a cycle ergometer ranges from 15%–25%, depending on work rate (9, 11, 20, 23, 28).

To compute gross efficiency during cycle ergometer or treadmill exercise requires measurement of work output and an appraisal of the subject's energy expenditure during the exercise. It should be emphasized that $\dot{V}O_2$ measurements must be made during steady state conditions. The work rate on the cycle ergometer or treadmill is calculated as discussed earlier and is generally expressed in kpm · min^{-1}. The energy expenditure during these types of exercise is usually estimated by first measuring $\dot{V}O_2$ (1 · min^{-1}) using open-circuit spirometry, and then converting it to kcal (i.e., 5 kcal = 1 1 O_2). In order to do the computation using the gross-efficiency formula, both numerator and denominator must be expressed in similar terms. Since the numerator (work output) is expressed in kpm, energy expenditure (kcal) must be converted to kpm (or vice versa) using the conversion factor found in table 6.1. Consider the following sample calculation of gross efficiency during submaximal steady state cycle ergometer exercise. Given:

Resistance against the cycle flywheel = 2 kp
Cranking speed = 50 rpm
Steady state $\dot{V}O_2$ = 1.5 1 · min^{-1}
Distance traveled per revolution = 6 m

Therefore:

Work rate = [(2 kp) × (50 rpm × 6 m/rev)]
= 600 kpm · min^{-1}
Energy
expenditure = 1.5 1 · min^{-1} ($\dot{V}O_2$) × 5 kcal · 1 $O_2$$^{-1}$
= 7.5 kcal · min^{-1}

Figure 6.5 Changes in gross efficiency during arm crank ergometry as a function of work rate.

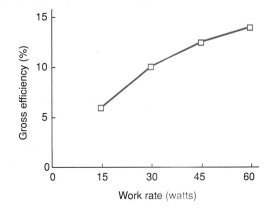

To convert kcal to kpm, multiply by 426.8 (table 6.1):

Energy
expenditure = 426.8 kg-m · kcal^{-1} × 7.5 kcal · min^{-1}
= 3,201 kpm · min^{-1}

Hence, gross efficiency $= \dfrac{600 \text{ kpm} \cdot \text{min}^{-1}}{3,201 \text{ kpm} \cdot \text{min}^{-1}} \times 100\%$
= 18.7%

Figure 6.5 depicts the changes seen in gross efficiency during arm ergometry exercise as a function of work rate. Note that efficiency tends to increase up to a point as the work rate increases (20, 23). This is because resting energy expenditure accounts for a large portion of the total energy expenditure at low exercise rates (11, 20). Therefore, as the work rate increases and the total body energy expenditure increases, resting energy expenditure contributes a smaller portion of the denominator and thus the ratio of work output to energy expenditure increases (gross efficiency increases).

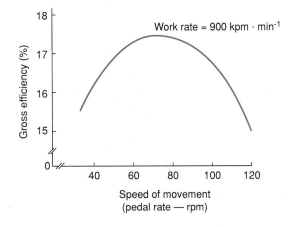

Figure 6.6 Effects of decreasing or increasing speed of movement on exercise efficiency. Note an optimum speed of movement for maximum efficiency at any given work rate.

Movement Speed and Efficiency

Research has shown that there is an "optimum" speed of movement for any given work rate. Recent evidence suggests that the optimum speed of movement increases as the power output increases (6). In other words, at higher power outputs, a greater speed of movement is required to obtain optimum efficiency. At low-to-moderate work rates, a pedaling speed of 40–60 rpm is generally considered optimum during arm or cycle ergometry (11, 19, 20, 22). Note that any change in the speed of movement away from the optimum results in a decrease in efficiency (figure 6.6). This decline in efficiency at low speeds of movement is probably due to inertia (20). That is, there may be an increased energy cost of performing work when movements are slow and the limbs involved must repeatedly stop and start. The decline in efficiency associated with high-speed movement (low work rates) may be because increasing speeds might augment muscular friction and thus increase internal work (4, 20).

Running Economy

As discussed previously, computation of work is not generally possible during horizontal treadmill running, and thus a calculation of exercise efficiency cannot be performed. However, the measurement of the steady state $\dot{V}O_2$ requirement (O_2 cost) of running at various speeds offers a means of comparing running economy (not efficiency) between two runners or groups of runners (13, 14, 18). Figure 6.7 compares the O_2 cost of running between a group of highly trained male and female distance runners. The similar slopes of the two lines suggests that running economy is comparable for highly trained men and women distance runners (14). A runner who exhibits poor running economy would require a higher $\dot{V}O_2$ (ml · kg^{-1} · min^{-1}) at any given running speed than an economical runner. Notice that the O_2 cost of running labeled on the ordinate (Y axis) is expressed as $\dot{V}O_2$ in ml · kg^{-1} · min^{-1}. Expressing $\dot{V}O_2$ as a function of the body weight is referred to as **relative $\dot{V}O_2$**, and is appropriate when describing the O_2 cost of weight-bearing activities such as running, climbing steps, walking, or ice skating.

Summary

1. An understanding of the terms work and power is necessary in order to compute human work output and the associated exercise efficiency:
    a. Work is defined as the product of force times distance:

    $$\text{Work} = \text{Force} \times \text{distance}$$

    b. Power is defined as work divided by time:

    $$\text{Power} = \text{Work} \div \text{time}$$

Figure 6.7 Comparison of the oxygen cost of horizontal treadmill running between highly trained men and women distance runners.

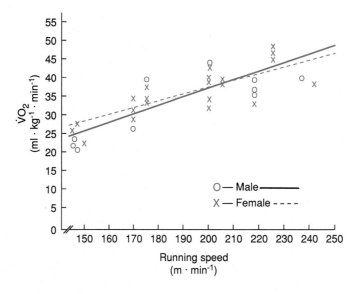

2. Measurement of energy expenditure at rest or during exercise is possible using either direct or indirect calorimetry. Direct calorimetry uses the measurement of heat production as an indication of metabolic rate. Indirect calorimetry estimates metabolic rate via measurement of oxygen consumption.
3. The energy cost of horizontal treadmill walking or running can be estimated with reasonable accuracy since the O_2 requirements of both walking and running increase as a linear function of speed.
4. The need to express the energy cost of exercise in simple terms has led to the development of the term MET. One MET is defined as the equivalent of resting $\dot{V}O_2$ (3.5 ml $\cdot$ kg^{-1} $\cdot$ min^{-1}).
5. Gross efficiency is defined as the mathematical ratio of work performed divided by the energy expenditure, and is expressed as a percent:

$$\text{Gross efficiency \%} = \frac{\text{Work output}}{\text{Energy expended}} \times 100$$

Although it is not possible to compute gross efficiency during horizontal running, the measurement of the O_2 cost of running (ml $\cdot$ kg^{-1} $\cdot$ min^{-1}) at any given speed offers a measure of running economy.

Study Questions

1. Define the following terms:
   a. work
   b. power
   c. percent grade
   d. relative $\dot{V}O_2$
   e. absolute $\dot{V}O_2$
   f. gross efficiency
2. Calculate the total amount of work performed in five minutes of exercise on the cycle ergometer given:

   Resistance on the flywheel = 2.5 kp
   Cranking speed = 60 rpm
   Distance traveled per revolution = 6 meters

3. Compute total work and power output per minute for ten minutes of treadmill exercise given:

> Treadmill grade $= 15\%$
> Horizontal speed $= 200 \text{ m} \cdot \text{min}^{-1}$
> Subject's weight $= 70 \text{ kg}$

4. Briefly, describe the procedure used to estimate energy expenditure using (a) direct calorimetry and (b) indirect calorimetry.

5. Compute the estimated energy expenditure during horizontal treadmill walking for the following examples:
   a. Treadmill speed $= 50 \text{ m} \cdot \text{min}^{-1}$
      Subject's weight $= 62 \text{ kg}$
   b. Treadmill speed $= 100 \text{ m} \cdot \text{min}^{-1}$
      Subject's weight $= 75 \text{ kg}$
   c. Treadmill speed $= 80 \text{ m} \cdot \text{min}^{-1}$
      Subject's weight $= 60 \text{ kg}$

6. Calculate the estimated O_2 cost of horizontal treadmill running for a 70-kg subject at 150, 200, and 235 $\text{m} \cdot \text{min}^{-1}$.

7. Calculate gross efficiency given:

> $\dot{V}O_2 = 1.5 \text{ l} \cdot \text{min}^{-1}$
> Work rate $= 600 \text{ kpm} \cdot \text{min}^{-1}$

Suggested Readings

American College of Sports Medicine. 1986. *Guidelines for Graded Exercise Testing and Exercise Prescription.* Philadelphia: Lea & Febiger.

Astrand, P., and K. Rodahl. 1986. *Textbook of Work Physiology.* New York: McGraw-Hill.

Consolazio, C., R. Johnson, and L. Pecora. 1963. *Physiological Measurements of Metabolic Function in Man.* New York: McGraw-Hill.

Daniels, J. 1985. A physiologist's view of running economy. *Medicine and Science in Sports and Exercise* 17:332–38.

Howley, E., and B. D. Franks. 1986. *Health/Fitness Instructors Handbook.* Champaign, Ill.: Human Kinetics Publishers.

Knuttgen, H. 1978. Force, power, and exercise. *Medicine and Science in Sports and Exercise.* 10:227–28.

References

1. American College of Sports Medicine. 1986. *Guidelines for Graded Exercise Testing and Exercise Prescription.* Philadelphia: Lea & Febiger.
2. Astrand, P., and K. Rodahl. 1986. *Textbook of Work Physiology.* New York: McGraw-Hill.
3. Brooks, G., and T. Fahey. 1984. *Exercise Physiology: Human Bioenergetics and its Applications.* New York: Macmillan.
4. Cavanagh, P., and R. Kram. 1985. Mechanical and muscular factors affecting the efficiency of human movement. *Medicine and Science in Sports and Exercise* 17:326–31.
5. ———. 1985. The efficiency of human movement— a statement of the problem. *Medicine and Science in Sports and Exercise* 17:304–8.
6. Coast, J., and H. G. Welch. 1985. Linear increase in optimal pedal rate with increased power output in cycle ergometry. *European Journal of Applied Physiology* 53:339–42.
7. Consolazio, C., R. Johnson, and L. Pecora. 1963. *Physiological Measurements of Metabolic Function in Man.* New York: McGraw-Hill.
8. Daniels, J. 1985. A physiologist's view of running economy. *Medicine and Science in Sports and Exercise.* 17:332–38.
9. Donovan, C., and G. Brooks. 1977. Muscular efficiency during steady-state exercise: effects of speed and work rate. *Journal of Applied Physiology* 43:431–39.
10. Fox, E., and D. Mathews. 1981. *The Physiological Basis of Physical Education and Athletics.* Philadelphia: Saunders College Publishing.
11. Gaesser, G., and G. Brooks. 1975. Muscular efficiency during steady-rate exercise: effects of speed and work rate. *Journal of Applied Physiology* 38:1132–39.
12. Grandjean, E. 1982. *Fitting the Task to the Man: An Ergonomic Approach.* New York: International Publications Service.
13. Hagan, R. et al. 1980. Oxygen uptake and energy expenditure during horizontal treadmill running. *Journal of Applied Physiology* 49:571–75.
14. Hopkins, P., and S. Powers. 1982. Oxygen uptake during submaximal running in highly trained men and women. *American Corrective Therapy Journal* 36:130–32.

15. Howley, E., and B. D. Franks. 1986. *Health/Fitness Instructor's Handbook*. Champaign, Ill.: Human Kinetics Publishers.

16. Knuttgen, H. 1978. Force, power, and exercise. *Medicine and Science in Sports and Exercise* 10:227–28.

17. Lakomy, H. 1986. Measurement of work and power output using friction-loaded cycle ergometers. *Ergonomics* 29:509–17.

18. Margaria, R. et al. 1963. Energy cost of running. *Journal of Applied Physiology* 18:367–70.

19. Michielli, D., and M. Stricevic. 1977. Various pedalling frequencies at equivalent power outputs. *New York State Medical Journal* 77:744–46.

20. Powers, S., R. Beadle, and M. Mangum. 1984. Exercise efficiency during arm ergometry: effects of speed and work rate. *Journal of Applied Physiology* 56:495–99.

21. Powers, S. et al. 1987. Measurement of oxygen uptake in the non-steady state. *Aviation, Space, and Environmental Medicine* 58:323–27.

22. Seabury, J., W. Adams, and M. Ramey. 1977. Influence of pedalling rate and power output on energy expenditure during bicycle ergometry. *Ergonomics* 20:491–98.

23. Shephard, R. 1982. *Physiology and Biochemistry of Exercise*. New York: Praeger.

24. Singleton, W. 1982. *The Body at Work*. London: Cambridge University Press.

25. Spence, A., and E. Mason. 1987. *Human Anatomy and Physiology*. Menlo Park, Calif.: Benjamin Cummings.

26. Stegeman, J. 1981. *Exercise Physiology: Physiological Bases of Work and Sport*. Chicago: Year Book Publishers.

27. Stuart, M. et al. 1980. Efficiency of trained subjects differing in maximal oxygen uptake and type of training. *Journal of Applied Physiology* 50:444–49.

28. Whipp, B., and K. Wasserman. 1969. Efficiency of muscular work. *Journal of Applied Physiology* 26:644–48.

7 The Nervous System: Structure and Control of Movement

Objectives

*B*y studying this chapter, you should be able to do the following:
1. Discuss the general organization of the nervous system.
2. Describe the structure and function of a nerve.
3. Draw and label the pathways involved in a withdrawal reflex.
4. Define depolarization, action potential, and repolarization.
5. Discuss the role of position receptors in the control of movement.
6. Describe the role of the vestibular apparatus in maintaining equilibrium.
7. Discuss the brain centers involved in voluntary control of movement.
8. Describe the structure and function of the autonomic nervous system.

Outline

Key Terms

action potential
afferent fibers
autonomic nervous system
axon
brain stem
cell body
central nervous system (CNS)
cerebrum
cerebellum
conductivity
dendrites
efferent fibers
EPSP
IPSP
irritability
kinesthesia
motor cortex
neuron
parasympathetic nervous system
peripheral nervous system (PNS)
proprioceptors
Schwann cells
sympathetic nervous system
synapses
reciprocal inhibition
resting membrane potential
vestibular apparatus

The nervous system provides the body with a rapid means of internal communication that allows us to move about, talk, and coordinate the activity of billions of cells. Thus, neural activity is critically important in the body's ability to maintain homeostasis. The purpose of this chapter is to present an overview of the nervous system, with emphasis on neural control of voluntary movement. We will begin with a brief discussion of the functions of the nervous system.

General Nervous System Functions

The nervous system is the body's means of perceiving and responding to events in the internal and external environments. Receptors capable of sensing touch, pain, temperature changes, and chemical stimuli send information to the **central nervous system (CNS)** concerning changes in our environment. The CNS may respond to these stimuli in several ways. The response may be involuntary movement (i.e., rapid removal of a hand from a hot surface), or alteration in the rate of release of some hormone from the endocrine system (chapter 5). In addition to integrating body activities and controlling voluntary movement, the nervous system is responsible for storing experiences (memory) and establishing patterns of response based on previous experiences (learning). A summary of the functions of the nervous system are as follows (6, 17):

1. Control of the internal environment (nervous system works with endocrine system).
2. Voluntary control of movement.
3. Programming of spinal cord reflexes.
4. Assimilation of experiences necessary for memory and learning.

Organization of the Nervous System

Anatomically, the nervous system can be divided into two main parts: the CNS and the **peripheral nervous system (PNS).** The CNS is that portion of the nervous system contained in the skull (brain) and the spinal cord; the PNS consists of nerve cells (**neurons**) outside the CNS (see figure 7.1).

The PNS can be further subdivided into two sections: (1) the sensory portion and, (2) the motor portion. The sensory division is responsible for transmission of neuron impulses from sense organs (receptors) to the CNS. Nerve fibers, which conduct information toward the CNS, are called **afferent fibers.** The motor portion of the PNS can be further subdivided into the somatic motor (which innervates skeletal muscle) and autonomic motor (which innervates involuntary effector organs like smooth muscle in the gut, cardiac muscle, and glands). Nerve fibers, which conduct impulses away from the CNS, are referred to as **efferent fibers.** The relationships between the CNS and the PNS are visualized in figure 7.2.

Structure of the Neuron

Neurons can be divided anatomically into three basic regions: (1) **cell body,** (2) **dendrites,** and (3) **axon** (see figure 7.3). The center of operation for the neuron is the cell body or soma, which contains the nucleus. Narrow, cytoplasmic attachments extend from the cell body and are called dendrites. Dendrites serve as a receptive area that can conduct electrical impulses toward the cell body. The axon carries the electrical message away from the cell body toward another neuron or effector organ. Axons may vary in length from a few millimeters to a meter (6). Each neuron has only one axon; however, the axon can divide into

Figure 7.1 Anatomical divisions of the nervous system.

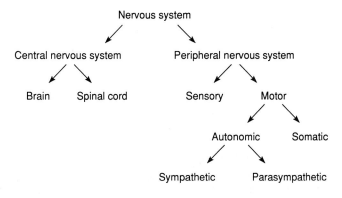

Figure 7.2 The relationship between the motor and sensory fibers of the peripheral nervous system (PNS) and the central nervous system (CNS).

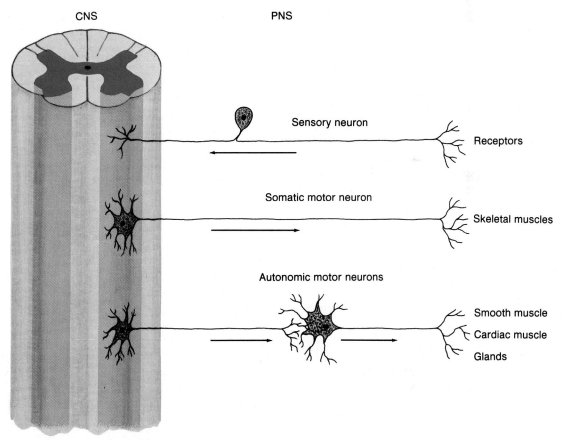

Figure 7.3 The parts of a neuron.

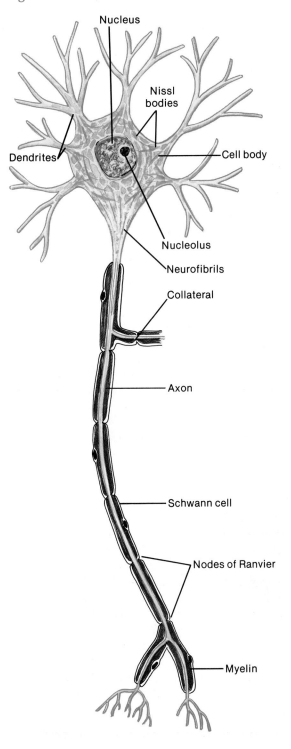

several collateral branches that terminate at other neurons, muscle cells, or glands (figure 7.3). Contact points between an axon of one neuron and another neuron are called **synapses** (see figure 7.4).

In large nerve fibers like those innervating skeletal muscle, the axons are covered with an insulating layer of cells called **Schwann cells** (figure 7.3). The membranes of Schwann cells contain a large amount of a lipid-protein substance called myelin, which forms a discontinuous sheath that covers the outside of the axon. The gaps or spaces between the myelin segments along the axon are called nodes of Ranvier and play an important role in neural transmission. In general, the larger the diameter of the axon, the greater the speed of neural transmission (6). Thus, those axons with large myelin sheaths conduct impulses more rapidly than small nonmyelinated fibers.

Electrical Activity in Neurons

Neurons are considered "excitable tissue" because of their specialized properties of irritability and conductivity. **Irritability** is the ability of the dendrites and neuron cell body to respond to a stimulus and convert it to a neural impulse. **Conductivity** refers to the transmission of the impulse along the axon. A nerve impulse can be thought of as an electrical signal carried the length of the axon. This electrical signal is initiated via some stimulus that causes a change in the normal electrical charge of the neuron.

Resting Membrane Potential

At rest, neurons are negatively charged on the inside of the cell with respect to the charge on the exterior of the cell. This negative charge is the result of an unequal distribution of charged ions (ions are elements with a positive or negative charge) across the cell membrane. Thus, a neuron is said to be polarized and this electrical charge difference is called the **resting membrane potential.** Cellular proteins, phosphate groups, and other nucleotides are negatively charged (anions) and are fixed inside the cell because they cannot penetrate the cell membrane. Since these negatively charged molecules are unable to leave the cell, they attract positively charged ions (cations) from the extracellular fluid. This results in an accumulation of a net positive charge on the outside surface of the membrane and a net negative charge on the inside surface of the membrane (6, 11).

Figure 7.4 An illustration of synaptic transmission. For a nerve impulse to continue from one neuron to another, it must cross the synaptic cleft at a synapse.

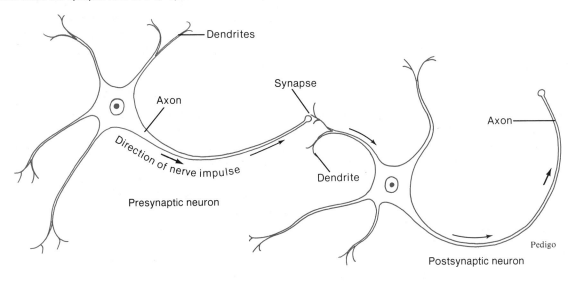

The permeability of the membrane to potassium, sodium, and other ions is regulated by proteins within the membrane that function as gates. Given that the concentration of potassium is high inside the cell and the concentration of sodium is high outside the cell, an alteration of the membrane's permeability to either potassium or sodium would result in a movement of these charged ions down their concentration gradients. At rest, the potassium gate is open much wider than the sodium gate, resulting in the net loss of positive charge from the inside of the membrane, making the resting membrane potential approximately −70 mv. To summarize, at rest the membrane potential of −70 mv is due primarily to the rapid diffusion of potassium out of the cell, caused by: (1) the higher permeability of the membrane for potassium than sodium, and (2) the concentration gradient for potassium from inside to outside the cell.

However, some sodium is always leaking into the cell at rest due to both its concentration gradient and the strong electrical attraction of −70 mv inside the membrane. If the potassium were to continue to diffuse out of the cell and sodium to continue to diffuse into the cell, the concentration gradients for these ions would decrease, and with it the membrane potential

of −70 mv. What prevents this from happening? The cell membrane has a sodium/potassium pump that uses energy from ATP to maintain the intracellular/ extracellular concentrations by pumping sodium out of the cell and potassium into the cell. Interestingly, this pump not only maintains the concentration gradients that are needed to maintain the resting membrane potential, but it also helps to generate the potential since it exchanges three sodium ions for every two potassium ions.

Action Potential

A neural message is generated when a stimulus of sufficient strength reaches the neuron membrane and opens sodium gates, which allows sodium ions to diffuse into the neuron, making the inside more and more positive (depolarizing the cell). When depolarization reaches a critical value called "threshold," the sodium gates open wide and an **action potential** or nerve impulse is formed (see figures 7.5 and 7.6). Once an action potential has been generated, a sequence of ionic exchanges occurs along the axon to propagate the nerve impulse. This ionic exchange along the neuron occurs in a sequential fashion at the nodes of Ranvier (figure 7.3).

Figure 7.5 An action potential is produced by an increase in sodium conductance into the neuron. As sodium enters the neuron the change becomes more and more positive and an action potential is generated. See text for details.

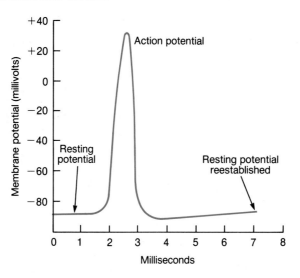

Figure 7.6 The bottom portion of this figure illustrates that when a neuron fiber is stimulated, sodium channels open, sodium ions (Na⁺) diffuse inward, and the membrane is depolarized (action potential is generated). The upper portion of this figure illustrates the repolarization of the nerve by the opening of potassium (K⁺) channels and K⁺ diffusing out.

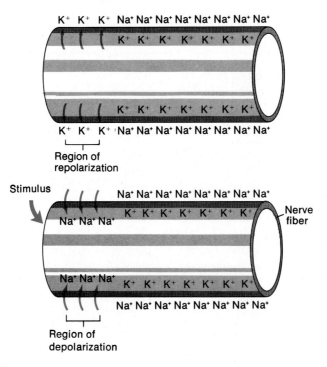

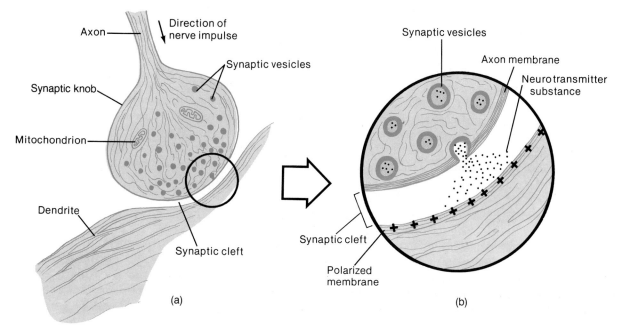

Figure 7.7 (*a*) When a nerve impulse reaches the synaptic knob at the end of an axon, (*b*) synaptic vesicles release a neurotransmitter substance that diffuses across the synaptic cleft.

Repolarization occurs immediately following depolarization resulting in a return of the resting membrane potential with the nerve ready to be stimulated again (figure 7.5). How does repolarization occur? Depolarization, with a slight time delay, causes a brief increase in membrane permeability to potassium. As a result, potassium leaves the cell, rapidly making the inside of the membrane more negative. (See top portion of figure 7.6.) Secondly, after the depolarization stimulus is removed, the sodium gates within the cell membrane close and sodium entry into the cell is slowed (therefore, few positive charges are entering the cell). The combined result of these activities quickly restore the resting membrane potential back to approximately -70 mv.

All-or-None Law

The development of a nerve impulse is considered to be an "all-or-none" response. This means that if a nerve impulse is initiated, the impulse will travel the entire length of the axon without a decrease in voltage. In other words, the neural impulse is just as strong after traveling the length of the axon as it was at the initial point of stimulation.

Another feature of the "all-or-none law" is that the strength of the action potential is fixed. That is, no matter how strong the stimulus, as long as it achieves threshold the magnitude of the action potential is constant.

Neurotransmitters and Synaptic Transmission

As mentioned previously, neurons communicate with other neurons at junctions called synapses. A synapse is a small gap (20–30 nanometers) between the synaptic knob of the presynaptic neuron and a dendrite of a postsynaptic neuron (see figure 7.7). Communication between neurons occurs via a process called synaptic transmission, and happens when sufficient amounts of a specific neurotransmitter are released from synaptic vesicles contained in the presynaptic neuron. The nerve impulse results in the synaptic vesicles releasing stored neurotransmitter into the synaptic cleft. (Neurotransmitters that cause depolarization of membranes are termed excitatory transmitters.) After release into the synaptic cleft, these neurotransmitters bind to "receptors" on the target membrane, which produces a series of graded depolarizations in the dendrites and cell body (1, 2, 11, 12, 16). These graded depolarizations are known as excitatory postsynaptic potentials (**EPSPs**). If sufficient amounts of the neurotransmitter are released, the postsynaptic neuron is depolarized to threshold and an action potential is generated.

A common neurotransmitter, which also happens to be the transmitter at the nerve/muscle junction, is acetylcholine. Upon release into the synaptic cleft, acetylcholine binds to receptors on the postsynaptic membrane and opens "channels," which allow sodium to enter the muscle cell. When enough sodium enters the postsynaptic membrane (muscle), depolarization results. In order to prevent chronic depolarization of the postsynaptic neuron, the neurotransmitter must be broken down into less active molecules via enzymes found in the synaptic cleft. In the case of acetylcholine, the degrading enzyme is called acetylcholinesterase. This enzyme breaks down acetylcholine into acetyl and choline and thus removes the stimulus for depolarization (6). Following break down of the neurotransmitter, the postsynaptic membrane repolarizes and is prepared to receive additional neurotransmitter and generate a new action potential.

Note that not all neurotransmitters are excitatory. In fact, some neurotransmitters have just the opposite effect of excitatory transmitters. These inhibitory transmitters cause a hyperpolarization (increased negativity) of the postsynaptic membrane. This hyperpolarization of the membrane is called an inhibitory postsynaptic potential (**IPSP**). The end result of an IPSP is that the neuron develops a more negative resting membrane potential, is pushed further from threshold, and thus resists depolarization. In general, whether a neuron reaches threshold or not is dependent on the ratio of the number of EPSPs to the number of IPSPs. For example, a neuron that is simultaneously bombarded by an equal number of EPSPs and IPSPs will not reach threshold and generate an action potential. On the other hand, if the number of EPSPs outnumber the IPSPs, the neuron is moved toward threshold and an action potential may be generated.

An interesting example of a neurotransmitter that can be both inhibitory and excitatory is acetylcholine. While acetylcholine produces depolarization of skeletal muscle, it causes a hyperpolarization of the heart, slowing the heart rate. This is because the combination of acetylcholine with receptors in the heart causes the opening of membrane channels that allow potassium to diffuse out of the cell. Thus, an outward diffusion of potassium produces a hyperpolarization of heart tissue and therefore moves further away from the threshold potential.

Somatic Receptors and Reflexes

The term somatic refers to the outer (i.e., nonvisceral) regions of the body. The CNS receives a constant bombardment of messages from somatic receptors about changes in both the internal and external environment. These receptors are "sense organs" that "change" forms of energy in the "real world" into the energy of nerve impulses, which are conducted to the CNS by sensory neurons. Van De Graaff (21) has called these sense organs "windows for the brain." A complete discussion of sense organs is beyond the scope of this chapter, so we will limit our discussion to those receptors responsible for position sense. These receptors are called **proprioceptors** and include muscle spindles, Golgi tendon organs, and joint receptors. Muscle spindles and Golgi tendon organs are discussed in chapter 8, so our discussion will center around joint receptors.

Kinesthetic Receptors

The term **kinesthesia** means conscious recognition of the position of body parts with respect to each other as well as recognition of limb-movement rates (13, 14, 15). These functions are accomplished by extensive sensory devices in and around joints. There are three principle types of kinesthetic receptors: (1) free nerve endings, (2) Golgi-type receptors, and (3) pacinian corpuscles. The most abundant of these are free nerve endings, which are sensitive to touch and pressure. These receptors are stimulated strongly at the beginning of movement; they adapt (i.e., become less sensitive to stimuli) slightly at first, but then transmit a steady signal until the movement is complete (3, 7). A second position receptor, Golgi-type receptors (not to be confused with Golgi tendon organs found in muscle tendons), are found in ligaments around joints. These receptors are not as abundant as free nerve endings, but function in a similar manner (6, 17). Pacinian corpuscles are found in the tissues around joints and adapt rapidly following the initiation of movement. This rapid adaptation presumably helps detect the rate of joint rotation (6, 17). To summarize, the joint receptors work together to provide the body with a conscious means of recognition of the orientation of body parts as well as feedback relative to the rates of limb movement.

Reflexes

A reflex arc is the nerve pathway from the receptor to the CNS and from the CNS along a motor pathway back to the effector organ. Reflex contraction of skeletal muscles can occur in response to sensory input, and is not dependent on activation of higher brain centers. One purpose of a reflex is to provide a rapid means of removing a limb from a source of pain. Consider the case of a person touching a sharp object. The obvious reaction to this painful stimulus is to quickly remove the hand from the source of pain. This rapid removal is accomplished via reflex action. Again, the pathways for this neural reflex are as follows (10): (1) first, a sensory nerve (pain receptor) sends a nerve impulse to the spinal column; (2) secondly, interneurons within the spinal cord are excited and in turn stimulate motor neurons; (3) finally, the excited interneurons cause depolarization of specific motor neurons, which control the flexor muscles necessary to withdraw the limb from the point of injury. The antagonistic muscle group (i.e., extensors) are simultaneously inhibited via IPSP's. This simultaneous excitatory and inhibitory activity is known as **reciprocal inhibition** (see figure 7.8).

Another interesting feature of the withdrawal reflex is that the opposite limb is extended to support the body during the removal of the injured limb. This event is called the crossed-extensor reflex and is illustrated by the left portion of figure 7.8. Notice that the extensors are contracting as the flexors are inhibited.

Vestibular Apparatus and Equilibrium

The **vestibular apparatus,** an organ located in the inner ear, is responsible for maintaining general equilibrium. Although a detailed discussion of the anatomy of the vestibular apparatus will not be presented here, a brief discussion of the function of the vestibular apparatus is appropriate. The receptors contained within the vestibular apparatus are sensitive to any change in head position or movement direction (11). Movement of the head excites these receptors and nerve impulses are sent to the CNS regarding this change in position. Specifically, these receptors provide information about linear acceleration and angular acceleration. This mechanism allows us to have a sense of acceleration or deceleration when running or traveling by car. Further, a sense of angular acceleration helps us maintain balance when the head is turning or spinning (i.e., performing gymnastics or diving).

The neural pathways involved in control of equilibrium are outlined in figure 7.9. Any head movement results in stimulation of receptors in the vestibular apparatus, which transmits neural information to the cerebellum and the vestibular nuclei located in the brain stem. Further, the vestibular nuclei relays a message to the oculomotor center (controls eye movement) and to neurons in the spinal cord that control movements of the head and limbs. Thus, the vestibular apparatus controls head and eye movement during physical activity, which serves to maintain balance and visually track the events of movement. In summary, the vestibular apparatus is sensitive to the position of the head in space and to sudden changes in the direction of body movement. Its primary function is to maintain equilibrium and preserve a constant plane of head position. Failure of the vestibular apparatus to function properly would prevent accurate performance of any athletic task that requires head movement. Since most sporting events require at least some head movement, the importance of the vestibular apparatus is obvious.

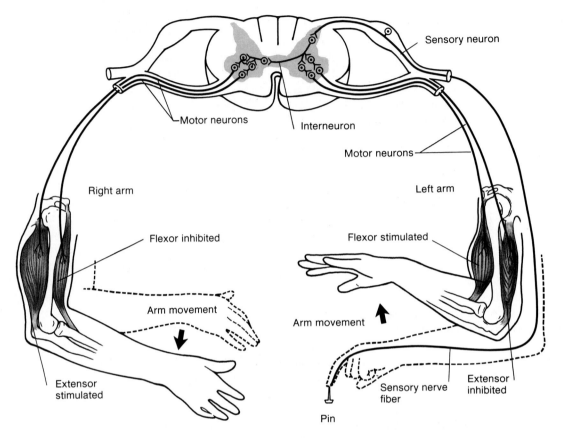

Figure 7.8 When the flexor muscle on one side of the body is stimulated to contract via a withdrawal reflex, the extensor on the opposite side also contracts.

Motor Control Functions of the Brain

The brain can be conveniently subdivided into three parts: the brain stem, cerebrum, and cerebellum. Figure 7.10 demonstrates the anatomical relationship between each of these components. Each of these structures make important contributions to the regulation of movement. The next several paragraphs will outline the brain's role in the regulation of performance of sports skills.

Brain Stem

The **brain stem** is located inside the base of the skull just above the spinal cord. It consists of a complicated series of nerve tracts and nuclei (clusters of neurons), and is responsible for many metabolic functions, cardiorespiratory control, and some highly complex reflexes. The major structures of the brain stem are the medulla, pons, and midbrain. In addition, there is a series of complex neurons scattered throughout the brain stem that is collectively called the reticular formation, which plays an important role in consciousness.

Figure 7.9 The role of the vestibular apparatus in maintainence of equilibrium and balance.

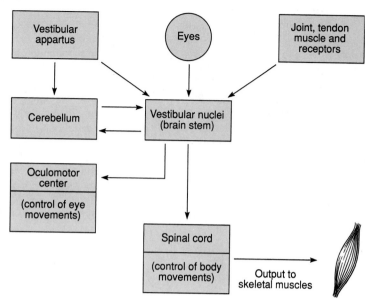

Figure 7.10 The anatomical relationship between the cerebrum, the cerebellum, and the brainstem.

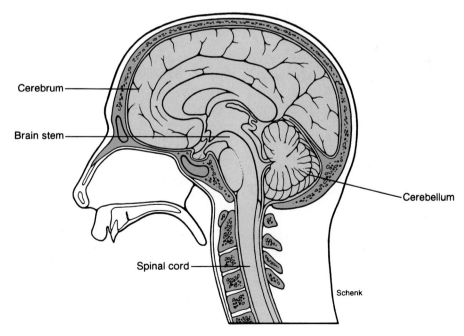

Box 7.1 Parkinson's Disease and Motor Function

Much of our present information concerning the regulation of motor control has come from those disorders involving various areas of the brain. When an area of the CNS malfunctions, the resulting impairment of motor control gives neuroscientists a better understanding of the function of the affected area. The basal ganglia is a series of clusters of neurons located in both cerebral hemispheres. One of the important functions of the basal ganglia is to aid in the regulation of movement. Parkinson's disease is a disorder of the basal ganglia, and results in a decrease in the synthesis of a neurotransmitter called dopamine. Dopamine's function in the basal ganglia appears to be one of inhibiting the amount of muscular activity as an aid in the control of various muscular activities. Since patients with Parkinson's disease have a reduction in the amount of discharge from the basal ganglia, this results in involuntary movement or tremors. Further, although Parkinson's patients can frequently carry out rapid movements normally, these individuals often have great difficulty in performing slow movements. This observation supports the concept that the basal ganglia is important in the conduct of slow voluntary movement. Treatment of Parkinson's disease is often accomplished by administering drugs that stimulate the production of the neurotransmitter, dopamine.

In general, the neuronal circuits in the brain stem are thought to be responsible for the control of eye movement and muscle tone, equilibrium, support of the body against gravity, and many special reflexes. One of the most important roles of the brain stem in control of locomotion is that of maintaining postural tone. That is, centers in the brain stem provide the nervous activity necessary to maintain normal upright posture and therefore support the body against gravity. It is clear that the maintainence of upright posture requires that the brain stem receive information from several sensory modalities (i.e., vestibular receptors, pressure receptors of the skin, vision). Damage to any portion of the brain stem results in impaired movement control (5, 11).

Cerebrum

The **cerebrum** is the large dome of the brain that is divided into right and left cerebral hemispheres. The outermost layer of the cerebrum is called the cerebral cortex and is composed of tightly arranged neurons. Although the cortex is only about one-fourth an inch thick, it contains over 8 million neurons. The cortex performs three very important motor behavior functions (6, 17): (1) organization of complex movement, (2) storage of learned experiences, and (3) the reception of sensory information. We will limit our discussion to the role of the cortex in the organization of movement. The portion of the cerebral cortex that is most concerned with voluntary movement is the **motor cortex.** Although the motor cortex plays a significant role in motor control, it appears that input to the motor cortex from subcortical structures (i.e., cerebellum, etc.) is absolutely essential for coordinated movement to occur (8, 17). Thus, the motor cortex can be described as the final relay point upon which subcortical inputs are focused. After the motor cortex sums these inputs the final movement plan is formulated and the motor commands are sent to the spinal cord. This "movement plan" can be modified by both subcortical and spinal centers, which supervise the fine details of the movement.

Cerebellum

The **cerebellum** lies behind the pons and medulla and has a convoluted appearance (figure 7.10). Although complete knowledge about cerebellar function is not presently available, much is known about the role of this structure in movement control. It is clear that the cerebellum plays an important role in coordinating and monitoring complex movement. This work is accomplished via connections leading from the cerebellum to the motor cortex, the brain stem, and the spinal cord. Evidence exists to suggest that the primary role of the cerebellum is to aid in the control of movement in response to feedback from proprioceptors (17). Further, the cerebellum may initiate fast, ballistic movements via its connection with the motor cortex (8). Damage to the cerebellum results in poor movement control and muscular tremor that is most severe during rapid movement.

Motor Functions of the Spinal Cord

One motor function of the spinal cord has already been discussed (withdrawal reflex). The precise role of spinal reflexes in the control of movement is still being debated. However, there is increasing evidence that normal motor function is influenced by spinal reflexes. In fact, some authors claim that reflexes play a major role in control of voluntary movements. These investigators believe that the events that underlie volitional movement are built on a variety of spinal reflexes (8, 19). Support for this idea comes from the demonstration that spinal reflex neurons are directly affected by descending neural traffic from the brain stem and cortical centers.

The spinal cord makes a major contribution in the control of movement by the preparation of spinal centers to perform the desired movement. The spinal mechanism by which a voluntary movement is translated into appropriate muscle action is termed "spinal tuning." Spinal tuning appears to operate in the following way. Higher brain centers of the motor system are concerned with only the general parameters of movement. The specific details of the movement are refined at the spinal cord level. In other words, although the general pattern of the anticipated movement is controlled by higher motor centers, additional refinement of this movement may occur by a complex interaction of spinal cord neurons and higher centers (17, 19). Thus, it appears that spinal centers play an important role in volitional movement.

Control of Motor Functions

Watching a highly skilled athlete perform a sports skill is exciting, but really does not give the observer an appreciation of the complex integration of many parts of the nervous system required to perform this act. A pitcher throwing a baseball seems to the observer to be accomplishing a simple act, but in reality this movement consists of a complex interaction of higher brain centers with spinal reflexes performed together with precise timing. How the nervous system produces a coordinated movement has been one of the major unresolved mysteries facing neurophysiologists for many decades. Although progress has been made toward answering the basic question of "how do humans control voluntary movement," much is still unknown about this process. Our purpose here will be to provide the reader with a simplistic overview of the brain and control of movement.

Traditionally, it was believed that the motor cortex controlled voluntary movement with little input from subcortical areas. Recent evidence suggests that this is not the case (8, 17). Although the motor cortex is the final executor of movement programs, it appears that the motor cortex does not give the initial signal to move, but rather ranks at the end of the chain of neurophysiological events involved in volitional movement (8). The first step in performing a voluntary movement begins in subcortical and cortical motivational areas, which play a key role in consciousness. This conscious "prime drive" sends signals to the so-called association areas of the cortex (not motor cortex), which forms a "rough draft" of the planned movement from a stock of stored subroutines. Information concerning the nature of the plan of movement is then sent to both the cerebellum and the basal ganglia (clusters of neurons located in the cerebral hemispheres) (see figure 7.11). These structures cooperate to convert the "rough draft" into precise temporal (timing) and spatial excitation programs (8). The cerebellum is possibly more important for making fast movements, while the basal ganglia is more responsible for slow or deliberate movements. From the cerebellum and basal ganglia the precise program is sent through the thalamus to the motor cortex, which forwards them down to spinal neurons for "spinal tuning"

Figure 7.11 Block diagram of the structures and processes leading to voluntary movement.

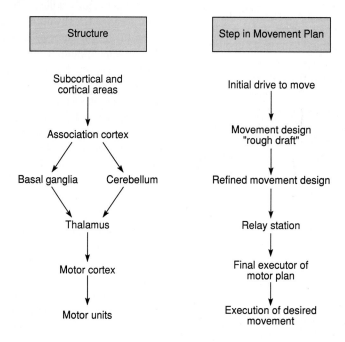

and finally to skeletal muscle. Feedback to the CNS from muscle receptors and proprioceptors allows for modification of motor programs if necessary. The ability to change movement patterns allows the individual to correct "errors" in the original movement plan.

To summarize, control of voluntary movement is complex and requires the cooperation of many areas of the brain as well as several subcortical areas. It should now be clear that the motor cortex does not by itself formulate the signals required to initiate voluntary movement. Instead the motor cortex receives input from a variety of cortical and subcortical structures. Finally, much is still unknown about the details of the control of complex movement, and this topic provides an exciting frontier for future research.

Autonomic Nervous System

The **autonomic nervous system** plays an important role in maintaining the constancy of the body's internal environment. In contrast to somatic motor nerves, autonomic motor nerves innervate effector organs, which are not usually under voluntary control. Autonomic motor nerves innervate cardiac muscle, glands, and smooth muscle found in airways, the gut, and blood vessels. In general, the autonomic nervous system operates below the conscious level, although some individuals apparently can learn to control some portions of this system. Although involuntary, it appears that the function of the autonomic nervous system is closely linked to emotion. For example, all of us have experienced an increase in heart rate following extreme excitement or fear. Further, secretions of digestive glands and sweat glands are affected by periods of excitement. It should not be surprising that participation in intense exercise results in an increase in autonomic activity.

Figure 7.12 A simple schematic demonstrating the neurotransmitters of the autonomic nervous system. Ach = acetylcholine; NE = norephinephrine; E = epinephrine. Note that the adrenal medulla releases both NE (80%) and E (20%) as hormones into the blood.

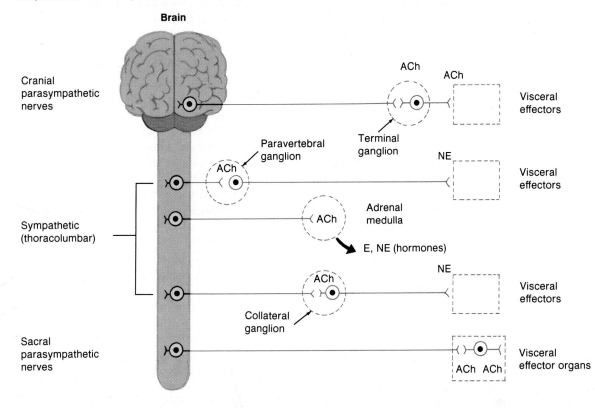

The autonomic nervous system can be separated both functionally and anatomically into two divisions: (1) **sympathetic** division and (2) **parasympathetic** division (see figure 7.12). In general, the sympathetic portion of the autonomic nervous system tends to activate an organ (i.e., increases heart rate), while parasympathetic impulses tend to inhibit it (i.e., slows heart rate). Therefore, the activity of a particular organ can be regulated according to the ratio of sympathetic/parasympathetic impulses to the tissue. In this way, the autonomic nervous system may regulate the activities of involuntary muscles and glands in accordance with the needs of the body (see chapter 5).

The sympathetic division of the autonomic nervous system has its cell bodies of the preganglionic neurons (a ganglion is a group of cell bodies outside of the CNS)

in the thoracic and lumbar regions of the spinal cord. These fibers leave the spinal cord and enter the sympathetic ganglia (figure 7.12). The neurotransmitter between the preganglionic neurons and postganglionic neurons is acetylcholine. Postganglionic sympathetic fibers leave these sympathetic ganglia and innervate a wide variety of tissues. The neurotransmitter released at the effector organ is primarily norepinephrine. Following sympathetic stimulation, norepinephrine is removed in a variety of ways. First, much of the norepinephrine is taken back up into the postganglionic fiber, while the remaining portion will be broken down into nonactive byproducts (9, 18).

The parasympathetic division of the autonomic nervous system has its cell bodies located within the brain stem and the sacral portion of the spinal cord.

Parasympathetic fibers leave the brain stem and the spinal cord and converge on ganglia in a wide variety of anatomical areas. Acetylcholine is the neurotransmitter in both preganglionic and postganglionic fibers. After parasympathetic nerve stimulation, acetylcholine is released and rapidly degraded by the enzyme acetylcholinesterase.

Summary

1. The nervous system is the body's means of perceiving and responding to events in the internal and external environments. Receptors capable of sensing touch, pain, temperature, and chemical stimuli send information to the CNS concerning changes in our environment. The CNS responds by either voluntary movement or a change in the rate of release of some hormone from the endocrine system, depending on which response is appropriate.

2. The nervous system is divided into two major divisions: (1) the central nervous system and (2) the peripheral nervous system. The central nervous system includes the brain and the spinal cord, whereas the peripheral nervous system includes the nerves outside the central nervous system.

3. Nerve cells are called neurons and are divided anatomically into the cell body, dendrites, and axon. Axons are covered by Schwann cells, with gaps between these cells called nodes of Ranvier.

4. Neurons are specialized cells that respond to physical or chemical changes in their environment. At rest, nerve cells are negatively charged in the interior when compared to the electrical charge outside the cell. This difference in electrical charge is called the resting membrane potential.

5. A neuron "fires" due to a stimulus changing the permeability of the membrane, allowing sodium to enter at a high rate, depolarizing the cell. When the depolarization reaches threshold, an action potential or nerve impulse is initiated. Repolarization occurs immediately following depolarization due to an increase in membrane permeability to potassium, and a decreased permeability to sodium.

6. Neurons communicate with other neurons at junctions called synapses. Synaptic transmission occurs when sufficient amounts of a specific neurotransmitter are released from the presynaptic neuron. Upon release, the neurotransmitter binds to a receptor on the postsynaptic membrane. An excitatory transmitter increases neuronal permeability to sodium and results in excitatory postsynaptic potentials (EPSPs). However, some transmitters are inhibitory and cause the neuron to become more negative (hyperpolarized). This hyperpolarization of the membrane is called an inhibitory postsynaptic potential (IPSP).

7. Proprioceptors are position receptors located in joint capsules, ligaments, and muscles. The three most abundant joint and ligament receptors are free nerve endings, Golgi-type receptors, and pacinian corpuscles. These receptors provide the body with a conscious means of recognition of the orientation of body parts as well as feedback relative to the rates of limb movement.

8. Reflexes provide the body with a rapid unconscious means of reacting to some stimuli.

9. The vestibular apparatus is responsible for maintaining general equilibrium and is located in the inner ear. Specifically, these receptors provide information about linear and angular acceleration.

10. Evidence exists to suggest that the spinal cord plays an important role in voluntary movement due to groups of neurons capable of controlling certain aspects of motor activity. The spinal mechanism by which a voluntary movement is translated into appropriate muscle action is termed spinal tuning.

11. The brain can be subdivided into three parts: the brain stem, the cerebrum, and the cerebellum.

12. The motor cortex controls motor activity with the aid of input from subcortical areas. The cerebellum receives feedback from proprioceptors after movement has begun and sends information to the cortex concerning possible corrections of that particular movement pattern. The basal ganglia are neurons involved in organizing complex movements and the initiation of slow movements. The premotor cortex operates in conjunction with the motor cortex to refine complex motor actions and may be important in acquisition of motor skills.

13. The autonomic nervous system is responsible for maintaining the constancy of the body's internal environment and can be separated into two divisions: (1) the sympathetic division and (2) the parasympathetic division. In general, the sympathetic portion (releasing norepinephrine) tends to excite an organ, while the parasympathetic portion (releasing acetlycholine) tends to inhibit the same organ.

Study Questions

1. Identify the location and functions of the central nervous system.
2. Draw a simple chart illustrating the organization of the nervous system.
3. Define synapses.
4. Define membrane potential and action potential.
5. Discuss an IPSP and an EPSP. How do they differ?
6. What are proprioceptors? Give some examples.
7. Describe the location and function of the vestibular apparatus.
8. What is meant by the term "spinal tuning"?
9. List the possible motor functions played by the brain stem, the motor cortex, and the cerebellum.
10. Describe the divisions and functions of the autonomic nervous system.

Suggested Readings

Eccles, J. C. 1973. *The Understanding of the Brain*. New York: McGraw-Hill.

Fox, S. I. 1987. *Human Physiology*. Dubuque, Ia.: Wm. C. Brown.

Henatsch, H., and H. Langer. 1985. Basic neurophysiology of motor skills in sport: a review. *International Journal of Sports Medicine* 6:2–14.

Hole, J. W. 1984. *Human Anatomy and Physiology*. Dubuque, Ia.: Wm. C. Brown.

Ito, M. Where are neurophysiologists going? 1986. *News in Physiological Sciences* 1:30–31.

Sage, G. H. 1984. *Motor Learning and Control: A Neuropsychological Approach*. Dubuque, Ia.: Wm. C. Brown.

References

1. Barchas, J. D. et al. 1978. Behavioral neurochemistry: neuroregulators and behavioral states. *Science* 200:964.
2. Barde, Y. A., D. Edgar, and H. Thoen. 1983. New neurotropic factors. *Annual Review of Physiology* 45:601.
3. Clark, F., and P. Burgess. 1975. Slowly adapting receptors in the cat knee joint: can they signal joint angle? *Journal of Neurophysiology* 38:1448–63.
4. Delong, M., and P. Strick. 1974. Relation of the basal ganglia, cerebellum, and motor cortex units to ramp and ballistic limb movements. *Brain Research* 71:327–35.
5. Eccles, J. C. 1973. *The Understanding of the Brain*. New York: McGraw-Hill.
6. Fox, S. I. 1987. *Human Physiology*. Dubuque, Ia.: Wm. C. Brown.
7. Goodwin, G., D. McCloskey, and P. Mathews. 1972. The contribution of muscle afferents to kinesthesia shown by vibration-induced illusions of movement and by the effects of paralyzing joint afferents. *Brain* 95:705–48.
8. Henatsch, H., and H. Langer. Basic neurophysiology of motor skills in sport: a review (1985). *International Journal of Sports Medicine* 6:2–14.
9. Hoffman, B., and R. Lefkowitz. 1980. Alpha and beta receptor subtypes. *New England Journal of Medicine* 302:1390.
10. Hole, J. W. 1984. *Human Anatomy and Physiology*. Dubuque, Ia.: Wm. C. Brown.

11. Kandel, E., and J. Schwartz, eds. 1981. *Principles of Neuroscience.* New York: Elsevier-North Holland Pub. Co.

12. Krieger, D. T., and J. B. Martin. 1981. Brain peptides. *New England Journal of Medicine* 304:876.

13. Mathews, P. 1977. Muscle afferents and kinesthesia. *British Medical Bulletin* 33:137–42.

14. ———. 1982. Where does Sherrington's muscle sense originate? *Annual Review of Neuroscience* 5:189–218.

15. O'Donovan, M. 1985. Developmental regulation of motor function. *Medicine and Science in Sports and Exercise* 17:35–43.

16. Redman, S. 1986. Monosynaptic transmission in the spinal cord. *News in Physiological Sciences* 1:171–74.

17. Sage, G. H. 1984. *Motor Learning and Control: A Neuropsychological Approach.* Dubuque, Ia.: Wm. C. Brown.

18. Stjarne, L. 1986. New paradigm: sympathetic neurotransmission by lateral interaction between secretory units? *News in Physiological Sciences* 1:103–6.

19. Smith, J. C., J. Feldman, and B. Schmidt. 1988. Neural mechanisms generating locomotion studied in mammalian brain stem–spinal cord in vitro. *FASEB Journal* 2:2283–88.

20. Snyder, S. H. 1980. Brain peptides as neurotransmitters. *Science* 209:976.

21. Van De Graaff, K. 1984. *Human Anatomy.* Dubuque, Ia.: Wm. C. Brown.

8 Skeletal Muscle: Structure and Function

Objectives

*B*y studying this chapter, you should be able to do the following:
1. Draw and label the microstructure of skeletal muscle.
2. Outline the steps leading to muscle contraction.
3. Define the terms isotonic and isometric.
4. Discuss the following terms: (1) simple twitch, (2) summation, and (3) tetanus.
5. Discuss the major biochemical and mechanical properties of the three human skeletal fiber types.
6. Discuss the relationship between skeletal muscle fiber types and performance.
7. List and discuss those factors that regulate the amount of force exerted during muscular contraction.
8. Graph the relationship between movement velocity and the amount of force exerted during muscular contraction.
9. Discuss the structure and function of a muscle spindle.
10. Describe the function of a Golgi tendon organ.

Outline

Key Terms

actin
ATPase
dynamic
end-plate potential
endomysium
epimysium
extensors
fasciculi
fast-twitch fibers
flexors
Golgi tendon organs (GTOs)
intermediate fibers
isometric
isotonic
motor neurons
motor unit
muscle spindle

myofibrils
myosin
neuromuscular junction
perimysium
sarcolemma
sarcomeres
sarcoplasmic reticulum
sliding filament theory
slow-twitch fibers
static
summation
terminal cisternae
tetanus
tonus
transverse tubules
tropomyosin
troponin
twitch

The human body contains over 400 voluntary skeletal muscles, which comprise between 40%–50% of the total body weight (16, 20, 23). Skeletal muscle performs three important functions: (1) force generation for movement, (2) force generation for postural support, and (3) heat production during periods of cold stress. The most obvious function of skeletal muscle is to enable an individual to move freely. Skeletal muscles are attached to bones by tough connective tissue called tendons. One end of the muscle is attached to a bone that does not move (origin), while the opposite end is fixed to a bone (insertion) that is moved during muscular contraction. A wide variety of different skeletal muscle movements are possible, depending on the type of joint and muscles involved. Muscles that decrease joint angles are called **flexors,** while muscles that increase joint angles are called **extensors.**

Given the role of skeletal muscles in determining sports performance, a thorough understanding of muscle structure and function is important to the physical educator, physical therapist, and sports scientist. It is the purpose of this chapter to discuss the structure and function of skeletal muscle.

Structure of Skeletal Muscle

Skeletal muscle is composed of several kinds of tissue. These include muscle cells themselves, nerve tissue, blood, and various types of connective tissue. Figure 8.1 displays the relationship between muscle and the various connective tissues. Individual muscles are separated from each other and held in position by several layers of connective tissue called fascia. In addition to fascia, there are three separate layers of connective

Figure 8.1 Connective tissue surrounding skeletal muscle.

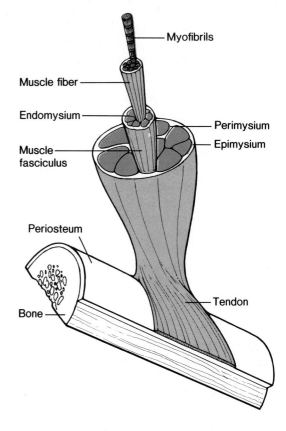

tissue found in skeletal muscle. The layer of connective tissue that closely surrounds skeletal muscle (located between the fascia and the muscle itself) is called the **epimysium.** As we move inward from the epimysium, connective tissue called the **perimysium** surrounds individual bundles of muscle fibers. These

Figure 8.2 The microstructure of muscle. Note that a skeletal muscle fiber contains numerous myofibrils, each consisting of units called sarcomeres.

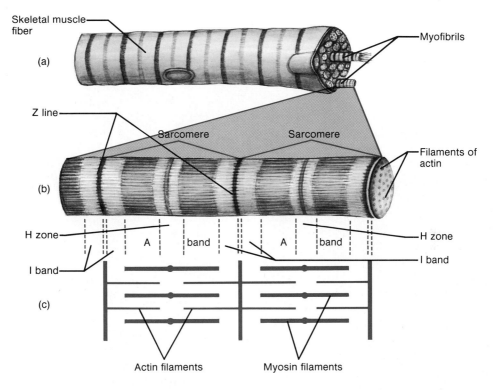

individual compartments of muscle cells are called **fasciculi.** Each muscle fiber within the fasciculus is surrounded by connective tissue called the **endomysium.**

Despite their unique shape, muscle cells have the same organelles that are present in other cells. That is, they contain mitochondria, lysosomes, etc. However, unlike most other cells in the body, muscle cells are multinucleated (i.e., many nuclei). One of the most distinctive features of the microscopic appearance of skeletal muscles is their striated appearance (see figure 8.2). These stripes are produced by alternating light and dark bands that appear across the length of the fiber.

Each individual muscle cell or fiber is a thin, elongated cylinder that generally extends the length of the muscle. The cell membrane in muscle is called the **sarcolemma.** Beneath the sarcolemma lies the sarcoplasm, which contains the cellular proteins, organelles, and myofibrils. **Myofibrils** are numerous threadlike structures that contain the contractile proteins (figure 8.2). In general, myofibrils contain two principal types of protein filaments: (1) thick filaments composed of the protein **myosin,** and (2) thin filaments composed of the protein **actin.** It is the arrangement of these two protein filaments that give skeletal muscle its striated appearance (figure 8.2). Located on the actin molecule itself are two additional types of protein, **troponin** and **tropomyosin.** These proteins make up a small portion of the muscle, but play an important role in regulation of the contractile process.

Figure 8.3 Within the sarcoplasm of muscle is a network of channels called the sarcoplasmic reticulum and the transverse tubules.

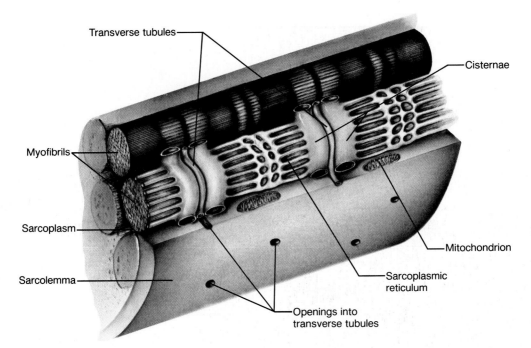

Myofibrils can be further subdivided into individual segments called **sarcomeres.** Sarcomeres are divided from each other by a thin sheet of connective tissue called a "Z line." Myosin filaments are located primarily within the dark portion of the sarcomere, which is called the "A band," while actin filaments occur principally in the lighter region of the sarcomere called "I bands" (figure 8.2). Note however, that the actin filaments overlap the myosin filaments and therefore are also found in the A band. In the center of the sarcomere there is a portion of the myosin filament with no overlap of the actin. This is the "H" zone.

Within the sarcoplasm of muscle is a network of membranous channels that surround each myofibril and run parallel with it. These channels are called the **sarcoplasmic reticulum** and are storage sites for calcium, which plays an important role in muscular contraction (see figure 8.3). Another set of membranous channels called the **transverse tubules** extend inward

from the sarcolemma and pass completely through the fiber. These transverse tubules pass between two enlarged portions of the sarcoplasmic reticulum called the **terminal cisternae.** All of these parts serve a function in muscular contraction and will be discussed in further detail later in this chapter.

Neuromuscular Junction

Each skeletal muscle fiber is connected to a fiber coming from a nerve cell. These nerve cells are called **motor neurons** and extend outward from the spinal cord. The motor neuron and all the muscle fibers it innervates is called a **motor unit.** Stimulation from motor neurons initiate the contraction process. The site where the motor neuron and muscle cell meet is called the **neuromuscular junction.** At this junction the sarcolemma forms a pocket that is called the "motor end plate" (see figure 8.4).

Figure 8.4 The connecting point between a motor neuron and a single muscle fiber is called the neuromuscular junction. The neurotransmitter acetylcholine is stored in synaptic vesicles at the end of the nerve fiber.

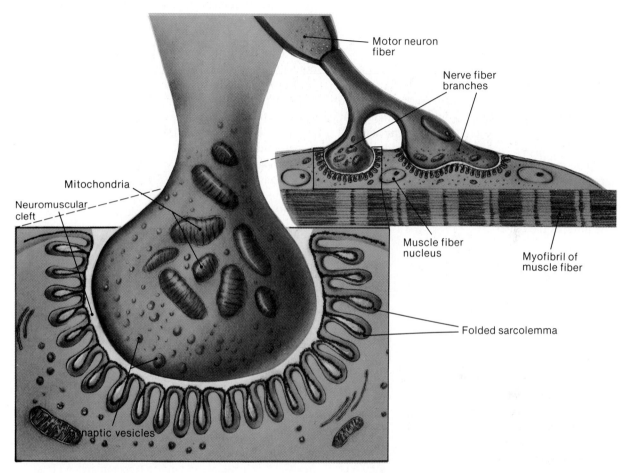

The end of the motor neuron does not physically make contact with the muscle fiber, but is separated by a short gap called the neuromuscular cleft. When a nerve impulse reaches the end of the motor nerve, the neurotransmitter acetylcholine is released and diffuses across the synaptic cleft to bind with receptor sites on the motor end plate. This causes an increase in the permeability of the sarcolemma to sodium, resulting in a depolarization called the **end-plate potential (EPP)**. The EPP is always large enough to exceed threshold, and the contractile process has begun.

Muscular Contraction

Muscular contraction is a complex process involving a number of cellular proteins and energy production systems. The final result is a sliding of actin over myosin, which causes the muscle to shorten and therefore develop tension. Although complete details of muscular contraction at the molecular level are not available, much is known about "how muscles contract." The process of muscular contraction is best explained by the **sliding filament theory** of contraction, and is discussed in the next several paragraphs (11, 24).

Overview of the Sliding Filament Theory

The step-by-step process of muscular contraction is illustrated in figure 8.5. Muscle fibers contract by a shortening of their myofibrils, which results in a reduction of distance from Z line to Z line. As the sarcomeres shorten in length, the A bands do not shorten but move closer together. However, note that the I bands do decrease in length. What causes the actin and myosin filaments to slide across each other during muscular contraction? Filament sliding occurs due to the action of the numerous cross-bridges extending out as "arms" from myosin and attaching on the actin filament. The "head" of the myosin cross-bridge is oriented in opposite directions on either end of the sarcomere (see figure 8.6). This orientation of cross-bridges is such that when they attach to actin on each side of the sarcomere they can pull the actin from each side towards the center.

Energy for Contraction

The energy for contraction comes from the breakdown of ATP by the enzyme **ATPase** (18, 21, 24). The bioenergetic pathways responsible for synthesis of ATP were discussed earlier in chapter 3. The breakdown of ATP to ADP $+$ Pi and the release of energy serves to energize the myosin cross-bridges. The ATP-released energy is used "to cock" the myosin cross-bridges, which in turn pull the actin molecules over myosin and thus shortens the muscle.

Note that a single contraction cycle or "power stroke" of all the cross-bridges in a muscle would shorten the muscle by only 1 percent of its resting length (11). Since muscles can shorten up to 60% of their resting length, it is clear that the contraction cycle must be repeated over and over again (11). In order for this to occur, the cross-bridges must detach from actin after each power stroke, resume their original position and then reattach to actin for another power stroke.

Regulation of Contraction

Relaxed muscles are easily stretched which demonstrates that at rest, actin and myosin are not attached. What regulates the interaction of actin and myosin and thus regulates muscle contraction? The regulation of contraction is a function of two regulatory proteins, troponin and tropomyosin, which are located on the actin molecule. The actin filament is formed from many smaller protein subunits arranged in a double row and twisted (figure 8.6a). Tropomyosin is a thin molecule that lies in a groove between the double row of actin. Attached directly to the tropomyosin is another type of protein, called troponin. Troponin and tropomyosin work together to regulate the attachment of the actin and myosin cross-bridges.

In a relaxed muscle, tropomyosin blocks the "active sites" on the actin molecule where the myosin cross-bridges must attach in order for contraction to occur. The "trigger" for contraction to occur is linked to the release of stored calcium (Ca^{++}) from the sarcoplasmic reticulum. Most of this Ca^{++} is stored within expanded portions of the sarcoplasmic reticulum known as the "terminal cisternae." In a relaxed muscle the concentration of Ca^{++} in the sarcoplasm is very low. However, when a nerve impulse arrives at the neuromuscular junction it travels down the transverse tubules to the sarcoplasmic reticulum and causes a release of Ca^{++}. Some of this Ca^{++} binds to troponin, which causes a position change in tropomyosin such that the "active sites" on the actin are uncovered (figure 8.6b and c). The energy released from the breakdown of ATP "cocks" the myosin cross-bridges. This energized cross-bridge then attaches to the active sites on actin and contraction occurs. Attachment of "fresh" ATP to the myosin cross-bridges allows the cross-bridge to detach and reattach to another active site on an actin molecule. This contraction cycle is repeated as long as free Ca^{++} is available to bind to troponin and ATP is available to provide the energy. The signal to stop contraction is the absence of the nerve impulse at the neuromuscular junction. When this occurs, an energy-requiring "Ca^{++} pump" located within the sarcoplasmic reticulum begins to move Ca^{++} back into the sarcoplasmic reticulum. This removal of Ca^{++} from troponin causes tropomyosin to move back to cover the binding sites on the actin molecule and cross-bridge interaction ceases.

Table 8.1 contains a step-by-step summary of the events that occur during muscular contraction. This process is often referred to as "excitation-contraction

Figure 8.5 The sliding filament theory of contraction. As contraction occurs, the Z lines are brought closer together. The A bands remain the same length, but the I and H bands get progressively narrower as shortening continues.

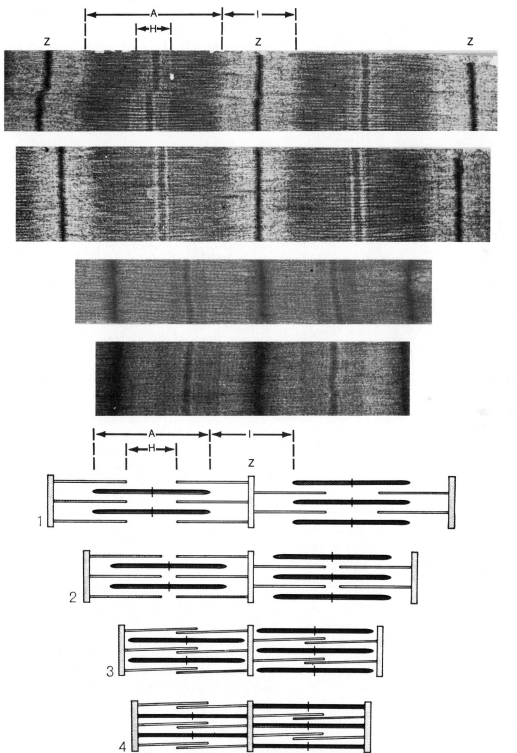

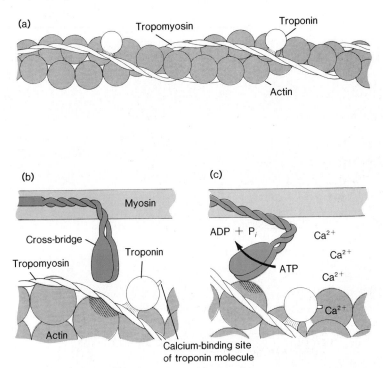

Figure 8.6 Proposed relationships between troponin, tropomyosin, myosin cross-bridges, and calcium. Note that when Ca⁺⁺ binds to troponin, tropomyosin is removed from the active sites on actin and cross-bridge attachment can occur.

coupling." Time spent learning the microstructure of muscle and the events that lead to contraction will pay dividends later as this material is important to a thorough understanding of exercise physiology.

Isometric and Isotonic Contractions

It is possible for skeletal muscle to exert force without the joint angle changing. This might occur when an individual pushes against the wall of a building (see figure 8.7). What happens here is that muscle tension increases but the wall does not move and therefore neither does the body part (e.g., arm) that applies the force. Contractions of this type are called **isometric** or **static.** Isometric contractions are common in the postural muscles of the body, which act to maintain a static body position during periods of standing or sitting.

In contrast, most types of exercise or sports skills involve contractions that result in movement of body parts. In this case, as in an isometric contraction, tension within the muscle increases but the joint angle changes as the body parts move. This type of contraction is termed **isotonic** or **dynamic** and is illustrated in figure 8.7.

The Simple Twitch

If a muscle is given a single stimulus, such as a brief electrical shock applied to the nerve innervating it, the muscle responds with a simple **twitch.** The movement of the muscle can be recorded on a special recording device and the time periods for contraction and relaxation studied. Figure 8.8 demonstrates the time course of a simple twitch. Notice that the twitch can be divided into three phases. First, immediately after the

Figure 8.7 (*a*) Isotonic contractions occur when a muscle contracts and shortens. (*b*) Isometric contractions occur when a muscle exerts force but does not shorten.

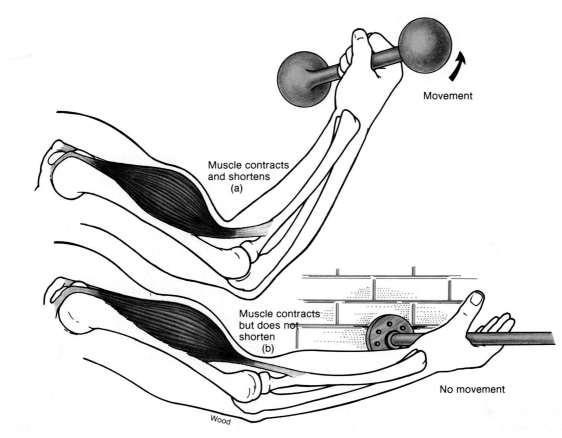

Movement

Muscle contracts and shortens (a)

Muscle contracts but does not shorten (b)

No movement

Wood

Figure 8.8 A recording of a simple twitch. Note the three time periods (latent period, contraction, and relaxation) following the stimulus.

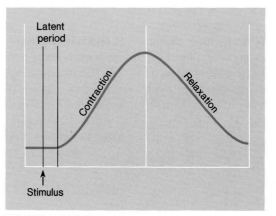

Latent period

Contraction

Relaxation

Stimulus

stimulus, there is a brief latent period (i.e., 0.005 second) prior to the beginning of muscle shortening. The second phase of the twitch is the contraction phase, which lasts approximately 0.04 sec. Finally, the muscle returns to its original length during the relaxation period, which lasts about 0.05 second and thus is the longest of the three phases.

The timing of the phases in a simple twitch varies among muscle fiber types (fiber types are discussed in the next section) and the force of contraction varies as well. This variability arises from differences in the responses of the individual fiber types that make up muscles. Individual muscle fibers behave much like individual neurons in that they exhibit all-or-none responses to stimulation. To contract, an individual muscle fiber must receive an appropriate amount of stimulation. However, fast-twitch fibers exert more force and contract in a shorter time period when stimulated than do slow-twitch fibers. Intermediate fibers exert a force that is somewhere between the force exhibited by fast- and slow-twitch fibers. The explanation for these observations is related to the fact that fast-twitch fibers contain more myofibrils and release Ca^{++} at a faster rate than do slow-twitch fibers (13, 15).

Fiber Types

Human skeletal muscle can generally be divided into three different types of fibers. These classifications are based on biochemical and performance characteristics of the individual muscle cells. Although some confusion exists concerning the nomenclature of fiber types, these three groups are often referred to as fast-twitch, intermediate, and slow-twitch fibers (7, 8, 12). Albeit some muscle groups are known to be composed of predominantly fast- or slow-twitch fibers, most muscle groups in the body contain a mixture of all three fiber types. The percentage of the respective fiber types contained in skeletal muscles is genetically determined and may play an important role in performance in both power and endurance events (10, 33).

Table 8.1 Summary of events that occur during the contractile process

1. Action potential in a motor neuron causes the release of acetylcholine into the synaptic cleft of the neuromuscular junction.
2. Acetylcholine binds with receptors on the motor endplate, producing an end-plate potential that exceeds threshold and leads to action potentials that are conducted down the transverse tubules deep into the muscle fiber.
3. When the action potential reaches the sarcoplasmic reticulum, Ca^{++} is released into the sarcoplasm. The Ca^{++} then binds to troponin, which causes a shift in the position of tropomyosin to uncover the "active sites" on the actin.
4. ATP is broken down to ADP + Pi + energy and the released energy is used to "cock" the myosin cross-bridge.
5. The "cocked" myosin cross-bridge attaches to the active site on actin and pulls the actin molecule over the myosin.
6. Attachment of "fresh" ATP to the myosin cross-bridges allows the cross-bridge to detach from actin and the contraction cycle is repeated as long as Ca^{++} is present.
7. When action potentials stop, the sarcoplasmic reticulum actively removes Ca^{++} from the sarcoplasm and tropomyosin again moves to its inhibitory position covering the active sites on the actin molecules.

Biochemical Characteristics of Skeletal Muscle

Fast-Twitch Fibers

Fast-twitch fibers (also called fast-glycolytic (FG) or Type IIb fibers) have a relatively small number of mitochondria, a limited capacity for aerobic metabolism, and are less resistant to fatigue than slow-twitch fibers (19, 30). However, fast-twitch fibers are rich in glycogen stores and glycolytic enzymes, which provide

Figure 8.9 Comparison of the rates with which maximum tension is developed in three different muscles. Muscle A is composed of fast-twitch fibers, muscle B is primarily composed of intermediate fibers, and muscle C is composed of slow-twitch fibers.

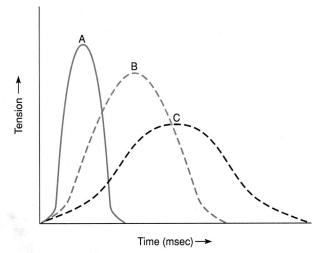

them with a large anaerobic capacity (28). In addition, fast-twitch fibers contain more myofibrils and ATPase than slow-twitch fibers, and are therefore able to contract more rapidly and develop more force than the slow-twitch fibers. The speed of contraction differences between slow- and fast-twitch fibers is illustrated in figure 8.9.

Slow-Twitch Fibers

Slow-twitch fibers (also called slow-oxidative (SO) or Type I fibers) contain larger numbers of mitochondria and are surrounded by more capillaries than fast-twitch fibers. In addition, slow-twitch fibers contain higher concentrations of the red pigment myoglobin than fast-twitch fibers. Myoglobin is similar to hemoglobin in the blood in that it binds O_2, but it also acts as a "shuttle" mechanism for O_2 between the cell membrane and the mitochondria. The high concentration of myoglobin, the large number of capillaries, and the high content of mitochondrial enzymes provide slow-twitch fibers with a high capacity for aerobic metabolism and a high resistance to fatigue.

Interestingly, the rate at which action potentials are conducted along the motor neurons that innervate slow-twitch fibers is slower than that of fast-twitch fibers. For example, the action potential conduction rate of motor neurons innervating fast-twitch fibers is 80–90 meters/second, while the conduction rate for slow-twitch fibers is only 60–70 meters/second (28). In fact, it is the motor neuron that determines the characteristic of the muscle fiber at the other end. When motor nerves innervating fast-twitch fibers and slow-twitch fibers are experimentally switched, the two muscle fiber types begin to reverse characteristics (28). That is, the fast-twitch fibers become slow-twitch fibers and the slow-twitch fibers become fast-twitch fibers. Therefore, all of the muscle fibers that are innervated by the same motor neuron (motor unit) are of the same type.

Table 8.2 *Characteristics of human skeletal muscle fiber types*

	Slow (Type I)	Intermediate (Type IIa)	Fast (Type IIb)
Diameter	Small	Intermediate	Large
Z-line thickness	Wide	Intermediate	Narrow
Glycogen content	Low	Intermediate	High
Resistance to fatigue	High	Intermediate	Low
Capillaries	Many	Many	Few
Myoglobin content	High	High	Low
Twitch rate	Slow	Fast	Fast
ATPase activity	Low	High	High
Predominant energy system	Aerobic	Combination	Anaerobic

Table 8.3 *Typical muscle fiber composition in elite athletes representing different sports and nonathletes*

Sport	% Slow-Twitch Fibers	% Fast-Twitch Fibers
Distance running	60–90	10–40
Track sprinters	25–45	55–75
Weight lifting	45–55	45–55
Shot putters	25–40	60–75
Nonathletes	47–53	47–53

Data from references 32, 35, and 36.

Intermediate Fibers

The final classification of fiber types is referred to as **intermediate fibers** (also called fast oxidative glycolytic (FOG) or Type IIa fibers). As the name implies, these fibers contain biochemical and fatigue characteristics that are somewhere between fast-twitch and slow-twitch fibers. Conceptually, intermediate fibers are often thought to be a mixture of both slow- and fast-twitch fiber characteristics. However, it appears likely that intermediate fibers are not a single fiber type per se, but represent a continuum between fast-twitch and slow-twitch fibers. The general characteristics of slow-twitch, fast-twitch, and intermediate fibers are summarized in table 8.2.

Fiber Types and Performance

Descriptive studies have demonstrated several interesting facts concerning the percentages of fast and slow-twitch muscle fibers found in humans. First, there are no apparent sex or age differences in fiber distribution (28). Secondly, the average sedentary man or woman possesses approximately 45%–55% slow-twitch fibers. Thirdly, it is commonly believed that successful power athletes (e.g., sprinters, fullbacks, etc.) possess a large percentage of fast-twitch fibers, whereas endurance athletes generally are shown to have a high percentage of slow-twitch fibers (35). Table 8.3 presents some examples of the percentage of slow-twitch fibers found in successful athletes.

Box 8.1 How Are Skeletal Muscle Fibers Typed?

The relative percentage of fast-twitch, slow-twitch, or intermediate fibers contained in a particular muscle can be estimated by removing a small piece of muscle (via a procedure called a biopsy) and performing histochemical staining of the individual muscle cells. Although several techniques exist, one of the most common procedures is to apply a stain that darkens muscle cells, which contain high concentrations of the enzyme ATPase. Since fast-twitch fibers contain large quantities of active ATPase, these fibers become dark, while slow-twitch fibers remain light in color. The shade of intermediate fibers tends to fall somewhere between the fast- and slow-twitch fibers. Hence, this technique provides a means of determining all three fiber types at the same time. Figure 8.10 is an example of a muscle cross section after histochemical staining showing fast-twitch, intermediate, and slow-twitch fibers.

One of the inherent problems with fiber typing in humans is that a muscle biopsy is usually only performed on one muscle group. Therefore, a single sample from one muscle may not be representative of the entire body. A further complication is that fiber types tend to be layered within muscle and thus a small sample of muscle taken from a single area of the muscle may not be truly representative of the total fiber population of the muscle biopsied (1, 34). Therefore, it is difficult to make a definitive statement concerning the whole body percentage of a particular fiber type based on the staining of a single muscle biopsy.

Figure 8.10 Histochemical staining of a cross-sectional area of muscle. The darker cells are fast-twitch fibers and the lightest-colored cells are slow-twitch fibers. Intermediate fibers are the cells with the gray appearance.

© Hans Hoppler, *Respiratory Physiology*, Volume 44, p. 94, 1981.

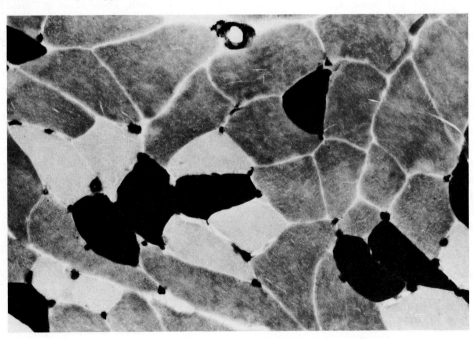

It is clear from table 8.3 that considerable variation in the percentage of various fiber types exists even among successful athletes competing in the same event or sport. In other words, two equally successful 10,000 meter runners might differ in the percentage of slow-twitch fibers that each possesses. For example, runner A might be found to possess 70% slow-twitch fibers, while runner B might contain 85% slow-twitch fibers. This observation demonstrates that an individual's muscle fiber composition is not the only variable that determines success in athletic events. In fact, it is generally believed that success in athletic performance is due to a complex interaction of psychological, biochemical, neurological, cardiopulmonary, and biomechanical factors (5, 6, 27).

Can specific types of training change a fast-twitch fiber to a slow-twitch fiber? The answer to this question is apparently no. Numerous researchers have studied this question and concluded that endurance training does not result in a complete conversion of fast-twitch fibers to slow-twitch fibers (3, 4, 14, 17, 22, 25, 27). However, endurance training does result in a marked improvement of the oxidative capacity of the three fiber types (4, 28, 29, 30). Conversely, training for increased strength and power results in an improvement of the anaerobic capacity of fast-twitch and intermediate fibers (35). Research continues in this area to determine the extent that training can alter the biochemical properties of skeletal muscle.

Force Regulation in Muscle

The amount of force exerted during muscular contraction is dependent on a number of factors. These include the types and number of motor units recruited, the initial length of the muscle, and nature of the neural stimulation of the motor units (2, 8, 9, 15). First, variations in the strength of contraction within an entire muscle depends on the number of muscle fibers that are stimulated to contract (i.e., recruited). If only a few motor units are recruited, the force is small. If more motor units are stimulated the force is increased. Figure 8.11 illustrates this point. Note that as the stimulus is increased, the force of contraction is increased due to the recruitment of additional motor units.

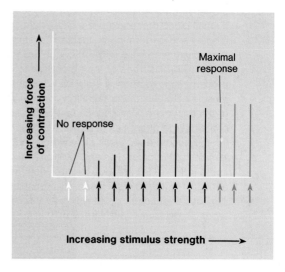

Figure 8.11 The relationship between increasing stimulus strength and the force of contraction. Weak stimuli do not activate many motor units and do not produce great force. In contrast, increasing the stimulus strength recruits more and more motor units and thus produces more force.

A second factor that determines the force exerted by a muscle is the initial length of the muscle at the time of contraction. There exists an "ideal" length of the muscle fiber. The explanation for the existence of an ideal length is related to the overlap between actin and myosin. For instance, when the resting length is longer than optimal, the overlap between actin and myosin is limited and few cross-bridges can attach. This concept is illustrated in figure 8.12. Note that when the muscle is stretched to the point where there is no overlap of actin and myosin, cross-bridges cannot attach and thus tension cannot be developed. At the other extreme, when the muscle is shortened to about 60% of its resting length, the Z lines are very close to the thick myosin filaments, and thus only limited additional shortening can occur.

A final factor that can affect the amount of force a muscle exerts upon contraction is the nature of the neural stimulation. Simple muscle twitches studied under experimental conditions reveal some interesting fundamental properties about how muscles function. However, normal body movements involve sustained

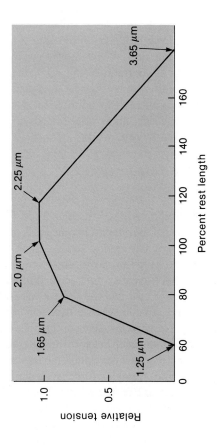

Figure 8.12 Length-tension relationships in skeletal muscle. Note that an optimal length of muscle exists, which will produce maximal force when stimulated. Lengths that are above or below this optimal length result in a reduced amount of force when stimulated.

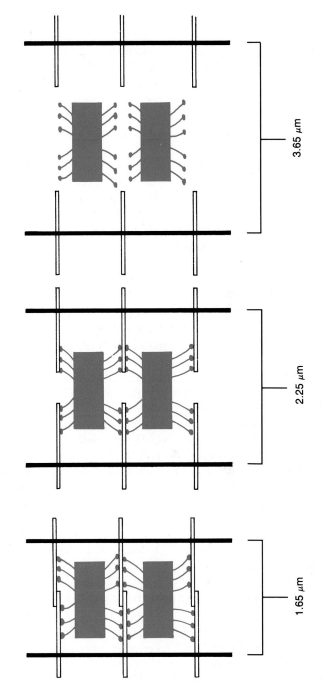

Figure 8.13 Recording showing the change from simple twitches to summation, and finally tetanus. Peaks to the left represent simple twitches, while increasing the frequency of the stimulus results in summation of the twitches, and finally tetanus.

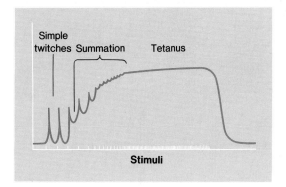

contractions that are not simple twitches. The sustained contractions involved in normal body movements can be closely replicated in the laboratory if a series of stimulations are applied to the muscle. The recording pictured in figure 8.13 represents what occurs when successive stimuli are applied to the muscle. (The first few contractions represent simple twitches.) Note that as the frequency of stimulations is increased, the muscle does not have time to relax between stimuli and the force appears to be additive. This response is called **summation** (addition of successive twitches). If the frequency of stimuli is increased further, individual contractions are blended together in a single sustained contraction called **tetanus.** A tetanic contraction will continue until the stimuli is stopped or the muscle fatigues.

Muscular contractions that occur during normal body movements appear to be tetanic contractions. These sustained contractions result from a series of rapidly repeated neural impulses conducted by the motor neurons that innervate those motor units involved in the movement. It is important to appreciate that in the body neural impulses to various motor units do not arrive at the same time as they do in the laboratory-induced tetanic contraction. Instead, various motor units are stimulated to contract at different times. Thus, some motor units are contracting while some are relaxing. This type of tetanic contraction results in a smooth contraction and aids in sustaining a coordinated muscle contraction.

Another important point is that skeletal muscles are never completely relaxed. That is, a small amount of neural activity to muscle normally exists even during periods of no movement, which results in a condition of sustained slight contraction. This minimal amount of neural activity to muscles is called **tonus.** Muscle tonus is maintained throughout life as long as the nerve supply to the muscle is intact. Tonus involves alternating periods of contraction and relaxation in different motor units within a muscle. The maintenance of tonus requires energy expenditure, but does not fatigue the muscle since these brief periods of contraction are followed by rest.

Force-Velocity/Power-Velocity Relationships

In most physical activities, muscular force is applied through a range of movement. For instance, an athlete throwing the shot put applies force against the shot over a specified range of movement prior to release. How far the shot travels is a function of both the speed of the shot upon release and the angle of release. Since success in many athletic events is dependent on speed, it is important to appreciate some of the basic concepts underlying the relationship between muscular force and the speed of movement. The relationship between speed of movement and muscular force is shown in figure 8.14. Two important points emerge from an examination of figure 8.14.

1. At any given velocity of movement, the peak force exerted is greater in muscles that contain a high percentage of fast-twitch fibers when compared to muscle that possess predominantly slow-twitch fibers. Further, at any given force of contraction, the speed of movement is greater in muscles that contain a high percentage of fast-twitch fibers when compared to muscle with slow-twitch fibers.

2. The peak force generated by muscle decreases as the speed of movement increases. Simply stated, the greatest amount of force is

Figure 8.14 Muscle force-velocity relationships. Note that at any given speed of movement, muscle groups with a high percentage of fast-twitch (FT) fibers exert more *force* than those with muscle groups that contain primarily slow-twitch (ST) fibers.

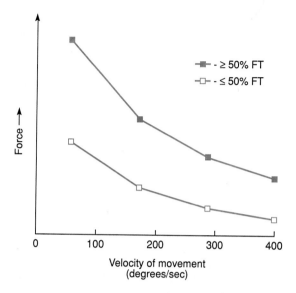

generated at the slowest speeds of movement. This principle holds true for both slow- and fast-twitch fibers.

The data contained in figure 8.14 also demonstrate that fast-twitch fibers are capable of producing greater peak muscular force at a faster speed than slow-twitch fibers. The biochemical mechanism to explain this observation is related to the fact that fast-twitch fibers contain higher quantities of active ATPase than do slow-twitch fibers (13, 15). Therefore, ATP is broken down more rapidly in fast-twitch fibers when compared to slow-twitch fibers. Further, calcium release from the sarcoplasmic reticulum is faster following neural stimulation in fast-twitch fibers when compared to slow-twitch fibers (15, 31).

The above discussion has practical importance for the coach, athlete, or physical educator. The message is simply that athletes that possess a high percentage of fast-twitch fibers would seem to have an advantage in power-type athletic events. This may explain why successful sprinters and weight lifters typically possess a relatively high percentage of fast-twitch fibers.

As might be expected, the fiber-type distribution in muscle influences the power-velocity curve (see figure 8.15). The peak power that can be generated by muscle is greater in muscle that contains a high percentage of fast-twitch fibers when compared with muscle that is largely comprised of slow-twitch fibers. Similar to the force-velocity curve, two important points should be retained from examination of the power-velocity curve:

1. At any given velocity of movement, the peak power generated is greater in muscle that contains a high percentage of fast-twitch fibers when compared to muscle with a high percentage of slow-twitch fibers. This difference is due to the aforementioned biochemical differences between fast- and slow-twitch fibers. Again, athletes who possess a high percentage of fast-twitch fibers can generate more power than athletes with predominantly slow-twitch fibers.

2. The peak power generated by any muscle increases with increasing velocities of movement up to a movement speed of 200–400 degrees/second. The reason for the plateau of power output with increasing movement speed is because muscular force decreases with increasing speed of movement (see figure 8.14). Therefore, with any given muscle group there is an optimum speed of movement that will elicit the greatest power output.

Receptors in Muscle

Skeletal muscle contains several types of sensory receptors. These include chemoreceptors, muscle spindles, and Golgi tendon organs. Chemoreceptors are specialized free nerve endings that send information to the central nervous system in response to changes in muscle pH, concentrations of extracellular potassium, and changes in O_2 and CO_2 tensions. Chemoreceptors may play a role in cardiopulmonary regulation during exercise and will be discussed in more detail in chapters 9 and 10.

Figure 8.15 Muscle power-velocity relationships. In general, the power produced by a muscle group increases as a function of velocity of movement. At any given speed of movement, muscles that contain a large percentage of fast-twitch (FT) fibers produce more *power* than those muscles that contain primarily slow-twitch (ST) fibers.

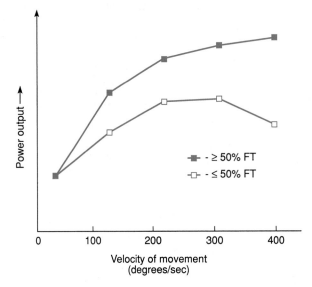

In order for the nervous system to properly control skeletal muscle movements it must receive continuous sensory feedback from the contracting muscle. This sensory feedback includes (1) information concerning the tension developed by a muscle and (2) an account of the muscle length. **Golgi tendon organs** provide the central nervous system with feedback concerning the tension developed by the muscle, while the **muscle spindle** provides sensory information concerning the relative muscle length. A discussion of each sensory organ follows.

Muscle Spindle

As previously stated, the muscle spindle functions as a length detector. Muscles that require the finest degree of control, such as the muscles of the hands, have the highest density of spindles. In contrast, muscles that are responsible for gross movements (e.g., quadriceps) contain relatively few spindles.

The muscle spindle is composed of several thin muscle cells (intrafusal fibers), which are surrounded by a connective tissue sheath. Like normal muscle fibers (called extrafusal fibers), muscle spindles insert into tendons on each end of the muscle. Therefore, muscle spindles run parallel with muscle fibers (see figure 8.16).

Muscle spindles contain two types of sensory nerve endings. The primary or annulospiral endings are located in the central region of the spindle and respond to dynamic changes in muscle length (figure 8.16). The second type of sensory endings is called the secondary or flower spray ending and is located near the end of the spindle. These sensory endings do not respond to rapid changes in muscle length, but provide the central nervous system with continuous information concerning static muscle length.

In addition to the sensory neurons, muscle spindles are innervated by gamma motor neurons, which stimulate the intrafusal fibers to contract simultaneously along with extrafusal fibers. Gamma motor neuron stimulation causes the central region of the intrafusal fibers to shorten, which serves to tighten the spindle. The need for contraction of the intrafusal fibers can be explained as follows. When skeletal muscles are shortened by motor-neuron stimulation, muscle spindles are passively shortened along with the skeletal

Figure 8.16 The structure of muscle spindles and their location in skeletal muscle.

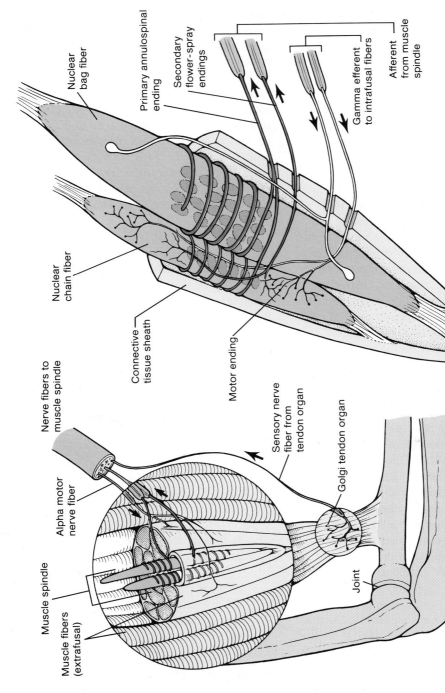

Nuclear bag fiber

Primary annulospinal ending

Secondary flower-spray endings

Gamma efferent to intrafusal fibers

Afferent from muscle spindle

Muscle spindle

Nuclear chain fiber

Connective tissue sheath

Motor ending

Nerve fibers to muscle spindle

Alpha motor nerve fiber

Sensory nerve fiber from tendon organ

Golgi tendon organ

Muscle spindle

Muscle fibers (extrafusal)

Joint

muscle fibers. If the intrafusal fibers did not compensate accordingly, this shortening would result in "slack" in the spindle and make them less sensitive. Therefore, their function as length detectors would be compromised.

Muscle spindles are responsible for the observation that rapid stretching of skeletal muscles results in a reflex contraction. This is called the stretch reflex and is present in all muscles, but is most dramatic in the extensor muscles of the limbs. The so-called "knee-jerk reflex" is often evaluated by the physician by tapping the patellar tendon with a rubber mallet. The blow by the mallet stretches the entire muscle and thus "excites" the primary nerve endings located in muscle spindles. The neural impulse from the muscle spindle synapses at the spinal cord level with a motor neuron, which then stimulates the extrafusal fibers of the extensor muscle, resulting in an isotonic contraction.

The functional importance of the muscle spindle is to assist in the regulation of movement and to maintain posture. This is accomplished by the muscle spindle's ability to detect and cause the central nervous system (CNS) to respond to changes in the length of skeletal muscle fibers. A practical example of how the muscle spindle assists in the control of movement can be appreciated by the following example. Suppose a student is holding a single book in front of him or her with the arm extended. This type of load poses a tonic stretch on the muscle spindle, which sends information to the CNS concerning the final length of the extrafusal muscle fibers. If a second book is suddenly placed upon the first book, the muscles would be suddenly stretched (arm would drop) and a burst of impulses from the muscle spindle would alert the CNS about the change in muscle length (and thus load). The ensuing reflex would recruit additional motor units to raise the arm back to the original position. Generally, this type of reflex action results in an overcompensation. That is, more motor units are recruited that are needed to bring the arm back to the original position. However, immediately following the overcompensation movement, an additional adjustment rapidly occurs and the arm is quickly returned to the original position.

Golgi Tendon Organs

The Golgi tendon organs (GTOs) continuously monitor tension produced by muscle contraction. Golgi tendon organs are located within the tendon and thus are in series with the extrafusal fibers (figure 8.17). In essence, GTOs serve as "safety devices" that help prevent excessive force during muscle contractions. When activated, GTOs send information to the spinal cord via sensory neurons, which in turn excite inhibitory neurons (i.e., send IPSPs). This inhibitory disynaptic reflex (i.e., two synapses are involved) helps prevent excessive muscle contractions and provides a finer control over skeletal movements. This process is pictured in figure 8.17.

It seems likely that GTOs play an important role in the performance of strength activities. For instance, the amount of force that can be produced by a muscle group may be dependent on the ability of the individual to voluntarily oppose the inhibition of the GTO. It seems possible that the inhibitory influences of the GTO could be gradually reduced in response to strength training (36). This would allow an individual to produce a greater amount of muscle force, and in many cases improve sport performance.

Summary

1. The human body contains over 400 voluntary skeletal muscles, which comprise between 40%–50% of the total body weight. Skeletal muscle performs three major functions: (1) motion, (2) postural support, and (3) heat production during cold stress.
2. Individual muscle fibers are composed of hundreds of threadlike protein filaments called myofibrils. Myofibrils contain two major types of protein: (1) actin—the thin filaments and (2) myosin—the thick filaments. It is the arrangement of actin and myosin that give skeletal muscle its striated appearance.
3. Motor neurons extend outward from the spinal cord and innervate individual muscle fibers. The site where the motor neuron and muscle cell meet is called the neuromuscular junction.

Figure 8.17 The Golgi tendon organ. The Golgi tendon organ is located in series with muscle and serves as a "tension monitor" which acts as a protective device for muscle. See text for details.

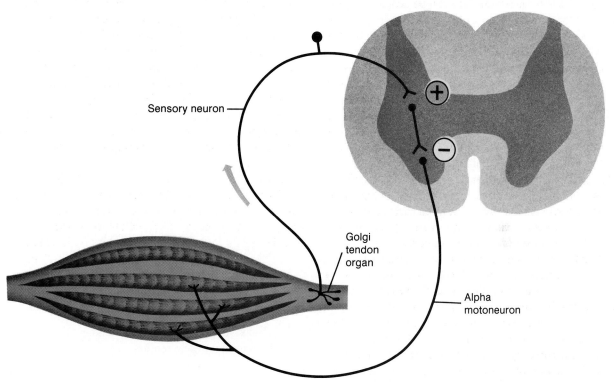

Sensory neuron

Golgi tendon organ

Alpha motoneuron

Acetylcholine is the neurotransmitter that stimulates the muscle fiber to depolarize, which is the signal to start the contractile process.

4. The sliding filament theory of contraction proposes that muscular shortening occurs by movement of the actin filament over the myosin filament. Muscular contraction is thought to occur in the following steps:

a. The nerve impulse travels down the transverse tubules and reaches the sarcoplasmic reticulum and Ca^{++} is released.

b. Ca^{++} binds to the protein troponin, which causes a position change in tropomyosin away from the "active sites"

on the actin molecule. The myosin cross-bridges then attach to the active sites on actin, which activates the enzyme ATPase. ATPase catalyzes the breakdown of ATP and the released energy is used to "cock" the myosin cross-bridges, which in turn pull the actin molecules over the myosin and thus shorten the muscle.

c. Muscular contraction occurs by multiple cycles of cross-bridge activity. Shortening will continue as long as energy is available and Ca^{++} is free to bind to troponin. When neural activity ceases at the neuromuscular junction, Ca^{++} is removed from the sarcoplasm and taken back into the sarcoplasmic reticulum by an energy-requiring process called the Ca^{++} pump.

5. Human skeletal muscle can be divided into three fiber types: (1) fast-twitch fibers, (2) intermediate fibers, and (3) slow-twitch fibers. Fast-twitch fibers are low in mitochondria, have a limited capacity for aerobic activity, but are well endowed with glycogen stores and ATPase. Further, fast-twitch fibers are not fatigue resistant, but have a large anaerobic capacity. In contrast, slow-twitch fibers are rich in mitochondria, are surrounded by capillaries, and contain a high capacity for aerobic activity. Intermediate fibers are thought to fall somewhere between fast- and slow-twitch fibers in their aerobic/anaerobic capacities.

6. The amount of force generated during muscular contraction is dependent on the following factors: (1) types and number of motor units recruited, (2) the initial muscle length, and (3) the nature of the motor units' neural stimulation.

7. The addition of muscle twitches is termed summation. When the frequency of neural stimulation to a motor unit is increased, individual contractions are fused together in a sustained contraction called tetanus.

8. The peak force generated by muscle decreases as the speed of movement increases. However, in general, the amount of power generated by a muscle group increases as a function of movement velocity.

9. The muscle spindle functions as a length detector in muscle. Golgi tendon organs continuously monitor the tension developed during muscular contraction. In essence, Golgi tendon organs serve as safety devices that help prevent excessive force during muscle contractions.

Study Questions

1. List the principal functions of skeletal muscles.
2. List the principal proteins contained in skeletal muscle.
3. Outline the contractile process. Use a step-by-step format illustrating the entire process, beginning with the nerve impulse reaching the neuromuscular junction.
4. Outline the mechanical and biochemical properties of human skeletal muscle fiber types.
5. Discuss those factors thought to be responsible for regulating force during muscular contractions.
6. Define the term summation.
7. Graph a simple muscle twitch and a contraction that results in tetanus.
8. Discuss the relationship between force and speed of movement during a muscular contraction.
9. Describe the general anatomical design of a muscle spindle and discuss its physiological function.
10. Discuss the function of Golgi tendon organs in monitoring muscle tension.

Suggested Readings

Armstrong, R., and H. Laughlin. 1985. Muscle function during locomotion in mammals. In (R. Giles, ed.) *Circulation, Respiration, and Metabolism,* 56–63. New York: Springer-Verlag.

Hole, J. 1987. *Human Anatomy and Physiology.* Dubuque, Ia.: Wm. C. Brown.

Hoppeler, H. 1986. Exercise-induced ultrastructure changes in skeletal muscle. *International Journal of Sports Medicine* 7:187–204.

Jones, N., N. McCartney, and A. McComas. 1986. *Human Muscle Power.* Champaign, Ill.: Human Kinetics Publishers.

Wilmore, J., and D. Costill. 1988. *Training for Sport and Activity.* Dubuque, Ia.: Wm. C. Brown.

References

1. Armstrong, R. et al. 1983. Differential inter- and intra-muscular responses to exercise: considerations in use of the biopsy technique. In (H. Knuttgen, J. Vogel, and J. Poormans, eds.) *Biochemistry of Exercise,* 775–80. Champaign, Ill.: Human Kinetics Publishers.

2. Armstrong, R., and H. Laughlin. 1985. Muscle function during locomotion in mammals. In (R. Giles, ed.) *Circulation, Respiration, and Metabolism,* 56–63. New York: Springer-Verlag.

3. Bagby, G., W. Sembrowich, and P. Gollnick. 1972. Myosin ATPase and fiber type composition from trained and untrained rat skeletal muscle. *Journal of Applied Physiology* 223:1415–17.

4. Baldwin, K. et al. 1972. Respiratory capacity of white, red, and intermediate muscle: Adaptive response to exercise. *Journal of Applied Physiology* 222:373–78.

5. Brooks, G., and T. Fahey. 1984. *Exercise Physiology: Human Bioenergetics and its Applications.* New York: John Wiley & Sons.

6. ———. 1987. *Fundamentals of Human Performance.* New York: John Wiley & Sons.

7. Buchthal, F., and H. Schmalbruch. 1970. Contraction times and fiber types in intact human muscle. *Acta Physiologica Scandanavica* 79:435–40.

8. Burke, R. 1986. The control of muscle force: Motor unit recruitment and firing pattern. In (N. Jones, N. McCartney, and A. McComas, eds.) *Human Muscle Power,* 97–105. Champaign, Ill.: Human Kinetics Publishers.

9. Carlson, F., and D. Wilkie. 1974. *Muscle Physiology.* Englewood Cliffs, N.J.: Prentice-Hall.

10. Costill, D., W. Fink, and M. Pollock. 1976. Muscle fiber composition and enzyme activities of elite distance runners. *Medicine and Science in Sports* 8:96.

11. Ebashi, S. 1976. Excitation-contraction coupling. *Annual Review of Physiology* 38:293–309.

12. Edgerton, V. et al. 1983. Muscle fiber activation and recruitment. In (H. Knuttgen, J. Vogel, and J. Poormans, ed.) *Biochemistry of Exercise,* 31–49. Champaign, Ill.: Human Kinetics Publishers.

13. Edgerton, V. et al. 1986. Morphological basis of skeletal muscle power output. In (N. Jones, N. McCartney, and A. McComas, eds.) *Human Muscle Power,* 43–58. Champaign, Ill.: Human Kinetics Publishers.

14. Edstrom, L., and L. Grimby. 1986. Effect of exercise on the motor unit. *Muscle and Nerve* 9:104–26.

15. Faulker, J., D. Claflin, and K. McCully. 1986. Power output of fast and slow fibers from human skeletal muscles. In (N. Jones, N. McCartney, and A. McComas, eds.) *Human Muscle Power,* 81–90. Champaign, Ill.: Human Kinetics Publishers.

16. Fox, S. 1987. *Human Physiology.* Dubuque, Ia.: Wm. C. Brown.

17. Gollnick, P., and B. Saltin. 1983. Hypothesis: Significance of skeletal muscle oxidative capacity with endurance training. *Clinical Physiology* 2:1–12.

18. Gollnick, P. 1985. Metabolism of substrates: energy substrate metabolism during exercise and as modified by training. *Federation Proceedings* 44:353–56.

19. Green, H. 1986. Muscle power: Fiber type recruitment, metabolism, and fatigue. In (N. Jones, N. McCartney, and A. McComas, eds.) *Human Muscle Power,* 65–79. Champaign, Ill.: Human Kinetics Publishers.

20. Hole, J. 1987. *Human Anatomy and Physiology.* Dubuque, Ia.: Wm. C. Brown.

21. Holloszy, J. 1982. Muscle metabolism during exercise. *Archives of Physical and Rehabilitation Medicine* 63:231–34.

22. Hoppeler, H. 1986. Exercise-induced ultrastructure changes in skeletal muscle. *International Journal of Sports Medicine* 7:187–204.

23. Johnson, L. 1983. *Biology.* Dubuque, Ia.: Wm. C. Brown.

24. Kodama, T. 1985. Thermodynamic analysis of muscle ATPase mechanisms. *Physiological Reviews* 65:468–540.

25. Larsson, L. 1982. Physical training effects on muscle morphology in sedentary males at different ages. *Medicine and Science in Sports and Exercise* 14:203.

26. Lowey, S. 1986. Cardiac and skeletal muscle myosin polymorphism. *Medicine and Science in Sports and Exercise* 18:284–91.

27. McArdle, W., F. Katch, and V. Katch. 1986. *Exercise Physiology: Energy, Nutrition, and Human Performance.* Philadelphia: Lea & Febiger.

28. Pette, D. 1980. *Plasticity of Muscle.* New York: Walter de Gruyter.

29. Pette, D. 1984. Activity-induced fast-to-slow transitions in mammalian muscle. *Medicine and Science in Sports and Exercise* 16:517–28.

30. Pette, D., and C. Spamer. 1986. Metabolic properties of muscle fibers. *Federation Proceedings* 45: 2910–14.

31. Ruegg, J. C. 1987. Excitation-contraction coupling in fast- and slow-twitch muscle fibers. *International Journal of Sports Medicine* 8:360–64.

32. Saltin, B. et al. 1977. Fiber types and metabolic potentials of skeletal muscles in sedentary man and endurance runners. *Annals of New York Academy of Sciences* 301:3–29.

33. Simoneau, J. et al. 1986. Inheritance of human skeletal muscle and anaerobic capacity adaptation to high-intensity intermittent training. *International Journal of Sports Medicine* 7:167–71.

34. Snow, D., and R. Harris. 1985. Thoroughbreds and greyhounds: Biochemical adaptations in creatures of nature and man. In (R. Giles, ed.) *Circulation, Respiration, and Metabolism,* 227–39. New York: Springer-Verlag.

35. Tesch, P., A. Thorsson, and P. Kaiser. 1984. Muscle capillary supply and fiber type characteristics in weight and power lifters. *Journal of Applied Physiology* 56:35–38.

36. Wilmore, J., and D. Costill, D. 1988. *Training for Sport and Activity.* Dubuque, Ia.: Wm. C. Brown.

9 *Circulatory Adaptations to Exercise*

Objectives

*B*y studying this chapter, you should be able to do the following:

1. Give an overview of the design and function of the circulatory system.
2. Describe the cardiac cycle and the associated electrical activity recorded via the electrocardiogram.
3. Discuss the pattern of redistribution of blood flow during exercise.
4. Outline the circulatory responses to various types of exercise.
5. Identify the factors that regulate local blood flow during exercise.
6. List and discuss those factors responsible for regulation of stroke volume during exercise.
7. Discuss the regulation of cardiac output during exercise.

Outline

Key Terms

arteries
arterioles
atrioventricular node (AV node)
autoregulation
capillaries
cardiac output
cardiac accelerator nerves
cardiovascular control center
central command
diastole
diastolic blood pressure
electrocardiogram (ECG)
intercalated discs
myocardium
pulmonary circuit
sinoatrial node (SA node)
stroke volume
systole
systolic blood pressure
vagus nerve
veins
venules

One of the major challenges to homeostasis posed by exercise is the increased muscular demand for oxygen; this demand may exceed resting needs by 15–25 fold during heavy exercise. The primary purpose of the cardiorespiratory system is to deliver adequate amounts of oxygen and remove wastes from body tissues. In addition, the circulatory system transports nutrients and aids in temperature regulation. It is important to note that the respiratory system and the circulatory system function together as a "coupled unit"; the respiratory system adds oxygen and removes carbon dioxide from the blood, while the circulatory system is responsible for delivery of oxygenated blood and nutrients to tissues in accordance with their needs. Stated another way, the "cardiopulmonary system" works to maintain oxygen and carbon dioxide homeostasis in body tissues.

In order to meet the increased oxygen demands of muscle during exercise, two major adjustments of blood flow must be made: (1) an increased **cardiac output** (i.e., increased amount of blood pumped per minute by the heart) and (2) a redistribution of blood flow from inactive organs to the active skeletal muscles. However, while the needs of the muscles are being met, other tissues, such as the brain, cannot be denied blood flow. This is accomplished by maintaining blood pressure, the driving force of the blood. A thorough understanding of the cardiovascular responses to exercise is important for the student of exercise physiology. Therefore, it is the purpose of this chapter to describe the design and function of the circulatory system and how it responds during exercise.

Organization of the Circulatory System

The human circulatory system is a closed loop that circulates blood to all body tissues. Circulation of blood requires the action of a muscular pump, the heart, that creates the "pressure head" needed to move blood through the system. Blood travels away from the heart in **arteries** and returns to the heart by way of **veins.** The system is considered "closed" because arteries and veins are continuous with each other through smaller vessels. Arteries branch extensively to form a "tree" of smaller vessels. As the vessels become microscopic they form **arterioles,** which eventually develop into "beds" of much smaller vessels called **capillaries.** Capillaries are the smallest and most numerous of blood vessels; all exchanges of oxygen, carbon dioxide, and nutrients between tissues and the circulatory system occur across capillary beds. Blood passes from capillary beds to small venous vessels called **venules.** As venules move back toward the heart they increase in size and become veins. Major veins empty directly into the heart. The mixture of venous blood from both the upper and lower body that accumulates in the right side of the heart is termed mixed venous blood. Mixed venous blood therefore represents an average of venous blood from the entire body.

Structure of the Heart
The heart is divided into four chambers and is often considered to be two-pumps-in-one. The right atrium and right ventricle form the right pump, while the left atrium and left ventricle combine to make the left pump (see figure 9.1). The right side of the heart is separated from the left side by a muscular wall called the interventricular septum. This septum prevents the mixing of blood from the two sides of the heart.

Figure 9.1 An anterior view of the heart.

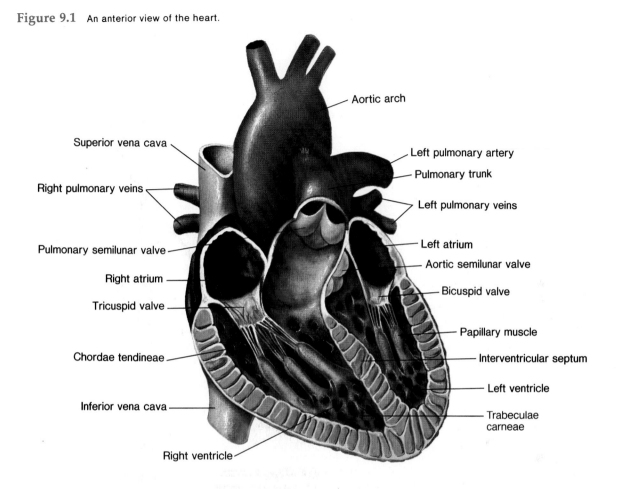

Blood movement within the heart is from the atria to the ventricles, and from the ventricles blood is pumped into the arteries. To prevent backward movement of blood, the heart contains four one-way valves. The right and left atrioventricular valves connect the atria with the right and left ventricles, respectively (figure 9.1). These valves are also known as the tricuspid valve (right atrioventricular valve) and the bicuspid valve (left atrioventricular valve). Backflow from the arteries into the ventricles is prevented by the pulmonary semilunar valve (right ventricle) and the aortic semilunar valve (left ventricle).

Pulmonary and Systemic Circuits

As mentioned previously, the heart can be considered as two-pumps-in-one. The right side of the heart pumps blood that is partially depleted of its oxygen content and contains an elevated carbon dioxide content as a result of gas exchange in the various tissues of the body. This blood is delivered from the right heart into the lungs through the **pulmonary circuit.** At the lungs, oxygen is loaded into the blood and carbon dioxide is released. This "oxygenated" blood then travels to the left side of the heart and is pumped to the various tissues of the body via the systemic circuit.

Figure 9.2 The heart wall is composed of three distinct layers: (1) epicardium, (2) myocardium, and (3) endocardium.

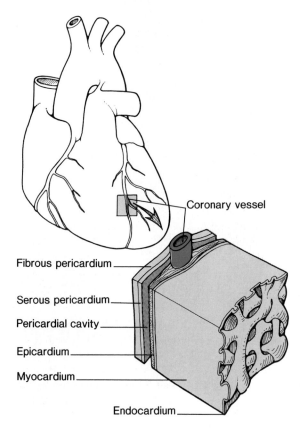

Coronary vessel

Fibrous pericardium

Serous pericardium

Pericardial cavity

Epicardium

Myocardium

Endocardium

Heart: Myocardium and Cardiac Cycle

In order to better appreciate how the circulatory system adjusts to the stress of exercise, it is important to understand elementary details of heart muscle structure as well as the electrical and mechanical activities of the heart.

Myocardium

The wall of the heart is composed of three layers: (1) an outer layer called the epicardium, (2) a muscular middle layer, the myocardium, and (3) an inner layer known as the endocardium (see figure 9.2). It is the **myocardium,** or heart muscle, that is responsible for contracting and forcing blood out of the heart. The myocardium receives its blood supply via the right and left coronary arteries. These vessels branch off the aorta and encircle the heart. The coronary veins run alongside the arteries and drain all coronary blood into a larger vein called the coronary sinus, which deposits blood into the right atrium.

Heart muscle differs from skeletal muscle in several important ways. First, unlike skeletal muscle cells, heart muscle cells are all interconnected via **intercalated discs.** These intercellular connections permit transmission of electrical impulses from one cell to another. Intercalated discs are nothing more than leaky membranes that allow ions to cross from one cell to another. Therefore, when one heart cell is depolarized

Figure 9.3 Increases in heart rate during exercise are achieved primarily through a decrease in the time spent in diastole; however, at high heart rates the length of time spent in systole also decreases.

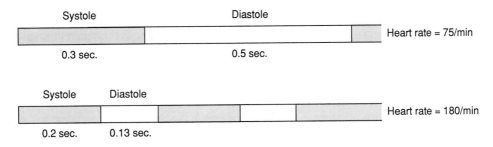

to contract, all connecting cells also become excited and contract as a unit. This arrangement is referred to as a "functional syncytium." Heart muscle cells in the atria are separated from ventricular muscle cells by a layer of connective tissue that does not permit transmission of electrical impulses. Hence, the atria contract separately from the ventricles.

A second difference between heart muscle cells and skeletal muscle cells is that heart muscle cannot be divided into different fiber types. The myocardium is thought to be a rather homogenous muscle that is similar in many ways to slow-twitch fibers found in skeletal muscle. That is, heart muscle cells are highly aerobic in nature, contain an extensive capillary supply, and have large numbers of mitochondria.

Heart muscle is similar to skeletal muscle in that it is striated (contains actin and myosin protein filaments) and contracts via the sliding filament theory of muscular contraction (chapter 8). In addition, like skeletal muscle, heart muscle can alter its force of contraction as a function of the degree of overlap between actin-myosin filaments. This length-tension relationship of the heart will be discussed later in the chapter.

Cardiac Cycle

The cardiac cycle refers to the repeating pattern of contraction and relaxation of the heart. The contraction phase is called **systole** and the relaxation period is called **diastole.** Generally, when these terms are used alone, they refer to contraction and relaxation of the ventricles. However, note that the atria also contract and relax; therefore, there is an atrial systole and diastole. Atrial contraction occurs during ventricular diastole and atrial relaxation occurs during ventricular systole. The heart thus has a two-step pumping action. The right and left atria contract together, which empties atrial blood into the ventricles. Approximately 0.1 seconds after the atrial contraction, the ventricles contract and deliver blood into both the systemic and pulmonary circuits.

At rest, contraction of the ventricles during systole ejects about two-thirds of the blood in the ventricles, leaving about one-third in the ventricles. The ventricles then fill with blood during the next diastole. A healthy twenty-one-year-old female might have an average resting heart rate of seventy-five beats per minute. This means that the total cardiac cycle lasts 0.8 seconds, with 0.5 seconds spent in diastole and the remaining 0.3 seconds dedicated to systole (see figure 9.3). If the heart rate increases from seventy-five beats per minute to 180 beats per minute (e.g., heavy exercise), there is a reduction in the time spent in both systole and diastole (13, 16). This point is illustrated in figure 9.3. Note that a rising heart rate results in a greater time reduction in diastole, while systole is less affected.

Pressure Changes during the Cardiac Cycle

During the cardiac cycle, the pressure within the heart chambers rises and falls. When the atria are relaxed, blood flows into them from the venous circulation. As these chambers fill, the pressure inside gradually increases. Approximately 70% of the blood entering the

Figure 9.4 Relationship between pressure, volume, and heart sounds during the cardiac cycle. Notice the change in ventricular pressure and volume during the transition from systole to diastole.

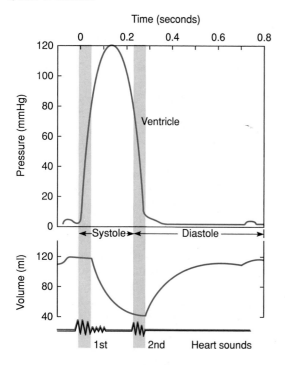

closing of the atrioventricular valves (first heart sound) and the closing of the aortic and pulmonary valves (second heart sound).

Arterial Blood Pressure

Blood exerts pressure throughout the vascular system, but is greatest within the arteries where it is generally measured and used as an indication of health. Blood pressure is created primarily by the action of the heart and is the force exerted by blood against the arterial walls.

Arterial blood pressure can be estimated by use of a sphygomomanometer (see Box 9.1). The normal blood pressure of an adult male is 120/80, while adult females tend to be lower (110/70). The larger number in the expression of blood pressure is the systolic pressure expressed in millimeters of mercury (mmHg). The lower number in the blood pressure ratio is the diastolic pressure again expressed in mmHg. **Systolic blood pressure** is produced as blood is ejected from the heart during ventricular systole. During ventricular relaxation (diastole), the arterial blood pressure decreases and represents **diastolic blood pressure.** The difference between systolic and diastolic blood pressure is called the "pulse pressure."

The average pressure during a cardiac cycle is called "mean arterial pressure." Mean arterial blood pressure is important because it determines the rate of blood flow through the systemic circuit.

Determination of mean arterial pressure is not easy. It is not a simple average of systolic and diastolic pressure since diastole generally lasts longer than systole. However, mean arterial pressure can be estimated in the following way:

$$\text{Mean arterial pressure} = \text{DBP} + .33 \text{ (pulse pressure)}$$

Here DBP is the diastolic blood pressure and the pulse pressure is the difference between systolic and diastolic pressures. Let's consider a sample calculation of mean arterial pressure at rest. For example, suppose

atria during diastole flows directly into the ventricles through the atrioventricular valves before the atria contract. Upon atrial contraction, atrial pressure rises and forces most of the remaining 30% of the atrial content into the ventricles.

Pressure in the ventricles is low while they are filling, but when the atria contract, the ventricular pressure increases slightly. Then as the ventricles contract, the pressure rises sharply, which closes the atrioventricular valves and prevents back-flow into the atria. As soon as ventricular pressure exceeds the pressure of the pulmonary artery and the aorta, the pulmonary and aortic valves open and blood is forced into both pulmonary and systemic circulations. Figure 9.4 illustrates the changes in ventricular pressure as a function of time during the resting cardiac cycle. Note the occurrence of two heart sounds that are produced by the

Box 9.1 Measurement of Arterial Blood Pressure

Arterial blood pressure is not usually measured directly but is estimated using an instrument called a sphygomomanometer (Box figure 9A). This device consists of an inflatable arm cuff connected to a column of mercury. The cuff can be inflated by a bulb pump, with the pressure in the cuff measured by the rising column of mercury. For example, a pressure of 100 mm of mercury (mm Hg) would be enough force to raise the column of mercury upward a distance of 100 mm.

Blood pressure is measured in the following way. The rubber cuff is placed around the upper arm so it surrounds the brachial artery. Air is pumped into the cuff so that the pressure around the arm exceeds arterial pressure. Since the pressure applied around the arm is greater than arterial pressure, the brachial artery is squeezed shut and blood flow is stopped. If a stethoscope is placed over the brachial artery (just below the cuff), no sounds are heard since there is no blood flow. However, if the air control valve is slowly opened to release air, the pressure in the cuff begins to decline and soon the pressure around the arm reaches a point that is equal to or just slightly below arterial pressure. At this point blood begins to spurt through the artery and a sharp sound can be heard through the stethoscope. The pressure (i.e., height of mercury column) at which the first tapping sound is heard represents systolic blood pressure.

As the cuff pressure continues to decline, a series of increasingly louder sounds can be heard. When the pressure in the cuff is equal to or slightly below diastolic blood pressure, the sounds heard through the stethoscope cease. Therefore, diastolic blood pressure represents the height of the mercury column when the sounds become abruptly muffled.

Box Figure 9.A   A sphygmomanometer is used to measure arterial blood pressure.

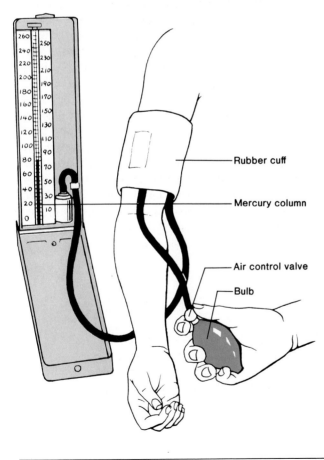

Rubber cuff

Mercury column

Air control valve

Bulb

an individual has a blood pressure of 120/80 mm Hg. The mean arterial pressure would be:

$$\text{Mean arterial pressure} = 80 \text{ mm Hg} + .33(120-80)$$
$$= 80 \text{ mm Hg} + 13$$
$$= 93 \text{ mm Hg}$$

Approximately 20% of all adults in the United States have hypertension, which is defined as blood pressure in excess of the normal range for the person's age and sex (13). Blood pressures above 140/90 are considered to be indicators of hypertension (13, 16). Hypertension is generally classified into one or two categories: (1) primary or essential hypertension and (2) secondary hypertension. The cause of primary hypertension is unknown. This type of hypertension constitutes 90% of all reported cases of hypertension in the United States. Secondary hypertension is a result of some known disease process and thus the hypertension is "secondary" to another disease. Box 9.2 discusses those factors that influence arterial blood pressure.

Electrical Activity of the Heart

Many myocardial cells have the unique potential for spontaneous electrical activity (i.e., each has an intrinsic rhythm). However, in the normal heart, spontaneous electrical activity is limited to a special region located in the right atrium. This region, called the **sinoatrial node** (SA node), serves as the pacemaker for the heart (see figure 9.5). Spontaneous electrical activity in the SA node occurs due to a decay of the resting membrane potential via inward diffusion of sodium during diastole. When the SA node reaches the depolarization threshold and "fires," the wave of depolarization spreads over the atria resulting in atrial contraction. The wave of atrial depolarization cannot directly cross into the ventricles but must be transported by way of specialized conductive tissue. This specialized conductive tissue radiates from a small mass of muscle tissue called the **atrioventricular node** (AV node). This node, located in the floor of the right atrium, connects the atria with the ventricles by a pair of conductive pathways called the right and left bundle branches (figure 9.5). Upon reaching the ventricles, these conductive pathways branch into smaller fibers called Purkinje fibers. The Purkinje fibers then spread the wave of depolarization throughout the ventricles.

A recording of the electrical changes that occur in the myocardium during the cardiac cycle is called an **electrocardiogram (ECG).** Analysis of ECG waveforms allows the physician to evaluate the heart's ability to conduct impulses and therefore determine if electrical problems exist. Further, analysis of the ECG during exercise is often used in the diagnosis of coronary artery disease (see Box 9.3). Figure 9.6 illustrates a normal ECG pattern. Notice that the ECG pattern contains several different deflections, or waves, during each cardiac cycle. Each of these distinct waveforms are identified by different letters. The P wave results from the depolarization of the atria, the QRS complex results from ventricular depolarization, and the T wave is due to ventricular repolarization. A step-by-step illustration of an ECG recording is given by figure 9.7. Note the formation of each new wave as a result of electrical activity in the heart.

Box 9.2 Factors That Influence Arterial Blood Pressure

Arterial blood pressure depends on a variety of factors, including cardiac output, blood volume, resistance to flow, and blood viscosity. These relationships are summarized in Box figure 9B. An increase in any of the above variables results in an increase in arterial blood pressure. Conversely, a decrease in any of the above variables causes a decrease in blood pressure.

How is blood pressure regulated? Acute (short-term) regulation of blood pressure is achieved by the sympathetic nervous system, while long-term regulation of blood pressure is primarily a function of the kidneys. The kidneys regulate blood pressure by their control of blood volume.

Pressure receptors (called baroreceptors) in the carotid artery and the aorta are sensitive to changes in arterial blood pressure. An increase in arterial pressure triggers these receptors to send impulses to the cardiovascular control center, which responds by decreasing sympathetic activity. A reduction in sympathetic activity may lower cardiac output and/or reduce vascular resistance, which in turn lowers blood pressure. Conversely, a decrease in blood pressure results in a reduction of baroreceptor activity to the brain. This causes the cardiovascular control center to respond by increasing sympathetic outflow, which raises blood pressure back to normal. For a complete discussion of blood-pressure regulation, see Rowell (36).

Box Figure 9.B Some factors that influence arterial blood pressure.

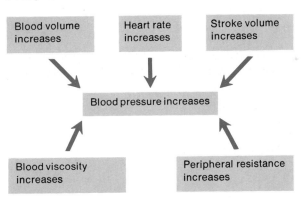

Figure 9.5 Conduction system of the heart.

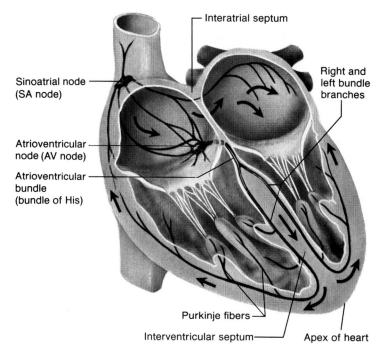

Interatrial septum

Sinoatrial node
(SA node)

Right and
left bundle
branches

Atrioventricular
node (AV node)

Atrioventricular
bundle
(bundle of His)

Purkinje fibers

Interventricular septum

Apex of heart

Figure 9.6 The normal electrocardiogram during rest.

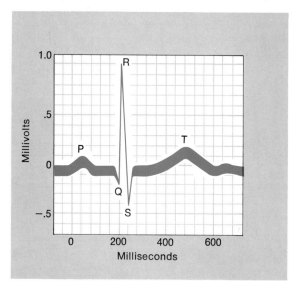

Box 9.3 Diagnostic Use of the ECG during Exercise

Cardiologists are physicians who specialize in diseases of the heart and vascular system. One of the diagnostic procedures commonly used to evaluate cardiac function is to make ECG measurements during an incremental exercise test (usually on a treadmill). This allows the physician to observe changes in blood pressure as well as changes in the patient's ECG during periods of stress.

The most common cause of heart disease is the collection of fatty plaque (called atherosclerosis) inside coronary vessels. This collection of plaque reduces blood flow to the myocardium. The adequacy of blood flow to the heart is relative—it depends on the metabolic demand placed on the heart. An obstruction to a coronary artery, for example, may allow sufficient blood flow at rest, but may be inadequate during exercise due to increased metabolic demand placed on the heart. Therefore, a graded exercise test may provide a means of performing a "stress test" to evaluate cardiac function.

An example of an abnormal exercise ECG is illustrated in Box figure 9C. Myocardial ischemia (reduced blood flow) may be detected by changes in the S-T segment of the ECG. Notice the depressed S-T segment in the picture on the right when compared to the normal ECG on the left. This S-T segment depression suggests to the physician that ischemic heart disease may be present and that additional diagnostic procedures may be warranted.

Box Figure 9.C Depression of the S-T segment of the electrocardiogram as a result of myocardial ischemia.

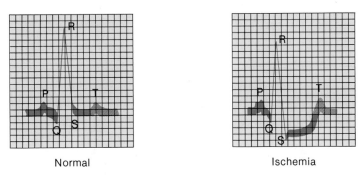

Normal   Ischemia

Cardiac Output

Cardiac output ($\dot{Q}$) is the product of the **stroke volume** (SV) (amount of blood pumped per heart beat) and the heart rate (HR):

$$\dot{Q} = SV \times HR$$

Thus, cardiac output can be increased due to a rise in either heart rate or stroke volume. During exercise in the upright position (e.g., running, cycling, etc.) the increase in cardiac output is due to both an increase in heart rate and stroke volume. Table 9.1 presents typical values at rest and during maximal exercise for heart rate, stroke volume, and cardiac output in both untrained and highly trained endurance athletes. The gender differences in stroke volume and cardiac output are due mainly to differences in body sizes between men and women (3) (see table 9.1).

Figure 9.7 An illustration of the relationship between the heart's electrical events and the recording of the ECG.

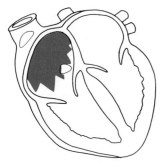

(a)

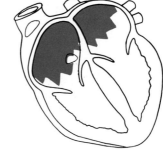

(b)

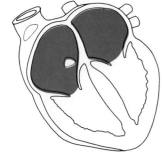

P

(c)

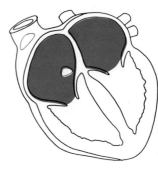

P-R interval

(d)

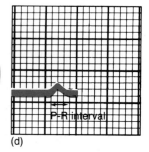

(e) QRS complex

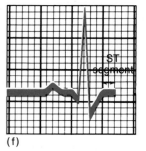

ST segment

(f)

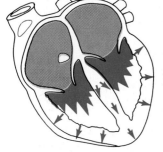

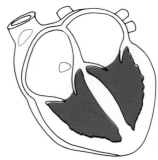

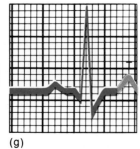

(g)

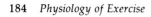

Table 9.1 *Typical resting and maximal exercise values for stroke volume (SV), heart rate (HR), and cardiac output (Q̇) for college-age untrained subjects and trained endurance athletes. (Body weights for males are 70 kg and 50 kg for females.)*

Subject	HR (beat/min)		SV (ml/beat)		Q̇ (l/min)
Rest					
Untrained Male	72	×	70	=	5.00
Untrained Female	75	×	60	=	4.50
Trained Male	50	×	100	=	5.00
Trained Female	55	×	80	=	4.50
Max Exercise					
Untrained Male	200	×	110	=	22.0
Untrained Female	200	×	90	=	18.0
Trained Male	190	×	180	=	34.2
Trained Female	190	×	125	=	23.9

Note that values are rounded off. Data from references 3, 13, and 36.

Venous Return during Exercise

Regardless of the mechanisms that regulate cardiac output during exercise, the heart can only pump the amount of blood that it receives. Therefore, cardiac output is ultimately dependent on the amount of venous blood returned to the right side of the heart. For example, a cardiac output of 20 liters per minute during exercise requires a matching venous return of 20 liters per minute. There are three principal mechanisms for increasing venous return during exercise: (1) constriction of the veins (venoconstriction), (2) pumping action of contracting skeletal muscle (muscle pump), and (3) pumping action of the respiratory system (respiratory pump).

1. *Venoconstriction.* Venoconstriction increases venous return by reducing the volume capacity of the veins to store blood. The end result of a reduced volume capacity in veins is to move blood back toward the heart. Venoconstriction occurs via a reflex sympathetic constriction of

smooth muscle in veins draining skeletal muscle, which is controlled by the cardiovascular control center (3, 16, 36).

2. *Muscle pump.* The muscle pump is a result of the mechanical action of rhythmic skeletal muscle contractions. As muscles contract, they compress veins and push blood back toward the heart. Between contractions, blood refills the veins and the process is repeated. Blood is prevented from flowing away from the heart between contractions by one-way valves located in large veins. During sustained muscular contractions (isometric exercise), the muscle pump cannot operate and venous return is reduced.

3. *Respiratory pump.* The rhythmic pattern of breathing also provides a mechanical pump by which venous return is promoted. The respiratory pump works in the following way. During inspiration, the pressure within the thorax (chest) decreases and abdominal

Figure 9.8 The activities of the S-A and A-V nodes can be altered by both the sympathetic and parasympathetic nervous systems.

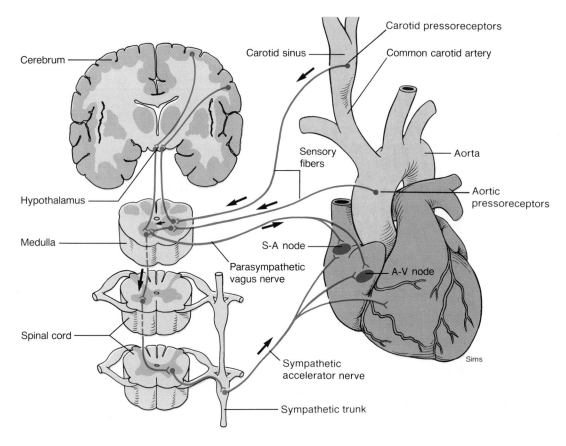

pressure increases. This creates a flow of venous blood from the abdominal region into the thorax and therefore promotes venous return. Although quiet breathing (rest) aids in venous return, the role of the respiratory pump is enhanced during exercise due to the greater respiratory rate and depth.

Regulation of Heart Rate

During exercise the quantity of blood pumped by the heart must change in accordance with the elevated skeletal muscle oxygen demand. Since the SA node controls heart rate, changes in heart rate often involve factors that influence the SA node. The two most prominent factors that influence heart rate are the parasympathetic and sympathetic nervous systems.

The parasympathetic fibers that supply the heart arise from neurons in the **cardiovascular control center** in the medulla oblongata and make up a portion of the **vagus nerve.** Upon reaching the heart, these fibers make contact with both the SA node and the AV node (see figure 9.8). When stimulated, these nerve endings release acetylcholine, which causes a decrease in the activity of both the SA and AV nodes due to hyperpolarization (i.e., moving the resting membrane potential further from threshold). The end result is a reduction of heart rate. Therefore, the parasympathetic nervous system acts as a braking system to slow down heart rate.

Even at rest, the vagus nerves carry impulses to the SA and AV nodes (13, 16). This is often referred to as "parasympathetic tone." As a consequence, parasympathetic activity can cause heart rate to increase or decrease. For instance, a decrease in parasympathetic tone to the heart can elevate heart rate, while an increase in parasympathetic activity causes a slowing of heart rate.

Studies have shown that the initial increase in heart rate during exercise, up to approximately 100 beats per minute, is due to a withdrawal of parasympathetic tone (36). At higher work rates, stimulation of the SA and AV nodes by the sympathetic nervous system is responsible for increases in heart rate (36). Sympathetic fibers reach the heart by means of the **cardiac accelerator nerves,** which innervate both the SA node and the ventricles (figure 9.8). Endings of these fibers release norepinephrine upon stimulation, which causes an increase in both heart rate and the force of myocardial contraction.

At rest, a normal balance between parasympathetic tone and sympathetic activity to the heart is maintained by the cardiovascular control center in the medulla oblongata. The cardiovascular control center receives impulses from various parts of the circulatory system relative to changes in important parameters (e.g., blood pressure, blood oxygen tension, etc.), and relays motor impulses to the heart in response to a changing cardiovascular need. For example, an increase in resting blood pressure above normal stimulates pressure receptors in the carotid arteries and the arch of the aorta, which in turn send impulses to the cardiovascular control center (figure 9.8). In response, the cardiovascular control center increases parasympathetic activity to the heart to slow the heart rate and reduce cardiac output. This reduction in cardiac output causes blood pressure to decline back toward normal.

Another regulatory reflex involves pressure receptors located in the right atrium. In this case, an increase in right atrial pressure signals the cardiovascular control center that an increase in venous return has occurred; hence, in order to prevent a backup of blood in the systemic venous system, an increase in cardiac output must result. The cardiovascular control center responds by sending sympathetic accelerator nerve impulses to the heart, which increases heart rate and

cardiac output. The end result is that the increase in cardiac output lowers right atrial pressure back to normal and venous blood pressure is reduced.

Finally, a change in body temperature can influence heart rate. An increase in body temperature above normal results in an increase in heart rate, while a lowering of body temperature below normal causes a reduction in heart rate (4, 13, 16, 24, 36, 37, 39). This topic will be discussed later in chapter 12.

Regulation of Stroke Volume

Stroke volume, at rest or during exercise, is regulated by three variables: (1) the end-diastolic volume (EDV), which is the volume of blood in the ventricles at the end of diastole; (2) the average aortic blood pressure; and (3) the strength of ventricular contraction.

EDV is often referred to as "preload" and influences stroke volume in the following way. Two physiologists, Frank and Starling, demonstrated that the strength of ventricular contraction was increased with an enlargement of EDV (i.e., stretch of the ventricles). This relationship has become known as the Frank-Starling law of the heart. The increase in EDV results in a lengthening of cardiac fibers, which improves the force of contraction in a manner similar to that seen in skeletal muscle (chapter 8). A rise in cardiac contractility results in an increase in the amount of blood pumped per beat. The principal variable that influences EDV is the rate of venous return to the heart. An increase in venous return results in a rise in EDV and therefore an increase in stroke volume. In contrast, a decrease in venous return lowers EDV and reduces stroke volume.

A second variable that affects stroke volume is the aortic pressure. In order to eject blood, the pressure generated by the left ventricle must exceed the pressure in the aorta. Therefore, aortic pressure (called afterload) represents a barrier to the ejection of blood from the ventricles. Stroke volume is thus inversely proportional to the afterload; that is, an increase in aortic pressure produces a decrease in stroke volume. However, it is noteworthy that afterload is minimized during exercise due to arteriole dilation. This arteriole dilation in the working muscles reduces afterload and makes it easier for the heart to pump a large volume of blood.

Figure 9.9 Factors that regulate cardiac output. Variables that stimulate cardiac output are shown by solid arrows, while factors that reduce cardiac output are shown by dotted arrows.

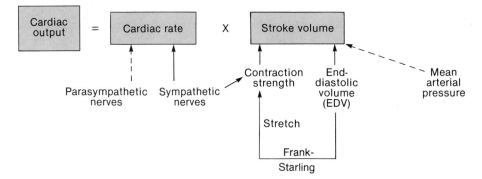

The final factor that influences stroke volume is the effect of circulating epinephrine/norepinephrine and direct sympathetic stimulation of the heart by cardiac accelerator nerves. Both of these mechanisms increase cardiac contractility by increasing the amount of calcium available to the myocardial cell (13, 16, 36).

In summary, cardiac output is the product of heart rate and stroke volume. Heart rate is determined by the interaction of the parasympathetic and sympathetic nervous systems. The parasympathetic nervous system serves to decrease heart rate, while the sympathetic nervous system accelerates heart rate. Stroke volume is determined by the interaction of EDV, sympathetic stimulation of the heart, and the mean arterial pressure. Figure 9.9 summarizes those variables that influence cardiac output during exercise.

Hemodynamics

One of the most important features of the circulatory system to remember is that the system is a continuous "closed loop." Blood flow through the circulatory system results from pressure differences between the two ends of the system. In order to understand the physical regulation of blood flow to tissues, it is necessary to appreciate the interrelationships between pressure, flow, and resistance. The study of these factors and the physical principles of blood flow is called hemodynamics.

Physical Characteristics of Blood

Blood is composed of two principle components: (1) plasma and (2) cells. Plasma is the "watery" portion of blood that contains numerous ions, proteins, and hormones. The cells that comprise blood are red blood cells (RBCs), platelets, and white blood cells. Red blood cells contain hemoglobin used for the transport of oxygen (see chapter 10). Platelets play an important role in blood clotting and white blood cells are important in preventing infection.

The percent of the blood that is comprised of cells is called the hematocrit. If an individual has a hematocrit of 40%, then 40% of the blood is cells and the remainder is plasma. On a percentage basis, RBC's comprise the largest fraction of cells found in blood. Therefore, the hematocrit is principally influenced by increases or decreases in RBC numbers. The average hematocrit of a normal college-age male is 42%, while the hematocrit of a normal college-age female averages approximately 38%. These values vary between individuals and are dependent on a number of variables.

Blood is several times more viscous than water, and this viscosity increases the difficulty with which blood flows through the circulatory system. One of the major contributors to viscosity is the concentration of RBCs found in the blood. Therefore, during periods of anemia (decreased RBCs), the viscosity of blood is lowered.

Figure 9.10 The flow of blood through the systemic circuit is dependent on the pressure difference (ΔP) between the aorta and the right atrium. In this illustration, the mean pressure in the aorta is 100 mm Hg, while the pressure in the right atrium is 0 mm Hg. Therefore, the "driving" pressure across the circuit is 100 mm Hg (100 − 0 = 100).

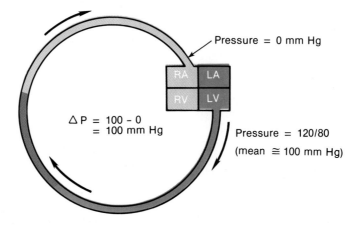

Pressure = 0 mm Hg

$\Delta P = 100 - 0$
$= 100$ mm Hg

Pressure = 120/80
(mean ≅ 100 mm Hg)

Conversely, an increase in hematocrit results in an elevation in blood viscosity. The potential influence of changing blood viscosity on performance will be discussed in chapter 25.

Relationships between Pressure, Resistance, and Flow

As mentioned earlier, blood flow through the vascular system depends in part on the difference in pressure at the two ends of the system. If the pressure at the two ends of the vessel are equal, there will be no flow. In contrast, if the pressure is higher at one end of the vessel than the other, blood will flow from the region of higher pressure to the region of lower pressure. The rate of flow is proportional to the pressure difference $(P_1 - P_2)$ between the two ends of the tube. Figure 9.10 illustrates the "pressure head" driving blood flow in the systemic circulatory system under resting conditions. Here the mean arterial pressure is 100 mm Hg (i.e., this is the pressure of blood in the aorta), while the pressure at the opposite end of the circuit (i.e., pressure in the right atrium) is 0 mm Hg. Therefore, the driving pressure across the circulatory system is 100 mm Hg (100 − 0 = 100).

It should be pointed out that the flow rate of blood through the vascular system is proportional to the pressure difference across the system, but is inversely proportional to the resistance. Inverse proportionality is expressed mathematically by the placement of this variable in the denominator of a fraction, since a fraction decreases when the denominator increases. Therefore, the relationship between blood flow, pressure, and resistance is given by the equation:

$$\text{Blood flow} = \frac{\Delta \text{ Pressure}}{\text{Resistance}}$$

where Δ pressure means the difference in pressure between the two ends of the circulatory system. Notice that blood flow can be increased by either an increase in blood pressure or a decrease in resistance. In practice, increases in blood flow during exercise are achieved by both a decrease in resistance and a rise in blood pressure.

What factors contribute to the resistance of blood flow? Resistance to flow is directly proportional to the length of the vessel and the viscosity of blood. However, the most important variable determining vascular resistance is the size of the blood vessel, since vascular resistance is inversely proportional to the fourth power of the radius of the vessel:

$$\text{Resistance} = \frac{\text{Length} \times \text{viscosity}}{\text{Radius}^4}$$

Figure 9.11 Pressure changes across the systemic circulation. Notice the large pressure drop across the small arteries and arterioles.

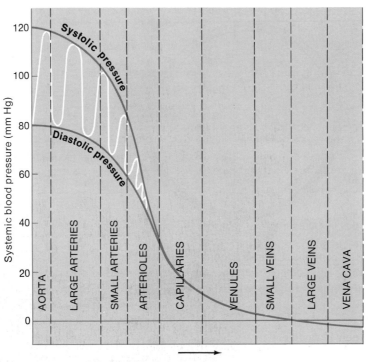

In words, an increase in either vessel length or blood viscosity results in a proportional increase in resistance. However, reducing the radius of a blood vessel by one-half would increase resistance sixteen-fold (i.e., $2^4 = 16$)!

Sources of Vascular Resistance

Under ordinary circumstances, the viscosity of blood and the length of the blood vessels are not manipulated in normal physiology. Therefore, the primary factor regulating blood flow through organs must be the radius of the blood vessel. Since the effect of changes in radius on changes in flow rate are magnified by a power of four, blood can be diverted from one organ system to another by varying degrees of vasoconstriction and vasodilation. This principle is used during heavy exercise to divert blood toward contracting skeletal muscle and away from less-active tissue. This concept will be discussed in detail in the next section.

The greatest vascular resistance in blood flow occurs in arterioles. This point is illustrated in figure 9.11. Note the large drop in arterial pressure that occurs across the arterioles; approximately 70%–80% of the decline in mean arterial pressure occurs across the arterioles.

Changes in Oxygen Delivery to Muscle during Exercise

During intense exercise, the metabolic need for oxygen in skeletal muscle may increase many times over the resting value (3). In order to meet this rise in oxygen demand, blood flow to the contracting muscle must increase. As mentioned earlier, increased oxygen delivery to exercising skeletal muscle is accomplished via two mechanisms: (1) an increased cardiac output and (2) a redistribution of blood flow from inactive organs to the working skeletal muscle.

Changes in Cardiac Output during Exercise

Cardiac output increases during exercise in direct proportion to the metabolic rate required to perform the exercise task. This is pointed out in figure 9.12. Note that the relationship between cardiac output and percent maximal oxygen uptake is linear. The increase in cardiac output during exercise in the upright position is achieved by both an increase in stroke volume and heart rate. However, note that stroke volume does not increase beyond a work load of approximately 40% of $\dot{V}O_2$ max (figure 9.12). Therefore, at work rates greater than 40% $\dot{V}O_2$ max the rise in cardiac output is achieved by increases in heart rate alone (3, 12, 15, 35). The examples presented in figure 9.12 for maximal heart rate, stroke volume, and cardiac output are typical values for a 70-kg active (but not highly trained) college-age male. See table 9.1 for examples of maximal stroke volume and cardiac output for trained men and women.

Maximal cardiac output tends to decrease in a linear fashion in both men and women after thirty years of age (15, 17). This is primarily due to a decrease in maximal heart rate with age (15). For example, since cardiac output equals heart rate times stroke volume, any decrease in heart rate would result in a decrease in cardiac output. The decrease in maximal heart rate with age can be estimated by the following formula:

$$\text{Max HR} = 220 - \text{age (years)}$$

According to this formula, a twenty-year-old subject might have a maximal heart rate of 200 beats per minute (220 − 20 = 200), whereas a fifty-year-old would have a maximal heart rate of 170 beats per minute (220 − 50 = 170). However, this is only an estimate and values can be actually 20 beats $\cdot$ min^{-1} higher or lower.

Changes in Arterial-Mixed Venous O_2 Content during Exercise

Note in figure 9.12 the change in the arterial-mixed venous oxygen difference (a-$\bar{v}$ O_2 diff) that occurs during exercise. The a-$\bar{v}$ O_2 difference represents the amount of O_2 that is taken up from 100 ml of blood by the tissues during one trip around the systemic circuit. An increase in the a-$\bar{v}$ O_2 difference during exercise is due to an increase in the amount of O_2 taken up and used for the oxidative production of ATP by skeletal muscle. The relationship between cardiac output ($\dot{Q}$), a-$\bar{v}$ O_2 diff, and oxygen uptake is given by the Fick equation:

$$\dot{V}O_2 = \dot{Q} \times (\text{a-}\bar{v}\ O_2\ \text{diff})$$

Simply stated, the Fick equation says that $\dot{V}O_2$ is equal to the product of cardiac output and the a-$\bar{v}$ O_2 diff. This means that an increase in either cardiac output or a-$\bar{v}$ O_2 diff would elevate $\dot{V}O_2$.

Redistribution of Blood Flow during Exercise

In order to meet the increased oxygen demand of the skeletal muscles during exercise it is necessary to increase muscle blood flow while at the same time reducing blood flow to less-active organs such as the liver, kidneys, and GI tract. Figure 9.13 points out that the change in blood flow to muscle and the splanchnic (pertaining to the viscera) circulation is dictated by the exercise intensity (metabolic rate). That is, the increase in muscle blood flow during exercise and the decrease in splanchnic blood flow change as a linear function of % $\dot{V}O_2$ max (35, 36).

Figure 9.14 illustrates the change in blood flow to various organ systems between resting conditions and during maximal exercise. Several important points need to be stressed. First, note that at rest, approximately 15%–20% of total cardiac output is directed toward skeletal muscle (3, 13, 36). However, during maximal exercise 80%–85% of total cardiac output goes to contracting skeletal muscle (27, 36, 42). This is necessary to meet the huge increase in muscle oxygen requirements during intense exercise. Second, notice that during heavy exercise the percent of total cardiac output that goes to the brain is reduced when compared to rest. However, the absolute amount of blood

Figure 9.12 Changes in blood pressure, stroke volume, cardiac output, heart rate, and the arterial-mixed venous oxygen difference as a function of relative work rates. See text for details.

Figure constructed from data from L. Rowell, "Human Cardiovascular Adjustments to Exercise and Thermal Stress," in *Physiological Reviews*, 54:75–159, 1974. Copyright © 1974 American Physiological Society, Bethesda, MD., and L. Rowell, *Human Circulation Regulation During Physical Stress*. Copyright © 1986 Oxford University Press, New York, NY.

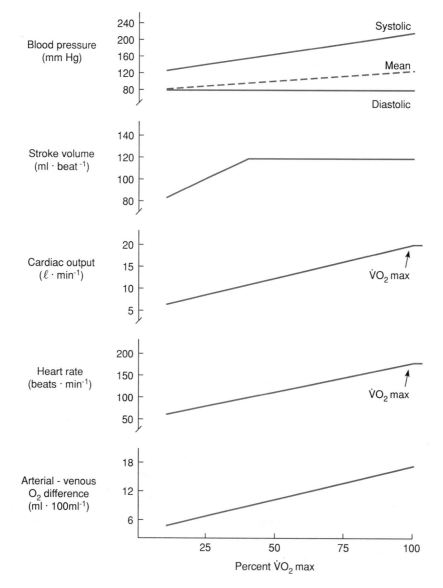

Figure 9.13 Changes in muscle and splanchnic blood flow as a function of exercise intensity. Notice the large increase in muscle blood flow as the work rate increases.

Figure constructed from data from L. Rowell, *Human Circulation Regulation During Physical Stress.* Copyright © 1986 Oxford University Press, New York, NY.

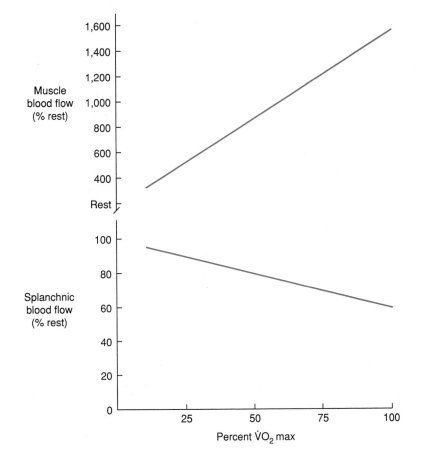

that reaches the brain is slightly increased above resting values (46). Further, although the percentage of total cardiac output that reaches the myocardium is the same during maximal exercise as it is at rest, the total coronary blood flow is increased due to the increase in cardiac output during heavy exercise. Finally, note the reduction in blood flow to the abdominal organs that occurs during exercise when compared to resting conditions.

Regulation of Local Blood Flow during Exercise

What regulates blood flow to various organs during exercise? Muscle as well as other body tissues have the unique ability to regulate their own blood flow in direct proportion to their metabolic needs. Blood flow to skeletal muscle during exercise is regulated in the following way. First, the arterioles in skeletal muscle have a high vascular resistance at rest. This is due to adrenergic sympathetic stimulation, which causes arteriole smooth muscle to contract (vasoconstriction). This

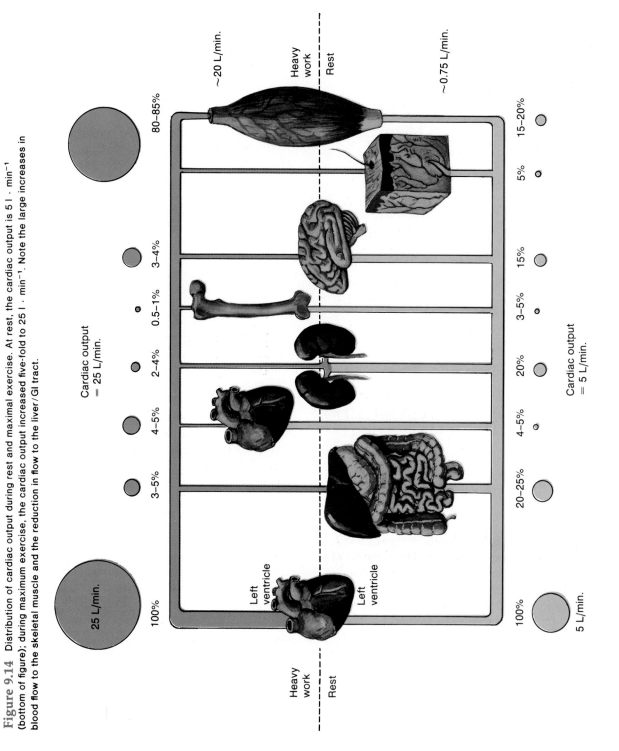

Figure 9.14 Distribution of cardiac output during rest and maximal exercise. At rest, the cardiac output is 5 l · min⁻¹ (bottom of figure); during maximum exercise, the cardiac output increased five-fold to 25 l · min⁻¹. Note the large increases in blood flow to the skeletal muscle and the reduction in blood flow to the liver/GI tract.

produces a relatively low blood flow to muscle at rest (4–5 ml per minute per 100 grams of muscle), but because muscles have a large mass, this accounts for 20%–25% of total blood flow from the heart.

Although controversy exists, it is speculated that at the beginning of exercise, the initial skeletal muscle vasodilation that occurs is due to a withdrawal of sympathetic outflow to arterioles in the working muscles. This initial vasodilation serves to "prime" the skeletal muscle for action. However, as the exercise progresses, vasodilation is maintained and increased by intrinsic metabolic control. This latter type of blood flow regulation is termed **autoregulation,** and is thought to be the most important factor in regulating blood flow to muscle during exercise. The high metabolic rate of skeletal muscle during exercise causes local changes such as decreases in oxygen tension, increases in CO_2 tension, extracellular potassium and adenosine concentrations, and a decrease in pH (increase in acidity). These local changes work together to cause vasodilation of arterioles feeding the contracting skeletal muscle (27, 42). Vasodilation reduces the vascular resistance and therefore increases blood flow. As a result of these changes, blood delivery to contracting skeletal muscle during heavy exercise may rise fifteen-to-twenty times above rest (3, 4, 13, 40). Further, arteriole vasodilation is combined with "recruitment" of capillaries in skeletal muscle. At rest, only 5%–10% of the capillaries in skeletal muscle are open at any one time; however, during intense exercise almost all of the capillaries in contracting muscle may be open (13, 36).

While the vascular resistance in skeletal muscle decreases during exercise, vascular resistance to flow in the visceral organs increases. This occurs due to an increased adrenergic sympathetic output to these organs, which is regulated by the cardiovascular control center. As a result of the reduction in visceral vasodilation during exercise (i.e., resistance increases), blood flow to the viscera may decrease to only 20%–30% of resting values (36, 37).

Circulatory Responses to Exercise

The changes in heart rate and blood pressure that occur during exercise reflect the type and intensity of exercise performed, the duration of exercise, and the environmental conditions under which the work was performed. For example, heart rate and blood pressure, at any given oxygen uptake, are higher during arm work when compared to leg work. Further, exercise in a hot/humid condition results in higher heart rates when compared to the same exercise in a cool environment. The next several sections discuss the cardiovascular responses to exercise under varying conditions.

Emotional Influence
Submaximal exercise in an emotionally charged atmosphere results in higher heart rates and blood pressures when compared to the same work in a psychologically "neutral" environment (3, 41). If the exercise is maximal (e.g., 400-meter dash), high emotion elevates the pre-exercise heart rate and blood pressure but does not generally alter the peak heart rate or blood pressure observed during the exercise itself.

Transition from Rest to Exercise
At the beginning of exercise there is a rapid increase in heart rate, stroke volume, and cardiac output. It has been demonstrated that heart rate and cardiac output begin to increase within the first second after muscular contraction begins (41) (see figure 9.15). If the work rate is constant and below the lactate threshold, a steady state plateau in heart rate, stroke volume, and cardiac output is reached within two-to-three minutes. This response is similar to that observed in oxygen uptake at the beginning of exercise (chapter 4).

Recovery from Exercise
Recovery from short-term, low-intensity exercise is generally rapid. This is illustrated in figure 9.15. Notice that heart rate, stroke volume, and cardiac output all decrease rapidly back toward resting levels following

Figure 9.15 Changes in cardiac output, stroke volume, and heart rate during the transition from rest to submaximal constant intensity exercise and during recovery. See text for discussion.

Figure constructed from data from L. Rowell, "Human Cardiovascular Adjustments to Exercise and Thermal Stress," in *Physiological Reviews*, 54:75–159, 1974. Copyright © 1974 American Physiological Society, Bethesda, MD., and L. Rowell, *Human Circulation Regulation During Physical Stress*. Copyright © 1986 Oxford University Press, New York, NY.

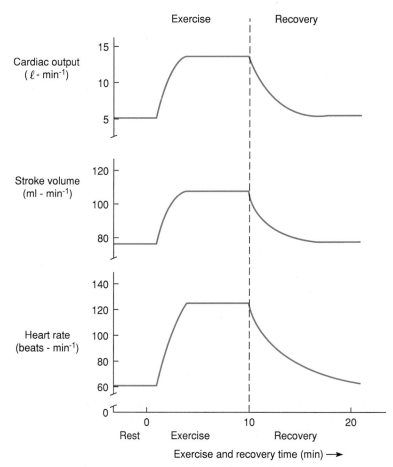

this type of exercise. Recovery speed varies from individual to individual, with well-conditioned subjects demonstrating better recuperative powers than untrained subjects. In regard to recovery heart rates, note that the slopes of heart-rate decay following exercise are generally the same for trained and untrained subjects. However, trained subjects recover faster following exercise since they don't achieve as high a heart rate as untrained subjects during a particular exercise.

Recovery from long-term exercise is much slower than the response depicted in figure 9.15. This is particularly true when the exercise was performed in hot/humid conditions, since an elevated body temperature delays the fall in heart rate during recovery from exercise (39).

Figure 9.16 Comparison of mean arterial blood pressures and heart rate during submaximal rhythmic arm and leg exercise.

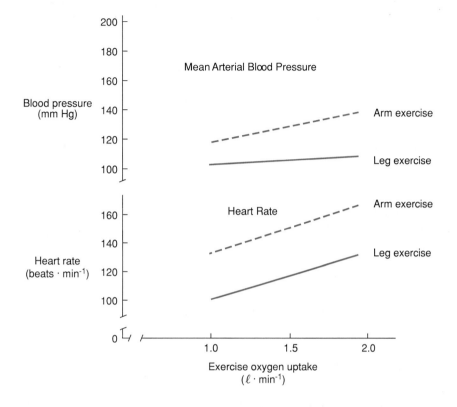

Incremental Exercise

The cardiovascular responses to incremental exercise are illustrated in figure 9.12. Heart rate and cardiac output increase in direct proportion to oxygen uptake. Further, blood flow to muscle increases as a function of oxygen uptake (figure 9.13). This insures that as the need to synthesize ATP to supply the energy for muscular contraction increases, the supply of O_2 reaching the muscle rises. However, both cardiac output and heart rate reach a plateau at 100 percent $\dot{V}O_2$ max (figure 9.12). This point represents a maximal ceiling for oxygen transport to exercising skeletal muscles, and is thought to occur simultaneously with the attainment of maximal oxygen uptake.

The increase in cardiac output during incremental exercise is achieved via a decrease in vascular resistance to flow and an increase in mean arterial blood pressure. The elevation in mean arterial blood pressure during exercise is due to an increase in systolic pressure, since diastolic pressure remains fairly constant during incremental work (figure 9.12).

Arm versus Leg Exercise

As mentioned earlier, at any given level of oxygen consumption, both heart rate and blood pressure are higher during arm work when compared to leg work (1, 2, 10, 25, 29, 34) (see figure 9.16). The explanation for the higher heart rate seems to be linked to a greater sympathetic outflow to the heart during arm work when compared to leg exercise (3). Additionally, isometric exercise also increases the heart rate above the expected value based on relative oxygen consumption (1, 2, 4, 21, 23, 25).

The relatively large increase in blood pressure for arm work is due to a vasoconstriction in the inactive muscle groups (3). For example, the larger the muscle group (e.g., legs) involved in performing the exercise, the more resistance vessels (arterioles) that are dilated. Therefore, this lower peripheral resistance is reflected in lower blood pressure (since cardiac output × resistance = mean pressure).

Intermittent Exercise

If exercise is discontinuous (e.g., interval training), the extent of the recovery of heart rate and blood pressure between bouts depends on the level of subject fitness, environmental conditions (temperature, humidity), and the duration and intensity of the exercise. With a relatively light effort in a cool environment, there is generally complete recovery between exercise bouts within several minutes. However, if the exercise is intense or the work is performed in a hot/humid environment, there is a cumulative increase in heart rate between efforts and thus recovery is not complete (40). The practical consequence of performing repeated bouts of light exercise is that many repetitions can be performed. In contrast, the nature of high-intensity exercise dictates that a limited number of efforts can be tolerated.

Prolonged Exercise

Figure 9.17 illustrates the change in heart rate, stroke volume, and cardiac output that occurs during prolonged exercise at a constant work rate. Note that cardiac output is maintained at a constant level throughout the duration of the exercise, however, stroke volume declines while heart rate increases (4, 7, 18, 24, 31, 37, 39, 40). Close examination of figure 9.17 demonstrates that the ability to maintain a constant cardiac output in the face of declining stroke volume is due to the increase in heart rate being equal in magnitude to the decline in stroke volume.

The increase in heart rate and decrease in stroke volume observed during prolonged exercise is often referred to as "cardiovascular drift" and is due to the influence of rising body temperature and dehydration (reduction in plasma volume) on venous return to the heart (see chapters 12 and 24). If prolonged exercise is performed in a hot/humid environment, the increase in heart rate and decrease in stroke volume is exaggerated even more than depicted in figure 9.17 (32, 33). In fact, it is not surprising to find near-maximal heart rates during submaximal exercise in the heat. For example, it has been demonstrated that during a 2.5-hour marathon race at a work rate of 70%–75% $\dot{V}O_2$ max, maximal heart rates may be maintained during the last hour of the race (11).

Regulation of Cardiovascular Adjustments to Exercise

The cardiovascular adjustments at the beginning of exercise are rapid. Within one second after the commencement of muscular contraction there is a withdrawal of vagal outflow to the heart, which is followed by an increase in sympathetic stimulation of the heart (36). At the same time there is a vasodilation of arterioles in active skeletal muscles and a reflexic increase in the resistance of vessels in less-active areas. The end result is an increase in cardiac output to insure that blood flow to muscle is matched to the metabolic needs (see figure 9.18). What is the signal to "turn on" the cardiovascular system at the onset of exercise? This question has puzzled physiologists for nearly 100 years. At present, a complete answer is not available. However, recent advances in understanding cardiovascular control has led to the development of the "central command theory" (5, 8, 9, 29, 43).

The term **central command** refers to a motor signal developed within the brain. The central command theory of cardiovascular control argues that the initial cardiovascular changes at the beginning of exercise are due to centrally generated cardiovascular motor signals, which set the general pattern of the cardiovascular response. However, it is commonly believed that cardiovascular activity can be and is modified by muscle chemoreceptors, muscle mechanoreceptors, and pressure-sensitive receptors (baroreceptors) located within the carotid arteries and the aortic arch. Muscle chemoreceptors are sensitive to increases in muscle metabolites (e.g., potassium, lactic acid, etc.) and send messages to higher brain centers to "fine-tune" the cardiovascular responses to exercise (6, 14, 20–28, 30). This is called "peripheral feedback."

Figure 9.17 Changes in cardiac output, stroke volume, and heart rate during prolonged exercise at a constant intensity. Notice that cardiac output is maintained by an increase in heart rate to offset the fall in stroke volume that occurs during this type of work.

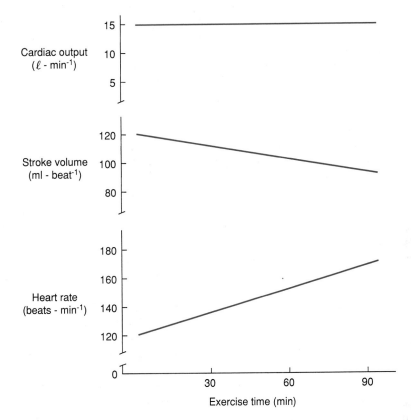

Figure 9.18 A summary of cardiovascular adaptations to exercise.

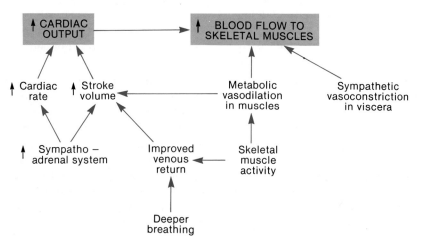

Figure 9.19 A summary of cardiovascular control during exercise. See text for discussion.

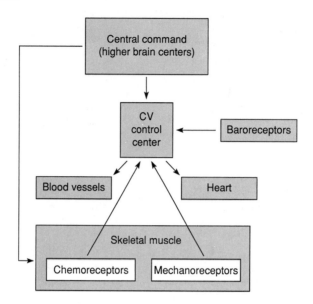

Muscle mechanoreceptors (e.g., muscle spindles, Golgi tendon organs) are sensitive to the force and speed of muscular movement. These receptors, like muscle chemoreceptors, send information to higher brain centers to aid in modification of the cardiovascular responses to a given exercise task (36, 38).

Finally, baroreceptors, which are sensitive to changes in arterial blood pressure, may also send afferent information back to the cardiovascular control center to add precision to the cardiovascular activity during exercise. These pressure receptors are important since they regulate arterial blood pressure around an elevated systemic pressure during exercise (36, 38).

In summary, the central command theory proposes that the initial signal to the cardiovascular system at the beginning of exercise comes from higher brain centers. However, fine-tuning of the cardiovascular response to a given exercise test is accomplished via a series of feedback loops from muscle chemoreceptors, muscle mechanoreceptors, and arterial baroreceptors (see figure 9.19). The fact that there appears to be some overlap between these three feedback systems during submaximal exercise suggests that redundancy

in cardiovascular control exists (36, 38). This is not surprising considering the importance of matching blood flow to the metabolic needs of exercising skeletal muscle. Whether or not one or many of these feedback loops becomes more important during heavy exercise is not presently known and poses an interesting question for future research.

Summary

1. The purposes of the cardiovascular system are: (1) transport of O_2 tissues and removal of wastes, (2) transport of nutrients to tissues, and (3) the regulation of body temperature.
2. The heart is two pumps in one. The right side of the heart pumps blood through the pulmonary circulation while the left side of the heart delivers blood to the systemic circulation.
3. The pacemaker of the heart is the SA node. SA node activity is modified by the parasympathetic nervous system (slows HR) and the sympathetic nervous system (increases HR).

4. Cardiac output is the product of heart rate and stroke volume ($\dot{Q} = HR \times SV$). Heart rate increases at the beginning of exercise due to a withdrawal of parasympathetic tone. At higher work rates the increase in heart rate is achieved via an increased sympathetic outflow to both the SA and AV nodes. Stroke volume is regulated via: (1) end-diastolic volume, (2) aortic blood pressure, and (3) the strength of ventricular contraction.

5. Venous return increases during exercise due to: (1) venoconstriction, (2) the muscle pump, and (3) the respiratory pump.

6. Blood flow through the vascular system is directly proportional to the pressure at the two ends of the system and inversely proportional to resistance:

$$\text{Blood flow} = \frac{\Delta \text{ Pressure}}{\text{Resistance}}$$

7. The most important factor determining resistance to blood flow is the radius of the blood vessel. The relationship between vessel radius, vessel length, blood viscosity, and flow is:

$$\text{Resistance} = \frac{\text{Length} \times \text{viscosity}}{\text{Radius}^4}$$

8. Oxygen delivery to exercising skeletal muscle increases due to: (1) an increased cardiac output, and (2) a redistribution of blood flow from inactive organs to the contracting skeletal muscles.

9. Cardiac output increases as a linear function of oxygen uptake during exercise. During exercise in the upright position, stroke volume reaches a plateau at approximately 40% of $\dot{V}O_2$ max; therefore, at work rates above 40% $\dot{V}O_2$ max the rise in cardiac output is due to increases in heart rate alone.

10. The changes in heart rate and blood pressure that occur during exercise are a function of the type and intensity of exercise performed, the duration of exercise, and the environmental conditions.

11. The "central command theory" of cardiovascular control during exercise proposes that the initial signal to "drive" the cardiovascular system at the beginning of exercise comes from higher brain centers. However, the cardiovascular response to a given exercise task is fine-tuned by feedback from muscle chemoreceptors, muscle mechanoreceptors, and arterial baroreceptors to the cardiovascular control center.

Study Questions

1. What are the major purposes of the cardiovascular system?
2. Briefly, outline the design of the heart. Why is the heart often called "two pumps in one"?
3. Outline the cardiac cycle and the associated electrical activity recorded via the electrocardiogram.
4. Graph the heart rate, stroke volume, and cardiac output response to incremental exercise.
5. What factors regulate heart rate during exercise? Stroke volume?
6. How does exercise influence venous return?
7. What factors determine local blood flow during exercise?
8. Graph the changes that occur in heart rate, stroke volume, and cardiac output during prolonged exercise. What happens to these variables if the exercise is performed in a hot/humid environment?
9. Compare heart rate and blood pressure responses to arm and leg work at the same oxygen uptake. What factors might explain the observed differences?
10. Explain the central command theory of cardiovascular regulation during exercise.

Suggested Readings

Brengelmann, G. 1983. Circulatory adjustments to exercise and heat stress. *Annual Review of Physiology* 45:191–212.

Fox, E., R. Bowers, and M. Foss. 1988. *Physiological Basis of Physical Education and Athletics*. Philadelphia: W. B. Saunders Company.

Ozolin, P. 1986. Blood flow in the extremities of athletes. *International Journal of Sports Medicine* 7:117–22.

McArdle, W., F. Katch, and V. Katch. 1986. *Exercise Physiology: energy, nutrition, and human performance*. Philadelphia: Lea & Febiger.

Rowell, L. 1986. *Human circulation regulation during physical stress*. New York: Oxford Press.

Weber, K., and J. Janicki. 1986. Cardiopulmonary exercise testing: physiological principles and clinical applications. Philadelphia: W. B. Saunders Company.

References

1. Asmussen, E. 1981. Similarities and dissimilarities between static and dynamic exercise. *Circulation Research* 48 (Suppl. 1):3–10.

2. Astrand, P. et al. 1965. Intra-arterial blood pressure during exercise with different muscle groups. *Journal of Applied Physiology* 20:253–57.

3. Astrand, P., and K. Rodahl. 1986. *Textbook of Work Physiology*. New York: McGraw-Hill.

4. Brengelmann, G. 1983. Circulatory adjustments to exercise and heat stress. *Annual Review of Physiology* 45:191–212.

5. Dormer, J., and H. L. Stone. 1982. Fastigial nucleus and its possible role in the cardiovascular response to exercise. In (O. Smith, R. Galosy, and S. Weiss, eds.) *Circulation, Neurobiology and Behavior*. New York: Elsevier.

6. Duncan, G., R. Johnson, and D. Lambie. 1981. Role of sensory nerves in the cardiovascular and respiratory changes with isometric forearm exercise in man. *Clinical Science* 60:145–55.

7. Ekelund, L., and A. Holmgren. 1964. Circulatory and respiratory adaptation during long-term, non-steady state exercise, in the sitting position. *Acta Physiologica Scandanavica* 62:240–55.

8. Eldridge, F., D. Milhorn, and T. Waldrop. 1981. Exercise hyperpnea and locomotion: parallel activation from the hypothalamus. *Science* 211:844–46.

9. Eldridge, F. et al. 1985. Stimulation by central command of locomotion, respiration, and circulation during exercise. *Respiratory Physiology* 59:313–37.

10. Eston, R., and D. Brodie. 1986. Responses to arm and leg ergometry. *British Journal of Sports Medicine* 20:4–6.

11. Fox, E., and D. Costill. 1972. Estimated cardiorespiratory responses during marathon running. *Archives of Environmental Health* 24:315–24.

12. Fox, E., R. Bowers, and M. Foss. 1988. *Physiological Basis of Physical Education and Athletics*. Philadelphia: W. B. Saunders Company.

13. Fox, S. 1987. *Human Physiology*. Dubuque, Ia.: Wm. C. Brown.

14. Freund, P., S. Hobbs, and L. Rowell. 1978. Cardiovascular responses to muscle ischemia in man—dependency on muscle mass. *Journal of Applied Physiology* 45:762–67.

15. Gerstenblith, G., D. Renlund, and E. Lakatta. 1987. Cardiovascular response to exercise in younger and older men. *Federation Proceedings* 46:1834–39.

16. Guyton, A. 1986. *Textbook of Medical Physiology*. Philadelphia: W. B. Saunders Company.

17. Hagberg, J. 1987. Effect of training on the decline of $\dot{V}O_2$ max with aging. *Federation Proceedings* 46:1830–33.

18. Hartley, L. 1977. Central circulatory function during prolonged exercise. *Annals of New York Academy of Sciences* 301:189–94.

19. Hole, J. 1987. *Human Anatomy and Physiology*. Dubuque, Ia.: Wm. C. Brown.

20. Johansson, B. 1962. Circulatory responses to stimulation of somatic afferents. *Acta Physiologica Scandanavica* (Suppl. 198):1–91.

21. Kaufman, M. et al. 1983. Effects of static muscular contraction on impulse activity of groups III and IV afferents in cats. *Journal of Applied Physiology* 55:105–12.

22. Kaufman, M. et al. 1984. Effect of ischemia on responses of group III and IV afferents to contraction. *Journal of Applied Physiology* 57:644–50.

23. Kaufman, M. et al. 1984. Effects of static and rhythmic twitch contractions on the discharge of group III and IV muscle afferents. *Cardiovascular Research* 18:663–68.

24. Kenny, W. L. 1988. Control of heat-induced cutaneous vasodilation in relation to age. *European Journal of Applied Physiology* 57:120–25.

25. Kilbom, A., and T. Brunkin. 1976. Circulatory effects of isometric muscle contractions, performed separately and in combination with dynamic exercise. *European Journal of Applied Physiology* 36:7–27.

26. Kniffki, K., S. Mense, and R. Schmidt. 1981. Muscle receptors with fine afferent fibers which may evoke circulatory reflexes. *Circulation Research* 48 (Suppl. 1):25–31.

27. Laughlin, M. H., and R. Korthius. 1987. Control of muscle blood flow during sustained physiological exercise. *Canadian Journal of Applied Sports Sciences* 12 (Suppl.):775–835.

28. McCloskey, D., and J. Mitchell. 1972. Reflex cardiovascular and respiratory responses originating in exercising muscle. *Journal of Physiology* (London) 224:173–86.

29. Mitchell, J. et al. 1980. The role of muscle mass in the cardiovascular response to static contraction. *Journal of Physiology* (London) 309:45–54.

30. Paterson, D., and A. Morton. 1986. Maximal aerobic power, ventilatory and respiratory compensation thresholds during arm cranking and bicycle ergometry. *Australian Journal of Science and Medicine in Sport* 18:11–15.

31. Powers, S., E. Howley, and R. Cox. 1982. Ventilatory and metabolic responses to heat stress during prolonged exercise. *Journal of Sports Medicine and Physical Fitness* 22:32–36.

32. ———. 1982. A differential catecholamine response to prolonged exercise and passive heating. *Medicine and Science in Sports* 14:435–39.

33. Ridge, B., and F. Pyke. 1986. Physiological responses to combinations of exercise and sauna. *Australian Journal of Science and Medicine in Sports.* 18:25–28.

34. Rosiello, R., D. Mahler, and J. Ward. 1987. Cardiovascular responses to rowing. *Medicine and Science in Sports and Exercise* 19:239–45.

35. Rowell, L. 1974. Human cardiovascular adjustments to exercise and thermal stress. *Physiological Reviews* 54:75–159.

36. ———. 1986. *Human Circulation Regulation during Physical Stress.* New York: Oxford Press.

37. Rowell, L., L. Hermansen, and J. Blackmon. 1976. Human cardiovascular and respiratory responses to graded muscle ischemia. *Journal of Applied Physiology* 41:693–701.

38. Rowell, L. 1980. What signals govern the cardiovascular response to exercise? *Medicine and Science in Sports and Exercise* 12:307–15.

39. Rubin, S. 1987. Core temperature regulation of heart rate during exercise in humans. *Journal of Applied Physiology* 62:1997–2002.

40. Sawka, M., R. Knowlton, and J. Critz. 1979. Thermal and circulatory responses to repeated bouts of prolonged running. *Medicine and Science in Sports* 11:177–80.

41. Shephard, R. 1981. *Physiology and Biochemistry of Exercise.* New York: Praeger.

42. Sjogaard, G., G. Sauard, and C. Juel. 1988. Muscle blood flow during isometric activity and its relation to muscle fatigue. *European Journal of Applied Physiology* 57:327–35.

43. Smith, O., R. Rushmer, and E. Lasher. 1960. Similarity of cardiovascular responses to exercise and to diencephalic stimulation. *American Journal of Physiology* 198:1139–42.

44. Tibes, V. 1977. Reflex inputs to the cardiovascular and respiratory centers from dynamically working canine muscles. *Circulation Research* 41:332–41.

45. Wyss, C. et al. 1983. Cardiovascular responses to graded reductions in hindlimb perfusion in exercising dogs. *American Journal of Physiology* 245: H481–H486.

46. Zobl, E. et al. 1965. Effect of exercise on the cerebral circulation and metabolism. *Journal of Applied Physiology* 20:1289–93.

10 Respiration during Exercise

Objectives

*B*y studying this chapter, you should be able to do the following:

1. Explain the principal physiological function of the pulmonary system.
2. Outline the major anatomical components that make up the respiratory system.
3. List the major muscles involved in inspiration and expiration at rest and during exercise.
4. Discuss the importance of matching blood flow to alveolar ventilation in the lung.
5. Explain how gases are transported across the blood-gas interface in the lung.
6. Discuss the major transportation modes of O_2 and CO_2 in the blood.
7. Discuss the effects of increasing temperature, decreasing pH, and increasing levels of 2-3 DPG on the oxygen-hemoglobin dissociation curve.
8. Describe the ventilatory response to constant load steady state exercise. What happens to ventilation if the exercise is prolonged and performed in a high-temperature/humid environment?
9. Describe the ventilatory response to incremental exercise. What factors are thought to contribute to the alinear rise in ventilation at work rates above 50%–70% of $\dot{V}O_2$ max?
10. Identify the location and function of chemoreceptors and mechanoreceptors that are thought to play a role in the regulation of breathing.
11. Discuss the neural-humoral theory of respiratory control during exercise.

Outline

Key Terms

alveoli

anatomical dead space

aortic bodies

alveolar ventilation ($\dot{V}_A$)

Bohr effect

bulk flow

carotid bodies

deoxyhemoglobin

diaphragm

diffusion

external respiration

hemoglobin

internal respiration

myoglobin

oxyhemoglobin

partial pressure

pleura

residual volume (RV)

respiration

spirometry

tidal volume

total lung capacity (TLC)

ventilation

ventilatory threshold (Tvent)

vital capacity (VC)

The word **respiration** can be divided into two separate but related subdivisions: (1) **external respiration** and (2) **internal respiration.** External respiration refers to ventilation (breathing) and the exchange of gases (O_2 and CO_2) in the lungs. Internal respiration relates to O_2 utilization and CO_2 production by the tissues. This chapter will be concerned with external respiration, and the term "respiration" will be used in the text as a synonym for external respiration. Since the respiratory, or pulmonary, system plays a key role in maintaining blood-gas homeostasis (i.e., O_2 and CO_2 tensions) during exercise, an understanding of lung function during work is important for the student of exercise physiology. It is the purpose of this chapter to discuss the design and function of the respiratory system during exercise.

Function of the Lung

The primary purpose of the respiratory system is to provide a means of gas exchange between the external environment and the body. That is, the respiratory system provides the individual with a means of replacing O_2 and removing CO_2 from the blood. The exchange of O_2 and CO_2 between the lung and blood occurs as a result of ventilation and diffusion. The term **ventilation** refers to the mechanical process of moving air into and out of the lungs. **Diffusion** is the random movement of molecules from an area of high concentration to an area of lower concentration. Since O_2 tension in the lung is greater than that of the blood, O_2 moves from the lungs into the blood. Similarly, the tension of CO_2 in the blood is greater than the tension of CO_2 in the lungs, and thus CO_2 moves from the blood into the lung and is expired. Diffusion in the respiratory system occurs rapidly because there is a large surface area within the lungs and a very short diffusion distance between blood and gas in the lungs. The fact that the O_2 and CO_2 tension in the blood leaving the lung is almost in complete equilibrium with the O_2 and CO_2 tension found within the lung is testimony to the high efficiency of normal lung function.

The respiratory system also plays an important role in regulation of the acid-base balance during exercise (see chapter 11). Additionally, the lung filters toxic materials from the circulation and acts as a reservoir for blood.

Structure of the Respiratory System

The human respiratory system consists of a group of passages that filter air and transport it into the lungs where gas exchange occurs within microscopic air sacs called **alveoli.** The major components of the respiratory system are pictured in figure 10.1. The organs of the respiratory system include the nose, nasal cavity, pharynx, larynx, trachea, bronchial tree, and the lungs themselves. The anatomical position of the lungs relative to the major muscle of inspiration, the diaphragm, is pictured in figure 10.2. Note that both the right and left lungs are enclosed by a set of membranes called **pleura.** The visceral pleura adheres to the outer surface of the lung, whereas the parietal pleura lines the thoracic walls and the diaphragm. These two pleura are separated by a thin layer of fluid that acts as a lubricant, allowing a gliding action of one pleura on the other. The pressure in the pleural cavity (intrapleural pressure) is less than atmospheric and becomes even lower during inspiration, causing air

Figure 10.1 Major organs of the respiratory system.

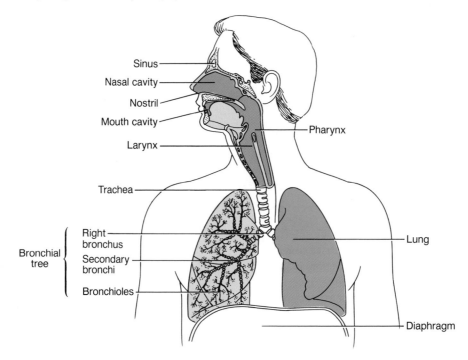

to inflate the lungs. The fact that intrapleural pressure is less than atmospheric is important since it prevents the collapse of the fragile air sacs within the lungs. More will be said about this later.

Conducting Zone

The air passages of the respiratory system are divided into two functional zones: (1) the conducting zone and (2) the respiratory zone (see figure 10.3). The conducting zone includes all those anatomical structures (e.g., trachea, bronchial tree, bronchioles) that air passes through en route to the respiratory zone. The region of the lung where gas exchange occurs is labeled as the respiratory zone and includes the respiratory bronchioles and alveolar sacs. Respiratory bronchioles are included in this region since they contain small clusters of alveoli.

Air enters the trachea from the pharynx (throat), which receives air from both the nasal and oral cavities. In general, humans breathe through the nose until ventilation is increased to approximately 20–30 liters per minute where the mouth becomes the primary passageway for air (20). In order for gas to enter or leave the trachea, it must pass through a valvelike opening called the glottis, which is located between the vocal cords.

The conducting zone of the respiratory system serves not only as a passageway for air, but also functions to humidify and filter the air as it moves toward the respiratory zone of the lung. Regardless of the temperature or humidity of the environment, the air that reaches the lung is warmed and is saturated with water vapor (34). This warming and humidification of air serves to protect body temperature and prevents the delicate lung tissue from desiccation (drying out).

Figure 10.2 Position of the lungs, diaphragm, and pleura.

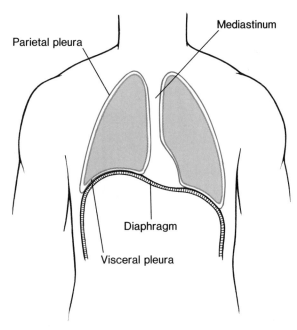

The role of the conducting zone and the respiratory zone in filtration of the inspired gas is critical in order to prevent lung damage due to the collection of inhaled particles in the respiratory zone. These filtration and cleaning processes are achieved via two principal means. First, mucus, secreted by the cells of the conducting zone, serves to trap small inhaled particles. This mucus is moved toward the oral cavity via tiny "fingerlike" projections called cilia. These cilia move in a wavelike fashion, which propels the mucus at a rate of 1–2 centimeters/minute. When a particle becomes trapped in the mucus, it is moved toward the pharynx via ciliary action, where it can be either swallowed or expectorated.

A second means of protecting the lung from foreign particles is by the action of cells called macrophages that reside primarily in the alveoli. These macrophages literally engulf particles that reach the alveoli. The cleansing action of both the cilia and macrophages has been shown to be hindered by cigarette smoke and certain types of air pollution (34).

The trachea branches into two primary bronchi (right and left) that enter each lung. The bronchial tree then branches several more times before forming bronchioles. Bronchioles are small branches of the segmental bronchi, which enter the basic units (lobules) of the lung. The bronchioles then branch several times before they become the alveolar ducts leading to the alveolar sacs (see figure 10.4).

Respiratory Zone

Gas exchange in the lungs occurs across about 300 million tiny (0.25–0.50 mm diameter) alveoli. The enormous number of these structures provides the lung with a large surface area for diffusion. It is estimated that the total surface area available for diffusion in the human lung is 60–80 square meters, or about the size of a tennis court. The rate of diffusion is further assisted by the fact that each alveolus is only one cell-layer thick, so that the total "blood-gas barrier" is only two cell-layers thick (alveolar cell and capillary cell) (see figure 10.5).

Figure 10.3 The conducting zones and respiratory zones of the pulmonary system.

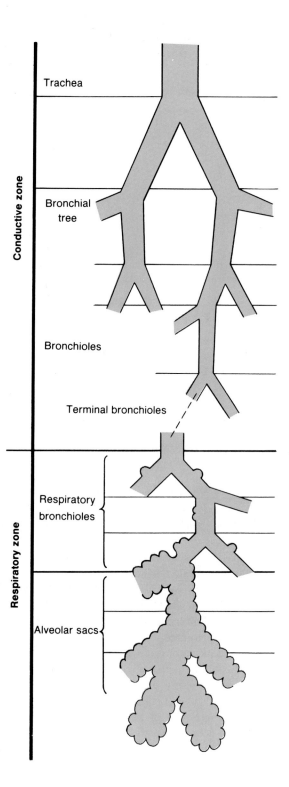

Trachea

Conductive zone

Bronchial tree

Bronchioles

Terminal bronchioles

Respiratory zone

Respiratory bronchioles

Alveolar sacs

Figure 10.4 The bronchial tree consists of the passageways that connect the trachea and the alveoli.

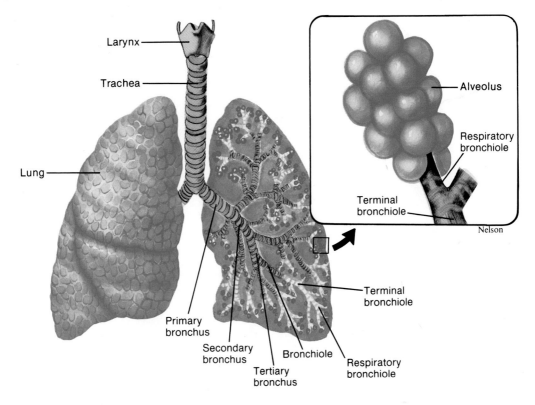

Larynx

Trachea

Lung

Alveolus

Respiratory bronchiole

Terminal bronchiole

Nelson

Primary bronchus

Secondary bronchus

Tertiary bronchus

Bronchiole

Respiratory bronchiole

Terminal bronchiole

Although the 300 million alveoli provide the ideal structure for gas exchange, the fragility of these tiny "bubbles" presents some problems for the lung. For example, because of the surface tension (pressure exerted due to the properties of water) of the liquid lining the alveoli, relatively large forces develop, which tend to collapse alveoli. Fortunately, some of the alveolar cells (called Type II, see figure 10.5) synthesize and release a material called surfactant, which lowers the surface tension of the alveoli and thus prevents their collapse.

Mechanics of Breathing

As previously mentioned, movement of air from the environment to the lungs is called pulmonary ventilation and occurs via a process known as **bulk flow.** Bulk flow refers to the movement of molecules along a passageway due to a pressure difference between the two ends of the passageway. Thus inspiration occurs due to the pressure in the lungs (intrapulmonary) being reduced below atmospheric pressure. Conversely, expiration occurs when the pressure within the lungs exceeds atmospheric pressure. The means by which this pressure change within the lungs is achieved will be discussed within the next several paragraphs.

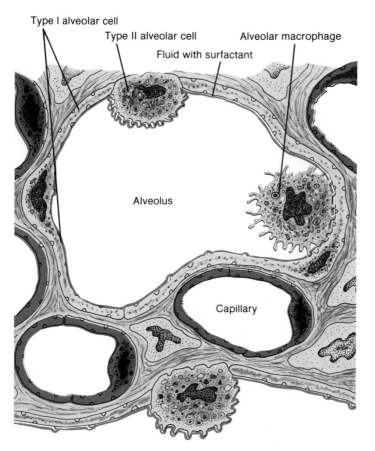

Type I alveolar cell

Type II alveolar cell   Alveolar macrophage

Fluid with surfactant

Alveolus

Capillary

Inspiration

The **diaphragm** is the most important muscle of inspiration (20, 22, 34). This thin dome-shaped muscle inserts into the lower ribs and is innervated by the phrenic nerves. When the diaphragm contracts, it forces the abdominal contents downward and forward. Further, the ribs are lifted outward (see figure 10.6). The outcome of these two actions is to reduce intrapleural pressure, which in turn causes the lungs to expand. This expansion of the lungs results in a reduction in intrapulmonary pressure below atmospheric, which allows airflow into the lungs.

During normal quiet breathing the diaphragm works alone to allow inspiration to occur. However, during exercise, accessory muscles of inspiration are called into play. These include the external intercostal muscles, pectoralis minor, the scalene muscles, and the sternomastoids. Collectively, these muscles assist the diaphragm in increasing the volume of the thorax, which aids in inspiration.

Expiration

Expiration is passive during normal quiet breathing. That is, no muscular effort is necessary for expiration to occur at rest. This is true because the lungs and

Figure 10.6 Diagram showing the action of diaphragm contraction on changing intrapulmonary pressure. The upper figure represents the period at the end of expiration where the diaphragm is relaxed and intrapleural pressure equals atmospheric pressure (i.e., no gas flow). The lower figure depicts the decrease in intrapleural pressure and resulting airflow into the lungs following diaphragm contraction.

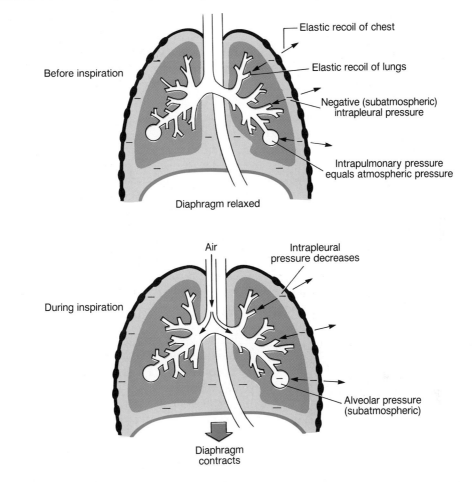

chest walls are elastic and tend to return to equilibrium position after expanding during inspiration. During exercise and voluntary hyperventilation, expiration becomes active. The most important muscles involved in expiration are those found in the abdominal wall which includes the rectus abdominus and the internal oblique. When these muscles contract, the diaphragm is pushed upward and the ribs are pulled downward and inward. This results in an increase in intrapulmonary pressure and expiration occurs.

Airway Resistance

At any given rate of airflow into the lungs, the pressure difference that must be developed depends on the resistance of the airways. Airflow through the airways of the respiratory system can be mathematically defined by the following relationships:

$$\text{Airflow} = \frac{P_1 - P_2}{\text{Resistance}}$$

where $P_1 - P_2$ is the pressure difference at the two ends of the airway, and resistance is the resistance to flow offered by the airway. In simple terms, airflow is increased any time there is an increase in the pressure gradient across the pulmonary system, or if there is a decrease in airway resistance. This same relationship for blood flow was discussed in chapter 9.

What factors contribute to airway resistance? By far the most important variable contributing to airway resistance is the diameter of the airway. Airways that are reduced in size due to disease (chronic obstructive lung disease, asthma, etc.) offer more resistance to flow than healthy, open airways. Recall from chapter 9 that if the radius of a blood vessel (or airway) is reduced by one-half, the resistance to flow is increased sixteen times! Therefore, one can easily understand the effect of obstructive lung diseases (i.e., exercise-induced asthma) on increasing the work of breathing, especially during exercise when pulmonary ventilation is ten to twenty times greater than at rest.

Pulmonary Ventilation

Prior to beginning a discussion of ventilation, it is helpful to define some commonly used pulmonary physiology symbols:

1. V is used to denote volume
2. $\dot{V}$ means volume per unit of time (generally one minute)
3. the subscripts $_{T, D, A, I, E}$ are used to denote tidal, dead space, alveolar, inspired, and expired, respectively.

Pulmonary ventilation refers to the movement of gas into and out of the lungs. The amount of gas ventilated per minute is the product of the frequency of breathing (f) and the amount of gas moved per breath (**tidal volume**):

$$\dot{V} = V_T \times f$$

In a 70-kg man the $\dot{V}$ at rest is generally around 7.5 liters/minute, with a tidal volume of 0.5 liters and a frequency of 15. During maximal exercise ventilation may reach 120–175 liters per minute, with a frequency of 40–50 and a tidal volume of approximately 3–3.5 liters.

It is important to understand that not all of the air that passes the lips reaches the alveolar gas compartment, where gas exchange occurs. Part of each breath remains in conducting airways (trachea, bronchi, etc.) and thus does not participate in gas exchange. This "unused" ventilation is called dead-space ventilation (V_D), and the space it occupies is known as **anatomical dead space.** The volume of inspired gas that reaches the respiratory zone is referred to as **alveolar ventilation ($\dot{V}_A$).** Thus total minute ventilation can be subdivided into dead space ventilation and alveolar ventilation:

$$\dot{V} = \dot{V}_A + \dot{V}_D$$

Note that pulmonary ventilation is not equally distributed throughout the lung. The basal (bottom) region of the lung receives more ventilation than the apex (top region), particularly during quiet breathing (34). This changes to some degree during exercise with the apical (top) regions of the lung receiving an increased percentage of the total ventilation (32).

Pulmonary Volumes and Capacities

Pulmonary volumes can be measured via a technique known as **spirometry.** Using this procedure, the subject breathes in a closed system in which the expired gas is trapped within a plastic or metal bell (spirometer) floating in water. When the subject expires, the bell moves upward, and upon inspiration the bell moves downward. Movements of the bell cause corresponding movements of a recording pen, which traces a record of breathing on a rotating drum recorder (see figure 10.7).

Figure 10.8 is a spirogram showing the measurement of tidal volumes during quiet breathing and the various lung volumes and capacities that are defined in table 10.1. Several of these terms require special mention. First, **vital capacity (VC)** is defined as the maximum amount of gas that can be expired after a maximum inspiration. Secondly, the **residual volume (RV)** is the volume of gas remaining in the lungs after a maximum expiration. Finally, **total lung capacity (TLC)** is defined as the amount of gas in the lungs after a maximum inspiration, and is the sum of the two lung volumes (VC + RV) just mentioned.

Figure 10.7 Photograph of a Collins (9 liter) spirometer used to measure lung volumes and capacities. (Courtesy of Warren E. Collins, Braintree)

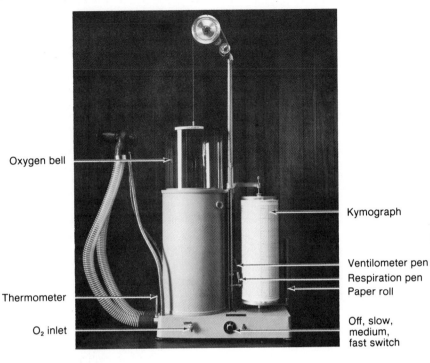

Figure 10.8 A spirogram showing lung volumes and capacities at rest.

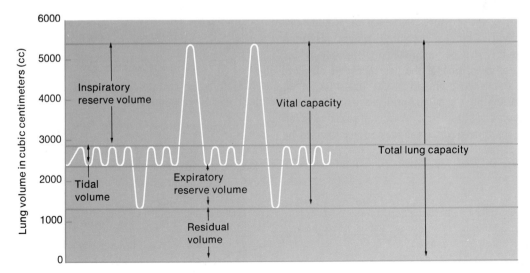

Table 10.1 Definitions of terms used to describe lung volumes and capacities

Term	Definitions
Lung Volumes	
Tidal volume	Volume of gas inspired or expired during unforced respiratory cycle
Inspiratory reserve	The volume of gas that can be inspired at the end of a tidal inspiration
Expiratory reserve	The volume of gas that can be expired at the end of a tidal expiration
Residual volume	The volume of gas left in the lungs after a maximal expiration
Lung Capacities	
Total lung capacity	The total amount of gas in the lungs at the end of a maximal inspiration
Vital capacity	The maximum amount of gas that can be expired after a maximum inspiration
Inspiratory capacity	The maximum amount of gas that can be inspired at the end of a tidal expiration
Functional residual capacity	The amount of gas remaining in the lungs after a normal quiet tidal expiration

Lung volumes are the four nonoverlapping components of the total lung capacity. Lung capacities are the sum of two or more lung volumes.

Diffusion of Gases

Prior to a discussion of diffusion of gases across the alveolar membrane into the blood, it is necessary to introduce the concept of **partial pressure.** According to Dalton's law, the total pressure of a gas mixture is equal to the sum of the pressures that each gas would exert independently. Thus, the pressure that each gas exerts independently can be calculated by multiplying the fractional composition of the gas times the absolute pressure (barometric pressure). Let's consider an example calculating the partial pressure of oxygen in air at sea level. The barometric pressure at sea level is 760 mm Hg (barometric pressure is the force exerted by the weight of the gas contained within the atmosphere). The composition of air is generally considered to be:

Gas	Percentage	Fraction
Oxygen	20.93	.2093
Nitrogen	79.04	.7904
Carbon dioxide	0.03	.0003
Total	100.0	

Therefore the partial pressure of oxygen (PO_2) at sea level can be computed as:

$$PO_2 = 760 \times .2093$$
$$PO_2 = 159 \text{ mm Hg}$$

In a similar manner, the partial pressure of nitrogen can be calculated to be:

$$PN_2 = 760 \times .7904$$
$$PN_2 = 600.7 \text{ mm Hg}$$

Since O_2, CO_2, and N_2 comprise almost 100% of the atmosphere, the total barometric pressure (P) can be computed as:

$$P \text{ (dry atmosphere)} = PO_2 + PN_2 + PCO_2$$

Diffusion of a gas across tissues is described by Fick's law of diffusion, which states that the rate of gas transfer is proportional to the tissue area, the diffusion coefficient of the gas, and the difference in the partial pressure of the gas on the two sides of the tissue, and is inversely proportional to the thickness:

$$V \text{ gas} = \frac{A}{T} \times D \times (P_1 - P_2)$$

where A is the area, T is the thickness of the tissue, D is the diffusion coefficient of the gas, and $P_1 - P_2$ is the difference in the partial pressure between the two sides of the tissue. In simple terms, the rate of diffusion for any single gas is greater when the surface area for diffusion is large and the "driving pressure" between the two sides of the tissue is high. In contrast, an increase in tissue thickness impedes diffusion. The lung is well designed for the diffusion of gases across the alveolar membrane into and out of the blood. First, the total surface area available for diffusion is large. Secondly, the alveolar membrane is extremely thin. The fact that the lung is an ideal organ for gas exchange is important since during maximal exercise the rate of O_2 uptake and CO_2 output may increase twenty to thirty times above that of rest.

The amount of O_2 or CO_2 dissolved in blood obeys Henry's law and is dependent on the temperature of blood, the partial pressure of the gas, and the solubility of the gas. Since the temperature of the blood does not change a great deal (i.e., 1–3° C during exercise), and the solubility of the gas remains constant, the major factor that determines the amount of dissolved gas is the partial pressure.

Figure 10.9 illustrates gas exchange via diffusion across the alveolar-capillary membranes and at the tissue level. Note that the PCO_2 and PO_2 of blood entering the lung are approximately 46 and 40 mm Hg, respectively. In contrast, the PCO_2 and PO_2 in alveolar gas are around 40 and 105 mm Hg, respectively. As a consequence of the difference in partial pressure across the blood-gas interface, CO_2 leaves the blood and diffuses into the alveolus, and O_2 diffuses from the alveolus into the blood. Blood leaving the lung has a PO_2 of approximately 100 mm Hg and a PCO_2 of 40 mm Hg.

Blood Flow to the Lung

The pulmonary circulation begins at the pulmonary artery, which receives venous blood from both the upper and lower body (recall that this is mixed venous blood). Mixed venous blood is then circulated through the pulmonary capillaries where gas exchange occurs, and this oxygenated blood is returned to the heart to be circulated throughout the body (see figure 10.10).

In the adult, the right ventricle of the heart (like the left) has an output of approximately 5 liters/minute. Therefore, the rate of blood flow throughout the pulmonary circulation is equal to that of the systemic circulation. The pressures in the pulmonary circulation are relatively low when compared to those in the systemic circulation (chapter 9). This low-pressure system is due to low vascular resistance in the pulmonary circulation (34). An interesting feature of pulmonary circulation is that during periods of increased pulmonary blood flow during exercise, the resistance in the pulmonary vascular system falls due to distension of vessels and the recruitment of previously unused capillaries. This decrease in pulmonary vascular resistance allows lung blood flow to increase during exercise with relatively small increases in pulmonary arterial pressure.

Figure 10.9 Partial pressures of O_2 (PO_2) and CO_2 (PCO_2) in blood as a result of gas exchange in the lung and gas exchange between capillaries and tissues.

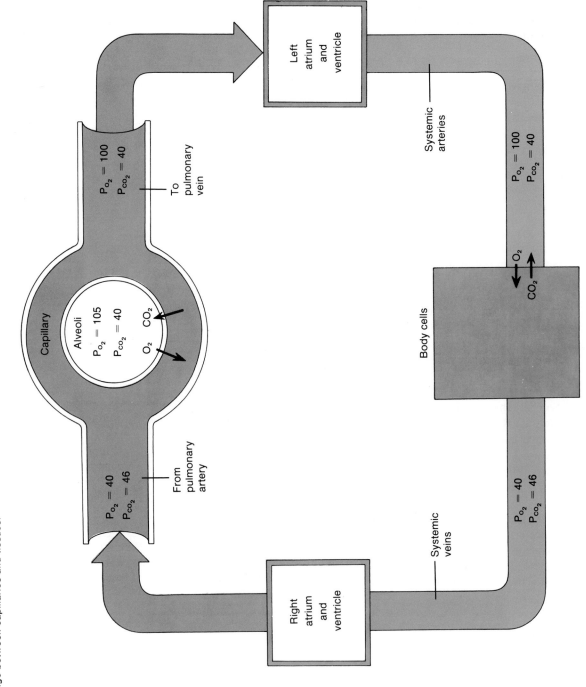

Figure 10.10 The pulmonary circulation is a low-pressure system that pumps mixed venous blood through the pulmonary capillaries for gas exchange. After completion of gas exchange, this oxygenated blood is returned to the left heart to be circulated throughout the body.

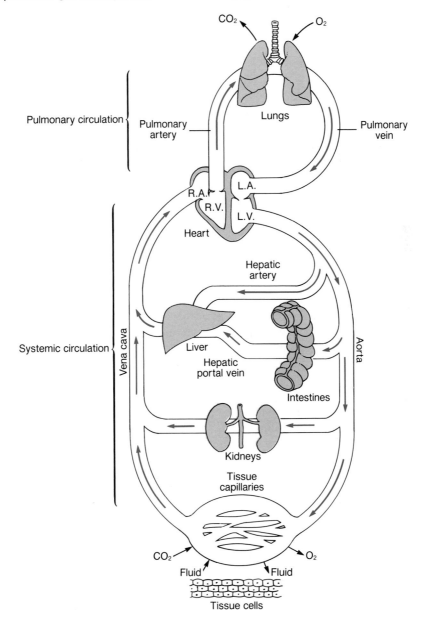

Figure 10.11 Regional blood flow within the lung. Note that there is a linear decrease in blood flow from the lower regions of the lung toward the upper regions.

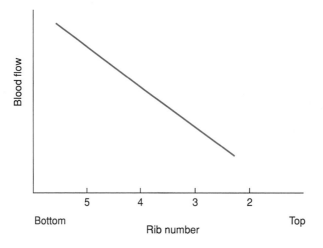

When standing, considerable inequality of blood flow exists within the human lung due to gravity. For example, in the upright position, blood flow decreases almost linearly from bottom to top, reaching very low values at the top (apex) of the lung (see figure 10.11). This distribution may be altered during exercise and with a change in posture. During light exercise, blood flow to the apex of the lung is increased. This is advantageous for improved gas exchange and will be discussed in the next section. When an individual lies supine, blood flow becomes uniform within the lung. In contrast, measurements of blood flow in humans suspended upside-down show that blood flow to the apex of the lung greatly exceeds that found in the base.

Ventilation-Perfusion Relationships

Thus far we have discussed pulmonary ventilation, blood flow to the lungs, and diffusion of gases across the blood-gas barrier in the lung. It seems reasonable to assume that if all these processes were adequate, normal gas exchange would occur in the lung. However, normal gas exchange requires a matching of ventilation to blood flow (perfusion). In other words, an alveolus can be well ventilated, but if blood flow to the alveolus does not adequately match ventilation, normal gas exchange does not occur. Indeed, mismatching of ventilation and perfusion is responsible for most of the problems of gas exchange that occur due to lung diseases.

The ideal ventilation-to-perfusion ratio (V/Q) is 1. That is, there is a one-to-one matching of ventilation to blood flow, which results in optimum gas exchange. Unfortunately, the V/Q ratio is generally not equal to 1 throughout the lung, but varies depending on the section of the lung being considered (22, 34). This concept is illustrated in figure 10.12, where the V/Q ratio at the apex and the base of the lung is calculated for resting conditions.

Let's discuss the (V/Q) ratio in the apex of the lung first. Here the ventilation (at rest) in the upper region of the lung is estimated to be 0.24 liters/minute, while the blood flow is considered to be 0.07 liters/minute. Thus, the V/Q ratio is 3.3 (i.e., 0.24/0.07 = 3.3). A large V/Q ratio represents a disproportionately high ventilation relative to blood flow, which results in poor gas exchange. In contrast, the ventilation at the base of the lung (figure 10.12) is 0.82 liters/minute, with a blood flow of 1.29 liters/minute (V/Q ratio = 0.82/ 1.29 = 0.63). A V/Q ratio less than 1 represents a

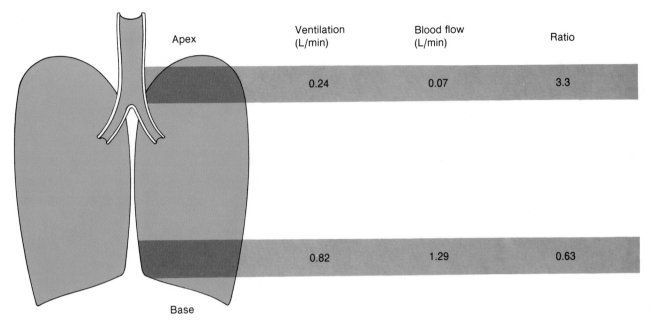

Figure 10.12 The relationship between ventilation and blood flow (ventilation/perfusion ratios) at the top (apex) and the base of the lung. The ratios indicate that the base of the lung is overperfused relative to ventilation and that the apex is underperfused relative to ventilation. This uneven matching of blood flow to ventilation results in less than perfect gas exchange.

Apex	Ventilation (L/min)	Blood flow (L/min)	Ratio
	0.24	0.07	3.3
	0.82	1.29	0.63

Base

greater blood flow than ventilation to the region in question. Although V/Q ratios less than 1 are not indicative of perfect conditions for gas exchange, in most cases V/Q ratios greater than 0.50 are adequate to meet the gas exchange demands at rest.

What effect does exercise have on the V/Q ratio? The complete answer to this question is not currently available. However, it appears that light exercise may improve the V/Q relationship, while heavy exercise results in V/Q inequality, and thus an impairment in gas exchange (32). Whether the increase in V/Q inequality is due to ventilatory inequality or perfusion inequality is not clear. The possible effects of this V/Q mismatch on blood gases will be discussed later in the chapter.

O$_2$ and CO$_2$ Transport in Blood

Although some O$_2$ and CO$_2$ are transported as dissolved gases in the blood, the major portion of O$_2$ and CO$_2$ transported via blood is done by O$_2$ combining with hemoglobin and CO$_2$ being transformed into bicarbonate (HCO$_3^-$). A complete discussion of how O$_2$ and CO$_2$ are transported in blood follows.

Hemoglobin and O$_2$ Transport
Approximately 99% of the O$_2$ transported in the blood is chemically bound to **hemoglobin,** which is a protein pigment contained in the red blood cells (erythrocytes). Each molecule of hemoglobin can transport four O$_2$ molecules. The binding of O$_2$ to hemoglobin forms **oxyhemoglobin,** while hemoglobin that is not bound to O$_2$ is referred to as **deoxyhemoglobin.**

Figure 10.13 The relationship between the partial pressure of O_2 in blood and the relative saturation of hemoglobin with O_2 is pictured here in the oxygen-hemoglobin dissociation curve. Notice the relatively steep portion of the curve up to PO_2 values of 40 mm Hg, after which there is a gradual rise to reach a plateau.

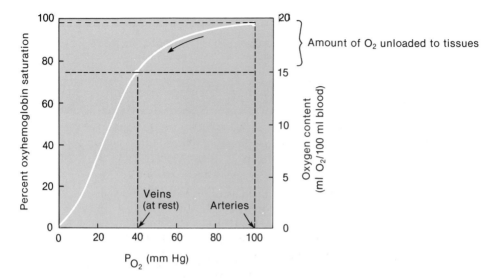

The amount of O_2 that can be transported per unit volume of blood is dependent on the concentration of hemoglobin. Normal hemoglobin concentration for a healthy male and female is approximately 150 grams and 130 grams, respectively, per liter of blood. When completely saturated with O_2, each gram of hemoglobin can transport 1.34 ml of O_2 (34). Therefore, the healthy male and female can transport approximately 201 ml and 174 ml of O_2, respectively, per liter of blood at sea level.

Oxyhemoglobin Dissociation Curve

The combination of O_2 with hemoglobin in the lung (alveolar capillaries) is sometimes referred to as "loading," and the release of O_2 from hemoglobin at the tissues is called "unloading." Loading and unloading is thus a reversible reaction:

$$\text{Deoxyhemoglobin} + O_2 \longleftrightarrow \text{Oxyhemoglobin}$$

The factors that determine the direction of this reaction are (1) the PO_2 of the blood and (2) the affinity or bond strength between hemoglobin and O_2. A high PO_2 drives the reaction to the right, while low PO_2 and a reduced affinity of hemoglobin for O_2 moves the reaction to the left. For example, a high PO_2 in the lungs results in an increase in arterial PO_2 and the formation of oxyhemoglobin. In contrast, a low PO_2 in the tissue results in a decrease of PO_2 in the systemic capillaries, which drives the reaction to the left and thus unloads O_2 to be used by the tissues.

The effect of PO_2 on the combination of O_2 with hemoglobin can be best illustrated by the oxyhemoglobin dissociation curve, which is presented in figure 10.13. This sigmoidal (S shaped) curve has several interesting features. First, the percent hemoglobin saturated with O_2 (% HbO_2) increases sharply up to an arterial PO_2 of 40 mm Hg. At PO_2 values above 40 mm Hg the increase in % HbO_2 rises slowly to a plateau around 90–100 mm Hg, at which the % HbO_2 is approximately 97%. At rest, the body's O_2 requirements are relatively low and only about 25% of the O_2 transported in the blood is unloaded to the tissues. In contrast, during intense exercise the mixed venous PO_2 may reach a value of 18–20 mm Hg, and the tissues may extract up to 90% of the O_2 carried by hemoglobin.

Figure 10.14 The effect of changing blood pH on the shape of the oxygen-hemoglobin dissociation curve. A decrease in pH results in a rightward shift of the curve (Bohr effect), while an increase in pH results in a leftward shift of the curve.

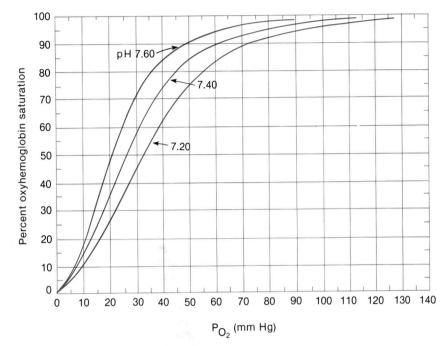

The shape of the oxyhemoglobin dissociation curve is well designed to meet human O_2 transport needs. The relatively flat portion of the curve (above a PO_2 of approximately 90 mm Hg) allows arterial PO_2 to oscillate from 90–100 mm Hg without a large drop in % HbO_2. This is important since there is a decline in arterial PO_2 with aging and upon ascent to altitude. At the other end of the curve (steep portion, 0–40 mm Hg), small changes in PO_2 result in a release of large amounts of O_2 from hemoglobin. This is critical during exercise where tissue O_2 consumption is high.

Effect of pH on O_2-Hb Dissociation Curve

In addition to the effect of blood PO_2 on O_2 binding to hemoglobin, a change in acidity, temperature, or red blood cell (RBC) levels of 2,3-diphosphoglyceric acid (2-3 DPG) can affect the loading/unloading reaction. First, let's consider the effect of changing blood acid-base status on hemoglobin's affinity for O_2. The strength of the bond between O_2 and hemoglobin is weakened by a decrease in blood pH (increased acidity), which results in increased unloading of O_2 to the tissues. This is represented by a "right" shift in the oxyhemoglobin curve and is called the **Bohr effect** (see figure 10.14). A right shift in the oxyhemoglobin dissociation curve might be expected during heavy exercise due to the rise in blood lactic acid levels observed in this type of work. After being produced in the muscle cell, lactic acid gives up a proton (H^+), which results in the decrease in pH. The mechanism to explain the Bohr effect is the fact that protons bond to hemoglobin, which reduces its O_2 transport capacity. Therefore, when there is a higher than normal concentration of H^+ in the blood (a condition called acidosis), there is a reduction in hemoglobin affinity for O_2. This facilitates the unloading of O_2 to the tissues during exercise since the acidity level is higher in muscles.

Figure 10.15 The effect of changing blood temperature on the shape of the oxygen-hemoglobin dissociation curve. An increase in temperature results in a rightward shift in the curve, while a decrease in blood temperature results in a leftward shift in the curve.

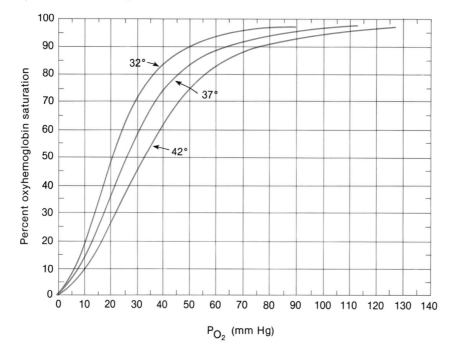

Temperature Effect on O_2-Hb Dissociation Curve

Another factor that affects hemoglobin affinity for O_2 is temperature. At a constant pH, the affinity of hemoglobin for O_2 is inversely related to blood temperature. A decrease in temperature results in a left shift in the oxyhemoglobin curve while an increase in temperature causes a right shift of the curve. This means that an increase in blood temperature weakens the bond between O_2 and hemoglobin which assists in the unloading of O_2 to muscle. Conversely, a decrease in blood temperature results in a stronger bond between O_2 and hemoglobin which hinders O_2 release. The effect of increasing blood temperature on the oxyhemoglobin dissociation curve is presented in figure 10.15.

2-3 DPG and the O_2-Hb Dissociation Curve

A final factor that can potentially affect the shape of the oxyhemoglobin dissociation is the concentration of 2-3 DPG found in red blood cells (RBCs). Red blood cells are unique in that they do not contain a nucleus or mitochondria. Therefore, they must rely on anaerobic glycolysis to meet the cell's energy needs. A by-product of RBC glycolysis is the compound 2-3 DPG, which can combine with hemoglobin and reduce hemoglobin's affinity for O_2 (i.e., right shift in oxyhemoglobin dissociation curve).

Red blood cell concentrations of 2-3 DPG are known to increase during exposure to altitude and in anemia (low blood hemoglobin) (34). However, reports in the literature about the acute effects of exercise on blood 2-3 DPG levels remain controversial. In an effort to resolve this issue, a group of Austrian researchers (35)

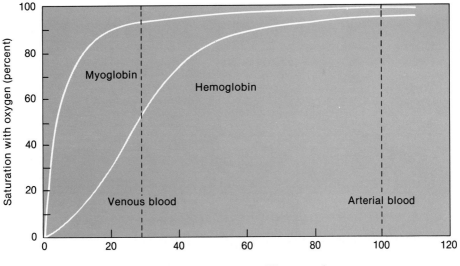

Figure 10.16 Comparison of the dissociation curve for myoglobin and hemoglobin. The steep myoglobin dissociation demonstrates a higher affinity for O_2 than hemoglobin.

performed a series of well-designed experiments that demonstrated that moderate exercise resulted in no change in blood levels of 2-3 DPG and that severe exercise resulted in a small decrease in blood 2-3 DPG. Therefore, although an increase in blood 2-3 DPG can alter $Hb\text{-}O_2$ affinity, it appears that exercise does not normally increase 2-3 DPG in the red blood cell. Therefore, the right shift in the oxyhemoglobin curve during heavy exercise is not due to changes in 2-3 DPG, but due to the degree of acidosis and blood temperature elevation.

O_2 Transport in Muscle

Myoglobin is a red pigment found primarily in skeletal muscle fibers and cardiac muscle (not in blood) and acts as a "shuttle" to move O_2 from the muscle cell membrane to the mitochondria. Myoglobin is found in large quantities in slow-twitch fibers (i.e., high aerobic capacity), but to a lesser degree in intermediate fibers, and only limited amounts can be found in fast-twitch fibers. Myoglobin is similar in structure to hemoglobin, but is about one-fourth the weight. The difference in structure between myoglobin and hemoglobin results in a difference in O_2 affinity between the two molecules. This point is illustrated in figure 10.16. Myoglobin has a greater affinity for O_2 than hemoglobin and therefore the myoglobin-O_2 dissociation curve is much steeper than that of hemoglobin's for PO_2 values below 20 mm Hg. The practical implication of the shape of the myoglobin-O_2 dissociation curve is that myoglobin discharges its O_2 at very low PO_2 values. This is important since the PO_2 in the mitochondria of contracting skeletal muscle may be as low as 1–2 mm Hg.

Myoglobin O_2 stores may serve as an "O_2 reserve" during transition periods from rest to exercise. At the beginning of exercise, there is a time lag between the onset of muscular contraction and an increased O_2 delivery to the muscle. Therefore, O_2 bound to myoglobin prior to the initiation of exercise serves to buffer

Figure 10.17 The three forms of CO_2 transport in blood. See text for discussion.

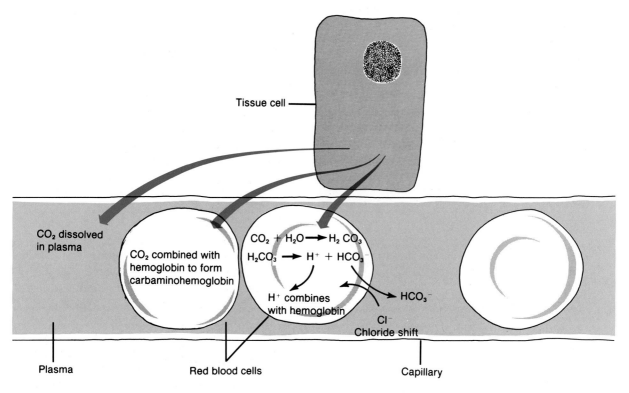

the O_2 needs of the muscle until the cardiopulmonary system can meet the new O_2 requirement. At the conclusion of exercise, myoglobin O_2 stores must be replenished and this O_2 consumption above rest contributes to the O_2 debt (chapter 4).

CO_2 Transport in Blood

Carbon dioxide is transported in the blood in three forms: (1) dissolved CO_2 (about 10% of blood CO_2 is transported this way), (2) CO_2 bound to hemoglobin (called carbamino-hemoglobin; about 20% of blood CO_2 is transported via this form), and (3) bicarbonate (70% of CO_2 found in blood is transported as bicarbonate (HCO_3^-)). The three forms of CO_2 transport in the blood are illustrated in figure 10.17.

Since most of the CO_2 that is transported in blood is transported as bicarbonate, this mechanism deserves special attention. Carbon dioxide can be converted to bicarbonate (within RBCs) in the following way:

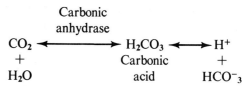

A high PCO_2 causes CO_2 to combine with water to form carbonic acid. This reaction is catalyzed by the enzyme carbonic anhydrase, which is found in RBCs. After formation, carbonic acid dissociates into a hydrogen ion and a bicarbonate ion. The hydrogen ion then binds to hemoglobin and the bicarbonate ion diffuses out of the RBC into the plasma (figure 10.17).

Since bicarbonate carries a negative charge (anion), the removal of a negatively charged molecule from a cell without replacement would result in an electrochemical imbalance across the cell membrane. This problem is avoided by the replacement of bicarbonate by chloride (Cl^-), which diffuses from the plasma into the RBC. This exchange of anions occurs in the RBC as blood moves through the tissue capillaries, and is called the "chloride shift" (figure 10.17).

When blood reaches the pulmonary capillaries, the PCO_2 of the blood is greater than that of the alveolus and thus CO_2 diffuses out of the blood across the blood-gas interface. At the lung, the binding of O_2 to Hb results in a release of the hydrogen ions bound to hemoglobin and promotes the formation of carbonic acid:

$$H^+ + HCO_3^- \longleftrightarrow H_2CO_3$$

Under conditions of low PCO_2 that exist at the alveolus, carbonic acid then dissociates into CO_2 and H_2O:

$$H_2CO_3 \longleftrightarrow CO_2 + H_2O$$

The release of CO_2 from the blood is summarized in figure 10.18.

Ventilation and Acid-Base Balance

The role of the pulmonary system in acid-base balance will be discussed in detail in chapter 11. Briefly, pulmonary ventilation can play a role in removing H^+ from the blood by the HCO_3^- reaction discussed above. For example, an increase in CO_2 in blood or body fluids results in an increase in hydrogen ion accumulation and thus a decrease in pH. In contrast, removal of CO_2 from blood or body fluids may decrease hydrogen ion concentration and thus increase pH. Recall that the CO_2-carbonic anhydrase reaction occurs as follows:

$$CO_2 + H_2O \longleftrightarrow H_2CO_3 \longleftrightarrow H^+ + HCO_3^-$$

Therefore, an increase in pulmonary ventilation causes exhalation of additional CO_2 and results in a reduction of blood PCO_2 and a lowering of hydrogen ion concentration. On the other side, a reduction in pulmonary ventilation would result in a buildup of CO_2 and an increase in hydrogen ion concentration (pH would decrease).

Ventilatory and Blood-Gas Responses to Exercise

Prior to a discussion of ventilatory control during exercise, it is useful to examine the ventilatory response to several different types of exercise.

Rest-to-Work Transitions

The change in pulmonary ventilation observed in the transition from rest to constant load submaximal exercise (i.e., below the lactate threshold) is pictured in figure 10.19. Note that ventilation increases abruptly at the beginning of exercise, followed by a slower rise toward a steady state value (8, 15, 16, 23, 42, 45).

Figure 10.19 also points out that arterial tensions of PCO_2 and PO_2 are relatively unchanged during this type of exercise (19, 21, 53). However, note that arterial PO_2 decreases and arterial PCO_2 tends to increase slightly in the transition from rest to steady state exercise (21). This observation suggests that the increase in alveolar ventilation at the beginning of exercise is not as rapid as the increase in metabolism.

Prolonged Exercise in a Hot Environment

Figure 10.20 illustrates the change in pulmonary ventilation during prolonged constant-load submaximal exercise (below the lactate threshold) in two different environmental conditions. The neutral environment represents exercise in a cool, low-relative-humidity environment (19° C, 45% relative humidity). The second condition represented in figure 10.20 is a hot/high-humidity environment, which hampers heat loss from the body. The major point to appreciate from figure 10.20 is that ventilation tends to "drift" upward during prolonged work. The mechanism to explain this increase in $\dot{V}_E$ during work in the heat is an increase in blood temperature, which directly affects the respiratory control center (36).

Another interesting point to gain from figure 10.20 is that although ventilation is greater during exercise in a hot/humid environment when compared to work in a cool environment, there is little difference in arterial PCO_2 between the two types of exercise. This finding suggests that the increase in ventilation seen during work in the heat is due to an increase in

Figure 10.18 Carbon dioxide is released from the blood in the pulmonary capillaries. At the time of CO_2 release in the lung there is a "reverse chloride shift" and carbonic acid dissociates into CO_2 and O_2.

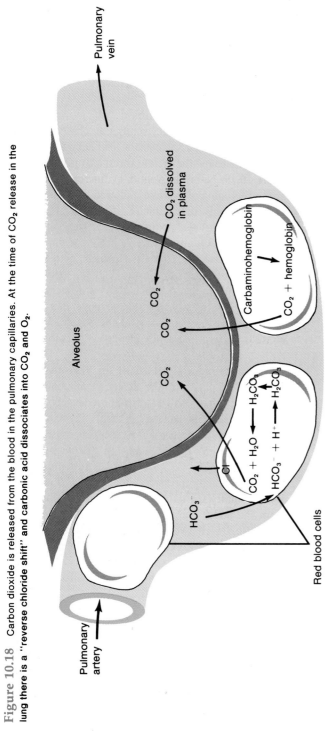

Figure 10.19 The changes in ventilation and partial pressures of O_2 and CO_2 in the transition from rest to steady state submaximal exercise.

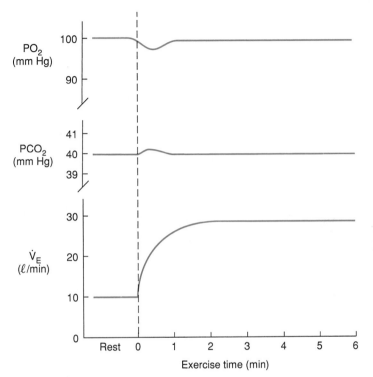

breathing frequency and dead-space ventilation (22). This type of breathing in humans in hot weather is similar to the "panting" observed in dogs and cats during warm conditions (22).

Incremental Exercise

The ventilatory response for an elite male distance runner and an untrained college student during an incremental exercise test is illustrated in figure 10.21. In both subjects, ventilation increases as a linear function of oxygen uptake up to 50%–75% of $\dot{V}O_2$ max, where ventilation begins to rise exponentially. This $\dot{V}_E$ "inflection point" has been called the **ventilatory threshold (Tvent)** (31, 38, 41).

An interesting point that emerges from figure 10.21 is the startling difference between the highly trained elite athlete and the untrained subject in arterial PO_2 during heavy exercise. The untrained subject is able to maintain arterial PO_2 within 10–12 mm Hg of the normal resting value, while the highly trained distance runner shows a decrease of 30–40 mm Hg at near-maximal work (18, 20, 22). This drop in arterial PO_2, often observed in the healthy, trained athlete, is similar to that observed in exercising patients who possess severe lung disease. However, do all healthy, elite endurance athletes develop low-arterial PO_2 values (low PO_2 is called hypoxemia) during heavy exercise? It appears that only about 50%–60% of highly trained endurance athletes ($\dot{V}O_2$ max 4.5 l/min or > 68 ml $\cdot$ kg $\cdot$ min^{-1}) show this marked hypoxemia (43). In addition, the degree of hypoxemia observed in these athletes during heavy work varies considerably among individuals (18, 39, 55). The reason for the subject differences is unclear.

Figure 10.20 Changes in ventilation and blood gas tensions during prolonged submaximal exercise in a hot/humid environment.

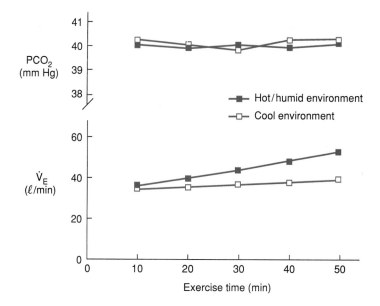

Control of Ventilation

Obviously, precise regulation of pulmonary gas exchange during rest and exercise is important in maintaining homeostasis by providing normal arterial O_2 content and maintenance of the acid-base balance

Perhaps the most important question concerning this exercise-induced hypoxemia is what factor(s) accounts for this failure of the pulmonary system? Unfortunately, a complete answer to this question cannot be provided. However, there is growing evidence that much of the decline in arterial PO_2 during heavy exercise in the elite athlete is due to diffusion limitations caused by a reduced amount of time that the RBC spends in the pulmonary capillaries. This short transit time for RBCs in the pulmonary capillary is probably due to high cardiac output achieved by these athletes during maximal exercise. This short RBC transit time may be less than the required time for gas equilibrium to be achieved between the lung and blood (18, 44, 56).

within the body. Although the control of breathing has been actively studied by physiologists for many years, many unanswered questions remain. Let's begin our discussion of ventilatory control during exercise with a review of ventilatory regulation at rest.

Ventilatory Regulation at Rest

As mentioned earlier, inspiration and expiration are produced by contraction and relaxation of the diaphragm during quiet breathing, and by accessory muscles during exercise. Contraction and relaxation of these respiratory muscles are directly controlled by somatic motor neurons in the spinal cord. Motor neuron activity, in turn, is directly controlled by the respiratory control center in the medulla oblongata and the pons area of the brain stem.

Respiratory Control Center

The initial drive to inspire or expire comes from neurons located in the medulla oblongata (labeled as the rhythmicity center in figure 10.22). Discharges from some of these neurons produce inspiration, while discharges from other neurons produce expiration. These

Figure 10.21 Changes in ventilation, blood gas tensions, and pH during incremental exercise in a highly trained male distance runner and an untrained male college student.

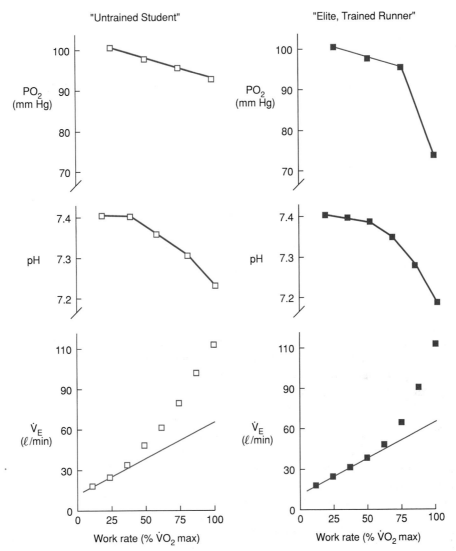

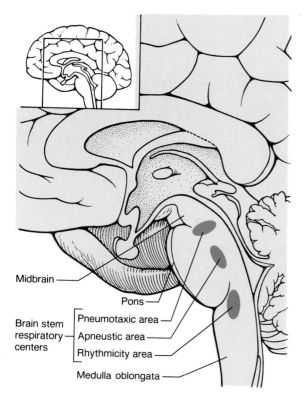

Figure 10.22 Locations of the brain stem respiratory control centers.

Midbrain

Pons

Brain stem respiratory centers
- Pneumotaxic area
- Apneustic area
- Rhythmicity area

Medulla oblongata

respiratory neurons act in a reciprocal way to produce a rhythmic pattern of breathing (47, 48). At rest, the cycle of inspiration and a passive expiration is built in, or intrinsic to the neural activity of the medulla. However, neural activity in the medulla can be modified by neurons located outside the respiratory rhythmicity center.

Two additional areas located in the pons that contribute to respiratory control are the "apneustic area" and the "pneumotaxic area." The apneustic area directly communicates with inspiratory neurons located in the rhythmicity center to stop inspiratory neuronal activity. Therefore, it is believed that the apneustic center functions as an "inspiratory cutoff switch" that terminates inspiration. Another group of respiratory neurons, the pneumotaxic area, functions to "fine tune" the activity of the apneustic area (figure 10.22). The practical function of the apneustic/pneumotaxic centers is that they work in concert to regulate the depth of breathing (34).

Input to the Respiratory Control Center

Several types of receptors are capable of modifying the actions of neurons contained in the respiratory control center. In general, input to the respiratory control center can be classified into two types: (1) neural and (2) humoral (blood-borne). Neural input refers to afferent or efferent input to the respiratory control center from neurons that are excited by means other than blood-borne stimuli. Humoral input to the respiratory control center refers to the influence of some blood-borne stimuli reaching a specialized chemoreceptor. This receptor reacts to the strength of the stimuli and sends the appropriate message to the medulla. A brief overview of each of these receptors will be presented prior to a discussion of ventilatory control during exercise.

Humoral Chemoreceptors

Chemoreceptors are specialized neurons that are capable of responding to changes in the internal environment. Traditionally, respiratory chemoreceptors are classified according to their location as being either "central chemoreceptors" or "peripheral chemoreceptors." The central chemoreceptors are located in the medulla (anatomically separate from the respiratory center) and are affected by changes in PCO_2 and H^+ of the cerebral spinal fluid (CSF). An increase in either PCO_2 or H^+ of the CSF results in the central chemoreceptors sending afferent input into the respiratory center to increase ventilation (19).

The peripheral chemoreceptors are located in the aortic arch and at the bifurcation of the common carotid artery. The receptors located in the aorta are called **aortic bodies** and those found in the carotid artery are **carotid bodies.** These peripheral chemoreceptors respond to increases in arterial H^+ concentrations and PCO_2 (1, 3, 10, 57). Additionally, the carotid bodies are sensitive to decreases in arterial PO_2. When comparing the relative importance of these two sets of peripheral chemoreceptors, it appears that the carotid bodies are the most prominent (19, 34).

Figure 10.23 Changes in ventilation as a function of increasing arterial PCO_2. Notice that ventilation increases as a linear function of increasing PCO_2.

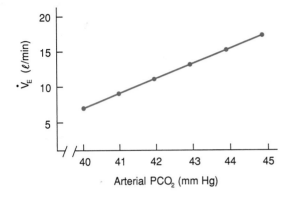

Arterial PCO_2 (mm Hg)

Figure 10.24 Changes in ventilation as a function of decreasing arterial PO_2. Note the existence of a "hypoxic threshold" for ventilation as arterial PO_2 declines.

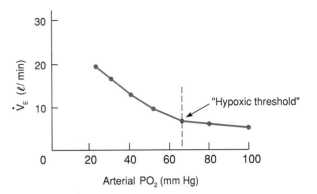

Arterial PO_2 (mm Hg)

Lung CO_2 Receptors

There is evidence that specialized chemoreceptors in the lungs of dogs, rabbits, and perhaps humans are sensitive to CO_2 and act to match ventilation with CO_2 return to the lungs (4, 9, 13, 28–30, 49, 51, 53, 55). In other words, an increase in CO_2 return to the lung stimulates lung receptors, which send a message to the respiratory control center to increase $\dot{V}_E$. This increase in $\dot{V}_E$ is hypothesized to be precisely matched to the amount of the CO_2 returned to the lung, and thus maintains arterial PCO_2 constant.

Effect of Blood PCO_2 and PO_2 on Ventilation

The effects of increases in arterial PCO_2 on minute ventilation can be seen in figure 10.23. Note that $\dot{V}_E$ increases as a linear function of arterial PCO_2. In general, a 1 mm Hg rise in PCO_2 results in a 2 liter/minute increase in $\dot{V}_E$ (34). The increase in $\dot{V}_E$ that results from a rise in arterial PCO_2 is likely due to CO_2 stimulation of both the carotid bodies and the central chemoreceptors (19).

In healthy individuals breathing at sea level, changes in arterial PO_2 have little effect on the control of ventilation (34). However, exposure to an environment with a barometric pressure much lower than sea level (i.e., high altitude), can alter arterial PO_2 and stimulate the carotid bodies, which in turn signal the respiratory center to increase ventilation. The relationship between arterial PO_2 and $\dot{V}_E$ is illustrated in figure 10.24. The point on the $PO_2/\dot{V}_E$ curve where $\dot{V}_E$ begins to rise rapidly is often referred to as the "hypoxic threshold" (hypoxic means low PO_2) (2). This hypoxic threshold usually occurs around an arterial PO_2 of 60–75 mm Hg. The chemoreceptors responsible for the increase in $\dot{V}_E$ following exposure to low PO_2 are the carotid bodies, since the aortic and central chemoreceptors in humans do not respond to changes in PO_2 (19, 34).

Neural Input to the Respiratory Control Center

Evidence obtained from animal experiments shows that neural input to the respiratory control center can come from both efferent and afferent pathways. For example, it has been demonstrated in cats that impulses from the motor cortex (i.e., central command) can control both skeletal muscle and drive ventilation in proportion to the amount of work being performed (24, 25). In short, neural impulses originating in the motor cortex may pass through the medulla and "spill over," causing an increase in $\dot{V}_E$ that is representative of the number of muscle motor units being recruited.

Afferent input to the respiratory control center during exercise may come from one of several peripheral receptors such as the muscle spindles, Golgi tendon organs, or joint pressure receptors (6, 33, 50). In addition, it is possible that special chemoreceptors located in muscle may respond to changes in potassium and H^+ concentrations and send afferent information to the respiratory control center. This type of input to the medulla is considered afferent neural information, since the stimuli is not humorally mediated. Finally, recent evidence suggests that the right ventricle of the heart contains mechanoreceptors that send afferent information back to the respiratory control center relative to increases in cardiac output (i.e., during exercise) (55). These mechanoreceptors might play important roles in providing afferent input to the respiratory control center at the onset of exercise.

Ventilatory Control during Submaximal Exercise

Respiratory physiologists have studied those factors that regulate breathing during exercise for over 100 years. However, at present, there is no clear agreement as to which factor(s) is most responsible for ventilatory control during work. In general, there are three schools of thought concerning the mechanisms that are responsible for regulation of breathing during exercise below the lactate threshold. The first school proposes that $\dot{V}_E$ during exercise is controlled primarily by either afferent neural feedback to the respiratory control center or efferent neural activity from higher brain centers (6, 7, 24, 33). A second school suggests that the changes in $\dot{V}_E$ that occur during exercise can all be traced to humoral stimuli (53, 57). The leading hypothesis in this area is based on experiments that suggest that CO_2-sensitive receptors in the lung provide the stimulus for ventilatory control (53). Finally, a third school proposes that ventilation during exercise is due to a combination of neural-humoral activity (17, 27).

Which of the above hypotheses is most accurate in explaining the precise regulation of alveolar ventilation to metabolic rate during light-to-moderate exercise? At present, it appears likely that ventilation is regulated by a combination of both humoral and neural input (neural-humoral hypothesis) to the medulla (17,

27, 40, 41, 44). There is convincing evidence that much of the drive to increase ventilation during exercise is due to neural input (both afferent and efferent) to the respiratory control center (6, 7, 24, 33, 50). However, the fact that arterial PCO_2 is tightly regulated during most types of submaximal exercise suggests that humoral chemoreceptors act to "fine tune" breathing to match the metabolic rate and thus maintain a rather constant arterial PCO_2 (11, 12, 53).

During prolonged exercise in a hot environment, ventilation can be influenced by additional factors other than those discussed above. For example, the drift upward in $\dot{V}_E$ seen in figure 10.20 may be due to a direct influence of rising blood temperature on the respiratory control center, and rising blood catecholamines (epinephrine and norepinephrine) stimulating the carotid bodies to increase $\dot{V}_E$ (36).

To summarize, ventilatory regulation during exercise is likely due to an interaction of both neural and humoral input to the respiratory control center. It seems likely that neural mechanisms provide the primary drive to breathe during exercise, with humoral chemoreceptors providing a means of precisely matching ventilation with the amount of CO_2 produced via metabolism. This apparent redundancy in mechanisms is not surprising when one considers the important role that respiration plays in sustaining life and maintaining a steady state during exercise (34). A summary of respiratory control during submaximal exercise appears in figure 10.25.

Ventilatory Control during Heavy Exercise

Controversy exists concerning the mechanism to explain the alinear rise in ventilation (ventilatory threshold) that occurs during an incremental exercise test. However, several factors may contribute to this rise. First, examination of figure 10.21 suggests that the alinear rise in both $\dot{V}_E$ and pH↓ often occur simultaneously. Since rising H^+ levels in blood have been shown to stimulate the carotid bodies and increase $\dot{V}_E$, it has been proposed that the rise in blood lactate, which occurs during incremental exercise, is the stimulus causing the alinear rise in $\dot{V}_E$ (i.e., ventilatory threshold). Based on this belief, it is common for researchers to estimate the lactate threshold noninvasively by measurement of the ventilatory threshold (5,

Figure 10.25 A summary of respiratory control during submaximal exercise. See text for details.

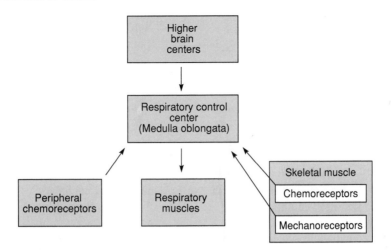

14, 54). However, several studies have shown that this technique is not perfect and that the ventilatory threshold and the lactate threshold do not always occur at the same work rate (26, 41).

What additional factors, other than rising blood lactate, might cause the alinear rise in $\dot{V}_E$ observed during incremental exercise? Certainly secondary factors, such as rising body temperature and blood catecholamines, might play a small contributory role to the increasing $\dot{V}_E$ during heavy exercise. Further, it is conceivable that afferent input to the respiratory control center might influence the ventilatory pattern during incremental exercise. For example, as exercise intensity increases, motor unit recruitment may occur in a nonlinear fashion and the associated efferent and afferent neural signal to the respiratory control center may signal the alinear rise in $\dot{V}_E$ seen at the ventilatory threshold (41).

In summary, it is logical to reason that the rise in blood lactate and reduction in blood pH observed at the lactate threshold can stimulate ventilation and thus may be the principal mechanism to "explain" the ventilatory threshold. However, secondary factors such as an increase in body temperature, rising blood catecholamines, and possible afferent neural influences might also contribute to ventilatory control during heavy exercise.

Summary

1. The primary function of the pulmonary system is to provide a means of gas exchange between the environment and the body. In addition, the respiratory system plays an important role in the regulation of the acid-base balance during exercise.

2. Anatomically, the pulmonary system consists of a group of passages that filter air and transport it into the lungs where gas exchange occurs within tiny air sacs called alveoli.

3. The major muscle of inspiration is the diaphragm. Air enters the pulmonary system due to intrapulmonary pressure being reduced below atmospheric (bulk flow). At rest, expiration is passive. However, during exercise expiration becomes active using muscles located in the abdominal wall (rectus abdominus and internal oblique).

4. The primary factor that contributes to airflow resistance in the pulmonary system is the diameter of the airway.

5. Gas moves across the blood-gas interface in the lung due to simple diffusion. The rate of diffusion is described by Fick's law and is proportional to the area for diffusion and the

difference in partial pressure across the membrane, and is inversely proportional to membrane thickness.

6. The pulmonary circulation is a low-pressure system with a rate of blood flow equal to that in the systemic circuit. In a standing position, most of the blood flow to the lung is distributed to the base of the lung due to gravitational force.

7. Efficient gas exchange between the blood and the lung requires proper matching of blood flow to ventilation (called ventilation-perfusion relationships). The ideal ratio of ventilation to perfusion is 1 since this ratio implies a perfect matching of blood flow to ventilation.

8. Over 99% of the O_2 transported in blood is chemically bonded with hemoglobin. The effect of the partial pressure of O_2 on the combination of O_2 with hemoglobin is illustrated by the s-shaped O_2-hemoglobin dissociation curve. An increase in body temperature and a reduction in blood pH results in a right shift in the O_2-hemoglobin dissociation curve and a reduced affinity of hemoglobin for O_2.

9. Carbon dioxide is transported in blood in three forms: (1) dissolved CO_2 (10% is transported in this way), (2) CO_2 bound to hemoglobin (called carboxyhemoglobin; about 20% of blood CO_2 is transported via this form), and (3) bicarbonate (70% of CO_2 found in blood is transported as bicarbonate (HCO_3^-).

10. At the onset of constant load submaximal exercise, ventilation increases rapidly, followed by a slower rise toward a steady state value. Arterial PO_2 and PCO_2 are maintained relatively constant during this type of exercise.

11. During prolonged exercise in a hot/humid environment, ventilation "drifts" upward due to the influence of rising body temperature on the respiratory control center.

12. Incremental exercise results in a linear increase in $\dot{V}_E$ up to approximately 50%–70% of $\dot{V}O_2$ max; at higher work rates, ventilation begins to rise exponentially. This ventilatory inflection point has been called the ventilatory threshold.

13. The respiratory control center is contained in the medulla oblongata. At rest, the normal breathing pattern is determined by intrinsic firing of inspiratory neurons. This intrinsic firing rate of respiratory neurons can be modified by neurons outside the medulla oblongata. The apneustic center and the pneumotaxic center (both located in the pons) work together to regulate the depth of breathing by acting as a cutoff switch for inspiratory neurons.

14. Input into the respiratory control center to increase ventilation may come from both neural and humoral sources. Neural input may come from higher brain centers, or it may arise from receptors in the exercising muscle. Humoral input may arise from central chemoreceptors, peripheral chemoreceptors, and/or lung CO_2 receptors. The central chemoreceptors are sensitive to increases in PCO_2 and decreases in pH. The peripheral chemoreceptors (carotid bodies are the most important) are sensitive to increases in PCO_2 and decreases in PO_2 or pH. Receptors in the lung that are sensitive to an increase in PCO_2 are hypothesized to exist.

15. Regulation of ventilation during submaximal exercise is due to both neural and humoral input to the respiratory control center. The primary drive to increase ventilation during exercise probably comes from neural afferents and/or efferents. The humoral role in this process is for the chemoreceptors to "fine tune" ventilation to match metabolism, which serves to closely regulate arterial PCO_2.

16. Controversy exists concerning the mechanism to explain the alinear rise in ventilation (ventilatory threshold) that occurs during an incremental exercise test. However, it appears that the rise in blood H^+ concentration that occurs during this type of exercise provides the principal stimulus to increase ventilation via stimulation of the carotid bodies.

Study Questions

1. What is the primary function of the pulmonary system? What secondary functions does it serve?
2. List and discuss the major anatomical components that make up the respiratory system.
3. What muscle groups are involved in ventilation during rest? During exercise?
4. What is the functional significance of the ventilation-perfusion ratio? How would a high V/Q ratio affect gas exchange in the lung?
5. Discuss those factors that influence the rate of diffusion across the blood-gas interface in the lung.
6. Graph the relationship between hemoglobin-O_2 saturation and the partial pressure of O_2 in the blood. What is the functional significance of the shape of the O_2-hemoglobin dissociation curve? What factors affect the shape of the curve?
7. Discuss the modes of transportation for CO_2 in the blood.
8. Graph the ventilatory response in the transition from rest to constant-load submaximal exercise. What happens to ventilation if the exercise is prolonged and performed in a hot/humid environment? Why?
9. Graph the ventilatory response to incremental exercise. Label the ventilatory threshold. What factor(s) might explain the ventilatory threshold?
10. List and identify the functions of the chemoreceptors that contribute to the control of breathing.
11. What neural afferents might also contribute to the regulation of ventilation during exercise?
12. Discuss the neural-humoral hypothesis of ventilatory control during exercise.

Suggested Readings

Dempsey, J. 1986. Is the lung built for exercise? *Medicine and Science in Sports and Exercise* 18:143–55.
Levitzky, M. 1987. *Pulmonary Physiology.* New York: McGraw-Hill.
Powers, S., and R. Beadle. 1985. Control of ventilation during submaximal exercise: A brief review. *Journal of Sports Sciences* 3:51–65.
———. 1985. Onset of hyperventilation during incremental exercise: A brief review. *Research Quarterly for Exercise and Sport* 56:352–60.

References

1. Allen, C., and N. Jones. 1984. Rate of change of alveolar carbon dioxide and the control of ventilation during exercise. *Journal of Physiology* (London) 355:1–9.
2. Asmussen, E. 1983. Control of ventilation in exercise. In (R. Terjung, ed.) *Exercise and Sport Science Reviews,* Vol. 2. Philadelphia: Franklin Press.
3. Band, D. et al. 1980. Respiratory oscillations in arterial carbon dioxide tension as a signal in exercise. *Nature* 283:84–85.
4. Banzett, R., H. Coleridge, and J. Coleridge. 1978. Pulmonary CO_2 ventilatory reflex in dogs: Effective range of CO_2 and vagal cooling. *Respiration Physiology* 34:121–34.
5. Beaver, W., K. Wasserman, and B. Whipp. 1986. A new method for detecting anaerobic threshold by gas exchange. *Journal of Applied Physiology* 60:2020–27.
6. Bennett, F. 1984. A role for neural pathways in exercise hyperpnea. *Journal of Applied Physiology* 56:1559–64.
7. Bennett, F., R. Tallman, and G. Grodins. 1984. Role of VCO_2 in control of breathing in awake exercising dogs. *Journal of Applied Physiology* 56:1335–37.
8. Bennett, F., and W. Fordyce. 1985. Characteristics of the ventilatory exercise stimulus. *Respiration Physiology* 59:55–63.
9. Beon, J., W. Kuhlmann, and M. Fedde. 1980. Control of respiration in the chicken: Effects of venous CO_2 loading. *Respiration Physiology* 39:169–81.

10. Bisgard, G. et al. 1982. Role of the carotid body in hyperpnea of moderate exercise in goats. *Journal of Applied Physiology* 52:1216–22.

11. Brice, A., et al. 1988. Ventilatory and $PaCO_2$ responses to voluntary and electrically induced leg exercise. *Journal of Applied Physiology* 64:218–25.

12. Brice, A. et al. 1988. Is the hyperpnea of muscular contractions critically dependent upon spinal afferents? *Journal of Applied Physiology* 64:226–33.

13. Brown, H., K. Wasserman, and B. Whipp. 1976. Effect of beta-adrenergic blockade during exercise on ventilation and gas exchange. *Journal of Applied Physiology* 41:886–92.

14. Caiozzo, V., et al. 1982. A comparison of gas exchange indices used to detect the anaerobic threshold. *Journal of Applied Physiology* 53:1184–89.

15. Casaburi, R. et al. 1977. Ventilatory and gas exchange dynamics in response to sinusoidal work. *Journal of Applied Physiology* 42:300–11.

16. Casaburi, R. et al. 1978. Ventilatory control characteristics of the exercise hyperpnea discerned from dynamic forcing techniques. *Chest* 73:280–83.

17. Dejours, P. 1964. Control of respiration in muscular exercise. In (W. Fenn, ed.) *Handbook of Physiology,* Section 3. Washington: American Physiological Society.

18. Dempsey, J. et al. 1982. Limitation to exercise capacity and endurance: Pulmonary system. *Canadian Journal of Applied Sports Sciences* 7:4–13.

19. Dempsey, J., G. Mitchell, and C. Smith. 1984. Exercise and chemoreception. *American Review of Respiratory Disease* 129:31–34.

20. Dempsey, J., and R. Fregosi. 1985. Adaptability of the pulmonary system to changing metabolic requirements. *American Journal of Cardiology* 55:59D-67D.

21. Dempsey, J., E. Vidruk, and G. Mitchell. 1985. Pulmonary control systems in exercise: Update. *Federation Proceedings* 44:2260–70.

22. Dempsey, J. 1986. Is the lung built for exercise? *Medicine and Science in Sports and Exercise* 18:143–55.

23. Dodd, S. et al. 1988. Effects of acute beta-adrenergic blockade on ventilation and gas exchange during the rest-to-work transition. *Aviation, Space, and Environmental Medicine* 59:255–58.

24. Eldridge, F., D. Millhorn, and T. Waldrop. 1981. Exercise hyperpnea and locomotion: Parallel activation from the hypothalamus. *Science* 211:844–46.

25. Eldridge, F. et al. 1985. Stimulation by central command of locomotion, respiration, and circulation during exercise. *Respiration Physiology* 59:313–37.

26. England, P. et al. 1985. The effect of acute thermal dehydration on blood lactate accumulation during incremental exercise. *Journal of Sports Sciences* 2:105–11.

27. Favier, R. et al. 1983. Ventilatory and circulatory transients during exercise: New arguments for a neurohumoral theory. *Journal of Applied Physiology* 54:647–53.

28. Green, J., and M. Sheldon. 1983. Ventilatory changes associated with changes in pulmonary blood flow in dogs. *Journal of Applied Physiology* 54:997–1002.

29. Green, J., and N. Schmidt. 1984. Mechanism of hyperpnea induced by changes in pulmonary blood flow. *Journal of Applied Physiology* 56:1418–22.

30. Green, J. et al. 1986. Effect of pulmonary arterial PCO_2 on slowly adapting stretch receptors. *Journal of Applied Physiology* 60:2048–55.

31. Hagberg, J. et al. 1982. Exercise hyperventilation in patients with McArdle's disease. *Journal of Applied Physiology* 52:991–94.

32. Hammond, M. et al. 1986. Pulmonary gas exchange in humans during exercise at sea level. *Journal of Applied Physiology* 60:1590–98.

33. Kao, F. 1963. An experimental study of the pathways involved in exercise hyperpnea employing cross-circulation techniques. In (D. Cunningham, ed.) *The Regulation of Human Respiration.* Oxford: Blackwell.

34. Levitzky, M. 1987. *Pulmonary Physiology.* New York: McGraw-Hill.

35. Mairbaurl, H. et al. 1986. Regulation of red cell 2,3–DPG and Hb-O_2-affinity during acute exercise. *European Journal of Applied Physiology* 55:174–80.

36. Powers, S., E. Howley, and R. Cox. 1982. Ventilatory and metabolic reactions to heat stress during prolonged exercise. *Journal of Sports Medicine and Physical Fitness* 22:32–36.

Powers, S. et al. 1983. Effects of caffeine ingestion on metabolism and performance during graded exercise. *European Journal of Applied Physiology* 50:301–7.

38. Powers, S. et al. 1983. Ventilatory threshold, running economy, and distance running performance. *Research Quarterly for Exercise and Sport* 54: 179–82.

39. Powers, S. et al. 1984. Hemoglobin desaturation during incremental arm and leg exercise. *British Journal of Sports Medicine* 18:212–16.

40. Powers, S., and R. Beadle. 1985. Control of ventilation during submaximal exercise: A brief review. *Journal of Sports Sciences* 3:51–65.

41. ———. 1985. Onset of hyperventilation during incremental exercise: A brief review. *Research Quarterly for Exercise and Sport* 56:352–60.

42. Powers, S. et al. 1985. Caffeine alters ventilatory and gas exchange kinetics during exercise. *Medicine and Science in Sports and Exercise* 18:101–6.

43. Powers, S. et al. 1988. Incidence of exercise-induced hypoxemia in the elite endurance athlete at sea level. *European Journal of Applied Physiology* 58: 298–302.

44. Powers, S., and J. Williams. 1987. Exercise-induced hypoxemia in highly trained athletes. *Sports Medicine* 4:46–53.

45. Powers, S. et al. 1987. Ventilatory and blood gas dynamics at onset and offset of exercise in the pony. *Journal of Applied Physiology* 62:141–48.

46. Powers, S., M. Stuart, and G. Landry. 1988. Ventilatory and gas exchange dynamics in response to head-down tilt with and without venous occlusion. *Aviation, Space, and Environmental Medicine* 59:239–45.

47. Richter, D. 1982. Generation and maintenance of the respiratory rhythm. *Journal of Experimental Biology* 100:93–107.

48. Richter, D., D. Ballantyne, and J. Remmers. 1986. How is the respiratory rhythm generated? A model. *News in Physiological Sciences* 1:109–11.

49. Sheldon, M., and J. Green. 1982. Evidence for pulmonary CO_2 sensitivity on ventilation. *Journal of Applied Physiology* 52:1192–97.

50. Tibes, V. 1977. Reflex inputs to the cardiovascular and respiratory centers from dynamically working canine muscles. *Circulation Research* 41:332–41.

51. Trenchard, D., N. Russell, and H. Raybould. 1984. Nonmyelinated vagal lung receptors and reflex effects on respiration in rabbits. *Respiration Physiology* 55:63–79.

52. Wasserman, K. et al. 1973. Anaerobic threshold and respiratory gas exchange during exercise. *Journal of Applied Physiology* 35:236–43.

53. Wasserman, K. et al. 1977. CO_2 flow to the lungs and ventilatory control. In (J. Dempsey and C. Reed, eds.) *Muscular Exercise and the Lung*. Madison, Wis.: University of Wisconsin Press.

54. Wasserman, K. 1984. The anaerobic threshold measurement to evaluate exercise performance. *American Review of Respiratory Disease* 129: 535–40.

55. Weissman, M. et al. 1982. Cardiac output increase and gas exchange at the start of exercise. *Journal of Applied Physiology* 52:236–44.

56. Williams, J., S. Powers, and M. Stuart. 1986. Arterial desaturation during heavy exercise in highly trained distance runners. *Medicine and Science in Sports and Exercise* 18:168–73.

57. Yamamoto, W., and M. Edwards. 1960. Homeostasis of carbon dioxide during intravenous infusion of carbon dioxide. *Journal of Applied Physiology* 15:807–18.

11 Acid-Base Balance during Exercise

Objectives

By studying this chapter, you should be able to do the following:
1. Define the terms acid, base, and pH.
2. Discuss the importance of acid-base regulation to exercise performance.
3. List the principle intracellular and extracellular buffers.
4. Explain the role of respiration in the regulation of acid-base status during exercise.
5. Outline acid-base regulation during exercise.
6. Discuss the principal ways that hydrogen ions are produced during exercise.

Outline

Key Terms

acidosis
acids
alkalosis
bases
buffers
hydrogen ions
ion
pH
respiratory compensation
strong acids
strong bases

*E*lectrolytes that release **hydrogen ions** are called acids (an **ion** is any atom that is missing electrons or has gained electrons). Substances that combine with hydrogen ions are termed bases. In physiology, the concentration of hydrogen ions is expressed in pH units. The pH of body fluids must be regulated (i.e., normal arterial blood pH = 7.40 ± .02) in order to maintain homeostasis. Regulation of the pH of body fluids is extremely important since changes in hydrogen ion concentrations can alter the rates of enzyme-controlled metabolic reactions and modify numerous other normal body functions. Therefore, acid-base balance is primarily concerned with the regulation of hydrogen ion concentrations. Heavy exercise can present a serious challenge to hydrogen ion control systems due to lactic acid production, and may limit performance in some types of intense activities (1, 2, 7, 8, 10, 12, 13, 15–19). Given the potential detrimental influence of hydrogen ion accumulation on exercise performance, it is important that the student of exercise physiology have an understanding of acid-base regulation.

Acids, Bases, and pH

In biological systems, one of the simplest, but most important ions is the hydrogen ion. The concentration of the hydrogen ion influences the rates of chemical reaction, the shape and function of enzymes as well as other cellular proteins, and the integrity of the cell itself (4, 6, 9, 20).

An **acid** is defined as a molecule that can liberate hydrogen ions and thus can raise the hydrogen ion concentration of an aqueous solution above that of pure water. In contrast, a **base** is a molecule that is capable of combining with hydrogen ions and therefore lowers the hydrogen ion concentration of the solution.

Acids that tend to give up hydrogen ions (ionize) more completely are termed **strong acids.** For example, lactic acid produced during heavy exercise as a result of glycolysis is a relatively strong acid. At normal body pH, lactic acid tends to liberate almost all of its hydrogen ions and therefore elevates the hydrogen ion concentration of the body.

Bases that ionize completely are defined as **strong bases.** The bicarbonate ions (HCO_3^-) are an example of a biologically important strong base. Bicarbonate ions are found in relatively large concentrations in blood and are capable of combining with hydrogen ions to form a weak acid called carbonic acid. The role of HCO_3^- in the regulation of acid-base balance during exercise will be discussed later in the chapter.

As stated earlier, the concentration of hydrogen ions is expressed in pH units. The **pH** of a solution is defined as the negative logarithm of the hydrogen ion concentration [H^+]. Recall that a logarithm is the exponent that indicates the power to which one number must be raised to obtain another number. For instance, the logarithm of 100 to the base 10 is 2. Thus, the definition of pH can be written mathematically as:

$$pH = -\log_{10}[H^+]$$

As an example, if the [H^+] = 40nM (0.000000040 M), then the pH would be 7.40.

A solution is considered neutral (in terms of acid-base status) if the concentration of H^+ and hydroxyl ions (OH^-) are equal. This is the case for pure water,

Figure 11.1 The pH scale. If the pH of arterial blood drops below the normal value of 7.4, the resulting condition is termed acidosis. In contrast, if the pH increases above 7.4, blood alkalosis occurs.

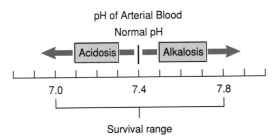

Figure 11.2 Acidosis results from an accumulation of acids or a loss of bases. Alkalosis results from a loss of acids or an accumulation of bases.

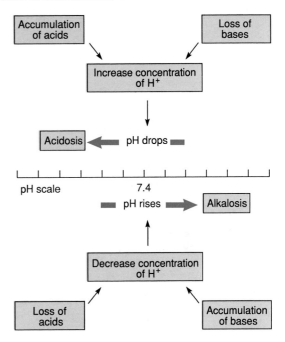

in which [H$^+$] and [OH$^-$] concentrations are both 0.00000010 M. Thus, the pH of pure water is:

$$pH \text{ (pure water)} = -\log_{10} [H^+]$$
$$= 7.0$$

Figure 11.1 shows the continuum of the pH scale. Note that as the hydrogen ion concentration increases, pH declines and the acidity of the blood increases, resulting in a condition termed **acidosis.** Conversely, as the hydrogen ion concentration decreases, pH increases and the solution becomes more basic (alkalotic). This condition is termed **alkalosis.** Conditions leading to acidosis or alkalosis are summarized in figure 11.2.

Hydrogen Ion Production during Exercise

Although small quantities of acids or bases are present in foods, the major threat to the pH of body fluids is acids formed in metabolic processes. These metabolic acids can be divided into three major groups (5, 14):

1. Volatile acids (e.g., carbon dioxide). Carbon dioxide, an end product in the oxidation of carbohydrates, fats, and proteins, can be regarded as an acid by virtue of its ability to react with water to form carbonic acid (H_2CO_3), which in turn dissociates to form H$^+$ and HCO$_3^-$:

$$CO_2 + H_2O \longleftrightarrow H_2CO_3 \longleftrightarrow H^+ + HCO_3^-$$

Because CO_2 is a gas and can be eliminated by the lungs, it is often referred to as a volatile acid. During the course of a day, the body produces large amounts of CO_2 due to normal metabolism. During exercise, metabolic production of CO_2 increases and therefore adds an additional "volatile acid" load on the body.

2. Fixed acids (e.g., sulfuric acid and phosphoric acid). Sulfuric acid is a product of the oxidation of certain amino acids, while phosphoric acid is formed in the metabolism of various phospholipids and nucleic acids. In contrast to CO_2, both sulfuric acid and phosphoric acid are nonvolatile and therefore are referred to as fixed acids. The production of fixed acids varies with the diet and is not greatly influenced by acute exercise. Hence, fixed acids are not a major contributor of hydrogen ions during heavy exercise.

Figure 11.3 Sources of hydrogen ions due to metabolic processes.

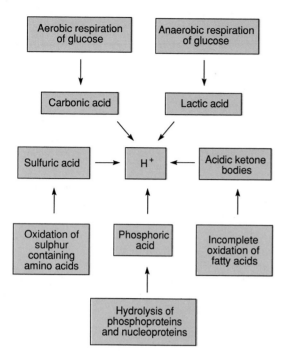

Importance of Acid-Base Regulation during Exercise

As discussed above, heavy exercise results in the production of large amounts of lactic acid by the contracting skeletal muscle. Lactic acid, a strong acid, ionizes and releases hydrogen ions. These hydrogen ions can exert a powerful effect on other molecules due to their small size and positive charge. Hydrogen ions exert their influence by attaching to molecules and thus altering their original size and shape (2, 7, 11). This change in size and shape may alter the normal function of the molecule (enzyme) and therefore influence metabolism in an important way.

An increase in the intramuscular hydrogen ion concentration can impair exercise performance in at least two ways. First, an increase in the hydrogen ion concentration reduces the muscle cell's ability to produce ATP by inhibiting key enzymes involved in both anaerobic and aerobic production of ATP (2, 7, 12). Second, hydrogen ions compete with calcium ions for binding sites on troponin, thereby hindering the contractile process (2, 7). This will be discussed again in chapter 19.

Acid-Base Buffer Systems

From the preceding discussion, it is clear that a rapid accumulation of hydrogen ions during heavy exercise can negatively influence muscular performance. Therefore, it is important that the body have control system(s) capable of regulating acid-base status to prevent drastic decreases or increases in pH. How does the body regulate pH? One of the most important means of regulating hydrogen ion concentrations in body fluids is by the aid of buffers. A **buffer** resists pH change by removing hydrogen ions when the hydrogen ion concentration increases, and releasing hydrogen ions when the hydrogen ion concentration falls.

Buffers often consist of a weak acid and its associated base (called a conjugate base). The ability of individual buffers to resist pH change is generally due to two factors. First, individual buffers differ in their intrinsic physiochemical ability to act as buffers. Simply stated, some buffers are better than others. A

3. Organic acids (e.g.. lactic acid). Organic acids, such as lactic acid and acetoacetic acid, are formed in the metabolism of carbohydrates and fats, respectively (chapters 3 and 4). Under normal resting conditions, both of these acids are further metabolized to CO_2 and therefore do not greatly influence the pH of body fluids. However, an exception to this rule is during heavy exercise (i.e., work above the lactate threshold). During periods of intense physical efforts, contracting skeletal muscles can produce large amounts of lactic acid, resulting in acidosis. In general, it appears that production of lactic acid during heavy exercise presents the greatest challenge to maintaining pH homeostasis during exercise. Some metabolic processes that serve as sources of hydrogen ions are illustrated in figure 11.3.

Table 11.1 Chemical acid-base buffer system

Buffer System	Constituents	Actions
Bicarbonate system	Sodium bicarbonate ($NaHCO_3$)	Converts strong acid into weak acid
	Carbonic acid (H_2CO_3)	Converts strong base into weak base
Phosphate system	Sodium phosphate ($Na_2HPO_4^-$)	Converts strong acid into weak acid
Protein system	COO^- group of a molecule	Accepts hydrogens in the presence of excess acid
	NH_3 group of a molecule	Accepts hydrogens in the presence of excess acid

second factor influencing buffering capacity is the concentration of the buffer present. The greater the concentration of a particular buffer, the more effective the buffer can be in preventing pH change.

Intracellular Buffers

The first line of defense in protecting against pH change during exercise is in the cell itself. The most common intracellular buffers are proteins and phosphate groups (14). Proteins contain several ionizable groups that are weak acids capable of accepting hydrogen ions. Weak phosphoric acids are found in relatively large concentrations in cells and also serve as an intracellular buffer system. In addition, bicarbonate in muscle has been demonstrated to be a useful buffer during exercise (11). A summary of the chemical action of intracellular buffer systems is presented in table 11.1.

Extracellular Buffers

The blood contains three principal buffer systems (11, 14): (1) proteins, (2) hemoglobin, and (3) bicarbonate. Blood proteins act as buffers in the extracellular compartment. Like intracellular proteins, these blood proteins contain ionizable groups that are weak acids and therefore act as buffers. However, because blood proteins are found in small quantities, their usefulness as a buffer during heavy exercise is limited.

In contrast, hemoglobin is a particularly important protein buffer and is a major blood buffer during resting conditions. In fact, hemoglobin has approximately six times the buffering capacity of plasma proteins due to its high concentration (14). Also contributing to the effectiveness of hemoglobin as a buffer is the fact that deoxygenated hemoglobin is a better buffer than oxygenated hemoglobin. As a result, once hemoglobin becomes deoxygenated in the capillaries, it is better able to bind hydrogen ions formed when CO_2 enters the blood from the tissues. Thus, hemoglobin helps to minimize pH changes caused by loading of CO_2 into the blood.

The bicarbonate buffer system is probably the most important buffer system in the body (14). This fact has been exploited by some investigators who have demonstrated that an increase in blood bicarbonate concentration (ingestion of bicarbonate) results in an improvement in performance in some types of exercise (1, 13) (see Box 11.1).

The bicarbonate buffer system involves the weak acid H_2CO_3, which undergoes the following dissociation reaction:

$$H_2O + CO_2 \longleftrightarrow H_2CO_3 \longleftrightarrow H^+ + HCO_3^-$$

The ability of carbonic acid (H_2CO_3) to act as a buffer is described mathematically by a relationship known as the Henderson-Hasselbalch equation:

$$pH = pKa + \log_{10}\left(\frac{HCO_3^-}{H_2CO_3}\right)$$

where pKa is the dissociation constant for H_2CO_3 and has a constant value of 6.1. In short, what the Henderson-Hasselbalch equation states is that the pH of a weak acid solution is determined by the ratio of the concentrations of the two forms of the buffer (ratio

Box 11.1 Sodium Bicarbonate Ingestion and Performance

Recent evidence suggests that performance in certain types of high-intensity exercise can be improved when athletes ingest sodium bicarbonate prior to exercise as a means of increasing blood-buffering capacity (1, 17). In general, these data suggest that boosting the blood-buffering capacity increases the time to exhaustion during exercise at intensities between 80%–120% $\dot{V}O_2$ max. It seems likely that if ingestion of sodium bicarbonate does improve physical performance, it does so by reducing the interference of hydrogen ions upon the intramuscular production of ATP and/or the contractile process itself.

The decision to use an ergogenic aid (performance aid) such as sodium bicarbonate must be considered in terms of both safety and the effectiveness of the procedure. Ingestion of sodium bicarbonate in small doses appears to be safe (1, 17); however, large doses of sodium bicarbonate produce diarrhea, vomiting, and in extreme cases could be fatal. Another important consideration for the use of any ergogenic aid is the legality. The International Olympic Committee has ruled that use of sodium bicarbonate during Olympic competition is illegal. (See chapter 23 for details.)

of bicarbonate to carbonic acid). The normal pH of arterial blood is 7.4 and the ratio of bicarbonate to carbonic acid is 20 to 1. Let's consider an example using the Henderson-Hasselbalch equation to calculate arterial blood pH. Normally the concentration of blood bicarbonate is 24 m Eq/L and the concentration of carbonic acid is 1.2 m Eq/L. Therefore, the blood pH can be calculated as follows:

$$
\begin{aligned}
pH &= pKa + \log_{10} 24/1.2 \\
&= 6.1 + \log_{10} 20 \\
&= 6.1 + 1.3 \\
pH &= 7.4
\end{aligned}
$$

Respiratory Influence on Acid-Base Balance

Recall that CO_2 is considered a volatile acid because it is the partial pressure of CO_2 in the blood that determines the concentration of carbonic acid. For example, according to Henry's law, the concentration of a gas in solution is directly proportional to its partial pressure. That is, as the partial pressure increases, the concentration of the gas in solution increases and vice versa.

Because CO_2 is a gas, it can be eliminated by the lungs and therefore the respiratory system is an important regulator of the amount of blood carbonic acid and pH. To better understand the role of the lungs in acid-base balance, let's reexamine the carbonic acid dissociation equation:

$$CO_2 + H_2O \longleftrightarrow H_2CO_3 \longleftrightarrow H^+ + HCO_3^-$$

This relationship demonstrates that when the amount of CO_2 in the blood increases, the amount of H_2CO_3 increases, which lowers pH by elevating the acid concentration of the blood (i.e., the reaction moves to the right). In contrast, when the CO_2 content of the blood is lowered (i.e., CO_2 is "blown off" by the lungs), the pH of the blood increases because less acid is present (reaction moves to the left). Therefore, the respiratory system provides the body with a rapid means of regulating blood pH by controlling the amount of CO_2 present in the blood.

Regulation of Acid-Base Balance via the Kidneys

Since the kidneys do not play an important part in acid-base regulation during short-term exercise, only a brief overview of the kidney's role in acid-base balance will be presented here. The principal means by which the kidneys regulate hydrogen ion concentration is by increasing or decreasing the bicarbonate concentration (3, 4, 5). When the hydrogen ion concentration increases in body fluids, the kidney responds by a reduction in the rate of bicarbonate excretion (bicarbonate concentration increases). Conversely, when the pH of body fluids rises (hydrogen ion concentration decreases), the kidneys increase the rate of bicarbonate excretion. Therefore, by changing the amount of buffer present in body fluids, the kidneys aid in the regulation of the hydrogen ion concentration. The kidney mechanism involved in regulating the bicarbonate concentration is located in a portion of the kidney called the "tubule," and acts through a series of complicated reactions and active transport across the tubular wall. For additional information on this topic, the student is referred to Fox (1987) in the suggested reading list.

Why is the kidney not an important regulator of acid-base balance during exercise? The answer lies in the amount of time required for the kidney to respond to an acid-base disturbance. In general, it takes several hours for the kidneys to react effectively in response to an increase in blood hydrogen ion (3, 4, 5). Therefore, the kidneys respond too slow to be of major benefit in the regulation of hydrogen ion concentration during exercise.

Regulation of Acid-Base Balance during Exercise

During the final stages of an incremental exercise test or during near-maximal exercise of short duration, there is a decrease in both muscle and blood pH primarily due to the increase in the production of lactic acid by the muscle (8). This point is illustrated in figure 11.4, where the changes in blood and muscle pH during an incremental exercise test are graphed as a function of % $\dot{V}O_2$ max. Note that muscle and blood pH follow similar trends during this type of exercise, but that muscle pH is always 0.4 to 0.6 pH units lower than blood pH. This is because muscle lactic acid concentration is higher than that of blood, and muscle buffering capacity is lower than that of blood.

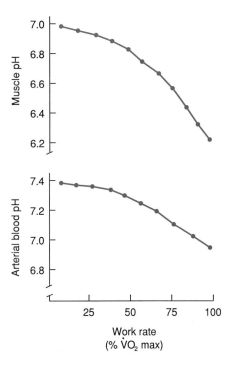

Figure 11.4 Changes in arterial blood pH and muscle pH during incremental exercise. Notice that arterial and muscle pH begin to fall together at work rates above 50% $\dot{V}O_2$ max.

The amount of lactic acid produced during exercise is dependent on: (1) the exercise intensity, (2) the amount of muscle mass involved, and (3) the duration of the work (3, 8). Exercise involving high-intensity leg work (e.g., running) may reduce arterial pH from 7.4 to a value of 7.0 within a few minutes (8, 10). Further, repeated bouts of this type of exercise may cause blood pH to decline even further to a value of 6.8 (8). This blood pH value is the lowest ever recorded and would present a life-threatening situation if it were not corrected within a few minutes.

How does the body act to regulate acid-base balance during exercise? Since the primary source of hydrogen ions produced during exercise is muscle lactic acid, it would seem reasonable that the first line of defense against a rise in acid production would reside in the muscle itself. This is indeed the case. It is estimated that intracellular proteins contribute as much as 60% of the cell's buffering capacity, with an additional 20%–30% of the total buffering capacity coming

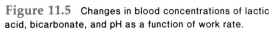

Figure 11.5 Changes in blood concentrations of lactic acid, bicarbonate, and pH as a function of work rate.

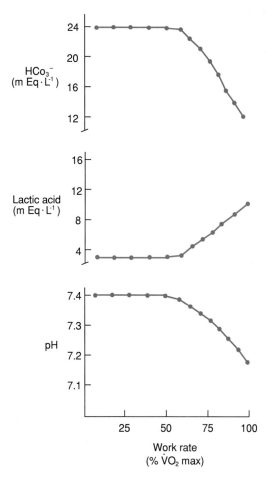

HCO_3^- (m Eq·L^{-1})

Lactic acid (m Eq·L^{-1})

pH

Work rate (% $\dot{V}O_2$ max)

incremental exercise. Note that as blood lactic acid concentration increases, blood bicarbonate concentration decreases proportionally. Also note that at approximately 50%–60% of $\dot{V}O_2$ max blood pH begins to decline due to the rise in acid production. This increase in blood hydrogen ion concentration stimulates the carotid bodies, which then signal the respiratory control center to increase alveolar ventilation (i.e., ventilatory threshold, chapter 10). An increase in alveolar ventilation results in the reduction of blood PCO_2 and therefore acts to reduce the acid load produced by exercise. The overall process of respiratory assistance in buffering lactic acid during exercise is referred to as **respiratory compensation** for metabolic acidosis.

Summary of Acid-Base Regulation during Exercise

Figure 11.6 outlines the process of buffering exercise-induced acidosis. The first line of defense against exercise-produced hydrogen ions is the chemical buffer systems of the intracellular compartment and the blood. These buffer systems act rapidly to convert strong acids into weak acids, and are therefore considered the body's first line of defense against pH shifts. Intracellular buffering occurs with the aid of cellular proteins, bicarbonate, and phosphate groups. Blood buffering of hydrogen ions occurs by bicarbonate, hemoglobin, and blood proteins, with bicarbonate playing the most important role. The second line of defense against pH shift during exercise is respiratory compensation for the metabolic acidosis.

from muscle bicarbonate (14). The final 10%–20% of muscle buffering capacity comes from intracellular phosphate groups.

Since the muscle's buffering capacity is limited, extracellular fluid (principally the blood) must possess a means of buffering hydrogen ions as well. The principal extracellular buffer and probably the most important buffer in the body is blood bicarbonate (14). Hemoglobin and blood proteins assist in this buffer process, but play only a minor role in blood buffering of lactic acid during exercise (14). Figure 11.5 illustrates the role of blood bicarbonate as a buffer during

Summary

1. Acids are defined as molecules that can liberate hydrogen ions, which raises the hydrogen ion concentration of an aqueous solution. Bases are molecules that are capable of combining with hydrogen ions.

2. The concentration of hydrogen ions in a solution is quantified by pH units. The pH of a solution is defined as the negative logarithm of the hydrogen ion concentration:

$$pH = -\log_{10} [H^+]$$

Figure 11.6 Lines of defense against pH change during intense exercise.

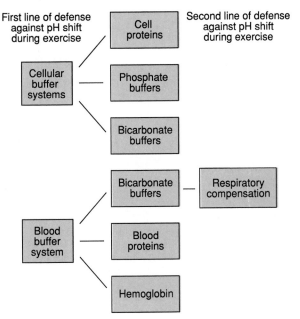

3. Metabolic acids can be subdivided into three major groups: (1) volatile acids (carbon dioxide), (2) fixed acids (sulfuric acid, phosphoric acid), and (3) organic acids (lactic acid).

4. Failure to maintain acid-base homeostasis during exercise can impair performance by inhibition of metabolic pathways responsible for production of ATP or by interference with the contractile process in the working muscle.

5. The body maintains acid-base homeostasis by buffer-control systems. A buffer resists pH change by removing hydrogen ions when the pH declines and by releasing hydrogen ions when the pH increases.

6. The principal intracellular buffers are proteins, phosphate groups, and bicarbonate. Primary extracellular buffers are bicarbonate, hemoglobin, and blood proteins.

7. Respiratory compensation for metabolic acidosis is the process of increasing alveolar ventilation, which lowers arterial PCO_2 and thus reduces blood H_2CO_3 concentration.

Study Questions

1. Define the terms acid, base, buffer, acidosis, alkalosis, and pH.
2. Graph the pH scale. Label the pH values that represent normal arterial and intracellular pH.
3. List and briefly discuss the three major groups of acids formed by the body.
4. Why is the maintenance of acid-base homeostasis important to physical performance?
5. What are the principal intracellular and extracellular buffers?
6. Discuss respiratory compensation for metabolic acidosis. What would happen to blood pH if an individual began to hyperventilate at rest? Why?
7. Briefly, outline how the body resists pH change during exercise.

Suggested Readings

Edwards, R. H. T. 1983. "Biochemical Bases of Fatigue in Exercise Performance: Catastrophe Theory of Muscular Fatigue." In *Biochemistry of Exercise.* Champaign, Ill.: Human Kinetics Publishers.

Fox, E., R. Bowers, and M. Foss. 1988. *The Physiological Basis of Physical Education and Athletics.* Philadelphia: Saunders College Publishing.

Fox, S. I. 1987. *Human Physiology.* Dubuque, Ia.: Wm. C. Brown.

Guyton, Arthur. 1986. *Textbook of Medical Physiology.* Philadelphia: W. B. Saunders Company.

Hultman, E., and K. Sahlin. 1980. Acid-base balance during exercise. (R. Hutton and D. Miller, eds.) *Exercise and Sport Science Reviews* 8:41–128. Philadelphia: Franklin Institute Press.

Vollestad, N., and O. M. Sejersted. 1988. Biochemical correlates of fatigue. *European Journal of Applied Physiology* 57:336–47.

References

1. Costill, D. et al. 1984. Acid-base balance during repeated bouts of exercise: Influence of bicarbonate. *International Journal of Sports Medicine* 5:228–31.

2. Edwards, R. H. T. 1983. "Biochemical Bases of Fatigue in Exercise Performance: Catastrophe Theory of Muscular Fatigue." In *Biochemistry of Exercise.* Champaign, Ill.: Human Kinetics Publishers.

3. Fox, E., R. Bowers, and M. Foss. 1988. *The Physiological Basis of Physical Education and Athletics.* Philadelphia: Saunders College Publishing.

4. Fox, S. I. 1984. *Human Physiology.* Dubuque, Ia.: Wm. C. Brown.

5. Guyton, Arthur. 1986. *Textbook of Medical Physiology.* Philadelphia: W. B. Saunders Company.

6. Hole, J. 1987. *Human Anatomy and Physiology.* Dubuque, Ia.: Wm. C. Brown.

7. Hultman, E., and J. Sjoholm. 1986. "Biochemical Causes of Fatigue." (N. Jones, N. McCartney, and A. McComes, eds.) *Human Muscle Power.* Champaign, Ill.: Human Kinetics Publishers.

8. Hultman, E., and K. Sahlin. 1980. Acid-base balance during exercise. (R. Hutton and D. Miller, eds.) *Exercise and Sport Science Reviews* 8:41–128. Philadelphia: Franklin Institute Press.

9. Johnson, L. 1983. *Biology.* Dubuque, Ia.: Wm. C. Brown.

10. Jones, N. et al. 1977. Effect of pH on cardiorespiratory and metabolic responses to exercise. *Journal of Applied Physiology* 43:959–64.

11. Jones, N. L. 1980. Hydrogen ion balance during exercise. *Clinical Science* 59:85–91.

12. Karlsson, J. 1979. Localized muscular fatigue: role of metabolism and substrate depletion. (R. Hutton and D. Miller, eds.) *Exercise and Sport Science Reviews* 7:1–42. Philadelphia: Franklin Institute Press.

13. Katz, A. et al. 1984. Maximal exercise tolerance after induced alkalosis. *International Journal of Sports Medicine* 5:107–10.

14. Laiken, N., and D. Fanestil. 1985. "Acid-Base Balance and Regulation of Hydrogen Ion Excretion." (J. West, ed.) *Physiological Basis of Medical Practice.* Baltimore: Williams and Wilkins.

15. McCartney, N., G. Heigenhauser, and N. Jones. 1983. Effects of pH on maximal power output and fatigue during short-term dynamic exercise. *Journal of Applied Physiology* 55:225–29.

16. Poortmans, J. 1983. "The Intramuscular Environment in Peripheral Fatigue." *Biochemistry of Exercise.* Champaign, Ill.: Human Kinetics Publishers.

17. Robertson, R. et al. 1987. Effect of induced alkalosis on physical work capacity during arm and leg exercise. *Ergonomics* 30:19–31.

18. Sahlin, K. 1983. "Effects of Acidosis on Energy Metabolism and Force Generation in Skeletal Muscle." *Biochemistry of Exercise.* Champaign, Ill.: Human Kinetics Publishers.

19. Sharpo, R. et al. 1986. Effects of eight weeks of bicycle ergometer sprint training on human muscle buffer capacity. *International Journal of Sports Medicine* 7:13–17.

20. Stewart, P. A. 1983. Modern quantitative acid-base chemistry. *Canadian Journal of Physiology and Pharmacology* 61:1444–64.

21. Vollestad, N., and O. M. Sejersted. 1988. Biochemical correlates of fatigue. *European Journal of Applied Physiology* 57:336–47.

12 *Temperature Regulation*

Objectives

By studying this chapter, you should be able to do the following:
1. Define the term homeotherm.
2. Present an overview of heat balance during exercise.
3. Discuss the concept of "core temperature."
4. List the principal means of involuntarily increasing heat production.
5. Define the four processes by which the body can lose heat during exercise.
6. Discuss the role of the hypothalamus as the body's thermostat.
7. Explain the thermal events that occur during exercise in both a cool/moderate and hot/humid environment.
8. List the physiological adaptations that occur during acclimatization to heat.
9. Describe the physiological responses to a cold environment.
10. Discuss the physiological changes that occur in response to cold acclimatization.

Outline

Key Terms

anterior hypothalamus
conduction
convection
evaporation
homeotherms
hyperthermia
hypothalamus
hypothermia
posterior hypothalamus
radiation

*B*ody core temperature regulation is critical because cellular structures and metabolic pathways are affected by temperature. For example, enzymes that regulate metabolic pathways are greatly influenced by temperature changes; an increase in body temperature above 45° C (normal core temperature is approximately 37° C) may destroy the protein structure of enzymes, resulting in death, while a decrease in body temperature below 34° C may cause a slowed metabolism and abnormal cardiac function (arrhythmias) (3, 9, 16). Hence, people and many animals live their entire lives only a few degrees from their thermal death point. Therefore it is clear that body temperature must be carefully regulated.

Animals who maintain a rather constant body core temperature are called **homeotherms.** The maintenance of a constant body temperature requires that heat loss must match the rate of heat production. To accomplish thermal regulation, the body is well equipped with both nervous and hormonal mechanisms that regulate metabolic rate as well as the amount of heat loss in response to body temperature changes. The temperature-maintenance strategy of homeotherms uses a "furnace" rather than a "refrigerator" to maintain body temperature at a constant level. That is, the body temperature is set near the high end of the survival range and is maintained fairly constant by continuous metabolic heat production coupled with a small but continual heat loss. The rationale for this strategy seems to be that temperature regulation by heat conservation and generation is very efficient, while man's cooling capacity is much more limited (13).

Because contracting skeletal muscles produce large amounts of heat, long-term exercise in a hot/humid environment presents a serious challenge to temperature homeostasis. In fact, many exercise scientists believe that overheating is the only serious threat to health that exercise presents to a healthy individual. It is the purpose of this chapter to discuss the principles of temperature regulation during exercise. The cardiovascular and pulmonary responses to exercise in a hot environment have already been discussed in chapters 9 and 10, respectively, and the influence of temperature on performance will be discussed in chapter 24.

Overview of Heat Balance during Exercise

The goal of temperature regulation is to maintain a constant deep-body temperature and thus prevent overheating or overcooling. If the core temperature is to remain constant, the amount of heat lost must match the amount of heat gained (see figure 12.1). Consistent with that, if heat loss is less than heat production, there is a net gain in body heat and therefore body temperature rises; if heat loss exceeds heat production, there is a net loss in body heat and body temperature decreases.

During exercise, body temperature is regulated by making adjustments in the amount of heat that is lost. One of the important functions of the circulatory system is to transport heat. Blood is very effective in this function since it has a high capacity to store heat. When the body is attempting to lose heat, blood flow is increased to the skin as a means of promoting heat loss to the environment. In contrast, when the goal of temperature regulation is to prevent heat loss, blood is directed away from the skin and toward the interior of the body to prevent additional heat loss.

Figure 12.1 Temperature homeostasis is maintained by an equal rate of body heat gain and heat loss.

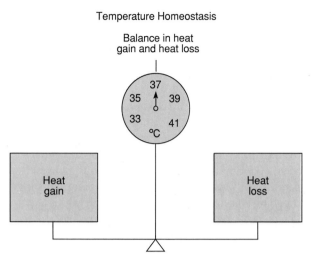

Temperature Homeostasis

Balance in heat
gain and heat loss

It is important to point out that within the body, temperature varies a great deal. That is, there is a gradient between deep-body temperature (i.e., deep central areas, including the heart, lungs, abdominal organs) and the "shell" (skin) temperature. In extreme circumstances (i.e., exposure to very cold temperatures), the core temperature may be 20° C higher than the shell. However, such large core-to-shell gradients are rare and the ideal difference between core and shell is approximately 4° C (1). Even within the core, temperature varies from one organ to another. Because large differences in temperature exist between one body part to another, it is important to be specific as to where body temperature is being measured. Therefore, the term "body temperature" is a misnomer and should be be replaced by more descriptive terms such as core temperature or skin temperature, depending on which temperature is being discussed (1).

Temperature Measurement during Exercise

Measurements of deep-body temperatures may be accomplished via mercury thermometers, or devices known as thermocouples or thermistors. One of the most common sites of core temperature measurement

is the rectum. Although rectal temperature is not the same as the temperature in the brain where temperature is regulated, it can be used to estimate changes in deep-body temperature during exercise. In addition, temperature measurements near the eardrum (called tympanic temperature) have been found to be a good estimate of the actual brain temperature. Another alternative is to measure the temperature of the esophagus as an indication of core temperature. Like rectal temperature, esophageal temperature is not identical to brain temperature, but offers a measure of deep-body temperature.

Skin temperature can be measured by placing temperature sensors (thermistors) on the skin at various locations. The mean skin temperature can be calculated by assigning certain factors to each individual skin measurement in proportion to the fraction of the body's total surface area that each measurement represents. For example, mean skin temperature (T_s) can be estimated by the following formula (14):

$$T_s = (T_{forehead} + T_{chest} + T_{forearm} + T_{thigh} + T_{calf} + T_{abdomen} + T_{back}) \div 7$$

where $T_{forehead}$, T_{chest}, $T_{forearm}$, T_{thigh}, T_{calf}, $T_{abdomen}$, and T_{back} represent skin temperatures measured on the forehead, chest, forearm, thigh, calf, abdomen, and back, respectively.

Overview of Heat Production/Heat Loss

As previously stated, the goal of temperature regulation is to maintain a constant core temperature. This regulation is achieved by controlling the rate of heat production and heat loss. When out of balance, the body either gains or loses heat. The temperature control center is an area in the brain called the **hypothalamus.** The hypothalamus works like a thermostat by initiating an increase in heat production when body temperature falls, and an increase in the rate of heat loss when body temperature rises. Temperature regulation is controlled by both physical and chemical processes. Let's begin our discussion of temperature regulation by introducing those factors that govern heat production and heat loss.

Figure 12.2 The body produces heat due to normal metabolic processes. Heat production can be classified as being either (1) voluntary or (2) involuntary.

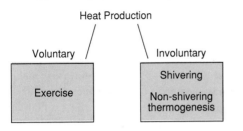

Heat Production

The body produces internal heat due to normal metabolic processes. At rest or during sleep, metabolic heat production is small; however, during intense exercise, heat production is large. Heat production can be classified as (1) voluntary (exercise) or (2) involuntary (shivering or biochemical heat production caused by the secretion of hormones such as thyroxin and catecholamines) (see figure 12.2).

Since the body is approximately 20%–25% efficient, 75%–80% of the energy expended during exercise is lost as heat. During heavy exercise, this can result in a large heat load. Indeed, work in a hot/humid environment serves as a serious test of the body's ability to lose heat.

Involuntary heat production by shivering is the primary means of increasing heat production during exposure to cold. Maximal shivering can increase the body's heat production by approximately fives times the resting value (3, 5). In addition, release of thyroxin from the thyroid gland can also increase metabolic rate. Thyroxin acts by increasing the metabolic rate of all cells in the body (11). Finally, an increase in blood levels of catecholamines (epinephrine and norepinephrine) can cause an increase in the rate of cellular metabolism (8). The increase in heat production due to the combined influences of thyroxin and catecholamines is called "nonshivering thermogenesis."

Heat Loss

Heat loss from the body may occur by four processes: (1) radiation, (2) conduction, (3) convection, and/or (4) evaporation. The first three of these heat loss mechanisms require a temperature gradient to exist between the skin and the environment. **Radiation** is heat loss in the form of infrared rays. This involves the transfer of heat from the surface of one object to the surface of another, with no physical contact being involved (i.e., sun transferring heat to the earth via radiation). At rest in a comfortable environment (i.e., room temperature = 21°–22° C), 60% of the heat loss occurs via radiation. This is possible because skin temperature will be greater than the temperature of surrounding objects (walls, floor, etc.), which causes a net loss of body heat due to the thermal gradient. Note that on a hot, sunny day (surface temperatures are greater than skin temperature) the body can also gain heat via radiation. Therefore, it is important to remember that radiation is heat transfer by infrared rays and can result in either heat loss or heat gain depending on the environmental conditions.

Conduction is defined as the transfer of heat from the body into the molecules of cooler objects in contact with its surface. In general, the body loses only small amounts of heat due to this process. An example of heat loss due to conduction is the transfer of heat from the body to a metal chair while a person is sitting on it. The heat loss occurs as long as the chair is cooler than the body surface in contact with it.

Convection is a form of conductive heat loss by the transmission of heat to either air or water molecules in contact with the body. In convective heat loss, air or water molecules are warmed and become less dense, rising away from the source of the heat and are replaced by cooler molecules. For example, a fan moving large quantities of air past the skin would increase the number of air molecules coming in contact with the skin and thus promote heat loss. Practically speaking, the amount of heat loss due to convection is dependent on the air flow over the skin. Therefore, under the same wind conditions, cycling at high speeds would improve convective cooling when compared to cycling at slow speeds or running. Swimming in cool water (water temperature less than skin temperature) also results in convective heat loss. In fact, water's effectiveness in cooling is many times greater than that of air.

The final means of heat loss is **evaporation.** Evaporation accounts for approximately 25% of the heat loss at rest, but under most environmental conditions is the most important means of heat loss during exercise. In evaporation, heat is transferred from the body to water on the surface of the skin. When this water gains sufficient heat (energy), it is converted to a gas (water vapor), taking the heat away from the body. Note that evaporation occurs due to a vapor pressure gradient between the skin and the air. Vapor pressure is the pressure exerted by water molecules that have been converted to gas (water vapor). Evaporative cooling during exercise occurs in the following way. When body temperature rises above normal, the nervous system stimulates sweat glands to secrete sweat onto the surface of the skin. As sweat evaporates, heat is lost to the environment, which in turn lowers skin temperature.

The amount of evaporation of sweat from the skin during exercise is dependent on three factors: (1) the temperature and relative humidity, (2) the convective currents around the body, and (3) the amount of skin surface exposed to the environment (1, 16). At high environmental temperatures, relative humidity is the most important factor by far in determining the rate of evaporative heat loss. High relative humidity reduces the rate of evaporation. In fact, when the relative humidity is near 100%, evaporation is limited. Therefore, cooling by way of evaporation is most effective under conditions of low humidity.

Why does high relative humidity reduce the rate of evaporation? The answer is linked to the fact that high relative humidity (RH) reduces the vapor pressure gradient between the skin and the environment. On a hot/humid day (e.g. RH = 80%–90%) the vapor pressure in the air is close to the vapor pressure on moist skin. Therefore, the rate of evaporation is greatly reduced. High sweat rates during exercise in a hot/high humidity environment result in useless water loss. That is, sweating per se does not cool the skin; it is evaporation that cools the skin (15).

Table 12.1 *The relationship between temperature and relative humidity (RH) on vapor pressure*

50% RH	
Temperature °C	Vapor Pressure (mmHg)
0	2.29
10	4.60
20	8.77
30	15.93

75% RH	
Temperature °C	Vapor Pressure (mmHg)
0	3.43
10	6.91
20	13.16
30	23.89

100% RH	
Temperature °C	Vapor Pressure (mmHg)
0	4.58
10	9.21
20	17.55
30	31.86

Let's explore in more detail those factors that regulate the rate of evaporation. The major point to keep in mind is that evaporation occurs due to a vapor pressure gradient. That is, in order for evaporative cooling to occur during exercise, the vapor pressure on the skin must be greater than the vapor pressure in the air. Vapor pressure is influenced by both temperature and relative humidity. This relationship is illustrated in table 12.1, which states that at any given relative humidity, a rise in temperature results in increased vapor pressure. Practically speaking, this means that less evaporative cooling occurs during exercise on a hot/humid day when compared to a cool/humid day. For example, an athlete running on a hot/humid day (e.g.,

Knowledge that evaporation of 1,000 ml of sweat results in 580 kcal of heat loss can be used to calculate the sweat and evaporation rate necessary to maintain a specified body temperature during exercise. Consider the following example: John Hothead is working on a cycle ergometer at a $\dot{V}O_2$ of 2.0 liters $\cdot$ min^{-1}, (energy expenditure of 10.0 kcal $\cdot$ min^{-1}). If John exercises for twenty minutes at this metabolic rate and is 20% efficient, how much evaporation would be necessary to prevent an increase in core temperature?[1] The total heat produced can be calculated as:

$$\text{Total energy expenditure} = 20 \text{ min} \times 10 \text{ kcal/min}$$
$$= 200 \text{ kcal}$$
$$\text{Total heat produced} = 200 \text{ kcal} \times .80^{[2]}$$
$$= 160 \text{ kcal}$$

The total evaporation necessary to prevent any heat gain would be computed as:

$$\frac{160 \text{ kcal}}{580 \text{ kcal/liter}} = \begin{array}{l} .275 \text{ liters (evaporation} \\ \text{necessary to prevent} \\ \text{heat gain)} \end{array}$$

[1] Assumes no other heat-loss mechanism is active.

[2] If efficiency is 20%, then 80%, or .80 of the total energy expenditure, must be released as heat.

---

air temperature $= 30°$ C; RH $= 100\%$) might have a mean skin temperature in the range of $33°$–$34°$ C. The vapor pressure on the skin would be approximately 35 mm Hg and the air vapor pressure would be around 32 mm Hg (table 12.1). This small vapor pressure gradient between the skin and air (3 mm Hg) would permit limited evaporation, and therefore little cooling would occur. In contrast, the same athlete running on a cool/humid day (e.g., air temperature $= 10°$ C; RH $= 100\%$) might have a mean skin temperature of $30°$ C. The vapor pressure gradient between the skin and air under these conditions would be approximately 21 mm Hg ($30 - 9 = 21$) (table 12.1). This relatively large skin-to-air vapor pressure gradient would permit a reasonably large evaporative rate, and therefore adequate body cooling would occur under these conditions.

How much heat can be lost via evaporation during exercise? Heat loss due to evaporation can be calculated in the following manner. The body loses 0.58 kcal of heat for each ml of water that evaporates (26). Therefore, evaporation of 1 liter of sweat would result in a heat loss of 580 kcal (1,000 ml $\times$ 0.58 kcal/ml $= 580$ kcal). See Box 12.1 for examples of additional heat loss calculations.

In summary, heat loss during exercise (other than swimming) in a cool/moderate environment occurs primarily due to evaporation. In fact, when exercise is performed in a hot environment (where air temperature is greater than skin temperature), evaporation is the only means of losing body heat. The means by which the body gains and loses heat during exercise are summarized in figure 12.3.

Body's Thermostat — Hypothalamus

As previously stated, the principal temperature regulatory center is located in the hypothalamus. The **anterior hypothalamus** is thought to be responsible for dealing with increases in body heat, while the **posterior hypothalamus** is responsible for reacting to a decrease in body temperature. In general, the hypothalamus operates much like a thermostat in your home—that is, it attempts to maintain a relatively

Figure 12.3 A summary of heat exchange mechanisms during exercise.

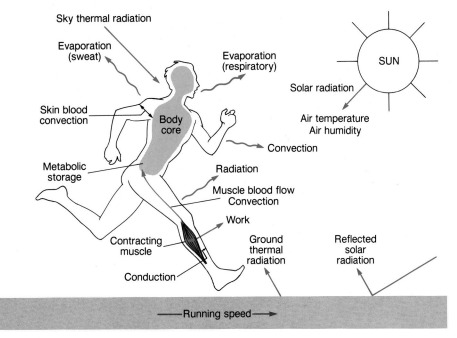

constant core temperature around some "set point." The set-point temperature in humans is approximately 37° C.

The input to the temperature-regulating centers in the hypothalamus comes from receptors in both the skin and the core. Changes in environmental temperature are first detected by thermal receptors (both heat and cold) located in the skin. These skin-temperature receptors transmit nerve impulses to the hypothalamus, which then initiates the appropriate response in an effort to maintain the body's set-point temperature. Further, heat-/cold-sensitive neurons are located in both the spinal cord and the hypothalamus itself, sensing changes in the core temperature.

An increase in core temperature above the set point results in the hypothalamus initiating a series of physiological actions aimed at increasing the amount of heat loss. First, the hypothalamus stimulates the sweat glands, which results in an increase in evaporative heat loss. In addition, the vasomotor control center withdraws the normal vasoconstrictor tone to the skin,

promoting increased skin blood flow and therefore allowing increased heat loss. Figure 12.4 illustrates the physiological responses associated with an increase in core temperature. When core temperature returns to normal, the stimulus to promote both sweating and vasodilation is removed. This is an example of a control system using negative feedback (chapter 2).

When cold receptors are stimulated in the skin or the hypothalamus, the thermoregulatory control center sets forth a plan of action to minimize heat loss and increase heat production. First, the vasomotor center directs peripheral blood vessels to vasoconstrict, which reduces heat loss (11). Second, if core temperature drops significantly, involuntary shivering begins. Additional responses include stimulation of the pilomotor center, which promotes piloerection (goosebumps). This piloerection reflex is an effective means of increasing the insulation space over the skin in fur-bearing animals, but is not an effective means of preventing heat loss in humans. Further, the hypothalamus indirectly increases thyroxin production and

Figure 12.4 A summary illustration of the physiological responses to an increase in "heat load."

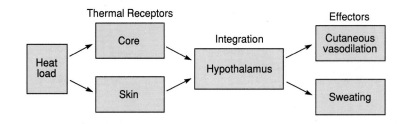

Response to a "Heat Load"

Figure 12.5. An illustration of the physiological responses to cold stress.

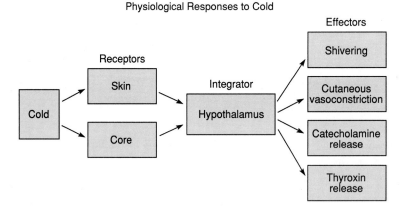

Physiological Responses to Cold

release, which increases cellular heat production (4). Finally, the posterior hypothalamus initiates the release of norepinephrine, which increases the rate of cellular metabolism (nonshivering thermogenesis). The physiological responses to a drop in core temperature are summarized in figure 12.5.

Shift in the Hypothalamic Thermostat Set Point due to Fever

A fever is an increase in body temperature above the normal range, and may be caused by a host of bacterial diseases or brain disorders. During a fever, certain proteins and other toxins secreted by bacteria can cause the set point of the hypothalamic thermostat to rise above the normal level. Substances that cause this effect are called pyrogens. When the set point of the hypothalamic thermostat is raised to a higher level than normal, all the mechanisms for raising body temperature are called into play (8). Within a few hours after the thermostat has been set to a higher level, the body core temperature reaches this new level due to heat conservation.

Thermal Events during Exercise

Now that an overview of how the hypothalamus responds to different thermal challenges has been presented, let's examine a brief scenario of the thermal events that occur during exercise in a cool/moderate environment (i.e., low humidity and room temperature). Heat production increases during exercise due

Figure 12.6 Heat exchange at rest and during cycle ergometer exercise at a variety of work rates. Note the steady increase in evaporative heat loss as a function of an increase in power output. In contrast, an increase in metabolic rate has essentially no influence on the rate of convective and radiative heat loss.

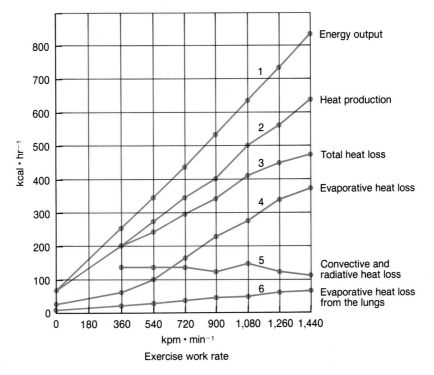

to muscular contraction and is directly proportional to the exercise intensity (see figure 12.6). The venous blood draining the exercising muscle distributes the excess heat throughout the body core. As core temperature increases, thermal sensors in the hypothalamus sense the increase in blood temperature, and the thermal integration center in the hypothalamus compares this increase in temperature with the set-point temperature and finds an error between the two (6, 16, 17). The response is to direct the nervous system to commence sweating and to increase blood flow to the skin (2). These acts serve to increase body heat loss and minimize the increase in body temperature. At this point, the internal temperature reaches a new, elevated steady state level (see figure 12.7). Note that this new steady state core temperature does not represent a change in the set-point temperature, as occurs in fever (6, 16, 17, 27). Instead, the thermal regulatory center attempts to return the core temperature back to resting levels, but is incapable of doing so in the face of the sustained heat production associated with exercise.

Figure 12.7 also illustrates the roles of evaporation, convection, and radiation in heat loss during constant-load exercise in a moderate environment. Notice the constant but small role of convection and radiation in heat loss during this type of exercise. This is due to a constant temperature gradient between the skin and the room. In contrast, evaporation plays the most important role in heat loss during exercise in this type of environment (19).

During constant-load exercise the core temperature increase is directly related to the exercise intensity and is independent of ambient temperature over a wide range of conditions (i.e., 8°–29° C with low relative humidity) (18). This point is illustrated in figure 12.8.

Figure 12.7 Changes in metabolic energy production, evaporative heat loss, convective heat loss, and radiative heat loss during twenty-five minutes of submaximal exercise in a cool environment.

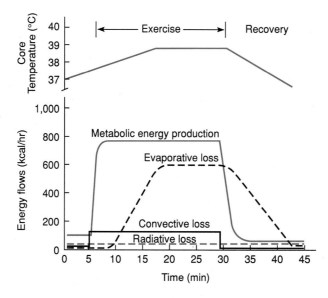

Figure 12.8 The relationship between metabolic rate and rectal temperature during arm (·) and leg (x) exercise.

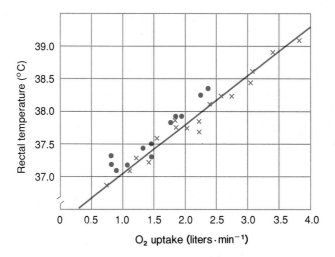

Figure 12.9 Heat exchange during exercise at different environmental temperatures. Notice the change in evaporative and convective/radiative heat loss as the environmental temperature increases. See text for discussion.

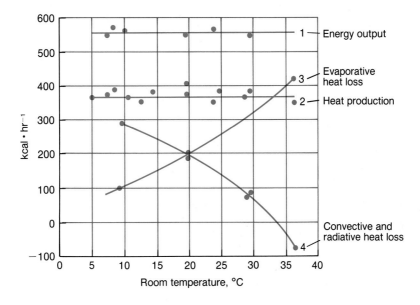

Notice the linear rise in core temperature as the metabolic rate increases. The fact that it is the exercise intensity and not the environmental temperature that determines the rise in core temperature during exercise suggests that the method of heat loss during continuous exercise is modified according to ambient conditions (18). This concept is presented in figure 12.9. Note that as the ambient temperature increases, the rate of convective and radiative heat loss decreases due to a decrease in the skin-to-room temperature gradient. This decrease in convective and radiative heat loss is matched by an increase in evaporative heat loss and core temperature remains the same (see figure 12.9).

Exercise in the Heat

Continuous exercise in a hot/humid environment poses a particularly stressful challenge to maintenance of normal body temperature and fluid homeostasis. High heat and humidity reduce the body's ability to lose heat by radiation/convection and evaporation, respectively. This inability to lose heat during exercise in a hot/humid environment results in a greater core temperature and a higher sweat rate (more fluid loss) when compared to the same exercise in a moderate environment (21–25). This point is illustrated in figure 12.10. Notice the marked differences in sweat rates and core temperatures during exercise between the hot/humid conditions and the moderate environment. The combined effect of fluid loss and high core temperature generally has a detrimental effect on performance in endurance events (see chapter 24) and increases the risk of **hyperthermia** (large rise in core temperature) and heat injury (see Box 12.2).

Although controversy exists, most women appear to be less heat tolerant than men (20). Factors contributing to women's limited heat tolerance include lower sweat rates and generally a higher percentage of body fat than men (a high percentage of body fat reduces heat loss). However, when women and men

Figure 12.10 Differences in core temperature and sweat rate during forty-five minutes of submaximal exercise in a hot/humid environment versus a cool environment.

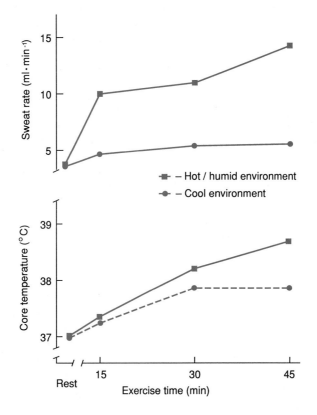

Heat Acclimatization

Regular exercise in a hot environment results in a series of physiological adjustments designed to minimize disturbances in homeostasis due to heat stress (this is referred to as heat acclimatization). The end result of heat acclimatization is a lower heart rate and core temperature both at rest and during submaximal exercise (7). The primary adaptations that occur during heat acclimatization are an increased plasma volume, earlier onset of sweating, higher sweat rate, reduced salt loss in sweat, and a reduced skin blood flow (7).

are matched for the same degree of heat acclimatization and similar body compositions, the gender differences in the physiological responses to thermal stress are small (20).

It is interesting that heat adaptation occurs rapidly, with almost complete acclimatization being achieved by seven to twelve days after the first exposure (2, 27).

Heat acclimatization results in a 10%–12% increase in plasma volume (3, 7). The increase in plasma volume is due to an increase in plasma proteins. This increased plasma volume maintains central blood volume, stroke volume, sweating capacity, and allows the body to store more heat with a smaller temperature gain.

As stated previously, heat adaptation results in an earlier onset of sweating. This means that sweating begins rapidly after the commencement of exercise, which translates into less heat storage at the beginning of exercise and a lower core temperature. In addition,

Box 12.2 Prevention of Heat Injuries

Heat injury may occur when the demands of the environment exceed the capabilities of the body's thermal regulatory mechanisms. The primary cause of heat injury is hyperthermia (high internal temperatures), and may result in heat stroke and death. Increases in body temperature of 2° C–3° C generally do not have any ill effects (1, 4). However, when internal temperatures rise above 40° C–41° C, central nervous system dysfunction may occur. The symptoms of heat stress are nausea, dizziness, reduction in sweat rate, and the general inability to think rationally. Above temperatures of 43° C–44° C there may be cellular damage resulting in permanent brain damage and perhaps death.

To prevent overheating during exercise, a maximum surface area should be exposed for evaporation (i.e., clothing shed). When clothing removal is not possible (e.g., football) frequent water breaks, coupled with rest periods to allow core temperature to decline, are useful in preventing heat injury. Once an athlete develops symptoms of heat injury, the two most obvious treatments are to remove the individual from the hot environment (stop exercising) and provide water or a balanced electrolyte drink. Rubbing the body with ice or submersion in cool water are an ideal means of reducing body temperature rapidly. See chapter 24 for details on the prevention of heat injuries.

Table 12.2 *A summary of the primary adaptations that occur as a result of heat acclimatization*

1. Increased plasma volume
2. Earlier onset of sweating
3. Higher sweat rate
4. Reduced sodium chloride loss in sweat
5. Reduced skin blood flow

heat acclimatization may increase the sweating capacity almost three-fold above the rate achievable prior to heat adaptation. Therefore, much more evaporative cooling is possible, which is a major advantage in minimizing heat storage during prolonged work. Finally, sweat losses of sodium and chloride are reduced following heat acclimatization due to an increased secretion of aldosterone (27). While this adaptation results in a reduction of electrolyte loss and aids in reducing electrolyte disturbances during exercise in the heat, it does not minimize the need to replace water loss, which is higher than normal (see chapters 23 and 24). A summary of heat-adaptive responses is presented in table 12.2.

Exercise in a Cold Environment

Exercise in a cold environment enhances an athlete's ability to lose heat and therefore greatly reduces the chance of heat injury. In general, the combination of metabolic heat production and warm clothing prevents the development of **hypothermia** (large decrease in core temperature) during short-term work on a cold day. However, exercise in the cold for extended periods of time (a long triathlon), or swimming in cold water, may overpower the body's ability to prevent heat loss, and hypothermia may result. In such cases, heat production during exercise is not able to keep pace with heat loss. This is particularly true during swimming in extremely cold water (e.g., < 15° C). Severe hypothermia may result in a loss of judgment, which increases the risk of further cold injury.

Individuals with a high percentage of body fat have an advantage over lean individuals when it comes to cold tolerance (11, 20). Large amounts of subcutaneous fat provide an increased layer of insulation from the cold. This additional insulation reduces the rate of heat loss and therefore improves cold tolerance. It is for this reason that women generally tolerate mild cold exposure better than men (20).

Participation in sports activities in the cold may present several other types of problems for the athlete. For example, hands exposed to cold weather become numb due to the reduction in the rate of neural transmission and reduced blood flow due to vasoconstriction. This results in a loss of dexterity and of course affects such skills as throwing and catching. In addition, exposed flesh is susceptible to frostbite, which may present a serious medical condition (3). Further details of a cold environment on performance will be presented in chapter 24.

Cold Acclimatization

In humans chronically exposed to cold (e.g., primitive societies, mountain climbers), there appears to be at least three physiological adaptations to cold exposure (10). First, cold adaptation results in a reduction in the mean skin temperature at which shivering begins. That is, people who are cold acclimatized begin shivering at a lower skin temperature when compared to unacclimatized individuals. The explanation for this observation is that cold-acclimatized individuals maintain heat production with less shivering by increasing nonshivering thermogenesis. They increase the secretion of norepinephrine, which results in an increase in metabolic heat production (3, 4, 10).

A second physiological adjustment that occurs due to cold acclimatization is that cold-adjusted individuals are able to maintain a higher mean hand-and-foot temperature during cold exposure when compared to unacclimatized persons. Cold acclimatization apparently results in improved intermittent peripheral vasodilation to increase blood flow (and heat flow) to both the hands and feet.

The third and final physiological adaptation to cold is the improved ability to sleep in cold environments. Unacclimatized people, when attempting to sleep in cold environments, will often shiver so much that sleep is impossible (3). In contrast, cold-acclimatized individuals have the ability to sleep comfortably in cold environments due to their elevated level of nonshivering thermogenesis. The exact time course of complete cold acclimatization is not clear. However, subjects placed in a cold chamber begin to show signs of cold acclimatization after one week (12).

In summary, cold acclimatization results in three principal physiological adaptations: (1) an increase in nonshivering thermogenesis, (2) improved peripheral circulation to maintain a higher hand-and-foot temperature, and (3) improved ability to sleep in the cold. The overall goal of these adaptations is to increase heat production and maintain core temperature, which will make the individual more comfortable during cold exposure.

Summary

1. Homeotherms are animals that maintain a rather constant body core temperature. In order to maintain a constant core temperature, heat loss must match heat gain.

2. Temperature varies a great deal within the body. In general, there is a thermal gradient from deep body temperatures (core temperature) to the shell (skin) temperature.

3. The body's thermostat is the hypothalamus. It works to maintain a constant core temperature (set point) by regulating the amount of heat loss due to involuntary heat production. The anterior hypothalamus is responsible for reacting to increases in core temperature, while the posterior hypothalamus governs the body's responses to a decrease in temperature.

4. Heat loss may occur due to: (1) conduction, (2) convection, (3) radiation, and (4) evaporation.

5. An increase in core temperature results in the anterior hypothalamus initiating a series of physiological actions aimed at increasing heat loss. These actions include: (1) the commencement of sweating, and (2) an increase in skin blood flow.

6. Cold exposure results in the posterior hypothalamus putting forth a plan of action designed to increase heat production and minimize heat loss.

7. During prolonged exercise in a moderate environment, core temperature will increase gradually above the normal resting value and will reach a plateau at approximately thirty to

forty-five minutes. However, during exercise in a hot/humid environment, core temperature does not reach a plateau, but will continue to rise. Long-term exercise in this type of environment increases the risk of heat injury.

8. Heat acclimatization results in: (1) an earlier onset of sweating during exercise, (2) a higher sweat rate, (3) a reduction in the amount of electrolytes lost in sweat, and (4) an increase in plasma volume.

9. Cold acclimatization results in three physiological adaptations: (1) improved ability to sleep in cold environments, (2) increased nonshivering thermogenesis, and (3) a higher intermittent blood flow to the hands and feet.

Study Questions

1. Define the following terms: (1) homeotherm, (2) hyperthermia, and (3) hypothermia.
2. Why does a significant increase in core temperature represent a threat to life?
3. Explain the comment that the term "body temperature" is a misnomer.
4. How is body temperature measured during exercise?
5. Briefly, discuss the role of the hypothalamus in temperature regulation. How do the anterior hypothalamus and posterior hypothalamus differ in function?
6. List and define the four avenues of heat loss. Which of these avenues plays the most important part during exercise in a hot/dry environment?
7. Discuss the two general categories of heat production in people.
8. What hormones are involved in biochemical heat production?
9. Briefly, outline the thermal events that occur during prolonged exercise in a moderate environment. Include in your discussion information concerning changes in core temperature, skin blood flow, sweating, and skin temperature.
10. List and discuss the physiological adaptations that occur during heat acclimatization.
11. How might exercise in a cold environment affect dexterity in such skills as throwing and catching?
12. Discuss the physiological changes that occur in response to chronic exposure to cold.
13. Calculate the amount of evaporation that must occur to remove 400 kcal of heat from the body.
14. How much heat would be removed from the skin if 520 ml of sweat evaporated during a thirty-minute period?

Suggested Readings

Gisolfi, C., and C. B. Wenger. 1984. Temperature regulation during exercise: Old concepts, new ideas. In (R. Terjung, ed.) *Exercise and Sport Science Reviews* 12:339–72.

Hole, J. 1987. *Human Anatomy and Physiology.* Dubuque, Ia.: Wm. C. Brown.

Hong, S., D. Rennie, and Y. Park. 1987. Humans can acclimatize to cold: a lesson from Korean divers. *News in Physiological Sciences* 2:79–82.

Wyndham, C. 1973. The physiology of exercise under heat stress. *Annual Review of Physiology* 35:193–220.

References

1. Astrand, P., and K. Rodahl. 1986. *Textbook of Work Physiology.* New York: McGraw-Hill.
2. Brengelmann, G. 1977. Control of sweating and skin blood flow during exercise. In *Problems with Temperature Regulation during Exercise.* (E. Nadel, ed.) New York: Academic Press.
3. Brooks, G., and T. Fahey. 1987. *Fundamentals of Human Performance.* New York: Macmillian.
4. Cabanac, M. 1975. Temperature regulation. *Annual Review of Physiology* 37:415–39.
5. Fox, S. 1987. *Human Physiology.* Dubuque, Ia.: Wm. C. Brown.
6. Gisolfi, C., and C. B. Wenger. 1984. Temperature regulation during exercise: Old concepts, new ideas. In (R. Terjung, ed.) *Exercise and Sport Science Reviews.* 12:339–72.
7. Gisolfi, C., and J. Cohen. 1979. Relationships among training, heat acclimation, and heat tolerance in men and women: The controversy revisited. *Medicine and Science in Sports* 11:56–59.

8. Guyton, A. C. 1986. *Textbook of Medical Physiology*. Philadelphia: W. B. Saunders Company.

9. Hole, J. 1987. *Human Anatomy and Physiology*. Dubuque, Ia.: Wm. C. Brown.

10. Hong, S., D. Rennie, and Y. Park. 1987. Humans can acclimatize to cold: A lesson from Korean divers. *News in Physiological Sciences* 2:79–82.

11. Horvath, S. 1981. Exercise in a cold environment. In *Exercise and Sport Science Review* 9:221–63.

12. Iampietro, P., D. Bass, and E. Buskirk. 1959. Diurnal oxygen consumption and rectal temperature of men during cold exposure. *Journal of Applied Physiology* 10:398–403.

13. Johnson, L. 1983. *Biology*. Dubuque, Ia.: Wm. C. Brown.

14. Kenney, W. 1988. Control of heat-induced cutaneous vasodilation in relation to age. *European Journal of Applied Physiology* 57:120–25.

15. McArdle, W., F. Katch, and V. Katch. 1986. *Exercise Physiology: Energy, Nutrition, and Human Performance*. Philadelphia: Lea & Febiger.

16. Nadel, E. 1979. Temperature regulation. In (R. Strauss, ed.) *Sports Medicine and Physiology*. Philadelphia: W. B. Saunders Company.

17. Nielson, B. 1969. Thermoregulation during exercise. *Acta Physicologica Scandanavica* (Suppl.) 323: 10–73.

18. Nielson, M. 1938. Die Regulation der Korpertemperatur bei Muskelarbeit. *Scandanavica Archives Physiology* 79:193.

19. Noble, B. 1986. *Physiology of Exercise and Sport*. St Louis: C. V. Mosby.

20. Nunneley, S. 1978. Physiological responses of women to thermal stress: A review. *Medicine and Science in Sports and Exercise* 10:250–55.

21. Powers, S., E. Howley, and R. Cox. 1982. A differential catecholamine response during prolonged exercise and passive heating. *Medicine and Science in Sports and Exercise* 6:435–39.

22. Powers, S., E. Howley, and R. Cox. 1985. Blood lactate concentrations during submaximal work under differing environmental conditions. *Journal of Sports Medicine and Physical Fitness* 25:84–89.

23. Powers, S., E. Howley, and R. Cox. 1982. Ventilatory and metabolic reactions to heat stress during prolonged exercise. *Journal of Sports Medicine and Physical Fitness* 22:32–36.

24. Robinson, S. 1963. Temperature regulation during exercise. *Pediatrics* 32:691–702.

25. Stolwijk, J., B. Saltin, and A. Gagge. 1968. Physiological factors associated with sweating during exercise. *Aerospace Medicine* 39:1101–05.

26. Wenger, C. B. 1972. Heat evaporation of sweat: Thermodynamic considerations. *Journal of Applied Physiology* 32:456–59.

27. Wyndham, C. 1973. The physiology of exercise under heat stress. *Annual Review of Physiology* 35:193–220.

13 Endurance Training: Effect on $\dot{V}O_2$ Max, Performance, and Homeostasis

Objectives

By studying this chapter, you should be able to do the following:

1. Explain the basic principles of training: overload and specificity.
2. Contrast cross-sectional with longitudinal research studies.
3. Indicate the typical change in $\dot{V}O_2$ max with endurance training programs, and the effect of the initial (pretraining) value on the magnitude of the increase.
4. State typical $\dot{V}O_2$ max values for various patient, sedentary, active, and athletic populations.
5. State the formula for $\dot{V}O_2$ max using heart rate, stroke volume, and the a-$\bar{v}$ O_2 difference; indicate which of the variables is most important in explaining the wide range of $\dot{V}O_2$ max values in the population.
6. Discuss, using the variables identified in objective 5, how the increase in $\dot{V}O_2$ max comes about for the sedentary subject who participates in an endurance training program.
7. Define preload, afterload, and contractility, and discuss the role of each in the increase in the maximal stroke volume that occurs with endurance training.
8. Describe the changes in muscle structure that are responsible for the increase in the maximal a-$\bar{v}$ O_2 difference with endurance training.
9. Describe how the capillary, myoglobin, and mitochondrial changes that occur in muscle as a result of an endurance training program are related to the following adaptations to submaximal exercise:
   a. a lower O_2 deficit
   b. an increased utilization of FFA and a sparing of blood glucose and muscle glycogen
   c. a reduction in lactate and H^+ formation
   d. an increase in lactate removal
10. Discuss how changes in "central command" and "peripheral feedback" following an endurance training program can lower the heart rate, ventilation, and catecholamine responses to a submaximal exercise bout.

Outline

Key Terms

A theme that has been used throughout this book is that there are automatic regulatory mechanisms operating at rest and during exercise to maintain homeostasis. Figure 13.1 identifies some of the variables that are maintained within narrow limits during exercise in spite of the tremendous demands placed on various tissues and organ systems. What has become clear is that participation in regular vigorous exercise increases the cardiovascular system's ability to deliver blood to the working muscles, and the muscle's capacity to produce energy aerobically. These changes occur in parallel and result in less disruption of the internal environment during exercise. This, of course, leads to improved performance.

The purpose of this chapter is to tie together much of what has been previously presented, rather than introduce new material. The title, Endurance Training: Effect on $\dot{V}O_2$ max, Performance, and Homeostasis, is a good one for this purpose since most tissues and organ systems are either directly or indirectly affected by endurance training programs. There is a need to discuss separately those physiological changes causing an increase in $\dot{V}O_2$ max from those associated with improvements in prolonged submaximal performance. $\dot{V}O_2$ max is most closely linked to the functional capacity of the cardiovascular system to deliver blood to the working muscles during maximal and supramaximal ($>100\%$ $\dot{V}O_2$ max) work, while maintaining mean arterial blood pressure. The ability to sustain long-term submaximal exercise is linked more to the maintenance of homeostasis due to specific structural and biochemical properties of working muscles (4, 20, 31). Before we begin a discussion of these topics, information about the principles of training and the design of research studies will be presented.

Principles of Training

The three principles of training include **overload, specificity,** and **reversibility.** These principles will be applied in chapters 16 and 17 for those training for fitness, and in chapters 21 and 22 for those training for performance.

Overload
Overload refers to the observation that a system or tissue must be exercised at a level beyond which it is presently accustomed in order for a training effect to occur. The system or tissue gradually adapts to this overload. This pattern of overload followed by adaptation continues until the system or tissue can no longer adapt. The typical variables that constitute the overload include the intensity, duration, and frequency (days per week) of exercise. The corollary of the overload principle, the principle of reversibility, simply indicates that the gains are quickly lost when the overload is removed (35).

Specificity
The training effect is specific to the muscle fibers involved in the activity. This may seem like an obvious statement in that one should not expect the arms to become trained during a ten-week jogging program. However, this also means that if an individual participates in a long, slow, distance running program that utilizes the slow-twitch muscle fibers, there is little or no training effect taking place in those fast-twitch fibers in the same muscle (20).

Specificity also refers to the types of adaptations occurring in muscle as a result of training. If a muscle is engaged in endurance types of exercise the primary adaptations are in capillary and mitochondria number,

Figure 13.1 Homeostatic variables maintained within narrow limits in spite of the challenge presented by exercise.

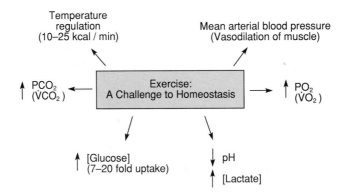

which increase the capacity of the muscle to produce energy aerobically (20, 35). If a muscle is engaged in heavy resistive training, the primary adaptations are in the contractile proteins; the mitochondrial and capillary density actually decrease (24). This high degree of specificity in the training effect raises the question of whether or not one type of training may interfere with the adaptations to the other.

Design of Training Programs

The effect of exercise training on various physiological systems has been studied using two different designs: cross-sectional and longitudinal. In cross-sectional studies the investigator examines groups differing in physical activity (e.g., cardiac patients, sedentary students, and world-class endurance athletes) and records the differences that exist in $\dot{V}O_2$ max, cardiac output, or fiber-type distribution. These studies are relatively inexpensive to conduct and provide good descriptive information about differences that exist between various populations. They are also useful in developing questions about how these differences came about, including hypotheses about the relative role of genetics versus training. Longitudinal studies examine *changes* in $\dot{V}O_2$ max, cardiac output, or fiber-type distribution occurring over the course of a training program. These studies control for the genetic factor since

the same subject is repeatedly tested, and allows one to investigate the *rate* at which the variables respond to training or detraining. Longitudinal studies are expensive and difficult to conduct due to the potential for subjects dropping out and the demand for all equipment and procedures to be maintained constant at all testing points in the study. Due to these constraints, only small numbers of subjects are used in these studies. The investigator must take special care that the subjects are representative of the population, and that they do not alter other life-style patterns (diet, smoking, etc.) that might influence the outcome of the study (3).

As we mentioned in the introduction, the effects of training on $\dot{V}O_2$ max will be discussed separately from that of performance and homeostasis. The application of this information in the design of training programs for fitness and performance is found in chapters 16, 17, 21, and 22.

Endurance Training and $\dot{V}O_2$ Max

Maximal aerobic power, $\dot{V}O_2$ max, is a reproducible measure of the capacity of the cardiovascular system to deliver blood to a large muscle mass involved in dynamic work (31). Chapter 4 introduced this concept, and chapters 9 and 10 showed how specific cardiovascular and pulmonary variables respond to graded exercise up to $\dot{V}O_2$ max. The following sections discuss

Figure 13.2 The percent improvement in $\dot{V}O_2$ max with endurance training is related to the initial $\dot{V}O_2$ max.

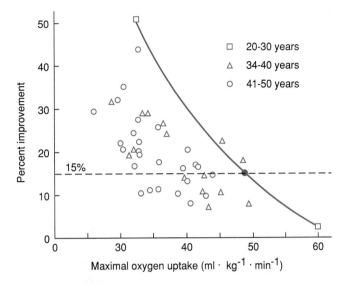

the effect of endurance exercise programs on the increase in $\dot{V}O_2$ max and the physiological changes bringing about that increase.

Training Programs and Changes in $\dot{V}O_2$ Max

Endurance training programs that increase $\dot{V}O_2$ max involve a large muscle mass in dynamic exercise (e.g., running, cycling, swimming, or cross-country skiing) for fifteen to sixty minutes per session, three to five times per week at an intensity of 50%–85% $\dot{V}O_2$ max (1). Details about how to design a training program for the average individual and the athlete are presented in chapters 16 and 21, respectively. While endurance training programs of two to three months duration cause an increase in $\dot{V}O_2$ max of about 15%, figure 13.2 shows the range of improvement to be as low as 2%–3% for those who start the program with high $\dot{V}O_2$ max values (9), and as high as 30%–50% for those with low initial $\dot{V}O_2$ max values (13, 19, 31, 32).

Table 13.1 shows that $\dot{V}O_2$ max can be less then 20 ml · kg^{-1} · min^{-1} in patients with severe cardiovascular and pulmonary disease, to more than 80 ml · kg^{-1} · min^{-1} in world-class distance runners and cross-country skiers. The extremely high $\dot{V}O_2$ max values measured in elite male and female endurance athletes has been ascribed to a genetic gift of a large cardiovascular capacity (3). Early work by Klissourus et al. (23) supported this idea with the observation that identical twins have very similar $\dot{V}O_2$ max values, while fraternal twins do not. Given that identical twins have identical genes, it was suggested that 93% of the variation in $\dot{V}O_2$ max values in the general population was due to genetics. On the surface that high estimate appears to be consistent with the small changes in $\dot{V}O_2$ max that occur with the training programs just mentioned, however, serious questions have been raised about this conclusion. A recent examination of this question suggests that we need to revise that estimate downward to a figure somewhat closer to 40% (5). While this estimate of the contribution of genetics to $\dot{V}O_2$ max is lower, it is clear that a genetic predisposition for possessing a high $\dot{V}O_2$ max value is still a prerequisite for values in the range of 60–80 ml · kg^{-1} · min^{-1}. Further, evidence exists that the sensitivity of the individual to the effect of the training program on $\dot{V}O_2$ max is also genetically determined (29).

Table 13.1 $\dot{V}O_2$ max values measured in healthy and diseased populations

Population	Males	Females
Cross-country skiers	84	72
Distance runners	83	62
Sedentary: young	45	38
Sedentary: middle-aged adults	35	30
Post myocardial infarction patients	22	18
Severe pulmonary disease patients	13	13

Values are expressed in ml · kg^{-1} · min^{-1}. Taken from Saltin and Astrand (34), Astrand and Rodahl (3), and Howley and Franks (21).

Consistent with these lower estimates of the genetic contribution to $\dot{V}O_2$ max are the observations that training for two to three years (13), or participation in severe interval training (19) can increase $\dot{V}O_2$ max by as much as 44%. The results of the latter study showed a linear increase in $\dot{V}O_2$ max over ten weeks of training, whereas most studies show a leveling off of the $\dot{V}O_2$ max values after only a few weeks of training. The much larger increase in $\dot{V}O_2$ max with this ten-week training program is related to a much higher intensity, frequency, and duration than is usually used in endurance exercise programs. What causes the $\dot{V}O_2$ max to increase as a result of an endurance exercise program?

$\dot{V}O_2$ Max: Cardiac Output and the Arteriovenous O_2 Difference

Since oxygen uptake is the product of systemic blood flow (cardiac output) and systemic oxygen extraction (arteriovenous oxygen difference), changes in $\dot{V}O_2$ max would have to be due to changes in one or more of the following variables on the right side of the equal sign.

$$\dot{V}O_2 \text{ max} = HR \text{ max} \times SV \text{ max} \times (a\text{-}\bar{v} \ O_2 \text{ difference}) \text{ max}$$

Cross-sectional comparisons of groups differing in their level of habitual physical activity have allowed scientists to identify the most important of these variables as the prime determinant of $\dot{V}O_2$ max. Such a comparison is presented in table 13.2, where values for $\dot{V}O_2$ max, maximal heart rate, maximal stroke volume, and the maximal a-$\bar{v}$ O_2 difference are presented for three groups of subjects: mitral stenosis patients (heart valve problem limiting stoke volume), normally active subjects, and finally, world class endurance athletes (31). The $\dot{V}O_2$ max is more than 100% greater for the normally active subjects compared to those with mitral stenosis, and again, almost 100% higher for the athletes as compared to the normally active subjects. What variable explains the tremendous differences in $\dot{V}O_2$ max values? Given that the maximal heart rate and the maximal a-$\bar{v}$ O_2 difference were virtually identical for the three groups, the only variable explaining the difference in $\dot{V}O_2$ max is the maximal stroke volume (43 ml versus 112 ml versus 205 ml).

Longitudinal studies provide a slightly different picture of how training causes an increase in $\dot{V}O_2$ max. Generally, maximal heart rate either remains the same or decreases with endurance training (13, 31). As a result, the increase in $\dot{V}O_2$ max is shared between the increase in the stroke volume and the systemic a-$\bar{v}$ O_2 difference. Studies reported by Saltin (32) in which young sedentary subjects trained for two to three months show that the sharing is about equal, half the gain due to SV changes and half to an increased oxygen extraction. When training is extended for years, the continued increase in $\dot{V}O_2$ max can be due to an increase in one factor more than the other. Data from Ekblom (13), shown in table 13.3, make this point. Subject LM's increase in $\dot{V}O_2$ max from the start was due primarily to an increase in stroke volume. The a-$\bar{v}$ O_2 difference changed only 9 milliliters per liter over the eighteen months of training. In contrast, subject IS, whose $\dot{V}O_2$ max increased 44% over fifty-one months, showed no change in maximal cardiac output from sixteen to fifty-one months, with the entire increase in $\dot{V}O_2$ max due to an expanded a-$\bar{v}$ O_2 difference. What causes the maximal stroke volume and the

Table 13.2 Physiological basis for differences in $\dot{V}O_2$ max in different populations

Population	$\dot{V}O_2$ max (ml · min^{-1})	=	Heart Rate (beats · min^{-1})	×	Stroke Volume (l · beat^{-1})	×	a-$\bar{v}$ O_2 Difference (ml O_2 · l^{-1})
Athletes	6,250	=	190	×	.205	×	160
Normally active	3,500	=	195	×	.112	×	160
Mitral stenosis	1,400	=	190	×	.043	×	170

From L. B. Rowell, *Human Circulation Regulation during Physical Stress.* Copyright © 1986 Oxford University Press, New York, N.Y.

Table 13.3 Longitudinal data on changes in maximal oxygen uptake

	$\dot{V}O_2$ max (l · min^{-1})	HR max (b · min^{-1})	Stroke Volume (ml · beat^{-1})	Cardiac Output (l · min^{-1})	a-$\bar{v}$ O_2 Difference (ml · l^{-1})
Subject LM					
Before training	3.58	206	124	25.5	140
Four months	4.38	210	143	28.1	142
Eighteen months	4.53	205	149	30.5	149
Subject IS					
Before training	3.07	205	122	23.9	126
Four months	3.87	205	134	26.2	131
Thirty-two months	4.36	185	151	27.6	158
Fifty-one months	4.41	186	146	26.6	166

From B. Ekblom, Effect of physical training on oxygen transport system in man, in *Acta Physiological Scandinavica.* Supplement 328, 1964. Copyright © 1969 Blackwell Scientific Publications Ltd., Oxford, England. Reprinted by permission.

maximal arteriovenous oxygen difference to increase as a result of endurance training? The answer is provided in the next two sections.

Stroke Volume

Stroke volume is equal to the difference between end diastolic volume (EDV) and end systolic volume (ESV). Figure 13.3 summarizes the factors increasing stroke volume: an increase in EDV due to an increase in ventricle size or an increase in venous return ("preload"), an increase in myocardial contractility (the force of contraction at a constant muscle fiber length, with other factors controlled), and a decrease in resistance to blood flow out of the heart ("afterload"). Each of these will be discussed relative to the increase in the maximal stroke volume that occurs with endurance training.

Figure 13.3 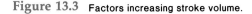 Factors increasing stroke volume.

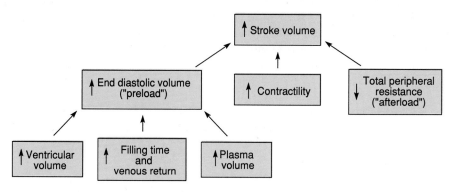

End Diastolic Volume (EDV). There is evidence that left ventricle size increases as a result of endurance training, with little change in ventricular wall thickness, while isometric exercises cause an increase in wall thickness, with little or no change in ventricular volume (11, 26, 30). This effect is believed to be due to the "volume loading" experienced by the heart *during exercise.* However, Rowell (31) raises the question that the increase in stroke volume that occurs with endurance training may simply be due to the chronic stretch of the myocardium *at rest* because of the increased filling time caused by the slower resting heart rate (**bradycardia**). Accompanying this increase in heart volume with endurance training is an increase in plasma volume, which would also increase preload. But the importance of the plasma volume change is probably small, and is difficult to evaluate. Overall, EDV increases as a result of an endurance training program, and according to the Frank-Starling mechanism (chapter 9), an increased stretch of the ventricle leads to an increase in stroke volume (31).

Cardiac Contractility. Cardiac contractility refers specifically to the strength of the cardiac muscle contraction when the fiber length (EDV), afterload (peripheral resistance), and heart rate are constant (since all affect contractility). While an acute exercise bout increases cardiac contractility due to the action of the sympathetic nervous system on the ventricle, it is difficult to conclude whether or not the inherent contractility of the heart changes with endurance training. The reason for this is that the factors that directly affect contractility (EDV, heart rate, and afterload) are themselves affected by endurance training (31). Blomqvist and Saltin (4) suggest that changes in contractility probably are not too important in explaining the increase in maximal stroke volume with endurance training. They base this belief on the observation that the fraction of the EDV ejected from the heart per beat (**ejection fraction**) is already so high in sedentary subjects prior to an endurance exercise program that there is not much to be gained by increasing contractility (30).

Afterload. Afterload refers to the peripheral resistance against which the ventricle is contracting as it tries to push a portion of the EDV into the aorta. If the heart contracts with the same force while the peripheral resistance decreases, a greater stroke volume will be realized. What is clear is that following an endurance training program, trained muscles offer less resistance to blood flow *during maximal work.* This decrease in resistance parallels the increase in maximal cardiac output so that mean arterial blood pressure is unchanged ($MAP = \dot{Q} \times TPR$). How does endurance training cause the decrease in the working muscle's resistance to facilitate a higher blood flow?

The increased blood flow through the trained muscle could be due to an increase in the local factors (H^+, CO_2, etc.) associated with the higher work rates achieved after an endurance training program, but it is not. This can be seen in the following example. Prior to training, a subject takes a graded exercise test while maximal values for $\dot{V}O_2$ max and $\dot{Q}$ are measured. On another day the same subject takes an exercise test set at a work rate equal to 120% of the $\dot{V}O_2$ max achieved on the previous test and, of course, measures the same value for $\dot{V}O_2$ max. This supramaximal ($>100\%$ $\dot{V}O_2$ max) test should have caused a higher concentration of local factors in the working muscles that would have facilitated vasodilation and increased muscle blood flow. However, if this vasodilation were to happen with the cardiac output already at its maximal value, mean arterial blood pressure would fall, with dire consequences (31). How is this fall in blood pressure prevented?

When an additional muscle mass is recruited to do the supramaximal work rate, other vascular beds would have to be vasoconstricted by the sympathetic nervous system to maintain blood pressure. Since the renal and splanchnic vascular beds are already maximally constricted at maximal work, the only possibility is to vasoconstrict some vascular beds in already active muscle when additional muscle groups are recruited to do the supramaximal work (31). Consequently, the increase in muscle blood flow during the maximal exercise test following an endurance training program is due to a reduction in the sympathetic vasoconstrictor activity to the arterioles of the trained muscles. This occurs simultaneously with the increase in maximal cardiac output, and this combination allows for the higher $\dot{V}O_2$ max at a constant mean arterial blood pressure, the homeostatic variable that appears to be closely regulated in maximal work (31).

Evidence supporting this explanation is found in studies where one-legged exercise is conducted. $\dot{V}O_2$ max measured during one-legged exercise on a cycle ergometer is equal to about 75%–80% of that measured during the regular two-legged test (9, 22). This is due to the greater arteriolar dilation achieved in the working muscles during one-legged exercise. If the same degree of vasodilation were to occur in each leg when both were exercising maximally, the muscle's *capacity for blood flow* would exceed the heart's ability to provide it, and blood pressure would fall. To counter this tendency during maximal two-legged work, some of the muscle mass must be vasoconstricted to maintain blood pressure (22, 31). This is why the two-legged $\dot{V}O_2$ max value is not the sum of the $\dot{V}O_2$ max values of each leg. In summary, during maximal work with trained muscles following an endurance training program there is a decrease in the resistance of that vascular bed to match the increase in maximal cardiac output to maintain blood pressure.

Arteriovenous O_2 Difference

While stroke volume causes 50% of the increase in $\dot{V}O_2$ max associated with an endurance exercise program in young sedentary subjects, O_2 extraction is responsible for the other 50% of the increase. The increase in the arteriovenous O_2 difference could be due to an elevation of the arterial oxygen content (higher hemoglobin or PO_2), or a decrease in the mixed venous oxygen content. Given that the hemoglobin concentration does not change with training and that the arterial PO_2 is usually sufficient to maintain arterial saturation of hemoglobin (chapter 10), the increase in the a-v̄ O_2 difference is not due to an increase in the arterial O_2 content (31).

The increased capacity of the muscle to extract O_2 following training is believed to be primarily due to the increase in capillary density, and secondarily to the increase in the myoglobin concentration and mitochondrial number (4, 20, 31). The increase in capillary density in trained muscle accommodates the increase in muscle blood flow during maximal exercise, decreases the diffusion distance to the mitochondria, and slows the rate of blood flow to allow time for diffusion to take place. Changes in capillary density parallel changes in leg blood flow and $\dot{V}O_2$ max with training (31). While increases in myoglobin and mitochondria favor O_2 transport from the capillary, the mitochondrial capacity of muscle far exceeds the capability of the heart to deliver O_2, making mitochondrial number *not* the factor limiting $\dot{V}O_2$ max (4, 20, 31).

Figure 13.4 provides a summary of the factors causing an increase in $\dot{V}O_2$ max with an endurance training program. The following paragraphs provide the detail:

1. In young, sedentary subjects 50% of the increase in $\dot{V}O_2$ max with endurance training

Figure 13.4 Summary of factors causing an increase in $\dot{V}O_2$ max with endurance training.

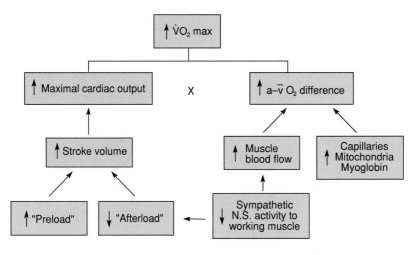

is due to an increase in maximal cardiac output due entirely to an increase in maximal stroke volume, with no change (or a small decrease) in maximal heart rate. The increase in maximal stroke volume is due to both an increase in preload and a decrease in afterload. The increased preload is primarily due to an increase in end diastolic ventricular volume. The decreased afterload is due to a decrease in the arteriolar constriction in the trained muscles, increasing maximal muscle blood flow with no change in the mean arterial blood pressure. The large differences in $\dot{V}O_2$ max values in the general population are due primarily to large differences in maximal stroke volume.

2. In young sedentary subjects 50% of the increase in $\dot{V}O_2$ max is due to an increase in the systemic a-$\bar{v}$ O_2 difference. This increase is accomplished by an increase in the capillary density of the trained muscles to accept the increase in maximal muscle blood flow. This allows for a sufficiently slow red blood cell transit time through the muscle, allowing enough time for oxygen diffusion, which is facilitated by the increase in myoglobin content and the number of mitochondria.

Endurance Training: Effects on Performance and Homeostasis

The ability to continue prolonged submaximal work is dependent on the maintenance of homeostasis during the activity. In the introduction to this chapter we mentioned that the increase in performance following an endurance training program was due more to biochemical and structural changes in the trained skeletal muscle than to a small increase in $\dot{V}O_2$ max. Endurance training causes rather large changes in the biochemical and structural characteristics of the working muscles. The muscles experience increases in the number of mitochondria (up to four-fold), myoglobin concentration, and capillary density (20). The increase in the mitochondria number is associated with increases in the enzymes involved in oxidative metabolism: Krebs cycle, fatty-acid (β-oxidation) cycle, and the electron transport chain. Changes also occur in the "shuttle system," used for moving NADH from the cytoplasm where it was produced in glycolysis to the mitochondria where it is used in the electron transport chain to produce ATP. Finally, changes occur in the types of LDH enzyme, which is involved in the conversion of pyruvate to lactate. It is the changes in these characteristics of muscle that "drive" or determine the overall physiological responses to a given submaximal

Figure 13.5 Influence of mitochondria number on the change in the ADP concentration needed to increase the $\dot{V}O_2$.

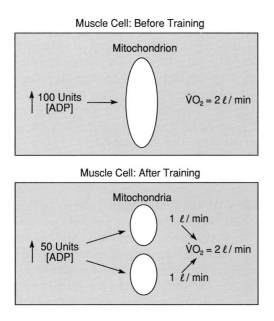

exercise bout. The following sections will describe how these biochemical and structural changes result in less disruption of crucial variables maintained by homeostatic mechanisms.

Biochemical Adaptations and the Oxygen Deficit

At the onset of exercise ATP is converted to ADP and Pi by the cross-bridges in order to develop tension. The increase in the ADP concentration in the cytoplasm is the immediate stimulus for ATP-producing systems to come into play to meet the ATP demands of the cross-bridges. Creatine phosphate responds immediately to this ATP need, followed by glycolysis and mitochondrial oxidative phosphorylation. The latter process provides all the ATP aerobically during the steady state phase of the work, with the mitochondrial oxygen consumption driven by the ADP concentration. Muscle cells with few mitochondria must have a high ADP concentration to stimulate the limited number of mitochondria to consume oxygen at a given rate (20).

How does endurance training affect these oxygen uptake responses at the onset of submaximal steady state work?

The steady state $\dot{V}O_2$ measured during a submaximal work test is not affected by endurance training. The mitochondria are still consuming the same number of O_2 molecules per minute. What is different, due to the large increase in mitochondria, oxidative enzymes, and the number of capillaries per muscle fiber, is how the ATP-producing chore is shared among the mitochondria. Figure 13.5 shows schematically that if a muscle cell has only one mitochondrion, an increase of 100 units in the ADP concentration is needed for the muscle to consume 2.0 liters of O_2 per minute. After training, when the number of mitochondria has doubled, the ADP concentration increases only half as much since each mitochondrion needs only half the stimulation to take up 1 liter of O_2 per minute. The increase in the capillary density and the myoglobin concentration in the muscle cell after endurance training are parallel changes that facilitate this process. In essence, after an endurance training program it takes less change in the ADP concentration to stimulate the mitochondria to take up the oxygen (20). Since less of a change in the ADP concentration is needed to stimulate the mitochondria, the rising ADP concentration at the onset of work (due to cross-bridges causing ATP → ADP + Pi) will cause oxidative phosphorylation to be activated earlier. This translates into a faster rise in the oxygen uptake curve at the onset of work, resulting in the steady state $\dot{V}O_2$ being achieved earlier (see figure 4.2) (18, 28). This faster rise in oxygen uptake at the onset of work means that the O_2 deficit is less: less creatine phosphate depletion and less lactate and H^+ formation (17).

The reason for the reduction in lactate and H^+ formation and creatine phosphate depletion is also linked to the lower ADP concentration in the muscle cell after the endurance training program. The lower ADP concentration results in less creatine phosphate depletion since the reaction for this is [ADP] + [CP] → [ATP] + [C]. The lower ADP concentration in the cell also results in less stimulation of glycolysis. Chapter 3 indicated that phosphofructokinase (PFK) is the enzyme in glycolysis that controls the rate at which glucose is

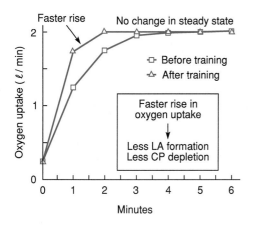

Figure 13.6 Endurance training reduces the O₂ deficit at the onset of work.

The increased number of mitochondria increases a muscle fiber's capacity to oxidize both carbohydrate and fat. However, the most dramatic change in muscle metabolism following training is in the increased utilization of fat, and the sparing of carbohydrate. This is due to an improved capacity to mobilize FFA from adipose tissue to muscle, an increased ability to transport FFA from the cytoplasm to the mitochondria of the muscle, and an increase in the fatty-acid (β-oxidation) cycle enzymes needed to degrade the FFA to acetyl-CoA units for the Krebs cycle (20). These points will now be discussed.

Mobilization of FFA

In the previous section we showed how the increased mitochondria number resulted in a lower ADP concentration needed to sustain a given oxygen uptake. This lower ADP concentration and higher CP concentration resulted in less stimulation of PFK, a reduced rate of glycolysis, and less lactate formation. While the emphasis in the previous section was on the events at the onset of work, the effects of the increased mitochondria number would hold for the duration of the exercise bout. The lower lactate production results in less blood lactate and, as described in figure 5.32, less inhibition of FFA mobilization from adipose tissue.

Plasma FFA provide half the fat oxidized by muscle during exercise, and the uptake of FFA by muscle is proportional to the FFA concentration in the plasma (27). The enhanced mobilization of FFA due to the lower blood lactate would favor the maintenance of the plasma FFA concentration at a time when the muscle is using FFA at a faster rate. The increase in capillary density at the muscle allows for both a slower muscle capillary blood flow during exercise and an increased surface area for the diffusion of FFA into the muscle. Lastly, the maintenance of a high cytoplasmic concentration of FFA acts to inhibit PFK activity to further reduce carbohydrate metabolism (20). All of these adaptations favor a reduced rate of carbohydrate oxidation, sparing the muscle glycogen and plasma glucose. Based on this discussion, one might expect the plasma FFA concentration to be higher after training since the adipose cell is not inhibited by a high blood lactate concentration; however that is not the case (6). How can that be?

metabolized, and that high levels of ADP and low levels of CP in the cell stimulate this enzyme to process glucose through the pathway. The reduced stimulation of glycolysis due to the lower ADP and higher CP concentrations following endurance training results in less reliance on anaerobic glycolysis to provide ATP at the onset of exercise (15, 17). The net result is a lower oxygen deficit, less depletion of creatine phosphate, and a reduction in lactate and H⁺ formation. Figure 13.6 shows that the biochemical adaptations following endurance training result in a faster rise in the oxygen uptake curve at the onset of work, with less disruption of homeostasis.

Biochemical Adaptations and the Plasma Glucose Concentration

Plasma glucose is the primary fuel of the nervous system and, as described in chapter 5, the majority of hormonal changes associated with fasting or exercise are aimed at maintaining this important homeostatic variable. How do the biochemical changes in muscle that occur as result of endurance training help maintain the blood glucose concentration during prolonged submaximal exercise? The answer is again found in the increases in mitochondrial number and capillary density that occur with endurance training.

Figure 13.7 Increased mitochondria number increases the rate of free-fatty-acid utilization, preserving plasma glucose.

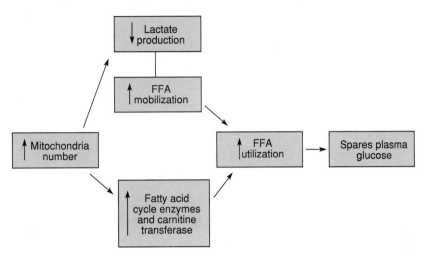

Transport of FFA from the Cytoplasm to the Mitochondria

The FFA are transported from the cytoplasm to the mitochondria by carnitine transferase, an enzyme associated with the mitochondrial membrane. This enzyme catalyzes the reaction of FFA and the carrier molecule, carnitine, which moves quickly across the mitochondrial membrane where the reaction is reversed, yielding the FFA for oxidation. The increase in the mitochondrial number with endurance training increases the surface area of the mitochondrial membranes and the amount of carnitine transferase such that FFA can move at a faster rate from the cytoplasm to the mitochondria for oxidation (33). The faster rate of transport from the cytoplasm to the mitochondria favors the diffusion of more FFA into the muscle cell from the plasma. This may explain why the plasma FFA concentration is not higher as a result of endurance training, even though fatty acids provide more fuel for working muscles.

Mitochondrial Oxidation of FFA

The increase in mitochondria number increases the enzymes involved in FFA oxidation, specifically, the fatty-acid (β-oxidation) cycle. This results in an increased rate at which acetyl-CoA molecules are formed from FFA for entry to the Krebs cycle, where citrate (the first molecule in the cycle) is formed. The high citrate level inhibits PFK activity in the cytoplasm and therefore reduces carbohydrate metabolism (20).

In summary, the lower lactate concentration at the same submaximal work rate following endurance training favors the mobilization of FFA from adipose tissue to maintain the plasma FFA concentration at a time when the muscle is increasing its rate of FFA uptake and oxidation. The combination of the increase in the density of capillaries and mitochondria per muscle fiber increases the surface area of the membranes and increases the amount of carnitine transferase needed for the movement of FFA from the plasma to the mitochondria. Lastly, the increases in the enzymes of the fatty acid cycle increase the rate of formation of acetyl-CoA from FFA for oxidation in the Krebs cycle. This increase in fat oxidation in endurance trained muscle spares both muscle glycogen and plasma glucose, the latter being a focal point of homeostatic regulatory mechanisms. These points are summarized in figure 13.7.

Figure 13.8 Increased mitochondria number decreases lactate and H+ formation to maintain the blood pH.

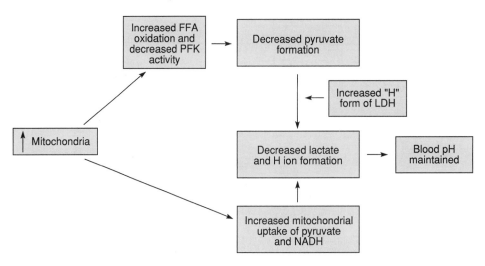

Biochemical Adaptations and Blood pH

The pH of blood is maintained near 7.40 ± .02 at rest. As described in chapter 11, acute and long-term challenges to the pH are met by responses of both the pulmonary and renal systems. How does endurance training result in less disruption of the blood pH during submaximal work? The answer relates to the reduced lactate and H+ formation following endurance training.

Lactate formation occurs when there is an accumulation of NADH and pyruvate in the cytoplasm of the cell where lactate dehydrogenase (LDH) is present:

$$[\text{pyruvate}] + [\text{NADH}] \xrightarrow[\text{LDH}]{} [\text{lactate}] + [\text{NAD}]$$

Anything that affects the concentration of pyruvate, NADH, or the type of LDH in the cell will affect the rate of lactate formation. We have already seen that the increased number of mitochondria can have a dramatic effect on pyruvate formation: the lower ADP concentration stimulates PFK less at the onset of work, and the increased capacity to use fats reduces the need for carbohydrate oxidation during prolonged work. If less carbohydrate is used, less pyruvate will be formed. In addition, the increase in mitochondria number increases the chance that pyruvate will be taken up by the mitochondria for oxidation in the Krebs cycle,

rather than being bound to LDH in the cytoplasm. All of these adaptations favor a lower pyruvate concentration and a reduction in lactate formation.

There are two additional biochemical changes in muscle due to endurance training that reduce lactate and, consequently, H+ formation. The NADH produced during glycolysis can react with pyruvate, as shown in the above equation, or it can be transported into the mitochondrion to be oxidized in the electron transport chain to form ATP (chapter 3). Endurance training increases the malate-aspartate shuttle system, which transports NADH into the mitochondrion (20). If the NADH formed in glycolysis is more quickly transported to the mitochondria, there will be less lactate and H+ formation. Lastly, endurance training causes a change in the type of LDH present in the muscle cell. This enzyme exists in five forms (isozymes): M_4, M_3H, M_2H_2, MH_3, and H_4. The H_4 or heart form of LDH has a low affinity for the available pyruvate. Endurance training shifts the LDH toward the H_4 form, making lactate and H+ formation less likely and the uptake of pyruvate by the mitochondria more likely. Figure 13.8 summarizes the effect these biochemical changes have on lactate formation and the production of H+ during submaximal work.

Figure 13.9 Changes in the blood lactate concentration are related to changes in lactate production and removal.

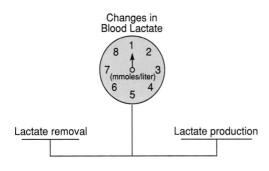

Biochemical Adaptations and Lactate Removal

Lactate accumulation in the blood is dependent on the balance between lactate production by working muscle and lactate removal by liver and other tissues. Figure 13.9 shows that the blood lactate concentration stays at 1 mmole/liter at rest and during light exercise when there is a balance between production and removal. As the exercise intensity increases, the blood lactate could rise due to an acceleration of lactate production, or to a reduction in the rate of removal by the liver and other tissues (7). As described in chapter 9, blood flow to nonworking muscles, kidney, liver, and GI tract decreases as exercise intensity increases, reducing the rate of lactate removal. How does endurance training affect blood flow to these tissues?

Endurance training causes an increase in the capillary density of the working muscles. This results in two changes favorable for oxygen transport to the mitochondria: a decrease in the distance from capillary to mitochondrion, and a decrease in the rate of blood flow through each capillary, allowing more time for the diffusion of oxygen to the mitochondria. As a result, the same submaximal work rate demands *less* blood flow to the working muscles after training. The muscle can extract more oxygen from each liter of blood (larger a-$\bar{v}$ O_2 difference) to achieve the same steady state $\dot{V}O_2$, with a lower blood flow.

Since the cardiac output for a given submaximal work rate is unchanged or only slightly decreased after training (13, 14), where is the blood flow now distributed that was formally going to the working muscles?

Two vascular beds that receive an increase in blood flow following training are the liver and the kidneys. Since the liver is a major site for lactate removal for gluconeogenesis, the blood lactate level is lower following an endurance training program due in part to the liver's increased ability to remove lactate. Figure 13.10 summarizes these events.

Endurance Training: Links between Muscle and Systemic Physiology

We have just described the importance of the local changes occurring in endurance-trained muscle on the maintenance of homeostasis during prolonged submaximal work. However, these same changes are also related to the lower heart rate, ventilation, and catecholamine responses measured during submaximal work following an endurance training program. What is the link between the changes in muscle and the improved heart rate and ventilation responses to exercise?

The following endurance training study illustrates the importance of the trained muscle in the body's overall response to a submaximal work bout. In this study each subject's left and right leg was tested separately on a cycle ergometer at a submaximal work rate prior to and during an endurance training program. Heart rate and ventilation were measured at the end of the submaximal exercise test, and a blood sample was obtained to monitor changes in lactate, epinephrine, and norepinephrine. During the study each subject *trained only one leg* for thirteen sessions, fifteen minutes a session, at an exercise intensity causing a heart rate of 170 beats per minute. At the end of each week of training the subject was tested at the same submaximal work rate used in the pretest. This procedure allowed the investigator to determine how fast the "training effect" occurred. Figure 13.11 shows that heart rate, ventilation, blood lactate, and plasma epinephrine and norepinephrine responses decreased throughout the study. Results such as these have been used to support the idea that the cardiovascular, pulmonary, and sympathetic nervous systems have each adapted to the exercise. However, that may not be quite true. At the end of this training program the "untrained" leg was trained for five consec-

Figure 13.10 Effect of endurance training on the redistribution of blood flow and lactate removal during exercise at a fixed submaximal workload.

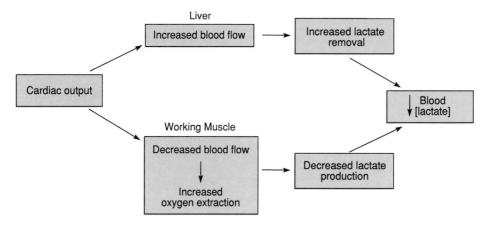

utive days at the same submaximal work rate used for the "trained leg." Physiological measurements were obtained during the exercise session on the first, third, and fifth days. If the cardiovascular, pulmonary, and sympathetic nervous systems had become "trained" as a result of the thirteen exercise sessions with the other leg, you might expect some "transfer" of the training effect when the untrained leg was tested. Interestingly, figure 13.11 shows that all the systems responded as if they had never been exposed to exercise (9). There was no transfer of the training effect from one leg to the other. This example shows that the heart rate, ventilation, and plasma catecholamine responses to prolonged submaximal exercise are determined, not by the specific adaptation of each organ or system, but by the training state of the specific muscle groups engaged in the exercise. How is this possible?

In chapter 10 the control of ventilation during exercise required a discussion of central and peripheral neural influences that could help explain the precise matching of ventilation with the increased oxygen demands of incremental exercise. This same approach will be taken here to explain how endurance training of specific muscle groups results in the decrease in cardiorespiratory and sympathetic nervous system responses to the same submaximal work rate. The output of the cardiovascular and respiratory control centers

is influenced by input from higher brain centers, where the motor task originates, as well as from the muscles carrying out the task. A decrease in recruitment of motor units or a reduction in input from the receptors in the working muscle reduces these physiological responses to the work task. Following a brief summary of "peripheral" and "central" control mechanisms, an attempt will be made to show how both are involved in the reduced physiological responses to submaximal exercise.

Peripheral Feedback

Rowell (31) indicates that Zuntz and Geppert were the originators of the idea that reflexes in working muscles might control or "drive" cardiovascular or pulmonary systems in proportion to the metabolic rate. A number of receptors have been examined that respond to chemical or physical changes in muscle that might signify work rate. The involvement of the muscle spindle and Golgi tendon organ received considerable attention as possible sites for these reflexes, given their ability to monitor changes in muscle length and tension development, respectively. However, the blocking of the afferent nerves from these receptors did not eliminate specific cardiovascular responses to muscle tension development (25, 31). Attention has now been directed to small-diameter nerve fibers (group III and

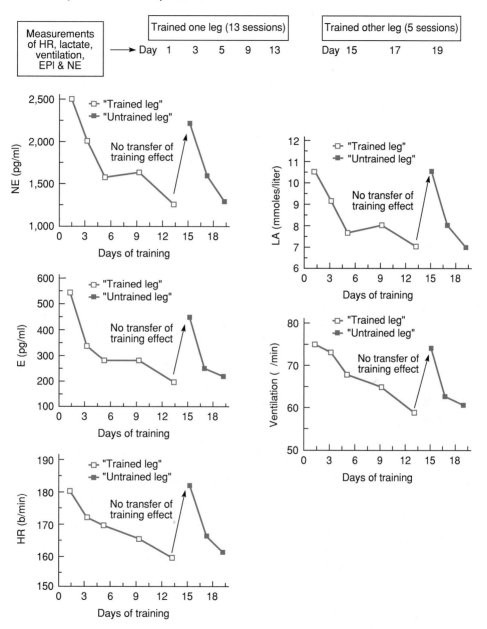

Figure 13.11 The lack of transfer of a training effect indicating the responses of the cardiovascular, pulmonary, and sympathetic nervous systems are more dependent on the trained state of the muscles involved in the activity rather than some specific adaptation in those systems.

Figure 13.12 Peripheral control mechanisms in muscle influence the heart rate, ventilation, and kidney and liver blood flow responses to submaximal work.

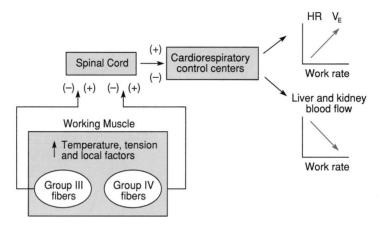

group IV fibers) that are responsive to both tension, temperature, and chemical changes in muscle. These fibers increase their rate of firing action potentials in proportion to changes in metabolic rate. Figure 13.12 shows schematically the neuronal circuitry for the reflex regulation of the cardiovascular and respiratory responses to exercise by these group III and group IV fibers.

Central Command

The general idea surrounding central control of the physiological response to exercise is presented in figure 13.13. Higher brain centers (motor cortex, basal ganglia, cerebellum—see chapter 7) prepare to execute a motor task and send action potentials through lower brain centers and spinal nuclei to influence the cardiorespiratory and sympathetic nervous system responses to exercise. As more motor units are recruited to develop the greater tension needed to accomplish a work task, larger physiological responses are required to sustain the metabolic rate of the muscles. For example, if some muscle fibers are prevented from contracting, additional muscle fibers must be recruited to maintain tension. This generates higher heart rate responses to the work task (2). How are these peripheral

and central controls related to the decreases in sympathetic nervous system activity, heart rate, and ventilation observed during submaximal exercise following an endurance training program?

The ability to perform a fixed submaximal exercise bout for a prolonged period of time is dependent on the recruitment of a sufficient number of motor units to meet the tension (work) requirements through oxidative phosphorylation. Prior to endurance training, more mitochondria-poor motor units must be recruited to carry out a work task at a given $\dot{V}O_2$. This results in a great "central" drive to the cardiorespiratory control centers that causes higher sympathetic nervous system, heart rate, and ventilation responses. The feedback from chemoreceptors at the untrained muscle would also stimulate the cardiorespiratory control center. With the increase in mitochondrial number following endurance training, local factors (H^+, adenosine compounds, etc.) do not change as much. This leads to less local stimulation of blood flow, and a reduced chemoreceptor input to the cardiorespiratory centers. In addition, the higher number of mitochondria allows the tension to be maintained with

Figure 13.13 Central control of motor unit recruitment, heart rate, ventilation, and liver and kidney blood flow responses to submaximal work.

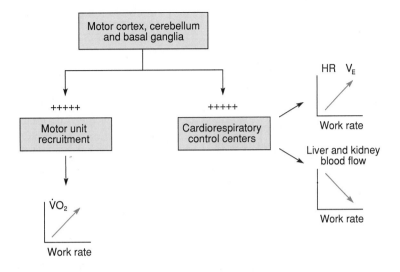

fewer motor units involved in the activity. This reduced "feed forward" input from the higher brain centers and reduced "feedback" from the muscle results in lower sympathetic nervous system output, heart rate, and ventilation responses to exercise (31).

Summary

1. The principle of overload states that for a training effect to occur a system or tissue must be challenged with an intensity, duration, or frequency of exercise to which it is unaccustomed. Over time the tissue or system adapts to this load. The reversibility principle is a corollary to the overload principle.

2. The principle of specificity indicates that the training effect is limited to the muscle fibers involved in the activity. In addition, the muscle fiber adapts specifically to the type of activity: mitochondrial adaptations to endurance training, and contractile protein adaptations to resistive weight training.

3. Cross-sectional training studies contrast the physiological responses of groups differing in habitual physical activity (e.g., sedentary versus runners). Longitudinal training studies examine the changes taking place over the course of a training program.

4. Endurance training programs that increase $\dot{V}O_2$ max involve a large muscle mass in dynamic activity for fifteen to sixty minutes per session, three to five times per week, at an intensity of 50%–85% $\dot{V}O_2$ max. While $\dot{V}O_2$ max increases about 15% as a result of an endurance training program, the range is 2%–50%, with the largest increases associated with those subjects with the smallest pretraining $\dot{V}O_2$ max values.

5. Genetic predisposition accounts for 40% of one's $\dot{V}O_2$ max value. Very strenuous and/or prolonged training can increase $\dot{V}O_2$ max 44%.

6. Fifty percent of the increase in $\dot{V}O_2$ max due to training is related to an increase in maximal stroke volume (maximal heart rate remains the same), and 50% is due to an increase in the a-$\bar{v}$ O_2 difference. The large differences in $\dot{V}O_2$ max in the normal population (2 versus 6 l · min^{-1}) are due to differences in maximal stroke volume.

7. The increase in stroke volume due to endurance exercise is related to a larger preload (EDV) and a reduced afterload related to a reduction in arteriolar constriction in the trained muscles.

8. The increase in the a-$\bar{v}$ O_2 difference is due to an increase in capillary number, and is facilitated by an increase in myoglobin and mitochondrial content.

9. Mitochondrial adaptations to endurance training include an increase in the enzymes involved in oxidative metabolism: Krebs cycle, fatty-acid (β-oxidation) cycle, and the electron transport chain.

10. Those mitochondrial adaptations result in the following:
    a. smaller O_2 deficit due to a more rapid increase in oxygen uptake at the onset of work
    b. an increase in fat metabolism that spares muscle glycogen and blood glucose
    c. a reduction in lacate and H^+ formation
    d. an increase in lactate removal

11. The biochemical changes in muscle due to endurance training influence the physiological responses to exercise. The reduction in "feedback" from chemoreceptors in the trained muscle and a reduction in the need to recruit motor units to accomplish a work task results in reduced sympathetic nervous system, heart rate, and ventilation responses to submaximal exercise.

Study Questions

1. Define the following principles of training: overload and specificity.

2. Give one example of a cross-sectional study and a longitudinal study.

3. Draw a graph of the percent change in $\dot{V}O_2$ max with endurance training programs, with the initial (pretraining) value on the x-axis.

4. What are typical $\dot{V}O_2$ max values for young men and women? Cardiac patients?

5. Given the formula for $\dot{V}O_2$ max using heart rate, stroke volume, and the a-$\bar{v}$ O_2 difference, which variable is most important in explaining the differences in $\dot{V}O_2$ max in different populations? Give a quantitative example.

6. Describe how the increase in $\dot{V}O_2$ max comes about for the sedentary subject who undertakes an endurance training program.

7. Explain the importance of preload, afterload, and contractility in the increase of the maximal stroke volume that occurs with endurance training.

8. What are the most important changes in muscle structure that are responsible for the increase in the maximal a-$\bar{v}$ O_2 difference that occurs with endurance training?

9. Describe how the capillary, myoglobin, and mitochondrial changes that occur in muscle as a result of an endurance training program are related to the following adaptations to submaximal exercise:
    a. a lower O_2 deficit
    b. an increased utilization of FFA and a sparing of blood glucose and muscle glycogen
    c. a reduction in lactate and H^+ formation
    d. an increase in lactate removal

10. Define "central command" and "peripheral feedback" and explain how changes in muscle as a result of endurance training can be responsible for the lower heart rate, ventilation, and catecholamine responses to a submaximal exercise bout.

Suggested Readings

Brooks, G., and T. Fahey. 1984. *Exercise Physiology: Human Bioenergetics and its Applications.* New York: John Wiley & Sons.

Fox, E. L., and D. K. Mathews. 1981. *The Physiological Basis of Physical Education and Athletics,* 3d ed. Philadelphia: W. B. Saunders Company.

McArdle, W. D., F. I. Katch, and V. L. Katch. 1986. *Exercise Physiology: Energy, Nutrition, and Human Performance,* 2d ed. Philadelphia: Lea & Febiger.

References

1. American College of Sports Medicine. 1984. The recommended quantity and quality of exercise for developing and maintaining fitness in healthy adults. In *Position Stands and Opinion Statements.* Indianapolis, Ind.: The American College of Sports Medicine.

2. Asmussen, E. et al. 1965. On the nervous factors controlling respiration and circulation during exercise. Experiments with curarization. *Acta Physiologica Scandinavica* 63:343–50.

3. Åstrand, P. O., and K. Rodahl. 1986. *Textbook of Work Physiology,* 3d ed. New York: McGraw-Hill Book Company.

4. Blomqvist, C. G., and B. Saltin. 1983. Cardiovascular adaptations to physical training. *Annual Review of Physiology* 45:169–89.

5. Bouchard, C. et al. 1986. Aerobic performance in brothers, dizygotic and monozygotic twins. *Medicine and Science in Sports and Exercise* 18:639–46.

6. Bransford, D. R., and E. T. Howley. 1979. Effects of training on plasma FFA during exercise. *European Journal of Applied Physiology* 41:151–58.

7. Brooks, G. A. 1985. Anaerobic threshold: review of the concept and directions for future research. *Medicine and Science in Sports and Exercise* 17:22–31.

8. Clausen, J. P. 1977. Effect of physical training on cardiovascular adjustments to exercise in man. *Physiological Reviews* 57:779–815.

9. Claytor, R. P. 1985. Selected cardiovascular, sympathoadrenal, and metabolic responses to one-leg exercise training. Dissertation, The University of Tennessee, Knoxville, Tenn.

10. Cronan, T. L., and E. T. Howley. 1974. The effect of training on epinephrine and norepinephrine excretion. *Medicine and Science in Sports* 6:122–25.

11. Ehsani, A. A., J. M. Hagberg, and R. C. Hickson. 1978. Rapid changes in left ventricular dimensions and mass in response to physical conditioning. *American Journal of Cardiology* 42:52–56.

12. Ekblom, B. et al. 1968. Effect of training on circulatory responses to exercise. *Journal of Applied Physiology* 24:518–28.

13. Ekblom, B. 1969. Effect of physical training on oxygen transport system in man. *Acta Physiologica Scandinavica* (Suppl.) 328:1–45.

14. Eldridge, F. L. et al. 1985. Stimulation by central command of locomotion, respiration, and circulation during exercise. *Respiratory Physiology* 59:313–37.

15. Favier, R. J. et al. 1986. Endurance exercise training reduces lactate production. *Journal of Applied Physiology* 61:885–89.

16. Felig, P. et al. 1982. Hypoglycemia during prolonged exercise in normal men. *The New England Journal of Medicine* 306:895–900.

17. Hagberg, J. M. et al. 1980. Faster adjustment to and recovery from submaximal exercise in the trained state. *Journal of Applied Physiology: Respiratory, Environmental, and Exercise Physiology* 48:218–24.

18. Hickson, R. C., H. A. Bomze, and J. O. Holloszy. 1978. Faster adjustment of O_2 uptake to the energy requirement of exercise in the trained state. *Journal of Applied Physiology: Respiratory, Environmental, and Exercise Physiology* 44:877–81.

19. ———. 1977. Linear increase in aerobic power induced by a strenuous program of endurance exercise. *Journal of Applied Physiology: Respiratory, Environmental, and Exercise Physiology* 42:372–76.

20. Holloszy, J. O., and E. F. Coyle. 1984. Adaptations of skeletal muscle to endurance exercise and their metabolic consequences. *Journal of Applied Physiology: Respiratory, Environmental, and Exercise Physiology* 56:831–38.

21. Howley, E. T., and B. D. Franks. 1986. *Health/Fitness Instructor's Handbook.* Champaign, Ill: Human Kinetics Publishers.

22. Klausen, K. et al. 1982. Central and regional circulatory adaptations to one-leg training. *Journal of Applied Physiology: Respiratory, Environmental, and Exercise Physiology* 52:976–83.

23. Klissouras, V. 1971. Heritability of adaptive variation. *Journal of Applied Physiology* 31:338–44.

24. MacDougall, J. D. 1986. Morphological changes in human skeletal muscle following strength training and immobilization. In (N. L. Jones, N. McCartney, and A. J. McComas, eds.) *Human Muscle Power,* chapter 17, 269–85.

25. Mitchell, J. H., and R. F. Schmidt. 1983. Cardiovascular reflex control by afferent fibers from skeletal muscle receptors. In (J. T. Shepherd, F. M. Abboud, and S. R. Geiger, eds.) *Handbook of Physiology. The Cardiovascular System. Peripheral Circulation and Organ Blood Flow,* 623–58. Bethesda, Md.: American Physiological Society.

26. Morganroth, J. et al. 1975. Comparative left ventricular dimensions in trained athletes. *Annals of Internal Medicine* 82:521–24.

27. Paul, P. 1975. Effects of long-lasting physical exercise and training on lipid metabolism. In (H. Howald and J. R. Poortmans, eds.) *Metabolic Adaptation to Prolonged Physical Exercise,* 156–87. Switzerland: Birkhauser Verlag Basel.

28. Powers, S. K., S. Dodd, and R. E. Beadle. 1985. Oxygen uptake kinetics in trained athletes differing in $\dot{V}O_2$ max. *European Journal of Applied Physiology* 54:306–8.

29. Prud'Homme, D. et al. 1984. Sensitivity of maximal aerobic power to training is genotype-dependent. *Medicine and Science in Sports and Exercise* 16:489–93.

30. Rerych, S. K. et al. 1980. Effects of exercise training on left ventricular function in normal subjects: A longitudinal study by radionuclide angiography. *American Journal of Cardiology* 45:244–52.

31. Rowell, L. B. 1986. *Human Circulation-Regulation during Physical Stress.* New York: Oxford University Press.

32. Saltin, B. 1969. Physiological effects of physical conditioning. *Medicine and Science in Sports* 1:50–56.

33. Saltin, B., and P. D. Gollnick. 1983. Skeletal muscle adaptability: Significance for metabolism and performance. In (L. D. Peachey, R. H. Adrian, and S. R. Geiger, eds.) *Handbook of Physiology,* Section 10: Skeletal Muscle, chapter 19. Baltimore: Williams and Wilkins Company.

34. Saltin, B., and P. O. Åstrand. 1967. Maximal oxygen uptake in athletes. *Journal of Applied Physiology* 23:353–58.

35. Saltin, B. et al. 1977. Fiber types and metabolic potentials of skeletal muscles in sedentary man and endurance runners. *Annals of the New York Academy of Science* 301:3–29.

Physiology of Health and Fitness

14 Factors Limiting Health and Fitness

Objectives

By studying this chapter, you should be able to do the following:
1. Contrast infectious with degenerative diseases as causes of death.
2. Describe health-related fitness using the wellness model.
3. Identify the three major categories of risk factors and examples of specific risk factors in each.
4. Describe the role of ''personal responsibility'' as a determinant of our well-being.
5. Describe in general terms what a Health Risk Appraisal (HRA) is, and the kinds of information that allows it to predict health risk.
6. Contrast the role of a HRA with that of a medical exam.
7. Describe the difference between primary and secondary risk factors for coronary heart disease (CHD).
8. Identify the major risk factors associated with CHD.
9. Explain why a high fat diet and inactivity do not appear as ''precursors'' of CHD in the HRA.
10. Summarize the 1990 Health Objectives for the Nation as they relate to physical fitness and exercise.
11. Summarize the 1990 Health Objectives for the Nation as they relate to nutrition.

Outline

Key Terms

atherosclerosis
degenerative diseases
infectious diseases
precursor
primary risk factor
secondary risk factor

The preface, in referring to this section of the book, stated the real need to separate fitness from performance when discussing the effects of exercise training. However, it is clear that there are factors other than exercise that limit a person's overall health and well-being. This chapter will present a review of these factors and point the way for the remainder of this section.

Wellness, Risk Factors, and Personal Responsibility

Figure 14.1 shows that during the course of the twentieth century the major causes of death in the United States have shifted from **infectious diseases** such as tuberculosis and pneumonia to **degenerative diseases** such as cancer and heart attacks, which are associated with various aspects of our life-style (9). This change is related to the appearance of better antibiotics on the one hand, and an increase in inappropriate health habits on the other. Interestingly, one of the problems we are now faced with is our definition of what "health" is. One attempt to deal with this is found in the concept of "wellness," introduced by Dunn in 1961, and popularized by Ardell (6). It is generally agreed that health means more than the simple absence of disease. In the wellness concept the absence of disease is the midpoint on a continuum going from premature death, due to degenerative diseases, to high-level wellness. High-level wellness in Ardell's original model (6) included physical fitness, proper nutrition, stress control, and self-responsibility. This latter point, self-responsibility, distinguishes wellness from the traditional medical model for health care and is the focal point of all health-related fitness programs. It is the recognition that the individual can and must exert control over various factors or forces that determine where he or she is on the wellness continuum. What are these forces that an individual must control in order to reduce the chance of premature death from life-style diseases?

In 1979 the surgeon general of the United States published a report, *Healthy People* (9), which addressed that question. The primary thrust of the report was that even though degenerative diseases have more complex causes than infectious diseases, many are preventable (9). Figure 14.2 shows the three major risk factor categories associated with health and disease, with specific risk factors identified under each. While some diseases (hemophilia and sickle-cell anemia) are primarily inherited, the vast majority of diseases result from an interaction of genetics and the individual's environment (9). The *inherited/biological factors* include age, gender, race, and the ease with which one might develop a disease. Nothing can be done about these risk factors; they are fixed and some people simply have a higher risk of certain degenerative diseases than others. However, what has become clear over the past forty years is that it is the *environmental and behavior risk factors* that are most influential in the early onset of degenerative diseases or death. Fortunately, it is these risk factors that are most susceptible to change, and this brings us back to the issue of personal responsibility as a major force determining one's well-being. Personal responsibility means more than getting sufficient exercise (see chapter 16), or eating the proper foods (see chapter 18). There is a need for people to speak out for clean air and water, to support community-wide blood pressure and serum cholesterol screenings, and to not drink and drive. How can you determine your risk of disease or early death?

Figure 14.1 Changes in the causes of death in the United States from 1900–1985. Please note the increase in death from cancer and heart disease, while the death rate from tuberculosis, influenza, and pneumonia decrease.
Source: National Center for Health Statistics, Division of Vital Statistics.

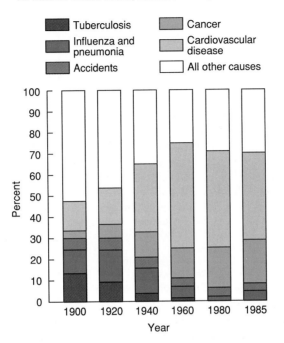

Deaths from Selected Causes as a Percent of
All Deaths: United States, Selected Years, 1900 to 1985

Figure 14.2 Major categories of risk factors with examples of each.
Source: U.S. Department of Health, Education, and Welfare, 1979, *Healthy People: The Surgeon General's Report on Health Promotion and Disease Prevention.*

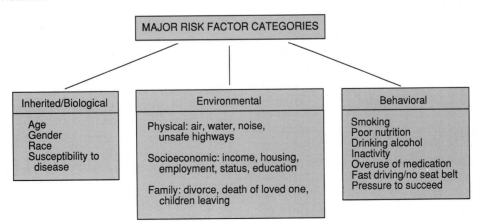

Table 14.1 Causes of death: groupings selected for Health Risk Appraisal

1. Mouth cancer	22. Rheumatic heart disease
2. Throat cancer	23. Hypertensive heart disease
3. Esophagus cancer	24. Heart attack
4. Stomach cancer	25. Stroke
5. Colon cancer	26. Arterial vascular disease
6. Rectal cancer	
7. Pancreas cancer	27. Pneumonia/influenza
8. Larynx cancer	28. Emphysema/chronic bronchitis
9. Lung cancer	29. Pneumoconiosis
10. Skin cancer and melanoma	
11. Breast cancer	30. Peptic ulcer
12. Cervix cancer	
13. Uterine cancer	31. Cirrhosis of the liver
14. Ovary cancer	
15. Prostate cancer	32. Kidney failure
16. Bladder cancer	
17. Brain cancer	33. Motor vehicle crash
18. Lymphoma	34. Pedestrian
19. Leukemia	35. Poisoning
	36. Fall
	37. Fire and flames
20. Diabetes mellitus	38. Drowning
	39. Other unintentional injury
21. Alcohol toxicity	
	40. Suicide
	41. Homicide/assault
	42. All other causes

Source: R. W. Amler, D. G. Moriarity, and E. B. Hutchins, eds., *Healthier People: The Carter Center of Emory University Health Risk Appraisal Program Guides and Documentation*, Atlanta, Ga.

Health Risk Appraisal

Over the past forty years epidemiological studies of entire communities (e.g., Framingham) have been carried out in order to study the relationship of various risk factors to the appearance of diseases (morbidity) or the age at death (mortality). In this way investigators can predict the likelihood that someone who smokes and has high serum cholesterol will die from cardiovascular disease compared to someone who does not have these risk factors (see Dawber for details about the Framingham study). This information has been used in the development of Health Risk Appraisals (HRAs), questionnaires that are used as part of health promotion/disease prevention programs. In one of the most recently developed HRAs, the investigators included forty-two causes of death. Forty-one of the forty-two accounted for 77% of all deaths in the United States from 1980–1982 (5).

Table 14.1 shows that the various forms of cancer are most heavily represented (numbers 1–19), followed by trauma (numbers 33–39), and circulatory diseases (numbers 22–26). However, as shown in table 14.2, circulatory diseases account for the greatest percentage of deaths.

Table 14.2 Leading causes of death in the United States: 1985 estimates

Causes	Total Number of Deaths	Percent of Total Deaths
1. Diseases of heart and blood vessels	991,332	47.6
2. Cancer	457,670	21.9
3. Accidents	92,070	4.4
4. Chronic obstructive pulmonary diseases	74,420	3.6
5. Pneumonia and influenza	66,630	3.2
6. All other causes	401,878	19.3

From: *1988 Heart Facts*. Copyright © 1988 American Heart Association, Dallas Tx.

The investigators selected twenty-three **precursors** (risk factors associated with the cause of death), depending on the quality of the evidence relating each to a disease. Evidence was classified as quantitative (A) when there was a strong numerical relationship between a risk factor and a disease (e.g., the incidence of lung cancer increased with the number of cigarettes smoked). When the relationship between risk factors and cause of death was not as strong, the evidence was classified as either semiquantitative (B), or qualitative (C). Each precursor was also classified as being modifiable (1), semi-modifiable (2), and fixed (3). Finally, the precursors were selected because of a presumed "cause and effect" relationship with the reason for death, rather than a simple statistical association. Table 14.3 shows nineteen causes of death, the precursors associated with each, the questions on the HRA dealing with those precursors, the quality of the evidence (A, B, or C), and the potential for modifying the precursor (1, 2, or 3). Please note the incredible frequency with which cigarettes and alcohol use appear on this list (5).

The Carter Center HRA is found in Appendix C, and is based on the above analysis. The important point to remember about an HRA is that it is primarily an educational and health promotion tool, and *not a substitute for a medical exam*. In addition, it is *not* designed for people who already have heart disease,

cancer, kidney disease, or other serious conditions (5). Further, the inventory contains a variety of questions that are known to be important to overall health, but are not included in the calculation of risk. This can be seen in an analysis of the risk factors associated with coronary heart disease (CHD).

Coronary Heart Disease

Coronary heart disease is associated with a gradual narrowing of the arteries serving the heart due to a thickening of the inner lining of the artery. This process, **atherosclerosis,** leads to heart attacks, which represent about 26% of all deaths in the United States (4). The risk factors associated with coronary heart disease have typically been divided into **primary** and **secondary,** where primary means that a factor in and of itself increases the risk of CHD, and secondary means that a certain factor increases the risk of CHD only if one of the primary factors is already present. These lists have evolved over time as more evidence has accumulated showing the association between various precursors and CHD. Table 14.4 shows a list of risk factors published in 1975, one from 1980, and finally one that represents current thinking (1, 2, 3, 4). The risk of CHD increases with the number of cigarettes smoked, the degree to which the blood pressure is elevated, and the quantity of cholesterol in the blood. In addition, the overall risk of CHD increases with the

Table 14.3 The Carter Center of Emory University Health Risk Appraisal Program

Precursors used by Healthier People to Compute Appraised Risk of Death from Nineteen Causes.*

No.	Cause of Death	Precursor(s)	Question No.(s)	Quality of Evidence	Precursor Modifiability
1	Mouth cancer	Smokeless tobacco	14	A	1
		Cigarettes	15–17	A	1
		Cigars	12	A	1
		Pipes	13	A	1
		Alcohol (drinks/wk)	23	A	1
2	Throat cancer	Smokeless tobacco	14	A	1
		Cigarettes	15–17	A	1
		Cigars	12	A	1
		Pipes	13	A	1
		Alcohol (drinks/wk)	23	A	1
3	Esophagus cancer	Cigarettes	15–17	A	1
7	Pancreas cancer	Cigarettes	15–17	A	1
8	Larynx cancer	Cigarettes	15–17	A	1
		Alcohol (drinks/wk)	23	A	1
9	Lung cancer	Cigarettes	15–17	A	1
11	Breast cancer	Mammography	26	A	1
		Menarche	24	A	3
		Age 1st birth	25	A	3
		Family Hx	27	A	3
12	Cervix cancer	Cigarettes	15–17	A	1
		Pap smear	29	A	1
		Hysterectomy	28	A	2
13	Uterine cancer	Hysterectomy	28	A	2
16	Bladder cancer	Cigarettes	15–17	A	1
20	Diabetes mellitus	Diabetes	6	A	3
24	Heart attack	Cigarettes	15–17	A	1
		Hypertension	7–9	A	1
		Obesity (MRW)	3–4	A	1
		Cholesterol	10	A	1
		HDL-Cholesterol	11	A	1
		Diabetes	6	A	3
		Male sex	1	A	3

Table 14.3 Continued

No.	Cause of Death	Precursor(s)	Question No.(s)	Quality of Evidence	Precursor Modifiability
25	Stroke	Cigarettes	15–17	A	1
		Hypertension	7–9	A	1
		Diabetes	6	A	3
		Male sex	1	A	3
27	Pneumonia/ influenza	Cigarettes	15–17	A	1
28	Emphysema/ chronic bronchitis	Cigarettes	15–17	A	1
30	Peptic ulcer	Cigarettes	15–17	A	1
31	Cirrhosis of liver	Alcohol (drinks/ wk)	23	A	1
32	Kidney failure	Diabetes	6	A	3
33	Motor vehicle traffic collision and non-collision	Speed	21	B	1
		Seat belts	20	B	1
		Drunk trips/mo	22	B	1
		Miles driven	18	B	2
		Vehicle size	19	B	2

MRW = Metropolitan relative weight
*Twenty-three additional causes of death used by healthier people have no "A" or "B" precursors and are computed as population age-sex rate only.
Quality of the Evidence is rated as quantitative (A), semiquantitative (B), and qualitative (C). The potential for changing a precursor is rated as modifiable (1), semi-modifiable (2), and fixed (3).
Source: R. W. Amler, D. G. Moriarity, and E. B. Hutchins, eds., *Healthier People: The Carter Center of Emory University Health Risk Appraisal Program Guides and Documentation,* Atlanta, Ga.

number of risk factors; that is, a person who has high blood pressure, high cholesterol, and smokes had about six times the risk of CHD as a person who has only one of these risk factors (7). What may be surprising is that a high saturated fat diet is not listed as a primary or secondary risk factor. You will also note in table 14.3 that diet and exercise were *not* selected as precursors of a heart attack in the analysis for the HRA. It does not mean that diet and exercise are not related to the overall risk of heart attack as predicted by the HRA. What has happened is that the effect of diet and exercise are "hidden" in the obesity and cholesterol precursors, both of which have been shown to be directly and independently affected by exercise and diet. The importance of diet and exercise is discussed in detail in chapters 16 and 18, respectively.

HRA Reports
The HRA is generally analyzed by computer to allow a comparison of the individual's risk with others. A printout may list the risk factors in the order of which change would yield the greatest benefit, and may also provide suggestions about how to initiate the changes. These latter recommendations could be general suggestions for diet, exercise, and car safety (wear seat belts), or specific suggestions about important medical exams that would be appropriate (e.g., Pap smear, routine serum cholesterol check). The information generated by HRAs can provide valuable information in the design of health promotion programs in schools, the workplace, or in the community to focus attention, personnel, and resources on the risk factors where the

Table 14.4 Risk factors for coronary heart disease

1975	1980	Current Thinking
Primary	**Primary**	**Primary (Major)**
Cigarette smoking	Cigarette smoking	Cigarette smoking
Hypertension	Hypertension	Hypertension
Hyperlipidemia	Hyperlipidemia	Elevated serum cholesterol and/or ratio of total to HDL cholesterol
		Abnormal resting ECG
		Diabetes*
Secondary	**Secondary**	**Secondary (Contributing)**
Family history of CHD	Family history of CHD	Family history of CHD[†]
Obesity	Obesity	Age, gender (male), Blacks
Physical inactivity	Physical inactivity	Obesity[‡]
Diabetes	Diabetes	Physical inactivity[‡]
Asymptomatic hyperglycemia	Hyperuricemia	Type A coronary-prone behavior
	Type A coronary-prone behavior	

* Listed as a secondary risk factor by the American Heart Association.
[†] Listed as major risk factor by the American Heart Association and the American College of Sports Medicine, but evaluated as being of minimal consequence by Caspersen and Heath (7).
[‡] Evidence is accumulating that suggests that these are primary risk factors.
From: American College of Sports Medicine (1, 2, 3), American Heart Association (4), and Caspersen and Heath (7).

greatest gains can be made. The U.S. government has clearly paid attention to the results of these HRAs in the development of long-range objectives for the nation.

Health Objectives for the 1990s

Following the publication of *Healthy People* in 1979 (9), the U.S. Department of Health and Human Services published *The 1990 Health Objectives for the Nation* (10). These objectives were based on the anal-ysis of health problems in the United States, and a recognition of what could be done to reduce their magnitude. These objectives, grouped by Preventive Health Services, Health Protection, and Health Promotion, are shown in table 14.5 (11). While it is beyond the scope of this chapter to go into the specific objectives associated with each of these, we feel that some detailed discussion concerning the nutrition and exercise objectives is appropriate.

Table 14.5 Health strategy targets

Preventive Health Services for Individuals
- High blood pressure control
- Family planning
- Pregnancy and infant health
- Immunization
- Sexually transmitted diseases

Health Protection for Population Groups
- Toxic agents and radiation control
- Occupational safety and health
- Accident prevention and injury control
- Fluoridation and dental health
- Surveillance and control of infectious diseases

Health Promotion for Population Groups
- Smoking and health
- Misuse of alcohol and drugs
- Nutrition
- Physical fitness and exercise
- Control of stress and violent behavior

Source: *The 1990 Health Objectives for the Nation: A Midcourse Review.* U.S. Department of Health and Human Services, 1986.

The objectives associated with Physical Fitness and Exercise (10) are presented in table 14.6. Several of these objectives call for an increase in aerobic physical activity for children (objectives a and b), and adults (objectives c and d). The proper intensity, duration, and frequency of exercise to bring about desired health benefits will be discussed in detail in chapter 16. Other objectives were directed at increasing both public (objective a) and physician (objective f) awareness of the proper quantity of exercise needed for health benefits, while another (objective g) encouraged an increase in corporate fitness programs. The last group of objectives focused on improvements in our ability to evaluate the fitness of children (objective h), monitor changes in fitness, job performance, and health care costs due to exercise programs (objectives i and j), and

finally, have data to monitor national trends in physical activity (objective k). It should be clear that regular physical activity is a normal and necessary part of a healthy life-style.

The nutrition objectives are listed in table 14.7. The first objective (objective a) under Improvement of Health Status included a reduction in iron deficiency anemia in women, the greatest nutritional deficiency disease problem in our country (see chapter 18). The nutrition objectives under Risk Reduction indicated a need to decrease weight through proper exercise and diet (objectives c and d), decrease serum cholesterol (objective e), and decrease salt intake (objective f). All of these problems will be discussed in chapter 18. The need to educate the public about diet and risk factors (objective i), proper food selection relative to fat, sugar, salt, and fiber (objective j), and the role of diet and exercise in weight control (objective k) was clearly spelled out. The 1990 objectives also specified a need for better labeling of foods (objective l), a reduction in sodium levels in food (objective m), an increase in the number of schools and workplaces following USDA/DHHS guidelines (objective u) (see chapter 18), that nutrition education be required in elementary and secondary schools (objective p), and that health-care providers should include nutrition education. The final objective (objective q) directs that a national nutrition status monitoring system be in place.

It is clear from these 1990 objectives that there is a strong belief that proper exercise and nutrition throughout life is needed for optimal health. Chapters 16 and 18 provide the details associated with recommended exercise and diet programs.

Summary

1. The causes of death in this country have shifted from infectious diseases to degenerative diseases.
2. Health-related fitness can be defined along the wellness model in which it is more than the absence of disease; it includes the elements of proper nutrition, exercise, stress control, and self-responsibility.

Table 14.6 The 1990 Health Objectives for the Nation — *physical fitness and exercise*

Risk Reduction

Objective a. By 1990, the proportion of children and adolescents ages 10 to 17 participating regularly in appropriate physical activities, particularly cardiorespiratory fitness programs which can be carried into adulthood, should be greater than 90 percent.

Objective b. By 1990, the proportion of children and adolescents ages 10 to 17 participating in daily school physical education programs should be greater than 60 percent.

Objective c. By 1990, the proportion of adults 18 to 64 participating regularly in vigorous physical exercise should be greater than 60 percent.

Objective d. By 1990, 50 percent of adults 65 years and older should be engaging in appropriate physical activity, e.g., regular walking, swimming, or other aerobic activity.

Public and Professional Awareness

Objective e. By 1990, the proportion of adults who can accurately identify the variety and duration of exercise thought to promote most effectively cardiovascular fitness should be greater than 70 percent.

Objective f. By 1990, the proportion of primary care physicians who include a careful exercise history as part of their initial examination of new patients should be greater than 50 percent.

Improvement of Services

Objective g. By 1990, the proportion of employees of companies and institutions with more than 500 employees offering employer-sponsored fitness programs should be greater than 25 percent.

Improvement of Surveillance and Evaluation

Objective h. By 1990, a methodology of systematically assessing the physical fitness of children should be established with at least 70 percent of children and adolescents ages 10 to 17 participating in such an assessment.

Objective i. By 1990, data should be available with which to evaluate short- and long-term health effects of participation in programs of appropriate physical activity.

Objective j. By 1990, data should be available to evaluate the effects of participation in programs of physical fitness on job performance and health care costs.

Objective k. By 1990, data should be available for regular monitoring of national trends and patterns of participation in physical activity, including participation in public recreation programs in community facilities.

Source: *Promoting Health / Preventing Disease: Objectives for the Nation.* Department of Health and Human Services, Fall 1980.

3. Risk factors can be divided into three categories: genetic/biological, environmental, and behavioral. The risks associated with the first category cannot be modified, but the risk factors in the latter two, which are responsible for the early onset of degenerative diseases, can be altered. This is where personal responsibility for health is directed.

4. A Health Risk Appraisal (HRA) is a questionnaire used as an educational tool in health promotion disease prevention programs. HRAs contain questions about risk factors (precursors) associated with disease and death, and on the basis of the quantity and kind of risk factors, an estimate of personal risk can be made.

Table 14.7 The 1990 Health Objectives for the Nation — *nutrition*

Improvement in Health Status

Objective a. By 1990, the proportion of pregnant women with iron deficiency anemia (as estimated by hemoglobin concentrations early in pregnancy) should be reduced to 3.5 percent.

Objective b. By 1990, growth retardation of infants and children caused by inadequate diets should have been eliminated in the United States as a public health problem.

Risk Reduction

Objective c. By 1990, the prevalence of significant overweight (120 percent of "desired" weight) among the U.S. adult population should be decreased to 10 percent of men and 17 percent of women, without nutritional impairment.

Objective d. By 1990, 50 percent of the overweight population should have adopted weight loss regimens, combining an appropriate balance of diet and physical activity.

Objective e. By 1990, the mean serum cholesterol level in the adult population 18 to 74 years of age should be at or below 200 milligrams per deciliter.

Objective f. By 1990, the mean serum cholesterol level in children aged 1 to 14 should be at or below 150 milligrams per deciliter (mg/dl).

Objective g. By 1990, the average daily sodium ingestion (as measured by excretion) for adults should be reduced to at least the three- to six-gram range.

Objective h. By 1990, the proportion of women who breast-feed their babies should be increased to 75 percent at hospital discharge and to 35 percent at six months of age.

Public and Professional Awareness

Objective i. By 1990, the proportion of the population which is able to correctly associate the principal dietary factors known or strongly suspected to be related to disease should exceed 75 percent for each of the following diseases: heart disease, high blood pressure, dental caries, and cancer.

Objective j. By 1990, 70 percent of adults should be able to identify the major foods which are: low in fat content, low in sodium content, high in calories, high in sugars, good sources of fiber.

Objective k. By 1990, 90 percent of adults should understand that to lose weight people must either consume foods that contain fewer calories or increase physical activity or both.

Improvement of Services

Objective l. By 1990, the labels of all packaged foods should contain useful calorie and nutrient information to enable consumers to select diets that promote and protect good health. Similar information should be displayed where nonpackaged foods are obtained or purchased.

Objective m. By 1990, sodium levels in processed food should be reduced by 20 percent from present levels.

Objective n. By 1985, the proportion of employee and school cafeteria managers who are aware of and actively promoting USDA/DHHS dietary guidelines should be greater than 50 percent.

Objective o. By 1990, all States should include nutrition education as part of required comprehensive school health education at the elementary and secondary levels.

Objective p. By 1990, virtually all routine health contacts with health professionals should include some element of nutrition education and nutrition counseling.

Improvement of Surveillance and Evaluation

Objective q. Before 1990, a comprehensive national nutrition status monitoring system should have the capability for detecting nutritional problems in special population groups, as well as for obtaining baseline data for decisions on national nutrition policies.

Source: *Promoting Health/Preventing Disease: Objectives for the Nation.* Department of Health and Human Services, Fall 1980.

5. The HRA is not a substitute for a medical exam, and its proper audience is *not* people who already have serious diseases.

6. A primary risk factor is one that exerts an independent effect on a disease, and a secondary risk factor is one that increases risk when another primary risk factor is present.

7. A high fat diet and inactivity may not appear as precursors of CHD on a HRA because their effects are already considered in the factors of high cholesterol and obesity.

8. The U.S. Department of Health and Human Services has stated specific health objectives related to exercise and nutrition that would reduce the nation's risk of heart and other diseases. In general, the objectives call for an increase in the number of persons doing aerobic exercise, and the selection of proper foods relative to dietary fat, sugar, salt, and fiber. In addition, special attention was made toward decreasing iron deficiency anemia in women, and the number of overweight persons, in general.

Study Questions

1. Contrast infectious diseases with degenerative diseases as causes of death.

2. What are the three major categories of risk factors? Provide examples within each category.

3. What does "personal responsibility mean in the wellness model of health care?

4. What is a health risk appraisal and how are the questions selected?

5. What is the difference between primary and secondary risks for coronary heart disease (CHD)? List examples of each.

6. Why does inactivity and a high fat diet not appear as "precursors" of CHD in a HRA?

7. Briefly summarize *The 1990 Health Objectives for the Nation* as they relate to exercise and nutrition.

Suggested Readings

Dawber, Thomas R. 1980. *The Framingham Study.* Cambridge, Mass.: Harvard University Press.

References

1. American College of Sports Medicine. 1975. *Guidelines for Graded Exercise Testing and Exercise Prescription.* Philadelphia, Pa.: Lea & Febiger.

2. ———. 1980. *Guidelines for Graded Exercise Testing and Exercise Prescription,* 2d ed. Philadelphia, Pa.: Lea & Febiger.

3. ———. 1986. *Guidelines for Exercise Testing and Prescription,* 3d ed. Philadelphia, Pa.: Lea & Febiger.

4. American Heart Association. 1988. *1988 Heart Facts.* Dallas: Author.

5. Amler, R. W., D. G. Moriarty, and E. B. Hutchins, eds. 1988. *Healthier People: The Carter Center of Emory University Health Risk Appraisal Program Guides and Documentation.* Atlanta: The Carter Center of Emory University.

6. Ardell, D. B. 1986. *High Level Wellness,* 2d ed. Berkeley, Calif.: Ten-Speed Press.

7. Caspersen, C. J., and G. W. Heath. 1988. The risk factor concept of coronary heart disease. In (S. N. Blair, P. Painter, R. R. Pate, L. K. Smith, and C. B. Taylor, eds.): *Resource Manual for Guidelines for Graded Exercise Testing and Prescription,* 111–25. Philadelphia: Lea & Febiger.

8. National Center for Health Statistics, Division of Vital Statistics, U.S. Public Health Service, Department of Health and Human Services.

9. U.S. Department of Health, Education and Welfare. 1979. *Healthy People: The Surgeon General's Report on Health Promotion and Disease Prevention.* Washington, D.C.: U.S. Government Printing Office. Stock No. 017–001–00416–2.

10. U.S. Department of Health and Human Services. Fall, 1980. *Promoting Health/Preventing Disease: Objectives for the Nation.* Washington, D.C.: U.S. Government Printing Office.

11. ———. 1986. *The 1990 Health Objectives for the Nation: A Midcourse Review.* Washington, D.C.: U.S. Government Printing Office.

15 Work Tests to Evaluate Cardiorespiratory Fitness

Objectives

*B*y studying this chapter, you should be able to do the following:
1. Identify the sequence of steps in the procedures for evaluating cardiorespiratory fitness (CRF).
2. Describe one maximal and one submaximal field test used to evaluate CRF.
3. Explain the rationale underlying the use of distance runs as estimates of CRF.
4. Identify the common measures taken during a graded exercise test (GXT).
5. Describe changes in the ECG that may take place during a GXT of subjects with ischemic heart disease.
6. List three criteria for having achieved $\dot{V}O_2$ max.
7. Contrast $\dot{V}O_2$ max with $\dot{V}O_2$ peak.
8. Estimate $\dot{V}O_2$ max from the last stage of a GXT and list the concerns about the protocol that may affect that estimate.
9. Estimate $\dot{V}O_2$ max by extrapolating a $HR/\dot{V}O_2$ relationship to the person's age-adjusted maximal HR.
10. Describe the problems with the assumptions made in the extrapolation procedure used in objective 9, and name the environmental and subject variables that must be controlled to improve such estimates.
11. Describe the rating of perceived exertion (RPE) and how it changes during a GXT.
12. Identify the criteria used to terminate the GXT.
13. Explain the reason why there are so many different GXT protocols and why the rate of progression through the test is of concern.
14. Describe a procedure used to set the initial work rate, and rate of progression on a cycle ergometer test.
15. Estimate $\dot{V}O_2$ max by either the extrapolation method (objective 9), or with use of the Åstrand and Ryhming nomogram, given a data set for the cycle ergometer or step.

Outline

Key Terms

angina pectoris
arrhythmias
conduction disturbances
double product

dyspnea
field test
myocardial ischemia
ST segment depression

*I*n chapter 14 we discussed the factors that limit health and fitness. One of those factors was a sedentary lifestyle, and according to the *1990 Health Objectives for the Nation* there is a need to increase physical activity to improve cardiorespiratory function (CRF). This implies that one can measure such changes in CRF. While most scientists believe that the function of the cardiorespiratory system is represented best by the measurement of $\dot{V}O_2$ max, others feel that the monitoring of heart rate (HR) and blood pressure (BP) at several submaximal work rates provides a more sensitive indicator of changes in CRF (34). You are already familiar with the use of a graded exercise test (GXT) to measure $\dot{V}O_2$ max; this chapter picks up on that theme and discusses the types of tests used to evaluate CRF. The type of test used depends on the fitness of the person being tested, the purpose of the test, and the facilities, equipment, and personnel available to conduct the test. The choice of the GXT would be different for a young, healthy child as compared to a sixty-year-old person with coronary heart disease (CHD) risk factors. The GXT might be used as a CRF test prior to entry into a fitness program, or it could be used as a diagnostic test by a cardiologist who evaluates a twelve-lead electrocardiogram for evidence of heart disease. Clearly, the type of personnel and equipment, and, of course, the cost would be very different in these two situations. Given such diversity, how should one begin the testing process?

Testing Procedures

Figure 15.1 shows a sequence of steps in a "decision tree," leading to participation in a fitness program. The first step in the evaluation of CRF is to identify those who might need a physician's clearance prior to taking an exercise test or participating in an exercise program. These procedures include obtaining written informed consent from the potential participant, a review of the person's health history, the administration of selected resting physiological measures, and then the use of submaximal or maximal GXTs (34). The exercise test can be stopped by the subject at any time, and the tester has the right to terminate any of the procedures if the subject displays abnormal responses or experiences symptoms suggestive of an inappropriate adaptation to the GXT (3). Depending on the outcome at each of these steps, the person might be admitted to a fitness program with little or no supervision, or referred for additional tests that might lead to an exercise program in which the participants are monitored and supervised. The following sections will explore these steps in more detail.

Informed Consent

The person being tested must understand all the procedures involved in the tests, the potential risks and benefits, that their data will be held confidential, and that the tests can be terminated at any time at the person's request. This information is stated in writing in a consent form that the potential participant signs before participating in any tests (34).

Figure 15.1 Decision tree in the evaluation of cardiorespiratory fitness.

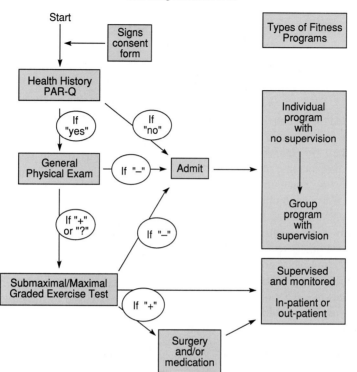

Screening Decision Tree

Review of the Health History

In chapter 14 a Health Risk Appraisal was used to develop an overall profile of health status with regard to a wide variety of factors. The health histories used to screen people for GXTs or fitness programs can be as simple as the Physical Activity Readiness Questionnaire (PAR-Q) shown in figure 15.2, or a detailed form such as the PAR_x which highlights absolute and relative contraindications for participating in exercise (see appendix D). An additional question added to various modifications of the PAR-Q asks about medication that might affect a person's response to exercise (e.g., an insulin-dependent diabetic or a cardiac patient taking the beta adrenergic blocker, propranolol) (23, 61). These forms are used to determine if a person needs consultation with a physician before taking a GXT, or before entering a fitness program. In general, persons who indicate that they have some form of coronary heart disease (CHD), or other major health problem, *must* be referred to a physician before taking a GXT or participating in a fitness program. For those with any primary risk factor (see chapter 14) for CHD, or any other major health problem, a physician-supervised GXT is recommended. The apparently healthy individuals who have no known major health problems or symptoms can be tested and can begin a graduated exercise program with minimal risk (3).

Figure 15.2 Physical Activity Readiness Questionnaire (PAR-Q). A self-administered questionnaire for adults.

PHYSICAL ACTIVITY READINESS QUESTIONNAIRE (PAR-Q)*
A Self-administered Questionnaire for Adults

PAR-Q & YOU

PAR-Q is designed to help you help yourself. Many health benefits are associated with regular exercise, and the completion of PAR-Q is a sensible first step to take if you are planning to increase the amount of physical activity in your life.

For most people physical activity should not pose any problem or hazard. PAR-Q has been designed to identify the small number of adults for whom physical activity might be inappropriate or those who should have medical advice concerning the type of activity most suitable for them.

Common sense is your best guide in answering these few questions. Please read them carefully and check the ☑ YES or NO opposite the question if it applies to you.

YES NO

☐ ☐ 1. Has your doctor ever said you have heart trouble?

☐ ☐ 2. Do you frequently have pains in your heart and chest?

☐ ☐ 3. Do you often feel faint or have spells of severe dizziness?

☐ ☐ 4. Has a doctor ever said your blood pressure was too high?

☐ ☐ 5. Has your doctor ever told you that you have a bone or joint problem such as arthritis that has been aggravated by exercise, or might be made worse with exercise?

☐ ☐ 6. Is there a good physical reason not mentioned here why you should not follow an activity program even if you wanted to?

☐ ☐ 7. Are you over age 65 and not accustomed to vigorous exercise?

If You Answered

YES to one or more questions

If you have not recently done so, consult with your personal physician by telephone or in person BEFORE increasing your physical activity and/or taking a fitness test. Tell him what questions you answered YES on PAR-Q, or show him your copy.

Programs

After medical evaluation, seek advice from your physician as to your suitability for:
- unrestricted physical activity, probably on a gradually increasing basis.
- restricted or supervised activity to meet your specific needs, at least on an initial basis. Check in your community for special programs or services.

NO to all questions

If you answered PAR-Q accurately, you have reasonable assurance of your present suitability for:
- A GRADUATED EXERCISE PROGRAM—A gradual increase in proper exercise promotes good fitness development while minimizing or eliminating discomfort.
- AN EXERCISE TEST—Simple tests of fitness (such as the Canadian Home Fitness Test) or more complex types may be undertaken if you so desire.

Postpone

If you have a temporary minor illness, such as a common cold.

*Developed by the British Columbia Ministry of Health. Conceptualized and critiqued by the Multidisciplinary Advisory Board on Exercise (MABE).
Reference PAR-Q Validation Report, British Columbia Ministry of Health, May, 1978.
*Produced by the British Columbia Ministry of Health and the Department of National Health & Welfare.

Resting Physiological Measures

The next step in the screening process requires that physiological measures be taken at rest prior to the GXT. Abnormal values would be a rationale for referral to a medical doctor. Heart rate and BP are *always* taken prior to a GXT, be it a submaximal fitness test or a diagnostic test taken to maximum. Diagnostic GXTs are *always* preceded by a resting ECG (3). In addition, a blood sample may be taken for analysis of blood lipids and glucose. Abnormal resting values for HR, BP, or the ECG would require medical consultation prior to taking the GXT. In centers that are using the GXT for diagnostic purposes, these abnormal values are expected in the populations they serve, and since a physician is present, decisions to proceed are made on the spot. However, in fitness centers where nonmedical personnel are involved, an abnormal response at rest requires medical referral before testing is conducted (34).

Submaximal Tests

If the resting values indicate that a person can proceed, a submaximal GXT can be used to evaluate CRF. HR and BP (and ECG where appropriate) are measured at each stage of the test that progresses from light work (~ 3 METs) to a predetermined end point such as 70%–85% of predicted maximal heart rate. A treadmill, cycle ergometer, or a bench can be used to impose the work rates, and these tests will be described in detail in subsequent sections. Abnormal responses (see later) would be a rationale for terminating the test and seeking medical advice about what additional tests may be required and what type of exercise program (supervised versus unsupervised) may be appropriate (34).

Maximal Tests

Instead of stopping the submaximal GXT at some predetermined end point (70%–85% maximal HR), the GXT can be taken to the point of volitional exhaustion, or to where specific signs (ECG or BP changes) or symptoms like chest pain (**angina pectoris**) or breathlessness (**dyspnea**) occur. In these cases HR, BP, and ECG are monitored throughout the test protocol, and CRF is based on the last work rate achieved. However, there are some maximal tests of CRF that are not "graded" and for which physiological measurements are not made during the test (e.g., Cooper's twelve-minute or 1.5-mile run (16), and the AAHPERD's 1-mile run (1). These latter **field tests** will now be considered in more detail, along with the Canadian Home Fitness Test (63), and a 1-mile walk test (42). This will be followed by a discussion of GXTs using the treadmill, cycle ergometer, and bench step.

Field Tests for Estimating CRF

Maximal Run Tests

Some field tests for CRF involve a measurement of how far a person can run in a set time (twelve to fifteen minutes), or how fast a person can run a set distance (1–2 miles). The advantages of such field tests include their moderately high correlation with $\dot{V}O_2$ max, the use of a natural activity, the large numbers of people who can be tested at one time, and the low cost. The disadvantages of using field tests include the difficulty of monitoring physiological responses, the importance that motivation plays in the outcome, and the fact that the test is not graded, but is a maximal effort. These field tests should be used only after a person has progressed through a program of exercise at lower intensities. The most popular field test for adults is Cooper's twelve-minute or 1.5-mile run (16), and for children twelve years or younger, the AAHPERD's 1-mile run (1). The aim is to determine the average velocity that can be maintained over the time or distance. These tests represent evolutionary changes from the original work of Balke (9), who showed that running tests of ten to twenty minutes duration provide reasonable estimates of $\dot{V}O_2$ max. The basis for the field tests is the linear relationship that exists between $\dot{V}O_2$ (ml $\cdot$ kg^{-1} $\cdot$ min^{-1}) and running speed, as shown in chapter 6. The duration of ten to twenty minutes represents a compromise that attempts to maximize the chance that the person is running at a speed demanding 90%–95% $\dot{V}O_2$ max, and minimize the contribution of energy coming from anaerobic sources. In distance runs of five minutes or less, anaerobic sources would be providing large amounts of energy, and $\dot{V}O_2$ max would probably be overestimated.

Table 15.1 Men's and women's aerobics fitness classifications

Men's

Category	Age (years)					
	13–19	20–29	30–39	40–49	50–59	60+
1. Very Poor	<35.0*	<33.0	<31.5	<30.2	<26.1	<20.5
2. Poor	35.0–38.3	33.0–36.4	31.5–35.4	30.2–33.5	26.1–30.9	20.5–26.0
3. Fair	38.4–45.1	36.5–42.4	35.5–40.9	33.6–38.9	31.0–35.7	26.1–32.2
4. Good	45.2–50.9	42.5–46.4	41.0–44.9	39.0–43.7	35.8–40.9	32.2–36.4
5. Excellent	51.0–55.9	46.5–52.4	45.0–49.4	43.8–48.0	41.0–45.3	36.5–44.2
6. Superior	>56.0	>52.5	>49.5	>48.1	>45.4	>44.3

*Values for oxygen uptake in $ml \cdot kg^{-1} \cdot min^{-1}$

Women's

Category	Age (years)					
	13–19	20–29	30–39	40–49	50–59	60+
1. Very Poor	<25.0*	<23.6	<22.8	<21.0	<20.2	<17.5
2. Poor	25.0–30.9	23.6–28.9	22.8–26.9	21.0–24.4	20.2–22.7	17.5–20.1
3. Fair	31.0–34.9	29.0–32.9	27.0–31.4	24.5–28.9	22.8–26.9	20.2–24.4
4. Good	35.0–38.9	33.0–36.9	31.5–35.6	29.0–32.8	27.0–31.4	24.5–30.2
5. Excellent	39.0–41.9	37.0–40.9	35.7–40.0	32.9–36.9	31.5–35.7	30.3–31.4
6. Superior	>42.0	>41.0	>40.1	>37.0	>35.8	>31.5

*Values for oxygen uptake in $ml \cdot kg^{-1} \cdot min^{-1}$
From: Kenneth H. Cooper, *The Aerobics Way*. Copyright © 1977 Bantam Books, Inc., New York, N.Y.

The method of calculating the $\dot{V}O_2$ when the running speed is known was described in detail in Box 6.2, and the formula is presented here again:

$$\dot{V}O_2 = 0.2 \ (m \cdot min^{-1}) + 3.5 \ (ml \cdot kg^{-1} \cdot min^{-1})$$

This formula provides reasonable estimates of $\dot{V}O_2$ max for adults, but would underestimate values for young children because of their relatively poor economy of running (21). On the other hand, this formula would overestimate the value for $\dot{V}O_2$ max for those who walk, running (21). On the other hand, this formula would overestimate the value for $\dot{V}O_2$ max for those who walk, since the net cost of walking is half that of running (see Box 6.1):

$$\dot{V}O_2 = 0.1 \ (m/min) + 3.5 \ (ml \cdot kg^{-1} \cdot min^{-1})$$

While Cooper (16) provides categories of $\dot{V}O_2$ max values by age and sex (see table 15.1), estimates of $\dot{V}O_2$ max based on distance runs are most useful when compared over time for the same individual, rather than between individuals. Variation in economy of running, motivation, and other factors makes such comparisons of estimated $\dot{V}O_2$ max values between individuals unreasonable (6, 62). In this light, distance swim and bicycle riding tests provide useful information about changes in an individual's CRF over time, even though estimates of $\dot{V}O_2$ max are not available at this time (17).

The formulas used for estimating $\dot{V}O_2$ max on a twelve-minute run are not very useful for prepubescent children since their economy of running is less than that of an adult (21). Investigators (43) worked around this problem by testing first, second, and third grade boys and girls with 800-, 1,200-, and 1,600-meter runs, and related performance to the measured $\dot{V}O_2$ max scores. They found the 1,600-meter run was the best predictor with good test/retest reliability (0.82 to 0.92) in children who were given instruction on paced running (43).

$\dot{V}O_2$ max (ml $\cdot$ kg^{-1} $\cdot$ min^{-1}) estimated in an endurance run test is not only influenced by the cardiovascular function of the individual, but also by the quantity of body fat carried along. It has been shown that differences in estimated $\dot{V}O_2$ max values between males and females can be explained, in part, by differences in % body fat (19, 20, 66). In a twelve-minute run test, performance was decreased 89 meters when body weight was experimentally increased by 5% to simulate an additional 5% fat (20). One should expect, then, that with a combined exercise and weight reduction program, CRF will increase due to both an increase in cardiovascular function and a decrease in % body fat.

In table 15.1 categories for $\dot{V}O_2$ max values were adjusted for age due to the observation that in the general population, $\dot{V}O_2$ max decreases with age. However, recent studies (35, 38, 69) have shown that in individuals who maintain their physical activity program and body weight over time, $\dot{V}O_2$ max does not decrease very much. This provides additional rationale for a regular evaluation of CRF by simple field tests, to keep track of small changes before they become big changes.

Walk Test

An alternative to the maximal run tests used to evaluate CRF is a 1-mile walk test in which the HR is monitored during the test (42). The equation used to predict $\dot{V}O_2$ max was based on one population of men and women, aged thirty to sixty-nine, and was then validated on another comparable population. The subject walks as fast as possible for one mile on a flat, measured track, and HR is measured at the end of the last lap. The following equation can be used to estimate $\dot{V}O_2$ max (ml $\cdot$ kg^{-1} $\cdot$ min^{-1}):

$$\dot{V}O_2 \text{ max} = 132.853 - 0.0769 \text{ (wt)} - 0.3877 \text{ (age)} + 6.315 \text{ (sex)} - 3.2649 \text{ (time)} - 0.1565 \text{ (HR)}$$

where (wt) is body weight in pounds, (age) in years, (sex) equals 0 for female and 1 for male, (time) is in minutes and hundredths of minutes, and (HR) is in beats $\cdot$ min^{-1} measured at the end of the last quarter mile.

This test appears to fill a void in the field tests available to estimate $\dot{V}O_2$ max since it uses a common activity and requires the simple measurement of HR. As a participant's fitness improves, the time required for the mile and/or the HR response decreases, increasing the estimated $\dot{V}O_2$ max.

Canadian Home Fitness Test

In contrast to the Cooper 1.5-mile run test and the 1-mile walk test, which require an all-out effort, the Canadian Home Fitness Test (CHFT) is a submaximal step test that uses the lowest two 8-inch steps found in a conventional staircase (63). The stepping cadence in this test is maintained by a long-playing record. Prior to the test the person completes the Physical Activity Readiness Questionnaire (PAR-Q) (figure 15.2) to determine if he or she should proceed. The first stage of the test requires the individual to step for three minutes at a rate equivalent to 65%–70% of the average $\dot{V}O_2$ max of the next oldest age group (remember $\dot{V}O_2$ max generally decreases with age). An immediate ten-second recovery pulse is counted, and if it does not exceed the maximum allowable, another three-minute step test at 65%–70% of the average $\dot{V}O_2$ max of the person's own age group is completed. Another pulse rate is then taken. Table 15.2 shows how physical fitness is evaluated as "undesirable," "minimal," or "recommended" (63). $\dot{V}O_2$ max can be estimated from the CHFT results (37).

Table 15.2 Physical fitness evaluation chart for the Canadian Home Fitness Test

10-Second Pulse Rate

Age (yr)	After First Three Minutes of Exercise	After Second Three Minutes of Exercise
15–19	If 30 or more, stop. You have an undesirable personal fitness level.	If 27 or more, you have a minimum personal fitness level. If 26 or less, you have the recommended personal fitness level.
20–29	If 29 or more, stop. You have an undesirable personal fitness level.	If 26 or more, you have a minimum personal fitness level. If 25 or less, you have the recommended personal fitness level.
30–39	If 28 or more, stop. You have an undesirable personal fitness level.	If 25 or more, you have a minimum personal fitness level. If 24 or less, you have the recommended personal fitness level.
40–49	If 26 or more, stop. You have an undesirable personal fitness level.	If 24 or more, you have a minimum personal fitness level. If 23 or less, you have the recommended personal fitness level.
50–59	If 25 or more, stop. You have an undesirable personal fitness level.	If 23 or more, you have a minimum personal fitness level. If 22 or less, you have the recommended personal fitness level.
60–69	If 24 or more, stop. You have an undesirable personal fitness level.	If 23 or more, you have a minimum personal fitness level. If 22 or less, you have the recommended personal fitness level.

From: R. J. Shephard et al., Development of the Canadian Home Fitness Test, in *Canadian Medical Association Journal* 114:675-79, 1976. Copyright © 1976 Canadian Medical Association, Ottawa, Canada.

Graded Exercise Tests: Measurements

Cardiorespiratory fitness is commonly measured using a treadmill, cycle ergometer, or a stepping bench. These tests are usually incremental, in which the work rate changes every two to three minutes until the subject reaches some predetermined end point, or when some pathological sign or symptom occurs. These GXT's can be maximal or submaximal, and the variables measured during the test can be as simple as HR and BP, or as complex as $\dot{V}O_2$; it depends on the purpose of the test, the facilities, equipment, and personnel involved (33). What follows is a brief summary of common measurements made during a GXT.

Heart Rate

Heart rate can be measured by palpation of the radial or carotid artery, using a stethoscope with the microphone on the chest wall, or by using surface electrodes that transmit the signal to an oscilloscope, electrocardiograph, or an integrated receiver that can display heart rate directly. In palpating the carotid artery, care must be taken not to use too much pressure, since this could slow the HR by way of the baroreceptor reflex. However, when people are trained in this procedure, reliable measurements can be obtained (55, 60). Heart rate is measured over a fifteen- to thirty-second time period *during* steady state exercise to obtain a reliable estimate of the HR. If using a *post-exercise* HR as an indication of the HR during exercise, the HR should be measured for ten seconds within the first fifteen seconds after stopping exercise because the HR changes rapidly at this time. The ten-second count is multiplied by 6 to express the HR in beats $\cdot$ min^{-1} (60).

Blood Pressure

Blood pressure is measured by auscultation as described in chapter 9. It is important to use the proper cuff size and a sensitive stethoscope to obtain correct values at rest and during work. In addition, if using an aneroid sphygmomanometer, it is important to calibrate it on a regular basis against the mercury sphygmomanometer (40). During the walking or cycling exercise test (BP cannot be reliably measured during a running test) the microphone of the stethoscope is placed below the cuff and over an area where the sound is the loudest (in many cases this will be in the intramuscular space on the medial side of the arm). The subject should not be holding onto the handlebar of the cycle or treadmill during the measurement. The first Korotkoff sound is taken as systolic BP, and the fourth sound (change in tone or muffling) is taken as diastolic BP (56). The HR can also be measured if the pressure is maintained just above the diastolic value. The following procedure can be used to obtain the HR and BP values during an exercise test: pump up cuff above the point where the pulse disappears, decrease pressure slowly (<5 mm Hg per second), and obtain systolic BP; decrease quickly to a value above diastolic BP and count HR for fifteen seconds; slowly decrease pressure and obtain the diastolic reading.

ECG

GXTs are used to diagnose CHD because exercise causes the heart to work harder and challenges the coronary arteries' ability to deliver sufficient blood to meet the oxygen demand of the myocardium. An estimate of the work (and O_2 demand) of the heart is the **double product,** the product of the HR, and the systolic BP (41, 54). As you already know, HR and systolic BP increase with exercise intensity such that myocardial oxygen demand increases throughout the test. The ECG is used as an indicator of the ability of the heart to function normally during these times of imposed work. During exercise the ECG can be measured with a single bipolar lead (CM$_5$), but a full twelve-lead arrangement is preferred (3). The ECG is evaluated for arrhythmias, conduction disturbances, and myocardial ischemia. **Arrhythmias** are irregularities in the normal electrical rhythm of the heart that can be localized to the atria (e.g., atrial fibrillation), the AV node (e.g., premature junctional contraction), or in the ventricles (e.g., premature ventricular contractions—PVCs). **Conduction disturbances** describe a defect in which depolarization is slowed or completely blocked (e.g., first degree AV block, or bundle branch block). **Myocardial ischemia** is defined as an inadequate perfusion of the myocardium relative to the metabolic demand of the ventricles. Since oxygen uptake by the myocardium is almost completely flow dependent, a flow limitation indicates an oxygen insufficiency. A *symptom* of myocardial ischemia is angina pectoris, which is pain or discomfort caused by a temporary ischemia; the pain could be located in the center of the chest, neck, jaw, shoulders, or radiate to the arms and hands (46). A *sign* associated with myocardial ischemia is a depression of the ST segment (chapter 9). Figure 15.3 shows three types of **ST segment depression.** People with upsloping or horizontal ST segment depression have similar life expectancies, but the prognosis for those with downsloping ST segment is worse (22). Interested readers are referred to Dubin's introductory text on ECG analysis (selected readings), and Ellestad's text on exercise electrocardiography (22).

Figure 15.3 Three types of ST-segment depression.

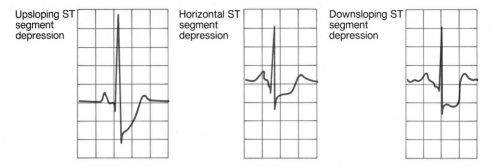

Upsloping ST segment depression

Horizontal ST segment depression

Downsloping ST segment depression

$\dot{V}O_2$ Max

The measurement of $\dot{V}O_2$ max represents the standard against which any estimate of CRF is compared (see chapters 6 and 20 for procedures). $\dot{V}O_2$ increases with increasing loads on a GXT until the maximal capacity of the cardiorespiratory system is reached. Commonly used criteria for having achieved $\dot{V}O_2$ max include a leveling off of the $\dot{V}O_2$ (<150 ml $\cdot$ min^{-1}, or < 2.1 ml $\cdot$ kg^{-1} $\cdot$ min^{-1}) even though a higher work rate is achieved (68), a lactate level of >8 mmoles $\cdot$ liter^{-1} (5), and the R exceeding 1.15 (36). While the majority ($>50\%$) of subjects will meet these criteria, some, especially the elderly (65) and postcoronary (39) subjects, will not. In addition, one should not expect a subject to meet all three of these standards (39, 65). For example, in one study (65) 20% of the women subjects who met the "leveling off" criterion did not even achieve an R of 1.00! These criteria are useful in that they give the investigator an objective indicator of the subjective effect of the subject. However, one should not expect all subjects to meet all the criteria on any single test.

$\dot{V}O_2$ max is a very reproducible measure on subjects following the same test protocol on the same piece of equipment. The value for $\dot{V}O_2$ max does not seem to be dependent on whether the test is a continuous GXT or a discontinuous GXT as long as it is conducted with the same work instrument (24, 47, 67). However, when $\dot{V}O_2$ max values are compared across protocols, some systematic differences appear (9). The highest value for $\dot{V}O_2$ max is usually measured with a running test up a grade on a treadmill followed by a walking test up a grade on a treadmill, and then on a cycle ergometer. In American populations walk test protocols yield values about 6% lower than a run test (47), and a cycle test is about 10%–11% lower than a run test (25, 47). Europeans show only a 5%–7% difference in this latter comparison (9, 32). In addition, an arm ergometer test will yield values equal to about 70% of the $\dot{V}O_2$ max measured with the legs (27, 59). These differences among tests have led to the convention to call $\dot{V}O_2$ max the standard value measured on a graded running test, and all other values, $\dot{V}O_2$ peak (58). It is important to recognize these differences when comparing one test to another, or when comparing the same subject over time with different ergometers. The actual measurement of $\dot{V}O_2$ max is crucial for research studies and in some clinical settings, however, it is unreasonable to suggest this as the standard to use as a measure of CRF in exercise programs.

Estimation of $\dot{V}O_2$ Max from Last Work Rate

Given the complexity and cost of the procedures involved in the measurement of $\dot{V}O_2$ max, it is no surprise that in many fitness and clinical settings $\dot{V}O_2$ max is estimated with equations that allow one to calculate $\dot{V}O_2$ from the last work rate achieved on the GXT. The equations outlined in chapter 6 allow such calculations, and in general the estimates are reasonable (50, 51). What is important in the use of these equations is that the work test is suited to the individual. If the increments in the GXT from one stage to the

Figure 15.4 Estimation of $\dot{V}O_2$ max from heart rate values measured during a series of submaximal work rates on a cycle ergometer. The test was stopped when the subject reached 85% of maximal HR. A line is drawn through the HR points measured during the test and is extrapolated to the age-adjusted estimate of maximal HR. Another line is dropped from that point to the x-axis, and the $\dot{V}O_2$ max is identified.

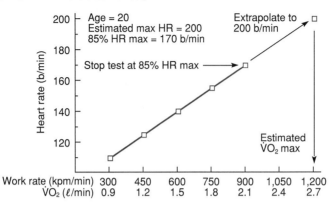

Work rate (kpm/min)	300	450	600	750	900	1,050	1,200
$\dot{V}O_2$ (ℓ/min)	0.9	1.2	1.5	1.8	2.1	2.4	2.7

next are too large relative to a person's CRF, or if the time for each stage is so short that a person might not be able to achieve the steady state oxygen requirement for that stage, then the equations will overestimate the person's $\dot{V}O_2$ max (26, 31, 50). As described in chapter 4, poorly fit individuals take longer to achieve the steady state at moderate to heavy work rates, and this increases the chance of an overestimation of $\dot{V}O_2$ max when using these formulas. This suggests that a more conservative protocol be used for low-fit individuals to allow them to reach a steady state at each stage. A recommended procedure is to use only the last completed stage of a test. However, independent of the proper matching of the protocol with the individual, one must remember that these are only *estimations*.

Estimation of $\dot{V}O_2$ Max from Submaximal HR Responses

Another common procedure used with GXT protocols is to estimate $\dot{V}O_2$ max on the basis of the subject's HR response to a variety of submaximal work rates (28). In these tests the HR is plotted against work rate (or estimated $\dot{V}O_2$) until the termination criterion of 70%–85% of age-adjusted maximal HR is reached. Figure 15.4 shows the HR response for a twenty year old who has taken a submaximal GXT on a cycle ergometer. Heart rate was measured at each work rate

until a value equal to 85% of estimated maximal HR was reached ($170 \text{ b} \cdot \text{min}^{-1}$). A line was drawn through the HR points and extrapolated to the estimated maximal HR, which is calculated by subtracting age from 220. Another line is dropped from that point to the x-axis, and the work rate or $\dot{V}O_2$ that would have been achieved if the individual had worked until maximal HR was reached is recorded (28). While this is a simple and commonly used procedure to estimate $\dot{V}O_2$ max, several potential problems exist.

The first problem relates to the formula used for estimating the maximal HR. These estimates have a standard deviation (SD) of about $11 \text{ beats} \cdot \text{min}^{-1}$ (44). A twenty year old's maximal HR might be estimated to be $200 \text{ beats} \cdot \text{min}^{-1}$, but if a person were out at ± 2 SD, the value would be 178 or 222 $\text{beats} \cdot \text{min}^{-1}$. For those who do maximal testing it is not uncommon to observe people having *measured* maximal HRs $\pm 20 \text{ beats} \cdot \text{min}^{-1}$ away from their age-adjusted estimate of maximal heart rate. Taking this as an example, what if the subject in figure 15.4 had a true maximal HR of only $180 \text{ beats} \cdot \text{min}^{-1}$ instead of the estimated $200 \text{ beats} \cdot \text{min}^{-1}$? The estimated $\dot{V}O_2$ max would be an overestimation of the correct value.

Further, a submaximal end point such as 85% of estimated maximal heart rate may be very light work for one individual and maximal work for another. The

Table 15.3 Rating of perceived exertion scales

Original Rating Scale		New Rating Scale	
6		0	Nothing at all
7	Very, very light	0.5	Very, very light (just noticeable)
8		1	Very light
9	Very light	2	Light (weak)
10		3	Moderate
11	Fairly light	4	Somewhat hard
12		5	Heavy (strong)
13	Somewhat hard	6	
14		7	Very heavy
15	Hard	8	
16		9	
17	Very hard	10	Very, very heavy (almost max)
18			
19	Very, very hard		
20			

From: G. A. V. Borg. Psychological bases of physical exertion, in *Medicine and Science in Sports and Exercise* 14:377-81, 1982. Copyright © 1982 American College of Sports Medicine, Madison, Wis. Reprinted by permission.

reason for this is related to the estimate of maximal heart rate (220 − age) mentioned earlier. If a thirty-year-old individual has a real maximum heart rate of 160 beats · min^{-1}, and the GXT takes the person to 85% of estimated maximal HR (220 − 30 = 190; 85% of 190 = 161 beats · min^{-1}), then the person would be taken to maximal HR.

Another problem with submaximal GXT protocols using the HR response as the primary indicator of fitness is that any variable that affects submaximal heart rate will affect the slope of the HR/$\dot{V}O_2$ line and, of course, the estimate of $\dot{V}O_2$ max. These variables would include: eating prior to the test, dehydration, elevated body temperature, temperature and humidity of the testing area, emotional state of the subject, medications that affect HR, and previous physical activity (8, 62). Clearly, if one is to use such protocols to estimate $\dot{V}O_2$ max, many environmental variables must be controlled.

As many problems as this approach has to the estimation of $\dot{V}O_2$ max, it is a useful one that provides appropriate feedback to participants in fitness programs. Following training, the HR response to any fixed submaximal work rate is lower, suggesting an increase in $\dot{V}O_2$ max when the HR/$\dot{V}O_2$ line is drawn through those HR points to the age-adjusted maximal HR. In this case, because the same individual is being tested over time, the 220 − age formula introduces only a constant and unknown error that will not affect the projection of the HR/$\dot{V}O_2$ line. Further, the low cost and ease of measurement make it a good test that can be used for education and motivation (61).

Rating of Perceived Exertion

Another common measurement made at each stage of the GXT is Borg's (12) Rating of Perceived Exertion (RPE). Table 15.3 lists his original and revised scales. The original scale used the rankings 6–20 to approximate the HR values from rest to maximum (60–200). The revised scale represents an attempt to provide a ratio scale of the RPE values. The RPE scores are good indicators of subjective effort and provide a quantitative way to track a person's progress through a GXT or an exercise session (14, 15, 29). This is helpful in knowing when a subject is approaching exhaustion, and the values can be used in prescribing exercise intensity (see chapter 16).

Termination Criteria

The reasons for stopping a GXT vary with the type of population being tested and the purpose of the test. The following list is adapted from the ACSM's *Guidelines for Exercise Testing and Prescription* (2, 3).

1. Subject requests to stop
2. Failure of monitoring system
3. $\dot{V}O_2$ max is reached, the normal end point for the apparently healthy individual
4. Abnormal signs and symptoms
   a. Dizziness, confusion, staggering, unsteadiness
   b. Angina, claudication (blockage of peripheral blood vessel), or other pain
   c. Nausea
   d. Labored breathing (dyspnea)
   e. Cyanosis or pallor
   f. Severe fatigue or distress
5. ECG changes
   a. ST segment displacement: 2 mm horizontal or downsloping, or elevation
   b. Ventricular arrhythmias: tachycardia, PVCs occurring every second or third beat, multifocal PVCs, R wave on T wave of PVCs
   c. Atrioventricular or ventricular conduction disturbances: onset of second- or third-degree heart block, exercise-induced left or right bundle branch block
6. Abnormal blood pressure responses
   a. Fall in systolic BP of 10 mm Hg, or failure of systolic BP to rise with increasing work after initial adjustment period
   b. Excessive blood pressure rise: systolic over 250 mm Hg; diastolic BP over 120 mm Hg
7. Heart rate response
   a. Unexplained low HR response to GXT (bradycardia)
   b. The age-adjusted maximal HR should not be used as the end point on a maximal GXT
   c. A percent of age-adjusted maximal HR (70%–85%) can be used to stop submaximal tests, or be used to alert the tester that subject is near maximum

Maximal versus Submaximal Tests

The decision to do a maximal or submaximal GXT is dependent on the reason for the test and the type of individual being tested. The submaximal test is useful for estimating CRF in a wide variety of populations, and provides useful information when used before and after a fitness program. However, for the asymptomatic individual the submaximal test may not provide a high enough work rate to cause ischemia in the coronary arteries that might be observed in changes in the ECG (3).

The objection to maximal tests for CRF evaluation, be they field tests or laboratory-controlled GXT protocols, is that they place a great deal of stress on a previously sedentary person. For example, no fitness instructor would exercise a sedentary person to maximum on the first day in a fitness program because of the soreness and personal discomfort that the person would experience. For this reason, and in spite of its shortcomings, a submaximal test might be the test of choice at the beginning of the fitness program, except when it is used in the diagnosis of CHD.

Graded Exercise Test: Protocols

The GXT protocols can be either submaximal or maximal, depending on the end points used to stop the test. The choice of the GXT should be based on the population (athletes, cardiac patients, children), purpose (estimate CRF, measure $\dot{V}O_2$ max, diagnose CHD), and cost (equipment and personnel) (33, 34). This section will discuss the selection of the test based on these factors and provide examples of common GXT protocols.

The choice of the GXT must consider the population being tested, given that the last stage in a GXT for cardiac patients might not even be a warm-up for a young athletic subject. Test protocols should vary in terms of the initial work rate, how large the increment in work rate will be between stages, and in the duration of each stage. In general, the GXT for a sedentary subject might start at 2–3 METs (1 MET = 3.5 ml · kg^{-1} · min^{-1}), progress at about 1 MET per stage, with each stage lasting two to three minutes to allow enough time for a steady state to be reached. For young active subjects, the initial work rate might be 6 METs, with increments of 2–3 METs per stage (56). Table 15.4 shows four well-known treadmill protocols and the populations for which they are suited. The National Exercise and Heart Disease protocol (53) is usually used with deconditioned subjects with the work rate increasing only 1 MET each three minutes. The Standard Balke protocol (11) starts at about 4 METs and progresses 1 MET each two minutes, and is suitable for most average sedentary adults. The Bruce protocol (13) starts at about 5 METs and progresses at 2–3 METs per stage. This protocol includes walking and running up a grade, and is not suitable for those at the low end of the fitness continuum. The last protocol shown is used by the fit and athletic populations, with the speed dependent on the fitness of the subject (8, 34).

As mentioned earlier, one of the most common approaches used in estimating $\dot{V}O_2$ max is to take the final stage in the test and apply the formula for converting grade and speed to $\dot{V}O_2$ in ml · kg^{-1} · min^{-1}. Nagle et al. (52), and Montoye et al. (50) have shown that apparently healthy individuals reach the new steady state requirement by 1.5 minutes or so of each stage up to moderately heavy work. These formulas give reasonable estimates of CRF if the test has been suited to the individual (31, 50). However, if the increments in the stages are too large, or if the time at each stage is too short, then the person might not be able to reach the oxygen requirement associated with that stage of the GXT. In these cases the formulas will overestimate the subject's $\dot{V}O_2$ max. This problem is more common with low-fit individuals and suggests that the more conservative tests be used to estimate the $\dot{V}O_2$ max based on grade and speed achieved.

Treadmill

Treadmill GXT protocols can accommodate the least to the most fit and use the natural activities of walking and running. Treadmills set the pace for the subject and provide the greatest potential load on the cardiovascular system. However, they are expensive, not portable, and make some measurements (BP and blood sampling) difficult (62). As mentioned previously, the type of treadmill test does influence the magnitude of the measured $\dot{V}O_2$ max, with the graded running test giving the highest value, the running test at 0% grade the next highest, and the walking test protocols the lowest (9, 47). There are also some limitations in the types of measurements that can be made, depending on whether walking or running is used. For example, during running tests measurement of BP is not possible, and there is more potential for artifact in the ECG tracing.

In order for estimates of $\dot{V}O_2$ to be obtained from grade and speed considerations, the grade and speed settings must be correct (33). In addition, there is a need for the subject to carefully follow the instructions of not holding onto the treadmill railing during the test if the estimates of $\dot{V}O_2$ are going to be reasonable, based on either the HR/$\dot{V}O_2$ line extrapolation to estimated maximal HR, or the use of the $\dot{V}O_2$ formula that uses the last speed/grade combination achieved (6, 57). For example, when a subject who was walking on a treadmill at 3.4 mph and 14% grade held onto the railing, the HR decreased 17 b · min^{-1} (6). This would result in an overestimation of the $\dot{V}O_2$ max, using either of the submaximal procedures just mentioned, and special equations would have to be developed if holding onto the handrail is allowed (48). Finally, with the treadmill there is no need to make adjustments to the $\dot{V}O_2$ calculation due to differences in body weight. Treadmill tests require the subject to carry his or her own weight, and the $\dot{V}O_2$ is therefore proportional to body weight (49).

In the following example of a submaximal GXT a forty-five-year-old male takes a Balke Standard Protocol (3 mph, 2.5% each two minutes), and the test is terminated at 85% of age-adjusted maximal HR (149 b · min^{-1}). Heart rate was measured in the last thirty

Table 15.4 Treadmill protocols

A—Protocol for Poorly Fit Subjects (53)

Stage*	METs	Speed (mph)	% Grade
1	2.5	2	0
2	3.5	2	3.5
3	4.5	2	7.0
4	5.5	2	10.5
5	6.5	2	14.0
6	7.5	2	17.5
7	8.5	3	12.5
8	9.5	3	15.0
9	10.5	3	17.5

*Stage lasts three min.

B—Protocol for Normal, Sedentary Subjects (11)

Stage*	METs	Speed (mph)	% Grade
1	4.3	3	2.5
2	5.4	3	5.0
3	6.4	3	7.5
4	7.4	3	10.0
5	8.5	3	12.5
6	9.5	3	15.0
7	10.5	3	17.5
8	11.6	3	20.0
9	12.6	3	22.5

*Stage lasts two min.

C—Protocol for Young, Active Subjects (13)

Stage*	METs	Speed (mph)	% Grade
1	5	1.7	10
2	7	2.5	12
3	9.5	3.4	14
4	13	4.2	16
5	16	5.0	18

*Stage lasts three min.

D—Protocol for Very Fit Subjects (8)

Stage*	METs	Speed (mph)	% Grade
1	12.9/18	7/10	2.5
2	14.1/19.8	7/10	5.0
3	15.3/21.5	7/10	7.5
4	16.5/23.2	7/10	10.0
5	17.7/24.9	7/10	12.5

*Stage lasts two min.; vigorous warm-up precedes test.

Figure 15.5 Estimation of V̇O$_2$ max from the heart rate values measured during different stages of a treadmill test.

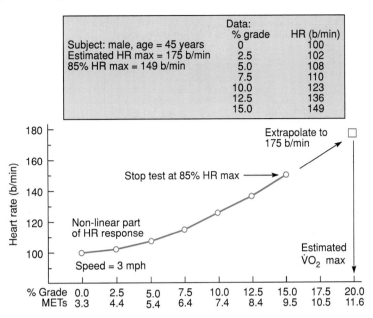

Data:		
	% grade	HR (b/min)
Subject: male, age = 45 years	0	100
Estimated HR max = 175 b/min	2.5	102
85% HR max = 149 b/min	5.0	108
	7.5	110
	10.0	123
	12.5	136
	15.0	149

seconds of each stage, and V̇O$_2$ max was estimated by the HR/V̇O$_2$ extrapolation to age-adjusted maximal HR (175 b · min^{-1}). Figure 15.5 shows the plot of the HR response at each stage, and the extrapolation to the person's estimated maximal heart rate. In the early stages of the test the HR does not increase in a predictable manner with increasing grade. This may be due to the changes in stroke volume that occur early in upright work (see chapter 9). The beginning stages also act as a warm-up and adjustment period for the subject. The HR response is usually quite linear between 110 b · min^{-1} and 85% maximal HR (7). The HR/V̇O$_2$ line is extrapolated to 175 b · min^{-1}, and a vertical line is dropped to the x-axis where the estimated V̇O$_2$ max is identified: 11.6 METs, or 40.6 ml · kg^{-1} · min^{-1}.

Cycle Ergometer

Cycle ergometers are portable, moderately priced work instruments that allow measurements to be easily made, but they are self-paced and result in some localized fatigue (62). On mechanically braked cycle ergometers (e.g., Monark) the work rate can be increased

by increasing the pedal rate or the resistance on the flywheel. Generally, the pedal rate is maintained constant during a GXT at a rate suitable to the populations being tested: 50–60 rpm for the low to average fit, 70–100 for the high fit and competitive cyclists (30). The pedal rate is maintained by having the subject attend to a metronome, or by providing some other source of feedback (visual analog or digital display of the rpm). The load on the wheel is increased in a sequential fashion to systematically overload the cardiovascular system. The starting work rate and the increment from one stage to the next would be dependent on the fitness of the subject and the purpose of the test, as mentioned earlier. The V̇O$_2$ can be estimated from a formula that gives reasonable estimates of the V̇O$_2$ up to work rates of about 1,200 kg-m · min^{-1} (2):

$$\text{V̇O}_2 \text{ (ml · min}^{-1}) = 2 \text{ ml · kg-m}^{-1} \times \text{kg-m · min}^{-1} + 300 \text{ ml · min}^{-1}$$

The cycle ergometer is different from the treadmill in that the body weight is supported by the seat, and the work rate is dependent only on the crank speed and

Figure 15.6 *The Y's Way to Physical Fitness* protocol used to select work rates for submaximal cycle ergometer testing of men and women.

Reprinted from *The Y's Way to Physical Fitness,* with permission of the YMCA of the USA, 101 N. Wacker Drive, Chicago, Ill. 60601.

(a) Guide to setting work loads for males on the bicycle ergometer

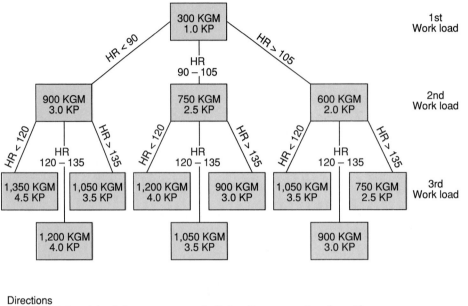

Directions

1. Set the 1st work load at 300 kgm/min (1.0 KP).
2. If HR in 3rd min is: Less than (<) 90, set 2nd load at 900 kgm (3 KP). Between 90 and 105, set 2nd load at 750 kgm (2.5KP). Greater than (>) 105, set 2nd load at 600 kgm (2.0 KP).
3. Follow the same pattern for setting 3rd and final load.
4. Note: if the 1st work load elicits a HR of 110 or more, it is used on the graph, and only <u>one</u> more work load will be necessary.

the load on the wheel. This means that for a small person the relative $\dot{V}O_2$ at any work rate is higher than for a big person. For example, if the work rate is 900 kg-m · min^{-1}, the estimated $\dot{V}O_2$ is 2,100 ml · min^{-1}; this represents a relative $\dot{V}O_2$ of 35 ml · kg^{-1} · min^{-1} for a 60-kg person, and only 23 ml · kg^{-1} · min^{-1} for a 90-kg person. In addition, the increments in the work rate, by demanding a fixed increase in the $\dot{V}O_2$ (e.g., an increment of 150 kg-m · min^{-1} is equal to a $\dot{V}O_2$ change of 300 ml · min^{-1}), forces the small and unfit subject to make larger cardiovascular adjustments than a large or high-fit subject. These facts have been taken into consideration by the American College of Sports Medicine (3) and the YMCA (28) in recommending

submaximal GXT protocols. The idea is to provide a means of obtaining a variety of HR responses to several submaximal work rates, but to do so in a way that keeps the test length down. The YMCA provides two protocols, one for women and one for men. Figure 15.6 shows the different "routes" followed depending on the subject's HR response. The YMCA protocol makes use of the observation that the relationship between $\dot{V}O_2$ and HR is a linear one between the HRs of 110 and 150 b · min^{-1}. For this reason the YMCA protocol requires the subject to work only one more work rate past the one that yields a HR $\geq$ 110 b · min^{-1}. As a general recommendation for all cycle ergometer tests, seat height is adjusted so that the knee is slightly

Figure 15.6 *Continued*

(b) Guide to setting work loads for females on the bicycle ergometer

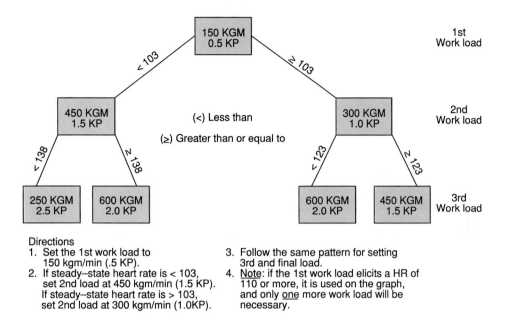

Directions
1. Set the 1st work load to 150 kgm/min (.5 KP).
2. If steady–state heart rate is < 103, set 2nd load at 450 kgm/min (1.5 KP). If steady–state heart rate is > 103, set 2nd load at 300 kgm/min (1.0KP).
3. Follow the same pattern for setting 3rd and final load.
4. Note: if the 1st work load elicits a HR of 110 or more, it is used on the graph, and only <u>one</u> more work load will be necessary.

bent when the foot is at the bottom of the pedal swing and parallel to the floor; the seat height is recorded for later testing. In the YMCA protocol each stage lasts three minutes and heart rate values are obtained in the last thirty seconds of the second and third minutes. If the difference in HR is <5 b · min^{-1} between the two time periods, a steady state is assumed; if not, an additional minute is added to that stage. A line then connects the two HR values and is extrapolated to the subject's estimated maximal HR. A vertical line is dropped to the x-axis and the estimated $\dot{V}O_2$ max value is obtained as described for the submaximal treadmill protocol.

Figure 15.7 shows the YMCA protocol for a thirty-year-old female. The first work rate chosen was 150 kg-m · min^{-1}, and a heart rate of 103 b · min^{-1} was measured. Following the YMCA protocol, the next load was 300 kg-m · min^{-1}. Because the HR was <123 for this work rate, the next work rate was increased to 600 kg-m · min^{-1}. A line was drawn through the two HR points greater than 100 b · min^{-1}, and

extrapolated to 190 b · min^{-1}. The estimated $\dot{V}O_2$ max for this woman was about 2.7 liters · min^{-1}.

In addition to this extrapolation procedure for estimating $\dot{V}O_2$ max, Åstrand and Ryhming (7) provide a method that requires the subject to complete just one work rate of about six minutes, demanding a HR between 125 and 170 b · min^{-1}. These investigators observed that at 50% $\dot{V}O_2$ max males had an average HR of 128, and females, 138 b · min^{-1}, and at 70% $\dot{V}O_2$ max the average HRs were 154 and 164 b · min^{-1}, respectively. These data were collected on young men and women, ages eighteen to thirty. The basis for the test is that if you know from a HR response that a person is at 50% $\dot{V}O_2$ max at a work rate equal to 1.5 l · min^{-1}, then the estimated $\dot{V}O_2$ max would be twice that, or 3.0 l · min^{-1}. A nomogram (see figure 15.8) is used to estimate the $\dot{V}O_2$ max based on the subject's HR response to one six-minute work rate. Because maximal HR decreases with increasing age, and the data were collected on young subjects, Åstrand

Figure 15.7 Example of the YMCA protocol used to estimate $\dot{V}O_2$ max.

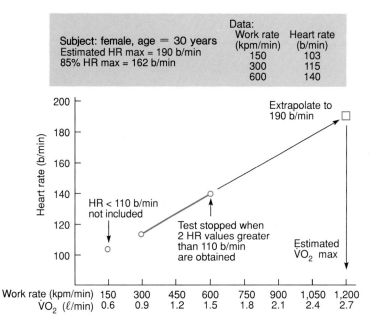

Subject: female, age = 30 years Estimated HR max = 190 b/min 85% HR max = 162 b/min	Data: Work rate (kpm/min)	Heart rate (b/min)
	150	103
	300	115
	600	140

(4) established correction factors with which one could multiply the estimated $\dot{V}O_2$ max taken from the nomogram to correct for the lower maximal HR.

Siconolfi et al. (64) presented a submaximal cycle ergometer test that is a modification of the YMCA protocol that uses the Åstrand and Ryhming (7) nomogram. It is presented here because the advantages of this test include (1) the requirement that the subject achieve only 70% of the estimated maximal HR, and (2) that the procedure was validated on men and women of ages twenty to seventy years. Men over age thirty-five and all women start the test at 150 kg-m · min⁻¹, and the work rate is increased that amount each two minutes until a HR ≥ 70% of estimated maximal HR is achieved; the subject continues for two or more minutes until a steady state HR is measured. Men under age thirty-five begin at 300 kg-m · min⁻¹ and increase that amount each two minutes as above. However, when the HR is between 60% and 70% of maximal HR, the work rate is increased

only 150 kg-m · min⁻¹. The Åstrand and Ryhming (7) nomogram is used as before (without the age correction), and the estimated $\dot{V}O_2$ max values are used in the following equations (64):

For males: $\dot{V}O_2$ (liters · min⁻¹) = 0.348 (X_1) − 0.035 (X_2) + 3.011

For females: $\dot{V}O_2$ (liters · min⁻¹) = 0.302 (X_1) − 0.019 (X_2) + 1.593

where $X_1 = \dot{V}O_2$ max from Åstrand and Ryhming nomogram, and X_2 = age in years. The test yields acceptable estimates of $\dot{V}O_2$ max and puts the subject under less stress by requiring that a HR of only 70% of the age-adjusted maximal HR be achieved.

Step Test

A step-test protocol can be used to estimate $\dot{V}O_2$ max in the same way that treadmill and cycle ergometer protocols were used. The step test requires inexpensive equipment, the step height does not have to be calibrated, everyone is familiar with the stepping exercise,

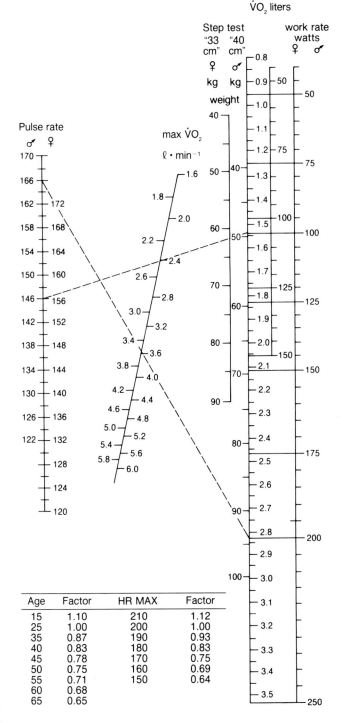

Figure 15.8 Nomogram for the estimation of $\dot{V}O_2$ max from submaximal HR values measured on either a cycle ergometer or step test. For the cycle ergometer the work rate in watts (1 watt = 6.1 kg $-$ m · min^{-1}) is shown on the two right-most columns, one for men and one for women. The results of a cycle ergometer test for a man who worked at 200 watts is shown. A dashed line is drawn between the 200-watt work rate and the HR value of 166 measured during the test. The estimated $\dot{V}O_2$ max is 3.6 liters · min^{-1}. The step test uses a rate of 22.5 lifts · min^{-1}, and two different step heights, 33 cm for women and 40 cm for men. The step test scale lists body weight for the subject and the results of a test on a 61-kg woman are shown. A dashed line is drawn between the 61 kg on the 33-cm scale and the HR value of 156 b · min^{-1} measured during the test. The estimated $\dot{V}O_2$ max is 2.4 liters · min^{-1}. These estimates of $\dot{V}O_2$ max are influenced by the person's maximal HR, which is known to decrease with age. A correction factor chosen from the accompanying table corrects these $\dot{V}O_2$ max values when either the maximal HR or age is known. Simply multiply the $\dot{V}O_2$ value by the correction factor.

Age	Factor	HR MAX	Factor
15	1.10	210	1.12
25	1.00	200	1.00
35	0.87	190	0.93
40	0.83	180	0.83
45	0.78	170	0.75
50	0.75	160	0.69
55	0.71	150	0.64
60	0.68		
65	0.65		

Figure 15.9 Use of a step test to predict $\dot{V}O_2$ max from a series of submaximal HR responses.

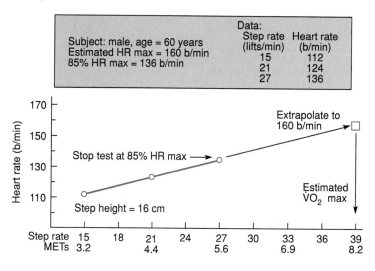

and the energy requirement is proportional to body weight, as is the treadmill (45). The work rate can be increased by increasing the step height, keeping the cadence the same, or by increasing the cadence, keeping the step height the same. The step height can be varied with a hand-cranking device (52), or by using a series of wooden steps with increments in step height of 10 cm. The rate of stepping is established with a metronome, and the stepping cadence has four counts: up, up, down, down. The subjects must step all the way up and down in time with the metronome. Figure 15.9 shows the results of a step test on a sixty-year-old man. In this step test the height of the step was kept constant, 16 centimeters, and the rate of stepping increased six lifts $\cdot$ min^{-1} each two minutes. The line drawn through the HR points is extrapolated to the estimated maximal HR, 160 b $\cdot$ min^{-1}, and a line is dropped to the horizontal axis to estimate the $\dot{V}O_2$ max.

The Åstrand and Ryhming (7) nomogram (figure 15.8) also accommodates a step test, using a rate of 22.5 lifts per minute (metronome = 90) and step heights of 40 cm for men and 33 cm for women. The principle is the same as described for their cycle ergometer protocol.

In summary, there are a variety of tests that can be used to estimate CRF. The usefulness of a test is a function of both the accuracy of the measurement and the ability to repeat the test on a routine basis to evaluate changes in CRF over time. It is this latter point that decreases the need that the test must be able to estimate the true $\dot{V}O_2$ max to the nearest ml $\cdot$ kg^{-1} $\cdot$ min^{-1}. In effect, if a person is taking a submaximal GXT on a regular basis and the HR response to a fixed work rate is decreasing over time, one could reasonably conclude that the person is making progress in the intended direction, independent of how accurate the estimate of $\dot{V}O_2$ max is.

Summary

1. Prior to an exercise test to evaluate cardiorespiratory fitness (CRF), a person completes a brief health history, resting measurements of HR and BP are taken, and an ECG is recorded. A decision to proceed is based on these measures, as well as the willingness of the person to take the exercise test (informed consent).

2. CRF can be estimated by maximal or submaximal exercise tests done in the "field" or in laboratories. Field tests include maximal distance run tests, 1-mile walk tests, and a step test that can be done at home.

3. The GXT is selected on the basis of the population (young/old; fit/unfit) such that the rate of progression allows a steady state to be achieved at most stages of the test. Failure to do so results in an overestimation of CRF.

4. The HR rate response to a variety of submaximal loads can be extrapolated to age-adjusted maximal HR (220 − age) to estimate CRF. This estimate of CRF may be inaccurate due to: (1) the estimate of maximal HR in which the standard deviation of the estimate is ± 11 b $\cdot$ min^{-1}, or (2) by environmental problems (room temperature, previous exercise, meal, emotion, etc.) that can affect the HR response.

5. The reasons for terminating an exercise test include the subject's request to stop, failure of the monitoring system, achieving $\dot{V}O_2$ max, appearance of abnormal signs (ECG, BP, HR), or symptoms (angina).

6. GXT procedures for a submaximal estimate of CRF are provided for the treadmill, cycle ergometer, and step.

Study Questions

1. What is the sequence of steps used in evaluating cardiorespiratory fitness?

2. What is a health or cardiac risk inventory? Name one currently in use and explain its purpose.

3. A forty-year-old man runs 1.5 miles (2,415 meters) in ten minutes. What is his estimated $\dot{V}O_2$ max? Is his value "normal"?

4. Draw an example of ST segment depression and describe its significance in the diagnosis of heart disease.

5. You are monitoring a GXT in which $\dot{V}O_2$ max is measured. How would you know if a person achieved $\dot{V}O_2$ max?

6. Given the following information collected during a treadmill test on a fifty-year-old man, estimate his $\dot{V}O_2$ max.

Work Rate	Heart Rate
3 METs	110
5 METs	125
7 METs	140

7. Given the assumption that the formula, 220 − age, can be used to estimate maximal heart rate, how far off could you be in your estimate of $\dot{V}O_2$ max in question 6?

8. What information do you gain by monitoring the RPE during a GXT?

9. List five reasons for stopping a GXT.

10. Should you use the same GXT protocol on all subjects? Why?

Selected Readings

Dubin, D. 1974. *Rapid Interpretation of EKGs*, 3d ed. Tampa, Fla.: Cover Publishing Company.

References

1. American Alliance for Health, Physical Education, Recreation and Dance. 1980. *Health-related physical fitness test manual*. Reston, Va.: Author.

2. American College of Sports Medicine. 1980. *Guideline Graded Exercise Testing and Exercise Prescription*, 2nd ed. Philadelphia: Lea & Febiger.

3. ———. 1986. *Guidelines for exercise testing and prescription*. Philadelphia: Lea & Febiger.

4. Åstrand, I. 1960. Aerobic work capacity in men and women with special reference to age. *Acta Physiologica Scandinavica* 49: Suppl. 169.

5. Åstrand, P. O. 1952. *Experimental studies of physical working capacity in relation to sex and age*. Copenhagen, Manksgaard.

6. ———. 1984. Principles of ergometry and their implications in sports practice. *International Journal of Sports Medicine* 5:102–5.

7. Åstrand, P. O., and I. Ryhming. 1954. A nomogram for calculation of aerobic capacity (physical fitness) from pulse rate during submaximal work. *Journal of Applied Physiology* 7:218–21.

8. Åstrand, P. O., and K. Rodahl. 1986. *Textbook of Work Physiology.* New York: McGraw-Hill Book Company.

9. Åstrand, P. O., and B. Saltin. 1961. Maximal oxygen uptake and heart rate in various types of muscular activity. *Journal of Applied Physiology* 16:977–81.

10. Balke, B. 1963. A simple field test for assessment of physical fitness. *Civil Aeromedical Research Institute Report* 63–66.

11. Balke, B. 1970. Advanced exercise procedures for evaluation of the cardiovascular system. Monograph. Milton, Wis.: The Burdick Corporation.

12. Borg, G. A. V. 1982. Psychological bases of physical exertion. *Medicine and Science in Sports and Exercise* 14:377–81.

13. Bruce, R. A. 1972. Multi-stage treadmill tests of maximal and submaximal exercise. In American Heart Association, *Exercise testing and training of apparently healthy individuals: a handbook for physicians.* New York: American Heart Association, 32–34.

14. Carton, R. L., and E. C. Rhodes. 1985. A critical review of the literature on ratings scales for perceived exertion. *Sports Medicine* 2:198–222.

15. Chow, R. J., and J. H. Wilmore. 1984. The regulation of exercise intensity by ratings of perceived exertion. *Journal of Cardiac Rehabilitation* 4:382–87.

16. Cooper, K. H. 1977. *The Aerobic Way.* New York: Bantam Books.

17. Cooper, M., and K. H. Cooper. 1972. *Aerobics for women.* New York: Evans.

18. Cumming, G. R., and L. M. Borysyk. 1972. Criteria for maximal oxygen uptake in men over 40 in a population survey. *Medicine and Science in Sports* 4:18–22.

19. Cureton, K. J., L. D. Hensley, and A. Tiburzi. 1979. Body fatness and performance differences between men and women. *Research Quarterly* 50:333–40.

20. Cureton, K. J. et al. 1978. Effect of experimental alterations in excess weight on aerobic capacity and distance running performance. *Medicine and Science in Sports* 10:194–99.

21. Daniels, J. et al. 1978. Differences and changes in $\dot{V}O_2$ among young runners 10–18 years of age. *Medicine and Science in Sports* 10:200–203.

22. Ellestad, M. 1980. *Stress Testing: Principles and Practice.* Philadelphia: F. A. Davis.

23. *Exercise and Your Heart.* 1981. U.S. Department of Health and Human Services. NIH Publication, No. 81–1677.

24. Falls, H., and L. D. Humphrey. 1973. A comparison of methods for eliciting maximal oxygen uptake for college women during treadmill walking. *Medicine and Science in Sports* 5:239–41.

25. Faulkner, J. A. et al. 1971. Cardiovascular responses to submaximum and maximum effort cycling and running. *Journal of Applied Physiology* 30:457–61.

26. Foster, C. et al. 1984. Prediction of oxygen uptake during exercise testing in cardiac patients and health volunteers. *Journal of Cardiac Rehabilitation* 4:537–42.

27. Franklin, B. A. 1985. Exercise testing, training and arm ergometry. *Sports Medicine* 2:100–119.

28. Golding, L. A., C. R. Myers, and W. E. Sinning. 1982. *The Y's Way to Physical Fitness.* Chicago: National Board of YMCA.

29. Gutmann, M. C. et al. 1981. Perceived exertion-heart rate relationship during exercise testing and training of cardiac patients. *Journal of Cardiac Rehabilitation* 1:52–59.

30. Hagberg, J. M. et al. 1981. Effect of pedaling rate on submaximal exercise responses of competitive cyclists. *Journal of Applied Physiology* 51:447–51.

31. Haskell, W. L. et al. 1982. Factors influencing estimated oxygen uptake during exercise testing soon after myocardial infarction. *American Journal of Cardiology* 50:299–304.

32. Hermansen, L., and B. Saltin. 1969. Oxygen uptake during maximal treadmill and bicycle exercise. *Journal of Applied Physiology* 26:31–37.

33. Howley, E. T. 1988. Exercise testing laboratory. In (S. N. Blair et al., eds.) *Resource Manual for Guidelines for Exercise Testing and Prescription,* Chapter 47. Philadelphia: Lea & Febiger.

34. Howley, E. T., and B. D. Franks. 1986. *Health/ Fitness Instructor's Handbook.* Champaign, Ill.: Human Kinetics Publishers.

35. Howley, E. T., H. J. Montoye, and F. J. Nagle. 1986. Minimal change in $\dot{V}O_2$ max with age in active subjects who maintain body weight. *Medicine and Science in Sports and Exercise* 18:521.

36. Issekutz, B., N. C. Birkhead, and K. Rodahl. 1962. The use of respiratory quotients in assessment of aerobic power capacity. *Journal of Applied Physiology* 17:47–50.

37. Jette, M. et al. 1976. The Canadian Home Fitness Test as a predictor of aerobic capacity. *Canadian Medical Association Journal* 114:680–83.

38. Kasch, F. W., J. P. Wallace, and S. P. Van Camp. 1985. Effects of 18 years of endurance exercise on the physical work capacity of older men. *Journal of Cardiopulmonary Rehabilitation* 5:308–12.

39. Kavanagh, T., and R. J. Shephard. 1976. Maximal exercise tests on "postcoronary" patients. *Journal of Applied Physiology* 40:611–18.

40. Kirkendall, W. M. et al. 1980. Recommendations for human blood pressure determination by sphygmomanometers. *Circulation* 62:1146A–55A.

41. Kitamura, K. et al. 1972. Hemodynamic correlates of myocardial oxygen consumption during upright exercise. *Journal of Applied Physiology* 32:516.

42. Kline, G. M. et al. 1987. Estimation of $\dot{V}O_2$ max from a one-mile track walk, gender, age, and body weight. *Medicine and Science in Sports and Exercise* 19:253–59.

43. Krahenbuhl, G. S. et al. 1978. Field testing of cardiorespiratory fitness in primary school children. *Medicine and Science in Sports and Exercise* 10:208–13.

44. Londeree, B. R., and M. L. Moeschberger. 1984. Influence of age and other factors on maximal heart rate. *Journal of Cardiac Rehabilitation* 4:44–49.

45. Margaria, R., P. Aghemo, and Rovelli. 1965. Indirect determination of maximal O_2 consumption in man. *Journal of Applied Physiology* 20:1070–73.

46. Martin, A. D. 1986. ECG and medications. In (E. T. Howley and B. D. Franks) *Health/Fitness Instructor's Handbook,* Chapter 12. Champaign, Ill.: Human Kinetics Publishers.

47. McArdle, W. D., F. I. Katch, and G. S. Pechar. 1973. Comparison of continuous and discontinuous treadmill and bicycle tests for max $\dot{V}O_2$. *Medicine and Science in Sports and Exercise* 5:156–60.

48. McConnell, T. R., and B. A. Clark. 1987. Prediction of maximal oxygen consumption during handrail-supported treadmill exercise. *Journal of Cardiopulmonary Rehabilitation* 7:324–31.

49. Montoye, H. J., and T. Ayen. 1986. Body size adjustment for oxygen requirement in treadmill walking. *Research Quarterly for Exercise and Sport* 57:82–84.

50. Montoye, H. J. et al. 1985. The oxygen requirement for horizontal and grade walking on a motor-driven treadmill. *Medicine and Science in Sports and Exercise* 17:640–45.

51. Montoye, H. J., T. Ayen, and R. A. Washburn. 1986. The estimation of $\dot{V}O_2$ max from maximal and sub-maximal measurements in males, age 10–39. *Research Quarterly for Exercise and Sport* 57: 250–53.

52. Nagle, F. J., B. Balke, and J. P. Naughten. 1965. Gradational step tests for assessing work capacity. *Journal of Applied Physiology* 20:745–48.

53. Naughton, J. P., and R. Haider. 1973. Methods of exercise testing. In (J. P. Naughton, H. K. Hellerstein, and L. C. Mohler, eds.) *Exercise Testing and Exercise Training in Coronary Heart Disease,* 79–91. New York: Academic Press.

54. Nelson, R. R. et al. 1974. Hemodynamic predictors of myocardial oxygen consumption during static and dynamic exercise. *Circulation* 50:1179–89.

55. Oldridge, N. B., W. L. Haskell, and P. Single. 1981. Carotid palpation, coronary heart disease and exercise rehabilitation. *Medicine and Science in Sports and Exercise* 13:6–8.

56. Pollock, M. L., J. H. Wilmore, and S. M. Fox. 1984. *Exercise in health and disease.* Philadelphia: W. B. Saunders Company.

57. Ragg, K. E. et al. 1980. Errors in predicting functional capacity from a treadmill exercise stress test. *American Heart Journal* 100:581–83.

58. Rowell, L. B. 1974. Human cardiovascular adjustments to exercise and thermal stress. *Physiology Reviews* 54:75–159.

59. Sawka, M. N. et al. 1983. Determination of maximal aerobic power during upper-body exercise. *Journal of Applied Physiology: Respiration, Environmental, and Exercise Physiology* 54:113–17.

60. Sedlock, D. A. et al. 1983. Accuracy of subject-palpated carotid pulse after exercise. *The Physician and Sportsmedicine* 11(4):106–16.

61. Sharkey, B. J. 1984. *Physiology of Fitness,* 2nd ed. Champaign, Ill.: Human Kinetics Publishers.

62. Shephard, R. J. 1984. Tests of maximal oxygen uptake: A critical review. *Sports Medicine* 1:99–124.

63. Shephard, R. J., D. A. Bailey, and R. L. Mirwald. 1976. Development of the Canadian home fitness test. *Canadian Medical Association Journal* 114:675–79.

64. Siconolfi, S. F. et al. 1982. Assessing $\dot{V}O_2$ max in epidemiologic studies: Modification of the Åstrand-Ryhming test. *Medicine and Science in Sports and Exercise* 14:335–38.

65. Sidney, K. H., and R. J. Shephard. 1977. Maximum and submaximum exercise tests in men and women in the seventh, eighth, and ninth decades of life. *Journal of Applied Physiology* 43:280–87.

66. Sparling, P. B., and K. J. Cureton. 1983. Biological determinants of the sex difference in 12-minute run performance. *Medicine and Science in Sports and Exercise* 15:218–23.

67. Stamford, B. A. 1976. Step increments versus constant load tests for determination of maximal oxygen uptake. *European Journal of Applied Physiology* 35:89–93.

68. Taylor, H. L., E. R. Buskirk, and A. Henschel. 1955. Maximal oxygen intake as an objective measure of cardiorespiratory performance. *Journal of Applied Physiology* 8:73–80.

69. Wallace, J. P. 1983. Physical conditioning: Intervention in aging cardiovascular function. In (A. R. Liss, ed.) *Intervention in the Aging Process, Part A: Quantitation, Epidemiology, and Clinical Research,* 307–23.

16 Training for Health and Fitness

Objectives

*U*pon completion of this chapter, you should be able to do the following:
1. Characterize physical inactivity as a coronary heart disease risk factor comparable to smoking, hypertension, and high serum cholesterol.
2. Contrast graphically the benefits to be gained versus the risks experienced with increasing physical activity.
3. Describe the risk of cardiac arrest for someone who engages in regular strenuous exercise.
4. Identify, generally, some of the 1990 health promotion/disease prevention objectives as they relate to physical activity, and describe the progress being made to achieve them.
5. Contrast "exercise" with "physical activity;" explain how both relate to lower risk of CHD and improvements in CRF.
6. Explain what "screening" and "progression" mean for a person wishing to initiate an exercise program.
7. Identify the optimal frequency, intensity, and duration of activity associated with improvements in CRF; why is more not necessarily better than less?
8. Calculate a target heart rate range by either the heart rate range or percent of maximal HR methods.
9. Explain why the appropriate sequence of physical activity for sedentary persons is walk → walk/jog → jog → games.
10. Explain how the target heart rate (THR) helps adjust exercise intensity in times of high heat, humidity, or while at altitude.

Outline

In chapter 14 we discussed a variety of risk factors related to cardiovascular and other diseases. Physical inactivity has long been considered only a secondary risk factor in the development of CHD—that is, an inactive life-style would increase a person's risk for CHD only if some other primary risk factors were present. This is no longer the case. Recent studies (25, 27, 35, 37) suggest that physical inactivity is a primary risk factor for coronary heart disease (CHD), similar to smoking, hypertension, and high serum cholesterol. Further, these studies show that regular vigorous physical activity is instrumental in reducing the risk of CHD in those who smoke or are hypertensive. This suggests that physical activity should be used along with other therapies to reduce the risk of CHD in those possessing other risk factors. There is little disagreement that regular physical activity is a necessary part of a healthy life-style (17). The only question is, how much?

In a recent symposium on the relationship of physical activity to health at the Center for Disease Control in Atlanta, a panel of distinguished scientists tried to deal with this question. A discussion of their findings is a good starting point in this chapter, which deals with training programs for health and fitness.

Physical Activity and Health

From a public health standpoint, the greatest health benefits would be obtained by having previously sedentary people become slightly active (34). This is shown schematically in figure 16.1, in which the health-related benefits of increasing physical activity is compared to the risks involved. The greatest benefits appear when the person moves from the sedentary existence and becomes moderately active (expending about 200–300 kcal at least every other day) *with less of an effect between those who are moderately active and those who are very active* (16). The 200–300 kcal is equivalent to walking 4–5 miles or jogging 2–3 miles. These benefits occur at a point where the overall risk associated with physical activity is relatively small. However, even though the risk of cardiac arrest in habitually active men is higher *during vigorous activity,* the overall (rest + exercise) risk of cardiac arrest in vigorously active men is only 40% of risk of sedentary men (36). Further, Paffenbarger (25, 27) found in his studies of longshoremen and Harvard alumni that the protective benefits of exercise were seen in those who were most active (expending > 2,000 kcal per week). The overall findings suggest (1) that those who are sedentary have much to gain by becoming habitually active in mild-to-moderate activities, and (2) those who exercise vigorously on a regular basis maintain a lower risk of CHD relative to less-active individuals with similar risk factors.

This positive relationship between physical activity and health has been accepted by the Department of Health and Human Services (HHS), which published, as is indicated in chapter 14, a variety of health promotion/disease prevention objectives in 1980 (11). These were ten-year objectives, stated in terms that could be evaluated along the way. The following is a selection of the objectives stating the 1990 goal:

1. The proportion of children and adolescents ages ten to seventeen participating regularly in appropriate physical activities—particularly cardiorespiratory fitness programs, which can be carried into adulthood—should be greater than 90%.

Figure 16.1 A theoretical description of the potential health benefits of physical activity compared to risks. The health-related benefits of physical activity increase dramatically with a small increase in physical activity when the risk of injury due to physical activity is low.

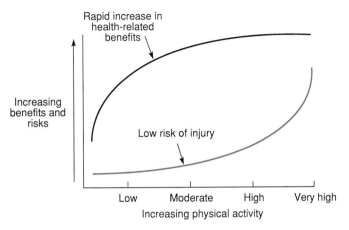

2. The proportion of children and adolescents ages ten to seventeen participating in daily school physical education programs should be greater than 60%.
3. The proportion of adults eighteen to sixty-four participating regularly in vigorous physical exercise should be greater than 60%.
4. Fifty percent of adults sixty-five and older should be engaging in appropriate physical activity, such as regular walking, swimming, or other aerobic activity.

In 1986 HHS published a "Midcourse Review" of how well the country was moving toward those objectives (12). Unfortunately, the findings indicated it was unlikely that we would be able to meet the 1990 objectives (12). It is clear that there is still much to be done in changing the activity habits of the young and old. This chapter provides some generally accepted steps to follow in achieving that goal.

However, before we start there is a need to distinguish between and among certain terms as they relate to physical activity, exercise, health, and fitness. **Physical activity** results in the expenditure of energy proportional to muscular work, and is related to **physical fitness. Exercise** represents a subset of physical activity that is planned and has as one of its goals to improve or maintain fitness components (6). In addition,

while physical fitness is usually associated with good health, this does not mean that a higher $\dot{V}O_2$ max due to an exercise program causes a lower risk of CHD. The cause of the lower risk of CHD may be because the physical activity can also change the distribution of cholesterol and increase fibrinolysis (clot dissolving) activity. So, both changes, an increase in $\dot{V}O_2$ max and a decrease in the risk of CHD, occur simultaneously, but by different mechanisms (16). This is an important distinction given that low levels of energy expenditure (slow walking) may be able to decrease the risk of CHD while causing little change in cardiorespiratory fitness (CRF), as defined by changes in $\dot{V}O_2$ max.

General Guidelines for Fitness Programs

In chapter 13 the concepts of overload and specificity were presented relative to the adaptations that take place with different training programs. While these principles apply here, what is important to remember is that it does not take very much exercise to achieve a health-related effect. This stands in marked contrast to the intensity of exercise needed to achieve performance goals (see chapter 21). This section will present the general guidelines associated with fitness programs, with particular emphasis on choosing the correct intensity (21).

Screening

The first thing to do if it has not already been done in the evaluation of CRF is to carry out some form of health status screening to decide who should begin an exercise program and who should obtain further consultation with a physician (see chapter 15 for details).

Progression

The emphasis in any health-related exercise program is to do too little rather than too much. By starting slowly and progressing from the easily accomplished activities to those that are more difficult, the chance of causing muscle soreness and of aggravating old injuries is reduced. The emphasis on slow-to-moderate walking as the primary activity early in the fitness program is consistent with this recommendation, and the participant must be educated to not move too quickly into the more demanding activities. Once the person can walk about 4 miles without fatigue, then the progression to a walk-jog and jogging program is a reasonable recommendation (21).

Warm-Up, Stretch, and Cool-Down, Stretch

Prior to the actual activity used in the exercise session, a variety of very light exercises and stretches are done to improve the transition from rest to the exercise state. While chapter 25 discusses warm-up as an ergogenic aid related to performance, the emphasis at the onset of an exercise session is to gradually increase the level of activity until the proper intensity is reached. Stretching exercises to increase the range of motion of the joints involved in the activity, as well as specific stretches to increase the flexibility of the lower back, are included in the warm-up. At the end of the activity session about five minutes of cool-down activities—slow walking and stretching exercises—are recommended to gradually return HR and BP toward normal. This part of the exercise session is viewed as important in reducing the chance of a hypotensive episode after the exercise session (21).

Exercise Prescription for CRF

The exercise program includes dynamic large muscle activities such as walking, jogging, running, swimming, cycling, rowing, and dancing. The CRF training effect of exercise programs is dependent on the proper frequency, duration, and intensity of the exercise sessions. An exercise program conducted three to five times per week, for fifteen to sixty minutes per session, at an intensity of about 50%–85% $\dot{V}O_2$ max, has been shown to cause appropriate CRF effects (1, 2). The combination of duration and intensity should result in the expenditure of about 200–300 kcal per session, and is consistent with achieving weight loss goals and reducing the risk factors associated with CHD (1, 2, 16, 30, 32).

Frequency

Improvements in CRF increases with the frequency of exercise sessions, with two sessions being viewed as less than adequate, and the gains in CRF leveling off after three to four sessions per week (2, 42). Gains in CRF can be achieved with a two days per week program, but the intensity has to be higher than the three days per week program, and participants might not achieve weight loss goals (29). The three to four days per week schedule includes a day off between sessions and reduces the scheduling problems associated with planned exercise programs. In addition, as figure 16.2 shows, higher frequencies are associated with higher rates of injuries (10, 31).

Duration

The duration has to be viewed together with intensity in that the total work accomplished per session (200–300 kcal) seems to be the most important variable associated with improvements in CRF once the minimal threshold of intensity is achieved (2). This is important given that many sedentary persons could more easily accomplish an exercise session of low intensity and long duration than the reverse, and achieve the health-related benefits of physical activity with minimal risk. For example, an 80-kg (176 lb) person

Figure 16.2 Effects of increasing the frequency, duration, and intensity of exercise on the increase in $\dot{V}O_2$ max in a training program. This figure demonstrates the increasing risk of orthopedic problems due to exercise sessions that are too long, or conducted too many times per week. The probability of cardiac complications increases with exercise intensity beyond that recommended for improvements in cardiorespiratory fitness.

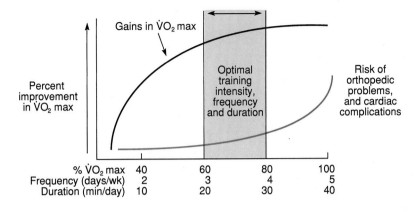

walking at about 3.5 mph would consume O_2 at the rate of 1 liter per minute. Given 5 kcal $\cdot$ l $O_2{}^{-1}$, the person is using 5 kcal $\cdot$ min^{-1}, and sixty minutes of walking would be required to expend 300 kcal. As the intensity of exercise increases, the duration needed to expend 300 kcal decreases. As figure 16.2 shows, doing strenuous exercise (75% $\dot{V}O_2$ max) beyond thirty minutes increases the risk of orthopedic problems.

Intensity

The intensity describes the overload on the cardiovascular system that is needed to bring about a training effect. Improvements in CRF occur when the intensity is between 50%–85% $\dot{V}O_2$ max. The intensity threshold for a training effect for those at the low end of the CRF continuum is about 50% $\dot{V}O_2$ max, when coupled with the right duration. Those at the top end of the CRF continuum can work at 85% $\dot{V}O_2$ max to achieve their goals. For most people, 60%–80% $\dot{V}O_2$ max seems to be a range sufficient to achieve CRF goals (1, 2). It would appear that in order for this information to be useful the exercise leader would have to know the energy requirements ($\dot{V}O_2$) of all the fitness activities so that a correct match could be made between the activity and the participant. Fortunately, because of the linear relationship between exercise intensity and HR, the exercise intensity can be set by using the HR values equivalent to 60%–80% $\dot{V}O_2$ max. The range of heart rate values associated with the exercise intensity needed to have a CRF training effect is called the **target heart rate (THR)** range. How do you determine the THR range?

Direct Method

Figure 16.3 shows the HR response of a twenty-year-old subject during a maximal GXT on a treadmill. The subject's $\dot{V}O_2$ max was 12 METs, so that 60% and 80% $\dot{V}O_2$ max is equal to about 7.2 and 9.6 METs, respectively. A line is drawn from each of these work rates up to the HR/$\dot{V}O_2$ line, and over to the y-axis where the HR values equivalent to these work rates are obtained. These HR values, 138–164 b $\cdot$ min^{-1}, represent the THR range, the proper intensity for a CRF training effect (1, 21).

Indirect Methods

The THR range can also be estimated by some simple calculations, knowing that the relationship between HR and $\dot{V}O_2$ is linear. The *heart rate reserve or Karvonen*

Figure 16.3 Target heart rate range determined from the results of an exercise stress test. The heart rate values measured at work rates equal to 60% and 80% $\dot{V}O_2$ max constitutes the THR Range.

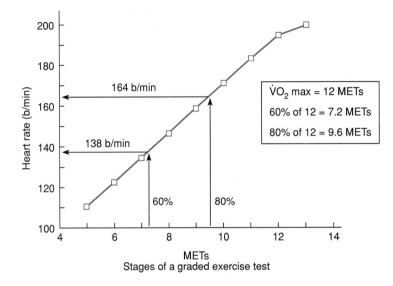

method of calculating a THR range has three simple steps (22):

1. Subtract resting HR from maximal HR to obtain HR reserve (HRR).
2. Take 60% and 80% of the HRR.
3. Add each HRR value to Resting HR to obtain the THR range.

For example:

1. If a subject has a maximal HR of 200 b · min⁻¹ and a resting HR of 60 b · min⁻¹, then the HRR is 140 b · min⁻¹ (200 − 60).
2. 60% × 140 b · min⁻¹ = 84 b · min⁻¹ and 80% × 140 b · min⁻¹ = 112 b · min⁻¹.
3. 84 b·min⁻¹ + 60 b·min⁻¹ = 144 b·min⁻¹ 112 b·min⁻¹ + 60 b·min⁻¹ = 172 b·min⁻¹. The THR range is 144–172 b · min⁻¹.

This method gives reasonable estimates of the exercise intensity because 60%–80% of the HRR is equal to about 60%–80% $\dot{V}O_2$ max.

The other indirect method of calculating the THR range is the *percentage of maximal HR* method. In this method you simply take 70% and 85% of maximal HR to obtain the THR range. In the following example the subject has a maximal HR of 200 b · min⁻¹. The THR range for this person is 140–170 b · min⁻¹ (70% × 200 = 140 b · min⁻¹; 85% × 200 = 170 b · min⁻¹). Seventy percent of maximal HR is equal to about 57% $\dot{V}O_2$ max, and 85% of maximal HR is equal to about 78% $\dot{V}O_2$ max, both within the intensity needed for CRF gains (18, 19, 20).

Table 16.1 lists the relationship between % $\dot{V}O_2$ max, % HRR, and % maximal HR. The intensity of exercise can be prescribed by the direct method, or by either of the indirect methods. Both of the indirect methods require knowledge of the maximal HR. If the maximal HR is measured during a maximal GXT, use it in the calculations. However, if you have to use the

Table 16.1 Relationship of percent of HR max, HRRᵃ, and % V̇O₂ max

% Max V̇O₂	% HRR	% Max HR
50	50	65
55	55	68
60	60	72
65	65	76
70	70	79
75	75	83
80	80	87
85	85	91
90	90	94

ᵃHRR is the difference between max HR and resting HR.
From: E. T. Howley and B. D. Franks, *Health/Fitness Instructor's Handbook.* Copyright © Human Kinetics Press, Inc., Champaign, Ill.

age-adjusted estimate of maximal HR (220 − age), remember the potential error, with the standard deviation of the estimate equal to ±11 b · min⁻¹. The estimated THR range is a *guideline* for exercise intensity and is meant to be used with other pieces of information (abnormal symptoms or signs) to determine if the exercise intensity is reasonable. In this regard, Borg's RPE scale can be used in prescribing exercise intensity for apparently healthy persons. Exercise perceived as "somewhat hard," 12–14 on the original RPE scale, approximates 70%–85% of maximal HR (1, 4, 8, 14, 15, 33). The RPE scale is helpful in that the participant will learn to associate the THR range with a certain whole-body perception of effort, decreasing the need for frequent pulse rate measurements. Remember, the intensity threshold needed to achieve CRF goals is lower for the less fit, and vice versa.

In order to determine if the subject is in the THR range during the activity, HR should be checked immediately after stopping, taking a ten-second pulse count within the first fifteen seconds. The pulse can be taken at the radial artery or the carotid artery, but if the latter is used, the participant should use only light pressure, since heavy pressure can actually slow the HR (33). Table 16.2 lists ten-second THRs appropriate for people of different ages and different percents of V̇O₂ max.

The proper intensity, frequency, and duration of exercise needed to have a CRF training effect were discussed in the previous section. However, there is a need for a sedentary individual to start slowly before exercising at the recommended intensities specified in the THR range.

Sequence of Physical Activity

The old adage that one should "walk before you run" is consistent with the way exercise should be recommended to sedentary persons, be they young or old. Once the person demonstrates an ability to do prolonged walking without fatigue, then controlled fitness exercises conducted at a reasonable intensity (THR) can be introduced. After that, and depending on the interest of the participant, a variety of fitness activities that are more gamelike can be included. This section will deal with this sequence of activities that can lead to a fit life (21).

Walking

The primary activity to recommend to someone who has been sedentary for a long period of time is walking. This recommendation is consistent with the introductory material on health benefits, and deals with the issue of injuries associated with more strenuous physical activity. In addition, there is good reason to believe that some subjects, especially the elderly, may use walking as their primary form of exercise. The emphasis at this stage is to simply get people active by providing an activity that can be done anywhere, anytime, and with anyone, young or old. In this way, the number of possible interfering factors that can result in the discontinuance of the exercise is reduced.

The person should choose comfortable shoes that are flexible, offer a wide base of support, with a fitted heel cup. There are a great number of "walking" shoes available, but a special pair of shoes is not usually required. The emphasis is on getting started; if walking becomes a "serious" activity, or if walking leads to

Table 16.2 Estimated ten-second THR[a]

Population	Intensity % $\dot{V}O_2$ max	Age (Years)						
		20	30	40	50	60	70	80
Inactive with several risk factors	50	22	21	20	18	17	16	15
	55	23	22	21	19	18	17	16
	60	24	23	22	20	19	18	17
Normal activity with few risk factors	65	25	24	23	21	20	19	18
	70	26	25	24	22	21	20	18
	75	28	26	25	24	22	21	19
	80	29	28	26	25	23	22	20
Very active with low risk	85	30	29	27	26	24	23	21
	90	31	30	28	27	25	24	22

[a]To be used only for people whose max HR is unknown.
From: E. T. Howley and B. D. Franks, *Health/Fitness Instructor's Handbook*. Copyright © 1986 Human Kinetics Press, Inc., Champaign, Ill.

hiking, then the investment would be reasonable. If weather is not to interfere with the activity, then proper selection of clothing is necessary. The participant should wear light, loose-fitting clothing in warm weather, and layers of wool or polypropylene in cold weather. For those who cannot bear the extremes in temperature and humidity out of doors, various shopping malls provide a good, controlled environment, with a smooth surface. Walkers should choose the areas in which they walk with care in order to avoid damaged streets, high traffic zones, and poorly lighted areas. Safety is important in any health-related exercise program (21).

A walking program is presented in Box 16.1 (21). The steps are rather simple, in that one does not progress to the next step unless he or she feels comfortable at the current step. The HR should be recorded as described above, but the emphasis is not on achieving the THR. Later on in the walking program, as one approaches higher walking speeds, he or she will attain the THR zone. Remember that walking, in spite of not being very strenuous by the THR zone scale, when combined with long duration, is an effective part of a

weight control and CHD risk factor reduction program (27). In addition, walking is an activity that many people find they can do every day; providing many opportunities to expend calories.

Jogging

Jogging begins when a person moves at a speed and form that results in a period of flight between foot strikes; this may be 3 or 4 mph, or 6 or 7 mph, depending on the fitness of the individual. As described in chapter 6, the net energy cost of jogging/running is about twice that of walking and, consequently, requires a greater cardiovascular response. This is not the only reason for the jogging program to follow a walking program; there is also more stress to joints and muscles due to the impact forces that must be tolerated during the push off and landing phases of the jogging (7).

The emphasis at the start of a jogging program is to make the transition from the walking program in such a way as to minimize the discomfort associated with the introduction of any new activity. This is accomplished by beginning with a jog-walk-jog program that eases the person into jogging by mixing in the

Box 16.1 Walking Program

Rules:

1. Start at beginning.
2. Be aware of new aches or pains.
3. Don't progress to next level if not comfortable.
4. Monitor heart rate and record it.
5. It would be healthful to walk at least every other day.

Day	Duration	Heart Rate	Comments
1	15 min		
2	20 min		
3	25 min		
4	30 min		
5	30 min		
6	30 min		
7	35 min		
8	40 min		
9	45 min		
10	45 min		
11	45 min		
12	50 min		
13	55 min		
14	60 min		
15	60 min		
16	60 min		
17	60 min		
18	60 min		
19	60 min		
20	60 min		

From E. T. Howley and B. D. Franks, *Health/Fitness Instructor's Handbook.* Copyright © 1986 Human Kinetics Publishers, Champaign, Ill.

lower energy cost and trauma associated with walking. The jogging speed is set according to the THR, with the aim to stay at the low end of the THR zone at the beginning of the program. As the participant adapts to jogging, the HR response for any jogging speed will decrease and jogging speed will have to be increased to stay in the THR zone. This is the primary marker that a training effect is taking place. Box 16.2 presents a jogging program with some simple rules to follow. Special attention is made to completing the walking program first, staying in the THR zone, and not progressing to the next level if not comfortable with the

Box 16.2 Jogging Program

Rules:

1. Complete the Walking Program before starting this program.
2. Begin each session with stretching and walking.
3. Be aware of new aches and pains.
4. Don't progress to next level if not comfortable.
5. Stay at low end of THR zone; record heart rate for each session.
6. Do program on a work-a-day, rest-a-day basis.

Level 1   Jog 10 steps, walk 10 steps. Repeat five times and take your heart rate. Stay within THR zone by increasing or decreasing walking phase. Do 20–30 minutes of activity.

Level 2   Jog 20 steps, walk 10 steps. Repeat five times and take your heart rate. Stay within THR zone by increasing or decreasing walking phase. Do 20–30 minutes of activity.

Level 3   Jog 30 steps, walk 10 steps. Repeat five times and take your heart rate. Stay within THR zone by increasing or decreasing walking phase. Do 20–30 minutes of activity.

Level 4   Jog 1 minute, walk 10 steps. Repeat three times and take your heart rate. Stay within THR zone by increasing or decreasing walking phase. Do 20–30 minutes of activity.

Level 5   Jog 2 minutes, walk 10 steps. Repeat two times and take your heart rate. Stay within THR zone by increasing or decreasing walking phase. Do 30 minutes of activity.

Level 6   Jog 1 lap (400 meters, or 440 yards) and check heart rate. Adjust pace during run to stay within the THR zone. If heart rate is still too high, go back to the Level 5 schedule. Do 6 laps with a brief walk between each.

Level 7   Jog 2 laps and check heart rate. Adjust pace during run to stay within the THR zone. If heart rate is still too high, go back to Level 6 activity. Do 6 laps with a brief walk between each.

Level 8   Jog 1 mile and check heart rate. Adjust pace during the run to stay within THR zone. Do 2 miles.

Level 9   Jog 2–3 miles continuously. Check heart rate at the end to ensure that you were within THR zone.

From E. T. Howley and B. D. Franks, *Health/Fitness Instructor's Handbook*. Copyright © 1986 Human Kinetics Publishers, Champaign, Ill.

current level. It should again be noted that jogging is not for everyone, and for those who are obese, or have ankle, knee, or hip problems, it might be a good activity to avoid. Two activities that reduce such stress are cycling (stationary or outdoor) and swimming (21). More on exercise for special populations in the next chapter.

Games, Sports, and Exercise to Music

As a person becomes accustomed to exercising at the THR range while jogging, or swimming, or cycling, more uncontrolled activities can be introduced that require higher levels of energy expenditure, but do so in a more intermittent fashion. Games (paddleball, racquetball, squash), sports (basketball, soccer), and various forms of exercise to music can keep a person's interest and make it more likely that the person will maintain a physically active life. These activities should be built on a walk-and-jogging base to reduce the chance that the participant will make poor adjustments to the activity. In addition, by having the habit of walking or jogging (swimming or cycling), when there is no one to play with or lead the class, the participant will still be able to maintain his or her habit of physical activity. In contrast to jogging, cycling, or swimming, it will be more difficult to stay in the THR range with these intermittent activities. It is more likely that the HR will move from below the threshold value to above the top end of the THR from time to time. This is to be expected, and is a normal response to activities that are intermittent in nature. It must be stressed, however, that when playing games it is important that the participants have some degree of skill and be reasonably well matched. If one is much better than the other, neither will have a good workout (24).

Environmental Concerns

It is important that the participant be educated about the effects of extreme heat and humidity, altitude, and cold on the adaptation to exercise. The THR range acts as a guide in that it provides feedback to the participant about the interaction of the environment and the exercise intensity. As the heat and humidity increase there is an increased need to circulate additional blood to the skin to dissipate the heat. As altitude increases there is less oxygen bound to hemoglobin and the person must pump more blood to the muscles to have the same oxygen delivery. In both of these situations the HR response to a fixed work bout will be higher. To counter that tendency and stay in the THR range, the subject should decrease the work rate. Exercise in most cold environments can be refreshing and safe if a person plans in advance and dresses accordingly. However, there are some temperature/wind combinations that should be avoided because of the inability to adapt to them. As mentioned previously, some people simply plan exercise indoors (shopping malls, health spas, home exercise) during those occasions so that their routine is not interrupted. These environmental factors will be considered in more detail in chapter 24.

Summary

1. Physical inactivity has been classified by some as a primary risk factor for coronary heart disease, and can reduce the overall risk of those who smoke or who are hypertensive.

2. In previously sedentary subjects small changes in physical activity result in large health benefits with only minimal risk.

3. Strenuous exercise increases the risk of a heart attack during the activity, but reduces the overall (rest and exercise) risk of such an event.

4. Several of the 1990 health promotion/disease prevention objectives relate to an increase in physical activity across the whole population; unfortunately, we have made little progress in achieving those objectives.

5. *Physical activity* results in energy expenditure proportional to muscular work, and *exercise* is a subset of physical activity where specific fitness goals have been identified.

6. Regular physical activity can increase $\dot{V}O_2$ max and decrease risk factors, but the first probably does not cause the second, which may be related more to a better lipid profile or an increased ability to dissolve blood clots.

7. A sedentary person needs to go through a health status screening prior to participating in exercise.

8. Exercise programs for previously sedentary persons should start with low-intensity activities (walking), and the person should not progress until he or she can walk about 4 miles comfortably.

9. The optimal characteristics of an exercise program are: intensity = 60%–80% $\dot{V}O_2$ max, frequency = three to four times per week; duration = minutes needed to expend about 200–300 kcal.

10. The THR range, taken as 60%–80% HRR, or 70%–85% of maximal HR, is a reasonable estimate of the proper exercise intensity.

11. The intensity threshold for a training effect is low ($\leq$ 50% $\dot{V}O_2$ max) for the deconditioned, and high ($\geq$ 80% $\dot{V}O_2$ max) for the very fit.

12. The THR acts as a guide to adjust exercise intensity in adverse environments such as high temperature and humidity, or altitude.

Study Questions

1. Is physical inactivity a primary or secondary risk factor for coronary heart disease? Explain.
2. From a public health standpoint, why is there so much attention paid to simply increasing a sedentary person's physical activity by a small amount rather than recommending strenuous exercise?
3. What is the risk of cardiac arrest for someone who participates in a regular physical activity program?
4. What is the difference between "exercise" and "physical activity"?
5. List the optimal frequency, intensity, and duration of exercise needed to achieve an increase in cardiorespiratory function.
6. For a person with a maximal heart rate of 180 beats · min^{-1} and a resting heart rate of 70 beats · min^{-1}, calculate a target heart rate range by the Karvonen method and the percent of maximal HR method.
7. Recommend an appropriate progression of activities for a sedentary person wishing to become fit.
8. Why is it important to monitor heart rate frequently during exercise in heat, humidity, and at altitude?

Suggested Reading

Howley, E. T., and B. Don Franks. 1986. *Health/Fitness Instructor's Handbook*. Champaign, Ill.: Human Kinetics Publishers.

References

1. American College of Sports Medicine. 1978. Position statement on the recommended quantity and quality of exercise for developing and maintaining fitness in healthy adults. *Medicine and Science in Sports and Exercise* 10:vii–x.
2. ———. 1986. *Guidelines for Exercise Training and Prescription*. Philadelphia: Lea & Febiger.
3. Badenhop, D. T. et al. 1983. Physiologic adjustments to higher- or lower-intensity exercise in elders. *Medicine and Science in Sports and Exercise* 15:496–502.
4. Birk, T. J., and C. A. Birk. 1987. Use of ratings of perceived exertion for exercise prescription. *Sports Medicine* 4:1–8.
5. Blair, S. N., D. R. Jacobs, and K. E. Powell. 1985. Relationships between exercise or physical activity and other health behaviors. *Public Health Reports* 100:172–80.
6. Caspersen, C. J., K. E. Powell, and G. M. Christenson. 1985. Physical activity, exercise, and physical fitness: Definitions and distinctions for health-related research. *Public Health Reports* 100:126–31.
7. Cavanagh, P. R. 1980. *The Running Shoe Book*. Mountain View, Calif.: Anderson World, Inc.
8. Chow, R. J., and J. H. Wilmore. 1984. The regulation of exercise intensity by ratings of perceived exertion. *Journal of Cardiac Rehabilitation* 4:382–87.
9. Couldry, W., C. B. Corbin, and A. Wilcox. 1982. Carotid vs. radial pulse counts. *The Physician and Sportsmedicine* 10:67–72.
10. Dehn, M. M., and C. B. Mullins. 1977. Physiologic effects and importance of exercise in patients with coronary artery disease. *Cardiovascular Medicine* 2:365.
11. Department of Health and Human Services. 1980. *Promoting health/preventing disease: Objectives for the nation*. Washington, D.C.: U.S. Government Printing Office.
12. ———. 1986. *The 1990 Health Objectives for the Nation: A Midcourse Review*. Washington, D.C.: U.S. Government Printing Office.

13. Dishman, R. K., J. F. Sallis, and D. R. Orenstein. 1985. The determinants of physical activity and exercise. *Public Health Reports* 100:158–71.

14. Gutmann, M. C. et al. 1981. Perceived exertion-heart rate relationship during exercise testing and training in cardiac patients. *Journal of Cardiac Rehabilitation* 1:52–59.

15. Hage, P. 1981. Perceived exertion: One measure of exercise intensity. *The Physician and Sportsmedicine* 9(9):136–43.

16. Haskell, W. L., H. J. Montoye, and D. Orenstein. 1985. Physical activity and exercise to achieve health-related physical fitness components. *Public Health Reports* 100:202–12.

17. Health Benefits of Exercise (Part 1 of 2). 1987. A round table. *The Physician and Sportsmedicine* 15(10):114–32.

18. Hellerstein, H. K., and R. Ader. 1971. Relationship between percent maximal oxygen uptake (% max $\dot{V}O_2$) and percent maximal heart rate (% MHR) in normals and cardiacs (ASHD). *Circulation* 43–44 (Suppl. II):76.

19. Hellerstein, H. K. et al. 1973. "Principles of Exercise Prescription for Normals and Cardiac Subjects." In (J. P. Naughton and H. K. Hellerstein, eds.) *Exercise Training in Coronary Heart Disease,* 129–67. New York: Academic Press.

20. Hellerstein, H. K., and B. A. Franklin. 1984. "Exercise Testing and Prescription." In (N. K. Wenger and H. K. Hellerstein, eds.) *Rehabilitation of the Coronary Patient,* 2nd ed., 197–284. New York: John Wiley and Sons.

21. Howley, E. T., and B. D. Franks. 1986. *Health/Fitness Instructor's Handbook.* Champaign, Ill: Human Kinetics Publishers.

22. Karvonen, M. J., E. Kentala, and O. Mustala. 1957. The effects of training heart rate: A longitudinal study. *Annals of Medicine Exp. Biol. Fenn* 35: 307–15.

23. Kopan, J. P., D. S. Siscovick, and G. M. Goldbaum. 1985. The risk of exercise: A public health view of injuries and hazards. *Public Health Report* 100: 189–95.

24. Morgans, L. F. et al. 1987. Heart rate responses during singles and doubles tennis competition. *The Physician and Sportsmedicine* 15(7):67–74.

25. Paffenbarger, R. S., and W. E. Hale. 1975. Work activity and coronary heart mortality. *New England Journal of Medicine* 292(March 13):545–50.

26. Paffenbarger, R. S., and R. T. Hyde. 1980. Exercise as protection against heart attack. *New England Journal of Medicine* 302:1026–27.

27. Paffenbarger, R. S., R. T. Hyde, and A. L. Wing. 1986. Physical activity, all cause mortality, and longevity of college alumni. *New England Journal of Medicine* 314(March 6):605–13.

28. ———. 1986. Physical activity and longevity of college alumni (letter). *New England Journal of Medicine* 315(August 7):399–401.

29. Pollock, M. L. et al. 1972. Effect of training two days per week at different intensities on middle-aged men. *Medicine and Science in Sports* 4:192–97.

30. Pollock, M. L. et al. 1975. Effects of mode of training on cardiovascular functions and body composition of adult men. *Medicine and Science in Sports and Exercise* 7:139–45.

31. Pollock, M. L. et al. 1977. Effects of frequency and duration of training on attrition and incidence of injury. *Medicine of Science in Sports* 9:31–36.

32. Pollock, M. L. 1978. How much exercise is enough? *The Physician and Sportsmedicine* 6:50–64.

33. Pollock, M. L., J. H. Wilmore, and S. M. Fox. 1984. *Exercise in Health and Disease.* Philadelphia: W. B. Saunders Company.

34. Powell, K. E., and R. S. Paffenbarger. 1985. Workshop on epidemiologic and public health aspects of physical activity and exercise: A summary. *Public Health Reports* 100:118–26.

35. Powell, K. E., P. D. Thompson, and C. J. Caspersen. 1987. Physical activity and the incidence of coronary heart disease. *Annals Review of Public Health* 8:253–87.

36. Siscovick, D. S. et al. 1984. The incidence of primary cardiac arrest during vigorous exercise. *New England Journal of Medicine* 311:874–77.

37. Siscovick, D. S. et al. 1984. Habitual vigorous exercise and primary cardiac arrest: Effect of other risk factors on the relationship. *Journal of Chronic Disease* 37:625–31.

38. Siscovick, D. S., R. E. LaPorte, and J. M. Newman. 1985. The disease-specific benefits and risks of physical activity and exercise. *Public Health Report* 100:180–88.

39. Smith, E. L., and C. Gilligan. 1983. Physical activity prescription for the older adult. *The Physician and Sportsmedicine* 11(8):91–101.

40. Stephens, T., D. R., Jacobs, and C. C. White. 1985. A descriptive epidemiology of leisure-time physical activity. *Public Health Reports* 100:147–58.

41. Taylor, C. B., J. F. Sallis, and R. Needle. 1985. The relation of physical activity and exercise to mental health. *Public Health Reports* 100:195–202.

42. Wenger, H. A., and G. J. Bell. 1984. The interactions of intensity, frequency and duration of exercise training in altering cardiorespiratory fitness. *Sports Medicine* 3:346–56.

17 Exercise for Special Populations

Objectives

*B*y studying this chapter, you should be able to do the following:

1. Describe the difference between Type I and Type II diabetes.
2. Describe the difference in how a "controlled" diabetic responds to exercise, as compared to one who is not in control.
3. Explain why exercise may complicate the life of a Type I diabetic, while being a recommended and primary part of a Type II diabetic's life-style.
4. Describe the changes in diet and insulin that might be made prior to a diabetic undertaking an exercise program.
5. Describe the sequence of events leading to an asthma attack, and how cromolyn sodium and β-adrenergic agonists act to prevent and/or relieve an attack.
6. Describe the cause of exercise-induced asthma, and how one may deal with this problem.
7. Contrast chronic obstructive pulmonary disease (COPD) with asthma in terms of causes, prognosis, and the role of rehabilitation programs in a return to "normal" function.
8. Identify the types of patient populations that one might see in a cardiac rehabilitation program, and the types of medications that these individuals may be taking.
9. Contrast the type of exercise test used for cardiac populations with the test used for the apparently healthy population.
10. Discuss the role of physical activity as a necessary part of an older individual's life-style; include comments on cardiorespiratory function and osteoporosis.
11. Compare the types of exercise programs that might be used for the three different classifications of the elderly.
12. Describe the guidelines for exercise programs for pregnant women.

Outline

Key Terms

arrhythmia
beta receptor agonist
coronary artery bypass graft surgery
  (CABGS)
cromolyn sodium
diabetic coma
immunotherapy
insulin shock

ketosis
mast cell
myocardial infarction
nitroglycerin
percutaneous transluminal coronary
  angioplasty
theophylline

Chapter 16 presented some recommendations for planning an appropriate exercise program for the apparently healthy individual. This chapter will extend that discussion with an examination of the special concerns that must be addressed when exercise is used for populations with specific diseases, disabilities, or limitations. However, the student of exercise science should recognize that this information is introductory in nature, and more detailed accounts are cited throughout the chapter.

Diabetes

Diabetes is a major health problem in the United States with more than 12 million having the disease and is the third largest cause of death by disease. Diabetes injures and kills indirectly by causing blindness, kidney disease, heart disease, stroke, and peripheral vascular disease leading to the amputation of the leg and foot (2). Diabetics are divided into two distinct groups on the basis of whether or not the diabetes is caused by lack of insulin (Type I), or a resistance to insulin (Type II). Type I, insulin-dependent diabetes develops primarily in young persons, and is associated with viral (flulike) infections. The warning signs, which develop quickly, consist of:

- frequent urination/unusual thirst
- extreme hunger
- rapid weight loss, weakness and fatigue
- irritability, nausea, and vomiting (2)

Since Type I diabetics do not produce adequate insulin they are dependent on exogenous (injected) insulin to maintain the blood glucose concentration within normal limits. Type II, noninsulin-dependent diabetes develops more slowly and later in life than does Type I diabetes. Type II diabetes represents about 90% of all diabetics (4), and is primarily linked to obesity. The increased mass of fat tissue results in a resistance to insulin, which is usually available in adequate amounts within the body. However, some Type II diabetics may require injectable insulin or an oral medication that stimulates the pancreas to produce additional insulin. The primary treatment of Type II diabetics includes diet and exercise to (1) reduce the body weight, and (2) help control the plasma glucose. Table 17.1 summarizes the differences between Type I and Type II diabetics (4, 8).

Exercise and the Diabetic

In chapter 5 we indicated that exercise increases the rate at which glucose leaves the blood, and in this way exercise has been viewed as a useful part of the treatment to maintain blood glucose control. However, this beneficial effect of exercise is dependent on whether or not the diabetic is in reasonable "control" before exercise begins. "Control" means that the blood glucose concentration is close to normal. Figure 17.1 shows the effect of a prolonged exercise bout on diabetics who were in "control" versus those who had not taken an adequate amount of insulin. A lack of insulin causes **ketosis,** a metabolic acidosis resulting from the accumulation of too many ketone bodies (short-chain fatty acids). The Type I diabetic who was in control shows a decrease in plasma glucose toward normal values during exercise, suggesting better control. On the other hand, those Type I diabetics who did not inject an adequate amount of insulin before exercise show an increase in plasma glucose (5). Why the difference in

Table 17.1 Summary of the differences between Type I and Type II diabetes

Characteristics	Type I Insulin-Dependent	Type II Noninsulin-Dependent
Another name	Juvenile-onset	Adult-onset
Proportion of all diabetics	~10%	~90%
Age at onset	<20	>40
Development of disease	Rapid	Slow
Family history	Uncommon	Common
Insulin required	Always	Common, but not always
Pancreatic insulin	None, or very little	Normal or higher
Ketoacidosis	Common	Rare
Body fatness	Normal/lean	Generally obese

From Berg (4) and Cantu (8).

response? The "controlled" diabetic has sufficient insulin such that glucose can be taken up into muscle during exercise, and counter the "normal" increase in glucose release from the liver due to the action of catecholamines and glucagon (see chapter 5). In contrast, the diabetic with inadequate insulin experiences only a small increase in glucose utilization by muscle, but has the "normal" increase in glucose release from the liver. This, of course, causes an elevation of the plasma glucose, resulting in a hyperglycemia.

Figure 17.2 summarizes these effects and adds one more (36). If an insulin-dependent diabetic starts exercise with too much insulin, the rate at which plasma glucose is used by muscle is accelerated, while glucose release from the liver is decreased. This causes a very dangerous hypoglycemic response. This information is crucial to understanding the use of exercise as part of a program to help diabetics control the blood glucose concentration. Further, it is the Type I diabetics who are primarily confronted with this problem, since the Type II noninsulin-dependent diabetics usually start with normal or slightly higher insulin levels (36). We will discuss each type of diabetes separately.

Type I Diabetes

For many years exercise was one part of the treatment for Type I diabetes, with insulin and diet being the other two (22). However, due to the information presented earlier, it is clear that if a diabetic is not in control prior to exercise, the ability to maintain a reasonable plasma glucose concentration may be compromised. The greatest concern is not the hyperglycemia and ketosis that can lead to **diabetic coma** when too little insulin is present; rather it is the possibility of hypoglycemia, which can lead to **insulin shock.** Richter and Galbo (36) and Kemmer and Berger (22) point out the difficulties a Type I diabetic has starting an exercise program: the person must maintain a regular exercise schedule in terms of intensity, frequency, and duration, as well as altering the diet and insulin. Such regimentation is difficult for some to follow, and given the variability in how a diabetic's blood glucose might respond to exercise on a day to day basis, the use of exercise as a primary tool in maintaining metabolic control has been diminished. Because metabolic control can be maintained by altering insulin and diet based on self-monitored blood glucose, exercise complicates this picture (22, 36). However, considering the

Figure 17.1 Effect of prolonged exercise on blood glucose and ketone body levels in normal subjects, diabetics in "control," and diabetics taking an inadequate amount of insulin (ketosis).

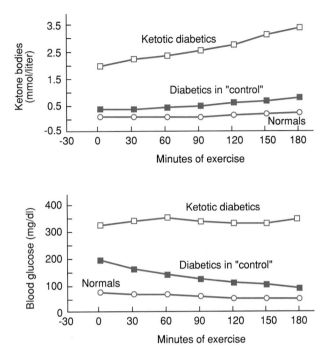

Figure 17.2 Effect of varied plasma insulin levels in Type I diabetics on glucose homeostasis during exercise.

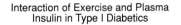

Interaction of Exercise and Plasma
Insulin in Type I Diabetics

Plasma insulin concentration	Liver glucose release	Glucose uptake by muscle	Blood glucose concentration
Normal or slightly decreased	⬆	⬆	→
Markedly decreased	⬆	↑	↑
Increased	↑	⬆	↓

importance of physical activity in an individual's life, a Type I diabetic should not be discouraged from participation in regular exercise—if they have no complications (22, 36).

The Type I diabetic should have a careful medical exam prior to starting an exercise program, and if over the age of thirty or has had diabetes for ten years or more, a graded diagnostic exercise test is recommended. This recommendation is based on the observation that strenuous exercise may accelerate or worsen retina, kidney, or peripheral nerve damage that is already present. The concern for the retina is related to the higher blood pressures developed during exercise, while the concern for the kidney is related to the decrease in blood flow to that organ with increasing intensities of exercise. The peripheral nerve damage may block signals coming from the foot such that serious damage may occur before it is perceived. Proper shoes for exercise, as well as the choice of the activity, are important (13).

The primary concern for the Type I diabetic starting an exercise program is adequate control of blood glucose, which should already exist. Once control exists, the increase in glucose uptake by the muscle must be balanced by an increase in carbohydrate intake and/or a decrease in the injected insulin. The decision is based on regular and frequent self-monitoring of the blood glucose concentration. Some basic guidelines to prevent hypoglycemia follow (13).

- For leisurely walk, no need to increase carbohydrate intake if blood glucose >100 mg · dl^{-1} (5.6 mM).
- For moderate activity with blood glucose of 100–180 mg · dl^{-1} (5.6–10 mM), 10–15 gm of carbohydrate is taken before exercise. If blood glucose is >180 (10 mM) and <300 mg · dl^{-1} (16.6 mM), no additional carbohydrate is needed. If >300 mg · dl^{-1}, exercise is not recommended until blood glucose is better controlled.
- For strenuous exercise of 1–2 hours with blood glucose in the normal range, consumption of 25–50 gm of carbohydrate is recommended before exercise.

- For prolonged exercise, including day-long hikes, insulin intake is decreased even though carbohydrate intake is increased. The decrease can be from 20%–75% of the normal dose (4).
- Additional carbohydrate should be consumed during recovery from exercise. Interestingly, hypoglycemia might occur following exercise if this is not done since dietary carbohydrate is also being used to replace the depleted muscle glycogen store.

In addition to these guidelines the diabetic should be reminded to increase fluid intake, carry a readily available form of carbohydrate and adequate identification, and exercise with someone who can help in an emergency.

Type II Diabetes

In contrast to the insulin-dependent diabetic whose life may be more complicated (in terms of blood glucose control) at the start of an exercise program, exercise is a primary recommendation for the Type II diabetic to help deal with both the obesity that is usually present, as well as to help control blood glucose. The combination of exercise and diet may be sufficient and thus, eliminate the need for insulin or an oral medication to stimulate insulin secretion (8). Because Type II diabetics represents about 90% of the whole population of diabetics, and that it occurs later in life (after 40 years of age), it is not uncommon to see such individuals in adult fitness programs. It is important for clear communication to exist between the participant and the exercise leader, in order to reduce the chance of a "surprise" hypoglycemic response.

Noninsulin-dependent diabetics do not experience the same fluctuations in blood glucose during exercise as do the Type I diabetics (13); however, those taking oral medication to stimulate insulin secretion may have to decrease their dosage to maintain a normal blood glucose concentration (36). Consistent with the recommendations for the Type I diabetic, clear identification and a readily available source of carbohydrate should be carried along. In addition, it would be much safer for a diabetic to exercise with a "buddy" who could help out if a problem developed.

As with all exercise programs for deconditioned individuals it is much more important to do too little than too much at the start of a program. By starting with light activity and gradually increasing the duration, exercise can be done each day. This will provide an opportunity to learn how to maintain adequate control of blood glucose while minimizing the chance of a hypoglycemic response. In addition, a "habit" of exercise will develop that is crucial if one is to realize the benefits. As the Type II diabetic adapts to light exercise, the option exists for more strenuous activity. The Type II diabetic secures a variety of benefits from participation in exercise: lower body fat and weight (see chapter 18), increased HDL cholesterol, increased sensitivity to insulin (decreasing the need), improved capacity for work, and an improved self-concept (4). These physiological changes should not only improve the prognosis of the Type II diabetic as far as control of blood glucose is concerned, they will reduce the overall risk associated with coronary heart disease (36).

Asthma

Asthma is a respiratory problem characterized by a shortness of breath accompanied by a wheezing sound. It is due to a constriction of the smooth muscle around the airways, a swelling of the mucosal cells, and a hypersecretion of mucous. The asthma can be caused by an allergic reaction, exercise, aspirin, dust, pollutants, and emotion, and can be divided into the following categories (30):

Extrinsic Asthma—allergen induced, mediated by an immune system reaction
Intrinsic Asthma—no allergic cause found
Aspirin-induced Asthma—10% of all asthmatics
Mixed Asthma—caused by more than one factor

Causes

An asthma attack is the result of an orderly sequence of events that can be initiated by a wide variety of factors. These events are important if we are to understand how certain medications prevent or relieve the asthmatic attack. Figure 17.3 summarizes these events. The focus of attention is on the **mast cell,** one of the cells that is part of tissue in the bronchial tubes. It is believed that a variety of factors such as dust, chemicals, antibodies, and exercise initiate the asthma attack by increasing Ca^{++} influx into the mast cell, causing a release of chemical mediators such as histimine, and a special chemical that attracts white blood cells. The mediators, in turn, (1) increase smooth muscle contraction (via an elevation of Ca^{++} in the muscle cell) leading to bronchoconstriction, (2) initiate a bronchoconstrictor reflex via the vagus nerve, and (3) cause an inflammation response (swelling of tissue). Given that the vast majority of people do not experience an asthmatic attack while being exposed to the above factors, a "sensitivity" or hyperirritability of the respiratory tract is a necessary prerequisite (30).

Prevention/Relief of Asthma

There are a variety of steps that can be taken to prevent the occurrence of an asthmatic attack, and provide relief should one occur. If a person is sensitive (allergic) to something then simple avoidance of the allergen will prevent the problem. If a person cannot avoid contact with the allergen, **immunotherapy** may be helpful in that the person becomes less sensitive to the allergen while being treated.

Drugs have been developed to deal with the mast cell, which is a focal point in the asthmatic response, as well as the bronchiolar smooth muscle that causes the decrease in airway diameter. **Cromolyn sodium** inhibits the chemical mediator release from the mast cell, probably by interfering with Ca^{++} influx into the cell. **Beta receptor agonists** (β_2-agonist) decrease chemical mediator release as well as cause a relaxation of bronchiolar smooth muscle by decreasing the Ca^{++} concentration in mast and smooth muscle cells. This effect is brought about through increased adenyl cyclase activity leading to an elevation of cytoplasmic cyclic AMP (see chapter 5). Finally, **theophylline,** a caffeine-like drug, aids in bronchiolar smooth muscle relaxation by inhibiting phosphodiesterase, the enzyme that inactivates cyclic AMP. The result is a higher cyclic AMP and lower Ca^{++} concentration in the cell. The effects of these drugs are summarized in figure 17.4. The net result is that both the inflammation response and the constriction of the bronchiolar smooth muscle are blocked.

Figure 17.3 Proposed mechanism by which an asthma attack is initiated.

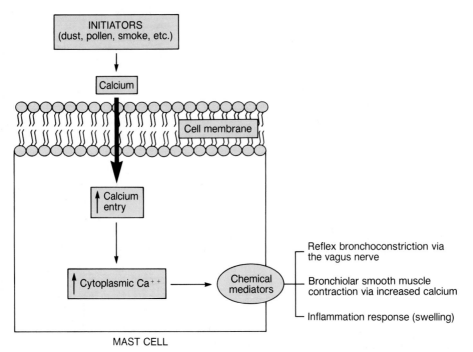

Figure 17.4 Mechanisms by which beta agonists, cromolyn sodium, and theophylline block the events that initiate or maintain an asthma attack.

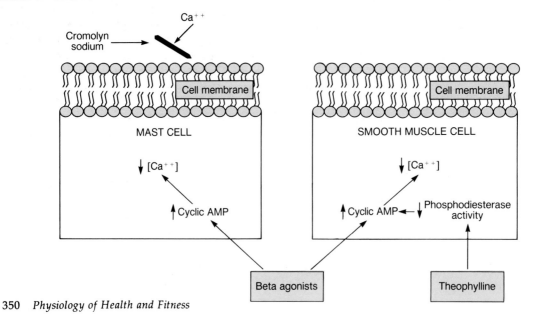

Exercise-Induced Asthma

A form of asthma that may be of particular interest to the reader is exercise-induced asthma (EIA). The asthmatic attack is caused by exercise and can occur five to fifteen minutes (Early Phase) or four to six hours (Late Phase) after exercise. Approximately 80% of asthmatics experience EIA, versus only 3%–4% of the nonallergic population (45). What is surprising is that sixty-seven members (11%) of the 1984 U.S. Olympic team had EIA and 41 of them (61%) won an Olympic medal (20, 45). Clearly, if anyone wondered whether or not EIA can be controlled, those results should dispell any doubts.

Numerous causes of EIA have been identified over the past 100 years. These included cold air, hypocapnia (low PCO_2), respiratory alkalosis, and specific intensities and durations of exercise. The focus of attention is now on the *cooling and drying* of the respiratory tract that occurs when large volumes of dry air are breathed during the exercise session (11, 38). Respiratory heat loss is related primarily to the rate of ventilation, with the humidity and the temperature of the inspired air being of secondary and tertiary importance. As you remember from chapter 10, when dry air is taken into the lungs it is moistened and warmed as it moves through the respiratory airways. In this way moisture is evaporated from the surface of the airways which is therefore cooled.

The proposed mechanism for how EIA is initiated takes us back to the mast cell mentioned earlier. When dry air removes water from the surface of the mast cell, an increase in osmolarity occurs. This increase in osmolarity triggers the influx of Ca^{++} that leads to the increased release of chemical mediators and the narrowing of the airways (11, 21, 38). This hypothesis has received strong support from data showing the EIA can be prevented when warm humidified air is breathed. What kind of circumstances bring on EIA?

The probability of an exercise-induced bronchospasm is related to the type of exercise, the time since the previous bout of exercise, the interval since medication was taken, and the temperature and humidity of the inspired air (38). It has been known since the late 1600s that certain types of exercise cause an attack more readily than others. Running was observed to cause more attacks than cycling or walking which, in turn, caused more than swimming. Interestingly, this old observation still finds support in studies where the temperature and the humidity of the inspired air is controlled. Running still caused more severe attacks than did swimming, even with O_2 consumption and V_E matched (38).

Generally, EIA is precipitated more with strenuous, long-duration exercise than the reverse (21, 38). One way to deal with this is to do short-duration exercise (<5 min) at low to moderate intensities. Further, when an exercise session occurs within sixty minutes of a previous EIA attack, the degree of bronchospasm is reduced (11). This suggests that a warm-up within an hour of more strenuous exercise would reduce the severity of an attack.

There was special concern for the athletes of the 1984 Olympic Games, given the high pollution index in Los Angeles, which can aggravate an EIA attack (33). As mentioned before, the fact that 61% of the athletes who experience EIA won Olympic medals suggests that procedures for preventing EIA with medication are pretty well worked out. Voy (45) reports that a simple questionnaire identified 90% of the athletes with EIA, even though only 52% were receiving treatment prior to the Olympics. The medications mentioned earlier were used to manage the condition to allow the athletes to go "all out."

For some of the athletes in which cromolyn sodium did not work, the β_2-agonists were used successfully. Pierson et al. (33) divides the pharmacological management of EIA into two categories: athletes with normal airway function, and those with abnormal function. A summary of these procedures follows:

Normal airway function

1. Use of β_2-agonists or Cromolyn sodium—ten minutes before competition
2. Rapid release theophylline—given at 5 mg $\cdot$ kg^{-1} one hour before exercise

Abnormal airway function

1. Sustained release theophylline—given at 12–20 mg $\cdot$ kg^{-1} $\cdot$ d^{-1}
2. Use of either β_2-agonist or cromolyn sodium—ten minutes before competition

The asthmatic who is simply participating in a fitness program should also follow a medication plan to *prevent* the occurrence of an EIA attack. The exercise session should include the conventional warm-up, with mild to moderate activity planned in five minute segments. Swimming is better than other types of exercise, given that air above the water tends to be warmer and contains more moisture. A scarf or face mask can be used when exercising outdoors in cold weather to help trap moisture. The participant should carry an inhaler with a β_2-agonist and use it at the first sign of wheezing (15). As with the diabetic, the buddy system is a good plan to follow in case a major attack occurs.

Chronic Obstructive Pulmonary Disease

Chronic obstructive pulmonary diseases (COPD) cause a reduction in airflow that can have a dramatic effect on daily activities. These diseases include chronic bronchitis, emphysema, and bronchial asthma, either alone or in combination. While asthma is a reversible problem, chronic bronchitis and emphysema are not. Chronic bronchitis is characterized by a persistent production of sputum due primarily to a thickened bronchial wall with excess secretions. In emphysema the elastic recoil of alveoli and bronchioles is reduced and those pulmonary structures are enlarged (6, 37). COPD is considerably different from the controlled asthmatic condition mentioned above. The patient with developing COPD perceives an inability to do normal activities without experiencing dyspnea, but, tragically, by the time this occurs the disease is already well advanced (6). COPD is characterized by a decreased ability to exhale and because of the narrowed airways, a "wheezing" sound is made. The person with COPD experiences a decreased capacity for work, which may influence employment, but he/she may also experience an increase in psychological problems, including anxiety (regarding the simple act of breathing) and depression (related to a loss of sense of self-worth).

It should be no surprise then that treatment of COPD includes more than simple medication and O_2 inhalation therapy. A typical COPD rehabilitation program focuses on the goal of the patient's ability for self-care, and to achieve that goal professionals are recruited to deal with the various manifestations of the disease process (31, 42). Figure 17.5 shows the number of medical and support personnel involved. The COPD patient receives education about the different ways to deal with the disease including breathing exercises, ways to approach the activities of daily living at home, and how to handle work-related problems. The latter can be so affected that new on-the-job responsibilities may have to be assigned, or if the person cannot meet the requirements, retirement may be the only outcome. In order to help deal with these problems counseling by psychologists and clergy may be needed for patient and family. The extent of these problems is directly related to the severity of the disease. Those with minimal disease may require the help of only a few of the professionals listed in figure 17.5, while others with severe disease may require the assistance of all. It is therefore important to understand that the rehabilitation program is very individualized (31, 42).

The exercise component of the rehabilitation program can follow the generally accepted exercise guidelines including the use of a target heart rate, the degree of dyspnea experienced, or can simply focus on an exercise goal of twenty to thirty minutes of light, continuous activity. Those who can proceed with the more traditional exercise rehabilitation program (THR, etc.) have relatively high maximal power outputs on an initial exercise test (6). For those at the low end of the scale, the exercise program advances on the basis of the patient's ability to do an additional five minutes of light exercise. End goals are very pragmatic: ability to do home or work activities, ability to climb two flights of stairs, etc. (6, 31). Generally, COPD patients achieve an increase in exercise tolerance without dyspnea and an increase in the sense of well-being, but without a reversal of the disease process (31, 37). The changes in the psychological variables are very important in the long run, given that the person's willingness to continue the exercise program is a major factor that will dictate the rate of decline during the course of the disease.

Figure 17.5 Model for rehabilitation of the patient with chronic obstructive pulmonary disease (COPD).

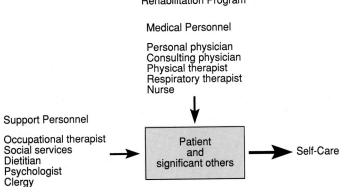

Cardiac Rehabilitation

Exercise training is now an accepted part of the therapy used to restore an individual who has some form of coronary heart disease (CHD). The details of how to structure such programs, from the first steps taken after being confined to a bed to the time of returning to work and beyond, are spelled out clearly in books such as *Exercise in Health and Disease* by Pollock, Wilmore, and Fox (34) and *Rehabilitation of the Coronary Patient* by Wenger and Hellerstein (49). This brief section will simply comment on various aspects of such programs.

Population

The persons served by cardiac rehabilitation programs include those who have experienced angina pectoris, myocardial infarctions (MI), coronary artery bypass graft surgery (CABGS), and angioplasty (12). Angina pectoris is the chest pain related to ischemia of the ventricle due to occlusion of one or more of the coronary arteries. The symptoms occur when the work of the heart (estimated by the double product: systolic blood pressure × HR) exceeds a certain value. **Nitroglycerin** is used to prevent an attack and/or relieve the pain by relaxing the smooth muscle in veins to reduce

venous return and the work of heart (29). Angina patients may also be treated with a beta blocker like propranolol (Inderal®), to reduce the HR and/or blood pressure such that the angina symptoms occur at a later stage into work. Exercise training supports this drug effect: as the person becomes trained, the HR response at any work rate is reduced. This allows the individual to take on more tasks without experiencing the chest pain.

Myocardial infarction patients have actual heart damage (loss of ventricular muscle) due to a prolonged occlusion of one or more of the coronary arteries. The degree to which left ventricular function is compromised is dependent on the mass of the ventricle permanently damaged. These patients are usually on medications to reduce the work of the heart (β-blocker), and control the irritability of the heart tissue so that dangerous **arrhythmias** (irregular heart rhythms) do not occur. Generally, these patients experience a training effect similar to those who do not have an MI (12).

Coronary artery bypass graft surgery (CABGS) patients have had surgery to bypass one or more blocked coronary arteries. In this procedure, superficial veins are taken from the leg and are used as arteries by sewing them onto existing coronary arteries above and below the blockage. The success of the surgery is dependent on the amount of heart damage that existed prior to surgery, as well as the success of the revascularization itself. In those who had chronic angina pectoris prior to CABGS, most find a relief of symptoms, with 50%–70% having no more pain. Generally, with an increased blood flow to the ventricle there is an improvement in both left ventricular function and the capacity for work (50). These patients benefit from systematic exercise training because most are deconditioned prior to surgery as a result of activity restrictions related to chest pain. The cardiac rehabilitation program also helps the patient differentiate angina pain from chest wall pain related to the surgery. The overall result is a smoother and less traumatic transition back to full function.

Some CHD patients undergo **percutaneous transluminal coronary angioplasty** to open occluded arteries. In this procedure the chest is not opened; instead, a balloon-tipped catheter (a long slender tube) is inserted into the coronary artery where the balloon is inflated to push the plaque back toward the arterial wall. These patients tend not to have as severe disease as those who undergo CABGS (43).

Testing

The testing of patients with CHD is much more involved than that presented for the apparently healthy person in chapter 15. There are classes of CHD patients for whom exercise or exercise testing is inappropriate and dangerous (1). The PAR$_x$ screening form, in appendix D, lists some absolute and relative contraindications for exercise. For those who can be tested, a 12-lead ECG is monitored at discrete intervals during the GXT, while a variety of leads are displayed continuously on an oscilloscope. Blood pressure, RPE, and various signs or symptoms are also noted. The criteria for terminating the GXT goes well beyond achieving a certain percentage of maximal HR, focusing instead on various pathological signs (e.g., ST-segment depression) and symptoms, such as angina pectoris (see chapter 15). On the basis of the response to the GXT the person may be referred for additional testing, such as the use of radioactive molecules to evaluate perfusion ([201] thallium) and the capacity of

the ventricle to eject blood ([99] technetium), or direct angiography, in which a dye that is opaque to x-rays is injected into the coronary arteries to determine the blockage directly (34).

Exercise Programs

The basic cardiac rehabilitative exercise program resembles the one mentioned earlier for apparently healthy persons in that warm-up with stretching, endurance exercise at a THR, and cool-down activities are included. However, the CHD patients, who are generally very deconditioned ($\dot{V}O_2$ max of ~ 20 ml $\cdot$ kg^{-1} $\cdot$ min^{-1}), require only light exercise to achieve their THR. In addition, because these patients are on a wide variety of medications that may decrease maximal heart rate, the THR zone is determined from their GXT results; the 220 − age formula cannot be used. The patients usually begin with intermittent low intensity exercise (one minute on, one minute off) and in time increase the duration of the work period. Given that CABGS and post-MI patients have had direct damage to their hearts, the exercise should facilitate, not interfere with, the healing process. As you might guess, given the nature of the patient and the risk involved, cardiac rehabilitation programs take place in hospitals and clinics where there is direct medical supervision and the capacity to deal with emergencies, should they occur. After a patient completes an eight- to twelve-week "Phase II" program, the person may continue in a "Phase III" program away from the hospital where there is less supervision, save the ability to respond to an emergency (34). What are the benefits of such programs to the patient with CHD?

Effects

There is no question that CHD patients have improved cardiovascular function as a result of an exercise program. This is shown in higher $\dot{V}O_2$ max values, higher work rates achieved without ischemia as shown by angina pectoris or ST-segment changes, and an increased capacity for prolonged submaximal work (34, 49). The improved lipid profile (lower total cholesterol and higher HDL cholesterol) is a function of more than the exercise alone given that weight loss and the saturated fat content of the diet can modify these variables (3, 32). It must be mentioned that a cardiac rehabilitation program should not be viewed simply as an exercise program. It is a multi-intervention effort involving exercise, medication, diet, and counseling.

Elderly

Maximal aerobic power decreases in the average population after the age of twenty at the rate of about 1% per year. As mentioned in chapter 16, this decrease is due to both inactivity and weight gain. Recent reports by Kasch et al. (19) and Wallace (48) show that not only can this decline be interrupted by a physical activity program, but middle-aged men who maintain their activity and body weight show no change in $\dot{V}O_2$ max over a ten to fifteen year period. Unfortunately, the vast majority of people experience the steady decline in $\dot{V}O_2$ max so that by sixty years of age their ability to engage comfortably in normal activities is reduced. This initiates a vicious cycle that leads to lower and lower levels of cardiorespiratory fitness, which may not allow them to perform daily tasks. In turn, this affects the elderly's quality of life and independence which may necessitate reliance of others (40). A physical activity program is useful, not only in dealing with this downward spiral of cardiorespiratory fitness, but with the osteoporosis that is related to the sudden hip fractures that can lead to more inactivity and death (40).

Osteoporosis is a loss of bone mass that primarily affects women over fifty years of age and is responsible for 1.2 million fractures annually. Type I osteoporosis is related to vertebral and distal radius fractures in fifty to sixty-five year olds, and is eight times more common in women than men. Type II osteoporosis, found in those ages seventy and above, results in hip, pelvic, and distal humerus fractures and is twice as common in women (18). The problem is more common in women over age fifty due to menopause and the lack of estrogen. Estrogen treatment, instituted early in menopause, may prevent bone loss. If estrogen is used years after menopause, lost bone cannot be replaced, but existing bone can be maintained (25). Given that prevention is better than treatment, attention is focused on adequate dietary calcium (16) and exercise (40).

Dietary calcium is important in preventing and treating osteoporosis. While the daily calcium requirement is 800 mg · d^{-1}, *most* women do not take in even 600 mg · d^{-1}. The extent of the problem may be even larger than just described, given that the requirements may actually be higher: 1,000 mg · d^{-1} for premenopausal women, and 1,500 mg · d^{-1} for early postmenopausal women (16). Consequently, women must focus attention on taking in an adequate amount of calcium as well as doing exercise to help maintain the integrity of their bones.

Bone structure is maintained by the force of gravity (upright posture), and the lateral forces due to muscle contraction. Weight-bearing activities (walking, jogging) are better than bicycling and swimming for maintaining spine and hip mineral, but for the low fit or those with previous fractures these latter activities are recommended (40). While we may know the exercise prescription needed to achieve cardiorespiratory fitness, such information is lacking relative to osteoporosis. However, two to three hours of exercise a week may reduce or reverse the bone mineral loss with age (40).

In making exercise recommendations for fitness, Smith (39) makes a distinction among the aged populations:

- young old—ages 55–75; $\dot{V}O_2$ max = 6–7 METs
- old old—age >75; $\dot{V}O_2$ max = 2–3 METs
- athletic old—age >55; $\dot{V}O_2$ max = 9–10 METs

The $\dot{V}O_2$ max values provide a focal point for a discussion of a physical activity program. Clearly, for the athletic old, their $\dot{V}O_2$ max allows for a variety of activities that would not be too different from the ordinary younger and more sedentary population. The average young old subject's $\dot{V}O_2$ max of 6–7 METs is similar to that of a cardiac patient, and progression through an exercise program would not be too different, compared to that patient population. However, those in the old old group have extremely low functional capacities, which demand creativity in terms of both exercise testing and prescription.

Stair-stepping provides an interesting substitute to traditional treadmill and cycle ergometer testing of the elderly. Smith and Gilligan's chair step test (40) requires that the person remain seated on a chair and alternate leg lifts such that the heel of the foot is raised 6, 12, or 18 inches and placed momentarily on a step. The recommended cadence used results in work stage increments of only 0.5 METs. While exercise prescription follows the procedures described in chapter 16, an exercise leader needs to implement unique, low intensity, controlled exercise. Exercises focus on the low end of the MET scale, using support (41). The old old individual does these exercises while lying, seated, or holding onto a chair while standing. The exercises include foot, leg, and arm movements that will increase flexibility and muscular endurance, and will expend calories. Given the rapid increase in the number of individuals in this age group, exercise leaders will be required to develop competence with such exercise programs.

In summary, the use of exercise programs for the elderly improves cardiorespiratory fitness and helps to maintain the integrity of bone. When this is coupled with the opportunity for socialization, it is easy to see why exercise is an important part of life from young children to old old "children."

Pregnancy

Pregnancy places special demands on a woman, due to the developing fetus' needs for calories, protein, minerals, vitamins, and of course, the physiologically stable environment needed to process these nutrients. It is against this background that the implementation of a fitness program must be evaluated. In much the same way that a diabetic, asthmatic, or cardiac patient would initiate an exercise program, the pregnant woman should begin with a thorough medical examination by her physician to rule out complications that would make exercise inappropriate, and to provide specific information about signs or symptoms to watch for during the course of the pregnancy. You might ask why there is such concern.

Interestingly, compared to our knowledge of how diabetics, asthmatics, and cardiac patients respond to exercise training, we know little about how the mother and fetus respond to such a program. In fact, according to Lotgering et al. (26, 27), the basic physiology of exercise related to pregnancy is not well

described. These authors provide a summary of information about how pregnancy affects the response of the mother to exercise, and how exercise affects various aspects of pregnancy. A good deal of the information is based on animal studies and the authors suggest caution in extrapolating to humans. In general, moderate exercise does not appear to interfere with oxygen delivery to the fetus, and the heart rate response of the fetus shows no signs of distress. On the basis of their review of human exercise studies, they conclude that among women in excellent condition prior to pregnancy, exercise does not appear to have any negative or positive effects on the fetus (26, 27). In one study in which a supervised exercise program (HR = 65%–70% $\dot{V}O_2$ max, three times/week, twenty-five minutes per session) was implemented twenty-two weeks into pregnancy and continued for thirteen weeks, the women had an 18% increase in $\dot{V}O_2$ max expressed in liters $\cdot$ min^{-1}, which because of the body weight gain equaled an 8% increase expressed in ml $\cdot$ kg^{-1} $\cdot$ min^{-1}. The control subjects showed a 10% decrease in the latter measure over this time period. There was no difference between the groups in regards to the delivery and health of the babies. What are reasonable recommendations to follow when a pregnant woman wishes to exercise?

Given the lack of research in this area, guidelines have been developing over the past decade, with disagreement voiced among specialists in obstetrics and gynecology (7, 14). For example, some believe, on the basis of research and clinical experience, that women should not start a new exercise program after becoming pregnant (7). In addition, due to the lack of research, others feel that it is difficult to support some fixed criteria (e.g., don't exercise over a HR of 140 b $\cdot$ min^{-1}). This statement is countered with the need to provide conservative guidelines that would most likely protect both mother and fetus (14). Table 17.2 lists the guidelines provided by the American College of Obstetricians and Gynecologists. The emphasis is on moderate exercise (HR $\leq$ 140 b $\cdot$ min) of short duration (fifteen minutes), that would not require a Valsalva maneuver. Coupled with short duration exercise, the plan recommends adequate hydration and not exercising in hot/humid weather in order to keep

Table 17.2 *American College of Obstetricians and Gynecologists Guidelines for Exercise During Pregnancy and Postpartum*

1. Regular exercise (at least three times per week) is preferable to intermittent activity. Competitive activities should be discouraged.
2. Vigorous exercise should not be performed in hot, humid weather or during a period of febrile illness.
3. Ballistic movements (jerky, bouncy motions) should be avoided. Exercise should be done on a wooden floor or a tightly carpeted surface to reduce shock and provide a sure footing.
4. Deep flexion or extension of joints should be avoided because of connective tissue laxity. Activities that require jumping, jarring motions, or rapid changes in direction should be avoided because of joint instability.
5. Vigorous exercise should be preceded by a five-minute period of muscle warm-up. This can be accomplished by slow walking or stationary cycling with low resistance.
6. Vigorous exercise should be followed by a period of gradually declining activity that includes gentle stationary stretching. Because connective tissue laxity increases the risk of joint injury, stretches should not be taken to the point of maximum resistance.
7. Heart rate should be measured at times of peak activity. Target heart rates and limits established in consultation with the physician should not be exceeded.
8. Care should be taken to gradually rise from the floor to avoid orthostatic hypotension. Some form of activity involving the legs should be continued for a brief period.
9. Liquids should be taken liberally before and after exercise to prevent dehydration. If necessary, activity should be interrupted to replenish fluids.
10. Women who have led sedentary life-styles should begin with physical activity of very low intensity and advance activity levels very gradually.
11. Activity should be stopped and the physician consulted if any unusual symptoms appear.

Pregnancy only
1. Maternal heart rate should not exceed 140 beats $\cdot$ min^{-1}.
2. Strenuous activities should not exceed 15 minutes in duration.
3. No exercise should be performed in the supine position after the fourth month of gestation is completed.
4. Exercises that employ the Valsalva maneuver should be avoided.
5. Calorie intake should be adequate to meet not only the extra energy needs of pregnancy, but also of the exercise performed.
6. Maternal core temperature should not exceed 38° C.

American College of Obstetricians and Gynecologists: Exercise During Pregnancy and the Postnatal Period (ACOG Home Exercise Programs). Washington, D.C., ACOG, 1985, p. 4. Reprinted by permission.

the body temperature below 38° C. High temperatures have been linked to tetrogenic damage to the fetus, but the effects of heat stress have not been systematically studied. Finally, exercises done in the supine position are not recommended after the fourth month of gestation (27). These are viewed as conservative guidelines and an appropriate place for the pregnant woman to start a discussion with her physician. However, it is recognized that those who were physically active before pregnancy can exercise safely at higher intensities and longer durations (7, 14).

Summary

1. Type I or insulin-dependent diabetes develops early in life and represents 10% of the diabetic population. Type II or insulin-resistant diabetes occurs later in life and is associated with obesity. Most cases of Type II diabetes can be controlled with diet and exercise alone.
2. If an "uncontrolled" Type I diabetic participates in exercise, the plasma glucose concentration may increase due to insufficient insulin. The liver's production of glucose

exceeds the muscle's ability to take up the glucose, so the plasma level increases. A Type I diabetic with an adequate amount of insulin shows a decrease in plasma glucose with exercise. If a diabetic has taken too much insulin, the exercise could precipitate a hypoglycemic response, with dire consequences.

3. A sedentary Type I diabetic has to juggle diet and insulin to stay in glucose balance. An exercise program complicates matters for the reasons mentioned above, and therefore, exercise is viewed as inappropriate as a normal means used to achieve "control." However, for those who have no complications, regular exercise is recommended in order for the diabetic to have as normal a life as possible.

4. The diabetic may have to increase carbohydrate intake and/or decrease the amount of insulin *prior to* activity in an attempt to maintain the glucose concentration close to normal *during* the exercise. The extent of these alterations is dependent on a number of factors, including the intensity and duration of the physical activity, the glucose concentration prior to the exercise, and the training state of the individual.

5. An asthmatic attack is brought on when an agent causes an increased influx of Ca^{++} into a mast cell in the respiratory tract, which, in turn, triggers the release of chemical mediators. These chemical mediators cause a reflex and calcium-mediated constriction of bronchiolar smooth muscle and an increase in the secretions into the airways. Cromolyn sodium and β-adrenergic agonists act to prevent this by preventing the entry of Ca^{++} into the mast cell, and by increasing the level of cyclic AMP in the mast and smooth muscle cells, respectively. The overall result is less chemical mediator release, less bronchiolar smooth muscle contraction, and a reduction in bronchiolar secretions.

6. Cooling and drying of the respiratory tract leads to an increase in the osmolarity of the fluid on the surface of a mast cell. This event is believed to be the central factor in the initiation of the asthmatic attack during exercise. Exercise of short duration, preceded by a warm-up, appears to reduce the chance of an attack. In addition, breathing warm, moist air can actually prevent the attack.

7. Chronic obstructive pulmonary disease (COPD) includes chronic asthma, emphysema, and bronchitis. These latter two diseases create changes in the lung that are irreversible, and result in a gradual deterioration of function. By the time a person can perceive a loss in function, the disease is well progressed. Rehabilitation is a multidisciplinary approach involving medication, breathing exercises, dietary therapy, exercise, and counseling. The programs are individually designed due to the variability in the extent of the illness, and the goals are very pragmatic in terms of the events of daily living and work.

8. Cardiac rehabilitation programs include a wide variety of patients, including those having angina pectoris, bypass surgery, myocardial infarctions, and angioplasty. These patients may be taking nitroglycerine to control angina symptoms, β-blockers to reduce the work of the heart, or antiarrhythmia medications to control dangerous heart rhythms.

9. The exercise tests for CHD patients include a 12-lead ECG, and are used for referral to other tests. The criteria for taking and stopping an exercise test are spelled out in detail, given the high risk of this population. Exercise programs bring about large changes in functional capacity in this population due to their low starting point. The programs are gradual and are based on their entry-level exercise tests and other clinical findings.

10. The elderly benefit from regular exercise that improves or maintains cardiorespiratory function. Exercise enables them to carry out activities associated with daily living, as well as maintain the integrity of bone. Older women have to be especially aware of the need to increase their calcium intake to help maintain their bone structure. Estrogen therapy may also be necessary.

11. The elderly are classified as young old (55–75 years; $\dot{V}O_2$ max = 6–7 METs), old old (>75 years; 2–3 METs), and athletic old (>55; $\dot{V}O_2$ max = 9–10 METs). The exercise programs vary dramatically based on the population. The athletic old can participate in many of the activities of the younger sedentary population. The young old can be involved in activities such as those found in cardiac rehabilitation programs. The old old need highly controlled activities that involve lying, sitting, and standing with support. The aim is to increase function with low risk of injury.

12. The guidelines for pregnant women are similar to those mentioned in chapter 16 with the following exceptions: don't exercise over a HR of 140 b · min⁻¹, keep durations to less than fifteen minutes during strenuous activities, keep maternal temperature below 38° C, don't do exercises in the supine position after the fourth month of gestation, and avoid the Valsalva maneuver.

Study Questions

1. What is the difference between Type I and Type II diabetes?
2. If a Type I diabetic does not take an adequate amount of insulin, what would happen to the blood glucose concentration during prolonged exercise? Why?
3. If exercise is helpful in controlling blood glucose, how could it complicate the life of a Type I diabetic?
4. Provide general recommendations regarding changes in insulin and diet for diabetics who are about to take a long hike.
5. How is exercise-induced asthma triggered, and how do medications reduce the chance of an attack?
6. What is COPD, and where does exercise fit in as a part of a rehabilitation program?
7. What are angina pectoris, CABGS, and angioplasty?
8. What additional measurements are made during a GXT of a cardiac patient, as compared to an apparently healthy individual?
9. Classify the elderly into three groups and describe exercise programs that might be consistent with each group.
10. What are the concerns about exercise during pregnancy, and what are the guidelines recommended for a pregnant woman who wishes to begin an exercise program?

Suggested Readings

Wenger, N. K., and H. K. Hellerstein. 1984. *Rehabilitation of the coronary patient.* 2d ed. New York: John Wiley & Sons.

Berg, K. E. 1986. *Diabetic's Guide to Health and Fitness.* Champaign, Ill.: Life Enhancement Publications.

References

1. American College of Sports Medicine. 1986. *Guidelines for Exercise Testing and Prescription.* Philadelphia: Lea & Febiger.
2. American Diabetes Association. 1985. Fact Sheet on Diabetes.
3. American Heart Association Committee Report. 1982. Rationale of the diet-heart statement of the American Heart Association. *Nutrition Today* (Sept./Oct.):16–20; (Nov./Dec.):15–19.
4. Berg, K. E. 1986. *Diabetic's Guide to Health and Fitness.* Champaign, Ill.: Life Enhancement Publications.
5. Berger et al. 1977. Metabolic and hormonal effects of muscular exercise in juvenile type diabetics. *Diabetologia* 13:355–65.

6. Berman, L. B., and J. R. Sutton. 1986. Exercise and the Pulmonary Patient. *Journal of Cardiopulmonary Rehabilitation* 6:52–61.

7. Caldwell, F., and T. Jopke. 1985. Questions and answers: ACSM 1985. *The Physician and Sportsmedicine* 13(8):145–51.

8. Cantu, D. C. 1982. *Diabetes and Exercise*. Ithaca, N.Y.: Movement Publications.

9. Clapp, J. F., and S. Dickstein. 1984. Endurance exercise and pregnancy outcome. *Medicine and Science in Sports and Exercise*. 16:556–62.

10. Collings, C. A., L. G. Curet, and J. P. Mullin. 1983. Maternal and fetal responses to a maternal aerobic exercise training program. *American Journal of Obstetrics and Gynecology* 145:702–7.

11. Eggleston, P. A. 1986. Pathophysiology of exercise-induced asthma. *Medicine and Science in Sports and Exercise* 18:318–21.

12. Franklin et al. 1986. Exercise prescription of the myocardial infarction patient. *Journal of Cardiopulmonary Rehabilitation* 6:62–79.

13. Franz, M. J. 1987. Exercise and the management of diabetes mellitus. *Journal of the American Dietetic Association* 87:872–80.

14. Gauthier, M. M. 1986. Guidelines for exercise during pregnancy: Too little or too much. *The Physician and Sportsmedicine* 14(4):162–69.

15. Gerhard, H., and E. N. Schachter. 1980. Exercise-induced asthma. *Postgraduate Medicine* 67:91–102.

16. Heaney, R. P. 1987. The role of calcium in prevention and treatment of osteoporosis. *The Physician and Sportsmedicine* 15(11):83–88.

17. Hedlund, L. R., and J. C. Gallagher. 1987. The effects of fluoride on osteoporosis. *The Physician and Sportsmedicine* 15(11):111–18.

18. Johnston, C. C., and C. Slemenda. 1987. Osteoporosis: An overview. *The Physician and Sportsmedicine* 15(11):65–68.

19. Kasch, F. W., J. P. Wallace, and S. P. Van Camp. 1985. Effects of 18 years of endurance exercise on the physical work capacity of older men. *Journal of Cardiopulmonary Rehabilitation* 5:308–12.

20. Katz, R. M. 1987. Coping with exercise-induced asthma in sports. *The Physician and Sportsmedicine* 15 (July):100–112.

21. Katz, R. M. 1986. Prevention with and without the use of medications for exercise-induced asthma. *Medicine and Science in Sports and Exercise* 18:331–33.

22. Kemmer, F. W., and M. Berger. 1983. Exercise and diabetes mellitus: Physical activity as a part of daily life and its role in the treatment of diabetic patient. *International Journal of Sports Medicine* 4:77–88.

23. Koivisto, V. A., and R. S. Sherwin. 1979. Exercise in diabetes: Therapeutic implications. *Postgraduate Medicine* 66:87–96.

24. Leon, A. S. et al. 1984. Exercise for diabetics: Effect of conditioning at constant body weight. *Journal of Cardiac Rehabilitation* 4:278–86.

25. Lindsay, R. 1987. Estrogen and osteoporosis. *The Physician and Sportsmedicine* 15(11):105–8.

26. Lotgering, F. K., R. D. Gilbert, and L. D. Longo. 1984. The interactions of exercise and pregnancy: A review. *American Journal of Obstetrics and Gynecology* 149:560–68.

27. Lotgering, F. K., R. D. Gilbert, and L. D. Longo. 1985. Maternal and fetal responses to exercise during pregnancy. *Physiological Reviews* 65:1–36.

28. Maehlum, S. 1984. Clinical application of exercise and training in diabetes mellitus. *International Journal of Sports Medicine* 5(Suppl.):47–48.

29. Martin, A. D. 1986. ECG and medications. In (E. T. Howley and B. D. Franks) *Health/Fitness Instructor's Handbook,* 185–98. Champaign, Ill.: Human Kinetics Publishers.

30. Middleton, E. 1980. A rational approach to asthma therapy. *Postgraduate Medicine* 67:107–23.

31. Miracle, V. A. 1986. Pulmonary exercise program: A model for pulmonary rehabilitation. *Journal of Cardiopulmonary Rehabilitation* 6:368–71.

32. *Physician and Sportsmedicine*. 1987. A Roundtable: Physiological adaptations to chronic endurance exercise training in patients with coronary artery disease. *Physician and Sportsmedicine* 15(9):129–56.

33. Pierson et al. 1986. Implications of air pollution effects on athletic performance. *Medicine and Science in Sports and Exercise* 18:322–27.

34. Pollock, M. L., J. H. Wilmore, and S. M. Fox. 1984. *Exercise in Health and Disease*. Philadelphia: W. B. Saunders Company.

35. Poortmans et al. 1986. Influence of the degree of metabolic control on physical fitness in Type I diabetic adolescents. *International Journal of Sports Medicine* 7:232–35.

36. Richter, E. R., and H. Galbo. 1986. Diabetes, insulin and exercise. *Sports Medicine* 3:275–88.

37. Shephard, R. J. 1976. Exercise and chronic obstructive lung disease. In (J. Keogle and R. S. Hutton, eds.) *Exercise and Sport Sciences Reviews* (Volume 4), 263–96. California: Journal Publishing Affiliates.

38. Sly, R. M. 1986. History of exercise-induced asthma. *Medicine and Science in Sports and Exercise* 18:314–17.

39. Smith, E. L. 1984. Special considerations in developing exercise programs for the older adult. In (J. D. Matarazzo et al. eds.) *Behavioral Health: A Handbook of Health-Enhancement and Disease Prevention,* 525–46. New York: John Wiley & Sons.

40. Smith, E. L., and C. Gilligan. 1987. Effects of inactivity and exercise on bone. *The Physician and Sportsmedicine* 15(11):91–102.

41. Smith, E. L., and K. G. Stoedefalke. 1978. Aging and Exercise. Copyright: Author.

42. Stockdale-Woolley, R., M. C. Haggerty, and P. M. McMahon. 1986. The pulmonary rehabilitation program at Norwalk Hospital. *Journal of Cardiopulmonary Rehabilitation* 6:505–18.

43. Tommaso, C. L., M. Lesch, and E. H. Sonnenblick. 1984. Alterations in cardiac function in coronary heart disease, myocardial infarction, and coronary bypass surgery. In (N. K. Wenger and H. K. Hellerstern, eds.) *Rehabilitation of the Coronary Patient,* 41–66. New York: John Wiley & Sons.

44. Vranic, M., and M. Berger. 1979. Exercise and diabetes mellitus. *Diabetes* 28:147–63.

45. Voy, R. O. 1986. The U. S. Olympic Committee experience with exercise-induced bronchospasm. 1984. *Medicine and Science in Sports and Exercise* 18:328–30.

46. Wahner, H. W. 1987. Diagnosis of osteoporosis. *The Physician and Sportsmedicine* 15(11):73–79.

47. Wahren, J., P. Felig, and L. Hagenfeldt. 1978. Physical exercise and fuel homeostasis in diabetes mellitus. *Diabetologia* 14:213–22.

48. Wallace, J. P. 1983. Physical conditioning: Intervention in aging cardiovascular function. In *Intervention in the Aging Process, Part A: Quantitation, Epidemiology, and Clinical Research,* 307–23. A. R. Liss, Inc.

49. Wenger, N. K., and H. K. Hellerstein. 1984. *Rehabilitation of the Coronary Patient.* 2d ed. New York: John Wiley & Sons.

50. Wenger, N. K., and J. W. Hurst. 1984. Coronary bypass surgery as a rehabilitative procedure. In (N. K. Wenger and H. K. Hellerstein, eds.) *Rehabilitation of the Coronary Patient,* 115–32. New York: John Wiley & Sons.

18 Body Composition and Nutrition for Health

Objectives

*B*y studying this chapter, you should be able to do the following:

1. Identify the U.S. Dietary Goals relative to (a) carbohydrates and fats as a percent of energy intake, (b) salt and cholesterol, and (c) saturated and unsaturated fats.
2. Contrast the Dietary Goals with the Dietary Guidelines.
3. Describe what is meant by the term Recommended Dietary Allowance, and contrast that with the U.S. Recommended Daily Allowance.
4. List the classes of nutrients.
5. Identify the fat- and water-soluble vitamins, what toxicity is, and which class of vitamins is more likely to cause this problem.
6. Contrast major minerals with trace minerals, and describe the role of calcium, iron, and sodium in health and disease.
7. Identify the primary role of carbohydrates, the two major classes, and the recommended changes in the American diet to improve health status.
8. Identify the primary role of fat, and the recommended changes in the American diet to improve health status.
9. Describe the Basic Four Food Groups; list some foods and the major nutrients represented in each group.
10. Describe the Exchange System of planning diets, and how it differs from the Basic Four Food Group approach.
11. Describe the limitation of the height/weight table in determining body composition.
12. Provide a brief description of the following methods of body composition: isotope dilution, photon absorptiometry, potassium-40, densitometry (underwater weighing), radiography, ultrasound, nuclear magnetic resonance, total body electrical conductivity, bioelectrical impedence analysis, and skinfold thickness.
13. Describe the two-component system of body composition and the assumptions made about the density values for the fat-free mass and the fat mass.
14. Explain the principle underlying the measurement of whole body density with underwater weighing, and why one must correct for residual volume and the volume of gas in the GI tract.
15. Explain why is there still an error of ±2.5% in the calculation of percent body fat with the underwater weighing technique.
16. Explain how a sum of skinfolds can be ''converted'' to a percent body fatness value, and why some formulas were ''population specific.''
17. List the recommended percent body fatness values for health and fitness for males and females, and explain the concern for both high and low values.
18. Discuss the reasons why the average weight at any height (fatness) has increased while deaths from cardiovascular diseases have decreased.
19. Distinguish between obesity due to hyperplasia and hypertrophy; discuss the effect of weight loss on fat cell number, the pattern of fat cell number increase in humans, and the prognosis for those with the hyperplasia form of obesity.

20. Describe the roles of genetics and environment in the appearance of obesity.
21. Explain the set point theory of obesity, and give an example of a physiological and behavioral control system.
22. Describe the pattern of change in body weight and dietary intake over the adult years.
23. Describe the pattern of weight loss on a low-calorie, low-carbohydrate diet; discuss the changes in body composition when weight is lost by diet alone versus diet plus exercise.
24. Discuss the effect of body fatness and diet on the BMR.
25. Define thermogenesis and how it is affected by both short- and long-term overfeeding; how might this affect the rate of weight gain in those who have a low rate of thermogenesis?
26. Explain how someone might minimize the effect of inactivity as a cause of obesity relative to the role of the BMR and thermogenesis.
27. Describe the effect of exercise on appetite and body composition.
28. Describe the difference between the *net* and *gross* caloric cost of physical activity.
29. Explain quantitatively why small differences in energy expenditure and dietary intake are important in weight gain over the years.

Outline

Key Terms

anorexia nervosa
atherosclerosis
basal metabolic rate (BMR)
bulimia
cholesterol
crude fiber
deficiency
dietary (edible) fiber
elements
energy wasteful systems
ferritin
food records
HDL cholesterol
hemosiderin
high-density lipoproteins (HDL)
ketosis
LDL cholesterol
lipoprotein
low-density lipoproteins (LDL)

major minerals
nutrient density
osteoporosis
provitamin
Recommended Dietary Allowances (RDA)
resting metabolic rate (RMR)
thermogenesis
toxicity
trace elements
transferrin
twenty-four-hour recall
U.S. Dietary Goals
U.S. Dietary Guidelines
U.S. Recommended Daily Allowances (U.S. RDA)
underwater weighing
whole body density

Chapter 14 described factors that limit health and fitness. These included hypertension, obesity, and elevated serum cholesterol. These three risk factors are linked to an excessive consumption of salt, total calories, and dietary fat, respectively. Clearly, knowledge of nutrition is essential to our understanding of health-related fitness. While chapter 3 described the metabolism of carbohydrates, fats, and proteins, this chapter will focus on the type of diet that should provide them. The first part of the chapter will present the nutritional goals for our nation, the nutrition standards and what they mean, a summary of the six classes of nutrients, and a way to evaluate our present diets and meet our nutritional goals. The second part of the chapter will discuss the role of exercise and diet in altering body composition. Nutrition related to athletic performance is covered in chapter 23.

Nutritional Goals

The American Heart Association (1) has focused our attention on the role of diet in the elevation of serum cholesterol, obesity, and the development of hypertension (1). Diet has also been linked to colon cancer and diabetes. In response to these problems a U.S. Senate Select Committee on Nutrition and Human Needs recruited experts to comment on and formulate **U.S. Dietary Goals** that would deal with diet-related problems (129). These goals, shown in figure 18.1, included the following:

1. Increase carbohydrate intake to represent 55%–60% of caloric intake.
2. Decrease fat consumption from 40% to 30% of caloric intake.
3. Decrease saturated fat intake to represent only 10% of caloric intake; increase polyunsaturated and monounsaturated fats to approximately 10% of caloric intake.
4. Reduce cholesterol intake to 300 mg per day.
5. Reduce sugar consumption to account for only 15% of total calories.
6. Reduce salt consumption by about 50%–85% to approximately 3 gm per day.

In order to achieve these goals the following changes in food selection and preparation were suggested:

1. Increase the intake of fruits, vegetables, and whole grains.
2. Increase consumption of poultry and fish, and decrease intake of meat.
3. Decrease intake of foods high in fat, and partially substitute polyunsaturated fat for saturated fat.
4. Substitute nonfat milk for whole milk.
5. Decrease consumption of butter fat, eggs, and other high-cholesterol sources.
6. Decrease consumption of sugar and foods high in sugar content.
7. Decrease consumption of salt and foods high in salt content.

Not everyone agreed with these specific quantitative goals and the strong statements that were made about the role of diet in the prevention and treatment of disease. The Select Committee subsequently published responses of scientists and medical doctors who disagreed with the stated dietary goals (128). The revised document encouraged weight reduction to attain "ideal weight," and recommended a reduction in the use of alcohol.

Figure 18.1 Dietary Goals for the United States. This figure lists the percentage of calories derived from fat, carbohydrate, and protein in the diet of the average American. The current diet contains too much fat, including saturated fat, and too little carbohydrate. Achievement of the goals of 30% fat and 58% carbohydrate would reduce the incidence of heart disease, as well as other diseases.

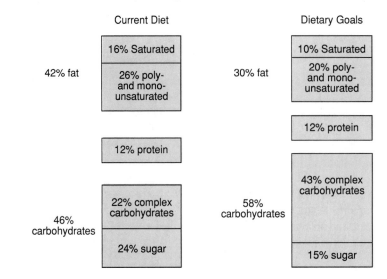

In 1980 the U.S. Departments of Agriculture and Health, Education and Welfare (97) published *Dietary Guidelines for Americans.* Rather than provide specific quantities to achieve for fat, cholesterol, salt, and carbohydrates as did the *Goals,* the *Guidelines* are more general statements aimed at people in good health. The following 1985 update on those guidelines shows little change over the previous five years (98).

- Eat a variety of foods.
- Maintain desirable weight.
- Avoid too much fat, saturated fat, and cholesterol.
- Eat food with adequate starch and fiber.
- Avoid too much sugar.
- Avoid too much sodium.
- If you drink alcoholic beverages, do so in moderation.

Each of these guidelines will be expanded in the following sections dealing with the essential nutrients, and body composition, and weight control.

Standards of Nutrition

Food provides the carbohydrates, fats, protein, minerals, vitamins, and water needed for life. The quantity of each nutrient thought to meet the needs of practically all healthy persons is stated in the **Recommended Dietary Allowances (RDA)** found in appendix E. The values for each nutrient vary due to gender, body size, whether or not long-bone growth is taking place, pregnancy, and lactation (96). Given the fact that individuals differ in their need for each nutrient, some requiring more than average and others less, the standards were set high enough to meet the needs of almost everyone (97.5% of the population), and also account for inefficient utilization by the body (96). For some vitamins and minerals the data used to set standards for specific population groups was considered inadequate, so values for these nutrients are referred to as "Estimated Safe and Adequate Intakes," rather than RDA's (see appendix F). The RDA does not set standards for carbohydrate and fat intake, but recommendations about these nutrients will be discussed shortly.

Table 18.1 Nutritional information on a can of tuna

Nutritional Information per Serving

Serving size:	2 oz. (including liquid)	Servings per container:	3.3	
Calories:	60	Fat:	Less than 1 gm	
Protein:	13 gm	Sodium:	310 mg	

Percentage of U.S. Recommended Daily Allowance per Serving

Protein:	25	Riboflavin (B_2):	2	Vitamin E:	2
Vitamin A:	*	Niacin:	35	Vitamin B_6:	15
Vitamin C:	*	Calcium:	*	Vitamin B_{12}:	25
Thiamin (B_1):	*	Iron:	4		

*Contains less than 2% of the U.S. RDA of these nutrients.

The RDA for caloric intake (energy) is not set at the same level as for the nutrients. Instead, the RDA for energy was simply set to meet the *average* caloric intake of each group (women, men, children, etc.) to reduce the chance that someone would gain weight while meeting the standard. The values for energy intake listed in appendix G assume an average level of physical activity (96), but, as we will discuss in more detail later in this chapter, there are many overweight individuals who may require less energy than is recommended due to their sedentary life-style. However, if an individual is consuming the recommended dietary allowance for energy and still gains weight, it is suggested that the person should increase his or her physical activity to achieve the desired weight rather than cut back on intake. The higher caloric intake will increase the chance that the person will meet the RDA for all the nutrients (96). How do you know how much of the RDA you have achieved?

The **U.S. Recommended Daily Allowances (U.S. RDA)** is a standard used in nutritional labeling that is based on the highest RDA for each nutrient (29). The U.S. RDA indicates what percent of these RDA standards is met by one serving of a product. The U.S. RDA can be used for males and females from age four to adults, except for pregnant and lactating women. Table 18.1 shows the U.S. RDA values from a label on a can of chunk light tuna packed in water. The package label indicates that a two-ounce serving will

provide 25% of the U.S. RDA standard for protein. This information is helpful in comparing products as well as in evaluating one's nutritional intake.

Classes of Nutrients

There are six classes of nutrients: water, vitamins, minerals, carbohydrates, fats, and proteins. In the following sections each nutrient will be described briefly and the primary food sources of each will be identified.

Water

Water is absolutely essential for life. While we can go without food for weeks, we would not survive long without water. The body is 50%–75% water, depending on age and body fatness, and a loss of only 3%–4% adversely affects aerobic performance. Larger losses can lead to death (93, 137). Under normal conditions without exercise, water loss equals about 2,300 ml/day, with most lost in urine. However, as higher environmental temperatures and heavy exercise are added, the water loss increases dramatically to 6–7 liters (51).

Under normal conditions the 2,300 ml of water per day is replaced with beverages (1,000–1,500 ml), solid food (500–1,000 ml), and the water derived from metabolic processes (250–400 ml) (29). Most people are surprised by the large volume of water contributed by "solid" food until they consider the following percentages of water in "solid" food: baked potato—75%, canned peas—77%, lettuce—96% (29). A general recommendation under ordinary circumstances is to consume 1 ml of water per kcal of energy expenditure (96). However, to avoid potential problems associated with dehydration, one should drink water *during* exercise; thirst is not an adequate stimulus to achieve water balance (see chapter 23).

Water weight can fluctuate depending on the body stores of carbohydrate and protein. Water is involved in the linkage between glucose molecules in glycogen and amino acid molecules in protein. The ratio is about 2.7 gms of water per gm of carbohydrate, and if an individual stores 454 gms (1 lb) of carbohydrate, body weight would increase by 3.7 lbs. Of course, when one diets and depletes this carbohydrate store, the reverse occurs. This results in an apparent weight loss of 3.7 lbs when only 1,816 kcal (454 gm of carbohydrate times 4 kcal/gm) have been lost. More on this later.

Vitamins

Vitamins have already been introduced in chapter 3 as organic catalysts involved in metabolic reactions. They are needed in small amounts and are not "used up" in the metabolic reactions. However, they are degraded (metabolized) like any biological molecule and must be replaced on a regular basis to maintain body stores. Several vitamins are in a precursor or **provitamin** form in foods, and are converted to the active form in the body. Carotene, called provitamin A, is good example. A chronic lack of certain vitamins can lead to **deficiency** diseases, and an excess of others can lead to a **toxicity** condition (29, 137). In our presentation, vitamins will be divided into the fat-soluble and water-soluble groups.

Fat-Soluble Vitamins

The fat-soluble vitamins include A, D, E, and K. These vitamins can be stored in large quantities in the body, thus a deficiency state takes longer to develop. However, because of their solubility, so much can be stored that a toxicity condition can occur. Vitamin D is regarded as the most toxic, and it is possible to achieve a level of toxicity with only four to five times the recommended dietary allowance (29, 55, 96). Toxicity, of

course, is far from a health-related goal. Table 18.2 summarizes the information on these vitamins, including RDA, dietary sources, function, and signs associated with deficiency or excess.

Water-Soluble Vitamins

The water-soluble vitamins include vitamin C and the B vitamins: thiamin (B-1), riboflavin (B-2), niacin, pyridoxine (B-6), folacin, B-12, pantothenic acid, and biotin. Most are involved in energy metabolism. You have already seen the role of niacin, as NAD, and riboflavin, as FAD, in the transfer of energy in the Krebs cycle and electron transport chain. Thiamin (as thiamine pyrophosphate) is involved in the removal of CO_2 as pyruvate enters the Krebs cycle. Vitamin B-6, folacin, B-12, pantothenic acid, and biotin are also involved as coenzymes in metabolic reactions. Vitamin C is involved in the maintenance of bone, cartilage, and connective tissue. Table 18.2 summarizes the information on these vitamins, including the RDA, function, dietary sources, and signs associated with deficiency or excess (29, 55, 124).

Minerals

Minerals are the chemical **elements,** other than carbon, hydrogen, oxygen, and nitrogen, associated with the structure and function of the body. We have already seen the importance of calcium in bone structure and in the initiation of muscle contraction, iron in O_2 transport on hemoglobin, and phosphorus in ATP. Minerals are important inorganic nutrients and are divided into two classes: (1) **major minerals** and (2) **trace elements.** The major minerals include calcium, phosphorous, potassium, sulfur, sodium, chloride, and magnesium, with whole-body quantities ranging from 35 gm for magnesium to 1,050 gm for calcium in a 70-kg man (29). The trace elements include iron, zinc, copper, iodine, manganese, selenium, chromium, molybdenum, cobalt, arsenic, nickle, fluoride, and vanadium. There are only 4 gm of iron and 0.0009 gm of vanadium in a 70-kg man. Like vitamins, some minerals taken in excess (e.g., iron and zinc) can be toxic. The following sections will focus attention on calcium, iron, and sodium.

Table 18.2 Key information about the vitamins

Vitamin	RDA for Healthy Adults	Major Dietary Sources	Major Functions	Signs of Severe, Prolonged Deficiency	Signs of Extreme Excess
Fat-Soluble					
A	Females: 800 RE, 4,000 IU[a] Males: 1,000 RE, 5,000 IU[a]	Fat-containing and fortified dairy products; liver; provitamin carotene in orange and deep green produce	Component of rhodopsin (Still under intense study)	Keratinization of epithelial tissues, including the cornea of the eye (xeropthalmia); night blindness; dry scaling skin; poor immune response	Damage to liver, kidney, bone; headache, irritability, vomiting, hair loss, blurred vision from pre-formed vitamin A. From carotene: yellowed skin
D	5µg (200 IU)	Fortified and full-fat dairy products, egg yolk	Promotes absorption and use of calcium and phosphorus	Rickets (bone deformities) in children; osteomalacia (bone softening) in adults	GI upset; cerebral, CV, kidney damage; lethargy
E	Females: eight α-tocopherol equivalents Males: ten α-tocopherol equivalents	Vegetable oils and their products; nuts, seeds; present at low levels in other foods	Antioxidant to prevent cell membrane damage; still under intense study	Possible anemia	In anemic children, blood abnormalities may develop
K	70–140 µg	Green leafy vegetables; meats	Aids in formation of certain proteins, especially those for blood clotting	Severe bleeding on injury; internal hemorrhage	Liver damage and anemia from high doses of the synthetic form menadione

Table 18.2 Continued

Vitamin	RDA for Healthy Adults	Major Dietary Sources	Major Functions	Signs of Severe, Prolonged Deficiency	Signs of Extreme Excess
Water-Soluble					
Thiamin (B-1)	Females: 1.1 mg Males: 1.5 mg	Pork, legumes, peanuts, enriched or whole grain products	Component of coenzyme used in energy metabolism	Beriberi (nerve changes, sometimes edema, heart failure)	?
Riboflavin (B-2)	Females: 1.3 mg Males: 1.7 mg	Dairy products, meats, eggs, enriched grain products, green leafy vegetables	Component of coenzyme used in energy metabolism	Skin lesions	?
Water-Soluble					
Niacin	Females: 14 niacin equivalents Males: 19 niacin equivalents	Nuts, meats; provitamin tryptophan in most proteins	Component of coenzyme used in energy metabolism	Pellagra (diarrhea, dermatitis, dementia, death)	Flushing of face, neck, hands; liver damage
B-6	Females: 2.0 mg Males: 2.2 mg	High protein foods in general, bananas, some vegetables	Component of coenzyme used in amino acid metabolism	Nervous and muscular disorders	Unstable gait, numb feet, poor hand coordination, abnormal brain function
Folacin	400 μg	Green vegetables, orange juice, nuts, legumes, grain products	Component of coenzyme used in DNA and RNA metabolism	Megaloblastic anemia (large, immature red blood cells); GI disturbances	Masks vitamin B-12 deficiency

Table 18.2 Continued

Vitamin	RDA for Healthy Adults	Major Dietary Sources	Major Functions	Signs of Severe, Prolonged Deficiency	Signs of Extreme Excess
B-12	3 µg	Animal products	Component of coenzyme used in DNA and RNA metabolism	Megaloblastic anemia; pernicious anemia when due to inadequate intrinsic factor; nervous system damage	?
Pantothenic acid	4–7 mg	Widely distributed in foods	Component of conezyme used in energy metabolism	Fatigue, sleep disturbances, nausea, poor coordination	?
Biotin	100–200 µg	Widely distributed in foods	Component of coenzyme used in energy metabolism	Fatigue, depression, muscular pain, dermatitis	?
C	60 mg	Fruits and vegetables, especially broccoli, cabbage, cantaloupe, cauliflower, citrus fruits, green pepper, strawberries	Maintains collagen; is an antioxidant; aids in detoxification; still under intense study	Scurvy (skin spots, bleeding gums, weakness); delayed wound healing; impaired immune response	GI upsets, confounds certain lab tests, poorer immune response

aLess accurate than RE values; to be used only until food composition tables are converted to RE values.
From Christian and Greger, *Nutrition for Living*. Copyright © 1985 Benjamin/Cummings Publishing Company, Menlo Park, Calif. Reprinted by permission.

Calcium

Calcium (Ca^{++}) and phosphorus combine with organic molecules to form the teeth and bones. The bones are a "store" of calcium that helps to maintain the plasma Ca^{++} concentration when dietary intake is inadequate (see parathyroid hormone in chapter 5). Bone is constantly turning over its calcium and phosphorus, so diet must replace what is lost. If the diet is deficient in calcium for a long period of time, loss of bone, or **osteoporosis,** can occur. This weakening of the bone due to the loss of calcium and phosphorous from its structure is more common in women than in men, and is accelerated at menopause. In 1980 it was estimated that there would be over 150,000 hip fractures annually in Caucasian women due to osteoporosis, with the medical cost exceeding $1 billion (102). Three major factors are implicated: dietary calcium intake, inadequate estrogen, and lack of physical activity (56, 114).

There is concern that the increase in osteoporosis in our society is related to an inadequate calcium intake. While the RDA for calcium is 800 mg/day, 50% of women over age thirty-five take in less than 500 mg/day (113). There is additional concern that the RDA of 800 mg/day should be increased to 1,000 mg/day for premenopausal women, and to 1,500 mg/day for early postmenopausal women (56). While menopause is the usual cause of a reduced secretion of estrogen, young, and extremely active female athletes are experiencing this problem associated with ammenorhea (22, 28). The decrease in estrogen secretion is associated with the acceleration of osteoporosis, and estrogen therapy has been used successfully in menopausal women to reduce the rate of bone loss (95). A third approach to deal with osteoporosis is based on the observation that exercise slows the rate of bone loss (2, 17, 91, 103). This has been shown in runners (17), as well as tennis players (91), and is viewed as an important reason for recommending regular moderate exercise in the elderly (see chapter 17).

Iron

Iron is an important part of hemoglobin and myoglobin, as well as in the cytochromes of the electron transport chain. To remain in iron balance males must absorb 1 mg/day, and females, 1.8 mg/day, the higher amount needed to replace that which is lost in the menses. The RDA is 10 mg/day for an adult male and 18 mg/day for an adult female because only 10% of dietary iron is absorbed. A 70-kg man has about 2,500 mg of iron in hemoglobin, 150 mg in myoglobin, 6–8 mg in enzymes, and about 3 mg bound to **transferrin,** the iron-transporting protein in plasma. In addition to this, iron is stored as **ferritin** or **hemosiderin** in the liver, spleen, and bone marrow. These iron stores may be 500–1,000 mg in men and less than 500 mg in women (54).

In spite of the higher need for iron, American women take in only 11 mg/day, while men take in 16 mg/day (29). This is due to higher caloric intakes in males than females. Since there is only 6 mg of iron per 1,000 kcal of energy in the American diet, a woman consuming 2,000 kcal/day would take in only 12 mg of iron. The male, consuming about 3,000 kcal/day, takes in 18 mg (54, 137). The diet provides iron in two forms, heme (ferrous) and nonheme (ferric). Heme iron, found primarily in meats, fish and organ meats, is absorbed better than nonheme iron, which is found in vegetables. However, the absorption of nonheme iron can be increased by the presence of meat, fish, and vitamin C (54, 137).

Anemia is a condition in which the hemoglobin concentration is low: less than 13 g/dl in men and less than 12 g/dl in women. This can be the result of a blood loss (e.g., blood donation or bleeding, or a lack of vitamins or minerals in the diet). The most common cause of anemia in North America is a lack of dietary iron (29). In fact, iron deficiency is the most common nutrient deficiency (137). In iron deficiency anemia more than the hemoglobin is affected. The iron bound to transferrin in the plasma is reduced and serum ferritin (an indicator of iron stores) is low (54). While children aged one to five, adolescents, young adult women and the elderly are more apt to develop anemia, it also occurs in competitive athletes. This latter point will be discussed in detail in chapter 23.

Sodium

Sodium is directly involved in the maintenance of the resting membrane potential and the generation of action potential in nerves (chapter 7) and muscles (chapter 8). In addition, sodium is the primary electrolyte determining the extracellular fluid volume. If sodium stores fall, the extracellular volume, including plasma, is decreased. This could cause major problems related to the maintenance of the mean arterial blood pressure (chapter 9) and body temperature (chapter 12).

The problem in our society is not with sodium stores that are too small, but just the opposite. Americans consume about 10–12 grams of salt each day, which exceeds the RDA of 2.7–8.2 grams. Some suggest that the RDA is too high and that the amount needed by a nonexercising individual may be as low as 0.5 gms/day (29). In addition, concern has been raised by the American Heart Association (1) that excess sodium intake can lead to hypertension in genetically susceptible individuals. This level of concern is shown in one of the *Dietary Guidelines for Americans,* namely, to avoid too much sodium. The following suggestions were made relative to that guideline (98):

- Learn to enjoy the flavors of unsalted foods.
- Cook without salt or with only small amounts of added salt.
- Try flavoring foods with herbs, spices, and lemon juice.
- Add little or no salt to table food.
- Limit your intake of salty foods such as potato chips, pretzels, salted nuts, popcorn, condiments (soy sauce, steak sauce, garlic salt), pickled foods, cured meat, some cheeses, and some canned vegetables and soups.
- Read food labels carefully to determine the amounts of sodium.
- Use lower sodium products, when available, to replace those you use with a higher sodium content.

Those involved in athletic competition, strenuous exercise, or work in the heat must be concerned about adequate sodium replacement. Generally, because these individuals consume more kcal of food (containing more sodium), this is usually not a problem. More on this in chapter 23.

The previous sections have focused attention on three minerals—calcium, iron, and sodium—because of their relationship to current medical and health-related problems. A summary of each of the minerals, their function, and food sources is presented in table 18.3.

Carbohydrates

Carbohydrates and fats are the primary sources of energy in the average American diet, representing 46% and 42% of the energy intake, respectively (96). Carbohydrates suffer a bad reputation from those on diets, especially when you consider that you would have to eat over twice as much carbohydrate as fat to consume the same number of calories (4 kcal/gm versus 9 kcal/gm). Carbohydrates can be divided into two classes, those that can be digested and metabolized for energy (sugars and starches), and those that are undigestible (fiber). The sugars are found in jellies, jam, fruit, soft drinks, honey, syrups, and milk, while the starches are found in cereals, flour, potatoes, and other vegetables (96).

Sugars and Starches

Carbohydrate is a major energy source for all tissues and a crucial source for two: red blood cells and neurons. The red blood cells depend exclusively on anaerobic glycolysis for energy, and the nervous system functions well only on carbohydrate. These two tissues can consume 180 grams of glucose per day (32). Given this need it is no surprise that the plasma glucose concentration is maintained within narrow limits by hormonal control mechanisms (chapter 5). During strenuous exercise the muscles could use 180 grams of glucose in less than one hour. As a result of these needs one might expect that carbohydrate would make up a large fraction of our energy intake. Currently 46% of energy intake is derived from carbohydrate (96), with the dietary goal being closer to 55%–60% (126). While the goal is to increase carbohydrate intake, one of the

Table 18.3 Key information about many essential minerals

Mineral	RDA for Healthy Adults	Major Dietary Sources	Major Functions	Signs of Severe, Prolonged Deficiency	Signs of Extreme Excess
Major Minerals					
Calcium	800 mg	Milk, cheese, dark green vegetables, legumes	Bone and tooth formation; blood clotting; nerve transmission	Stunted growth; maybe bone loss	Depressed absorption of some other minerals
Phosphorus	800 mg	Milk, cheese, meat, poultry, whole grains	Bone and tooth formation; acid-base balance; component of coenzymes	Weakness; demineralization of bone	Some forms depress absorption of some minerals
Magnesium	Females: 300 mg Males: 350 mg	Whole grains, green leafy vegetables	Component of enzymes	Neurological disturbances	Neurological disturbances
Sulfur	(Provided by sulfur amino acids)	Sulfur amino acids in dietary proteins	Component of cartilage, tendon, and proteins; acid-base balance	(Related to protein deficiency)	Excess sulfure amino acid intake leads to poor growth; liver damage
Sodium	1,100–3,300 mg[a]	Common salt, soy sauce, cured meats, pickles, canned soups, processed cheese	Body water balance; nerve function	Muscle cramps; reduced appetite	High blood pressure in genetically predisposed individuals
Potassium	1,875–5,625 mg[a]	Meats, milk, many fruits and vegetables, whole grains	Body water balance; nerve function	Muscular weakness, paralysis	Muscular weakness; cardiac arrest

Table 18.3 Continued

Mineral	RDA for Healthy Adults	Major Dietary Sources	Major Functions	Signs of Severe, Prolonged Deficiency	Signs of Extreme Excess
Chloride	1,700–5,100 mg[a]	Common salt, many processed foods (as for sodium)	Plays a role in acid-base balance; formation of gastric juice	Muscle cramps; reduced appetite; poor growth	Vomiting
Trace Minerals					
Iron	Females: 18 mg Males: 10 mg	Meats, eggs, legumes, whole grains, green leafy vegetables	Component of hemoglobin and enzymes	Iron deficiency, anemia, weakness, impaired immune function	Acute: shock, death Chronic: liver damage, cardiac failure
Iodine	0.15 mg	Marine fish and shellfish; dairy products; iodized salt; some breads	Component of thyroid hormones	Goiter (enlarged thyroid)	Iodide goiter
Fluoride	1.5–4.0 mg[a]	Drinking water, tea, seafood	Maintenance of tooth (and maybe bone) structure	Higher frequency of tooth decay	Mottling of teeth; skeletal deformation
Zinc	15 mg	Meats, seafood, whole grains	Component of enzymes	Growth failure; reproductive failure; impaired immune function	Nausea; vomiting; diarrhea; adversely affects copper metabolism
Selenium	0.05–0.2 mg[a]	Seafood, meat, whole grains	Component of enzyme; functions in close association with vitamin E	Muscle pain; maybe heart muscle deterioration	In animals; liver damage; depressed growth

Table 18.3 Continued

Mineral	RDA for Healthy Adults	Major Dietary Sources	Major Functions	Signs of Severe, Prolonged Deficiency	Signs of Extreme Excess
Copper	2–3 mg[a]	Seafood, nuts, legumes, organ meats	Component of enzymes	Anemia; bone changes	Liver and neurological damage
Cobalt	(Required as vitamin B-12)	Vitamin B-12 (animal products)	Component of vitamin B-12	Not reported except as vitamin B-12 deficiency	Diseases of red blood cells
Chromium	0.05–0.2 mg[a]	Brewers' yeast, liver, seafood, meat, some vegetables	Involved in glucose and energy metabolism	Impaired glucose metabolism	Lung, skin, and kidney damage (occupational exposures)
Manganese	2.5–5.0 mg[a]	Nuts, whole grains, vegetables and fruits	Component of enzymes	Abnormal bone and cartilage	Neuromuscular effects
Molybdenum	0.15–0.5 mg[a]	Legumes, cereals, some vegetables	Component of enzymes	Disorder in nitrogen excretion	Inhibition of enzymes; adversely affects cobalt metabolism

[a]Estimated safe and adequate daily dietary intake
From Christian and Greger, *Nutrition for Living.* Copyright © 1985 Benjamin/Cummings Publishing Company, Menlo Park, Calif. Reprinted by permission.

Dietary Guidelines for Americans is to avoid too much sugar. The following suggestions were made relative to that guideline (98).

- Use less of all sugars and foods containing large amounts of sugars, including white sugar, brown sugar, raw sugar, honey, and syrups. Examples include soft drinks, candies, cakes, and cookies.
- Remember, how often you eat sugar and sugar-containing foods is as important to the health of your teeth as how much sugar you eat. It will help to avoid eating sweets between meals.

- Read food labels for clues on sugar content. If the name sugar, sucrose, glucose, maltose, dextrose, lactose, fructose, or syrups appears first, then there is a large amount of sugar.
- Select fresh fruits or fruits processed without syrup or with light rather than heavy syrup.

Dietary Fiber
Dietary fiber is derived from cell walls and includes two insoluble forms, cellulose and hemicellulose, and two soluble forms, pectin and gum (38). Dietary fiber

cannot be digested and metabolized, and consequently provides a sense of fullness (satiation) during a meal without the additional calories (38). This fact has been used by bakeries who lower the number of calories per slice of bread by adding cellulose from wood (29)! Pectin and gum are used in food processing to thicken, stabilize, or emulsify the constituents of various food products (29). The percent of fiber in foods is expressed either as **crude fiber** or as **dietary (edible) fiber.** The crude fiber values are derived from a harsh chemical analysis that "digests" a food in a manner our digestive system cannot, and provides little useful information relative to human nutrition (29, 38). The dietary fiber values are based on mild chemical analyses or human fecal waste studies and are the best estimates of dietary fiber (29).

Dietary fiber has long been linked to optimal health. Fiber acts as a hydrated sponge as it moves along the large intestine, making constipation less likely by reducing transit time (29, 38). Vegetarian diets high in soluble fiber have been linked to lower serum cholesterol due to the loss of more bile (cholesterol-containing) acids in the feces. However, the fact that vegetarian diets are also lower in the percent of calories from fat, which can also lower serum cholesterol, makes the interpretation of the data more complicated (38). While a high fiber diet reduces the incidence of diverticulosis, a condition in which outpouchings (diverticula) occur in the colon wall, the role of fiber in colon cancer is still questionable (29, 38).

Given the broad role of dietary fiber in normal health, it is no surprise that the *Dietary Guidelines for Ameicans* recommends that Americans increase their intake of fiber. However, at this time no RDA exists for dietary fiber. The following recommendations accompanied the *Dietary Guidelines for Americans* in order to deal with the needs for more fiber and more complex carbohydrates:

- Choose foods that are good sources of fiber and starch, such as whole-grain breads and cereals, fruits, vegetables, and dry beans and peas.
- Substitute starchy foods for those that have large amounts of fats and sugars.

Fats

Dietary lipids include triglycerides, phospholipids, and **cholesterol.** If solid at room temperature, lipids are fats; if liquid, oils. Fats contain 9 kcal/gm, and represent 42% of the American diet, higher than the dietary goal of 30% (30).

Fat not only provides fuel for energy, it is important in the absorption of fat-soluble vitamins, cell membrane structure, hormone synthesis (steroids), insulation, and protection of vital organs (29). Most fat is stored in cells in adipose tissue, for subsequent release into the bloodstream as free fatty acids (chapter 4). Because of fat's caloric density (9 kcal/gm), we are able to carry a large energy reserve, with little weight. In fact, the energy content of one pound of adipose tissue, 3,500 kcal, is sufficient to cover the cost of running a marathon. The other side of this coin is that because of this very high caloric density it takes a long time to use the energy in that adipose tissue when on a diet.

The focus of attention in the medical community has been on the role of dietary fat in the development of **atherosclerosis,** a process in which the arterial wall becomes thickened, leading to a narrowing of the lumen of the artery. This is the underlying problem associated with coronary artery disease and stroke. While the specific cause is not known, it is believed that a variety of factors can damage the protective endothelial lining of the artery, allowing substances to build up and block the artery. The factors that can accelerate this process include elevated serum cholesterol and triglycerides, high blood pressure, and cigarette smoking (35). In the section on dietary goals, two of the recommendations dealt with this problem of atherosclerosis: a reduction in salt intake (see minerals), and a reduction in fat, saturated fat, and cholesterol. A reduction in each of the last three has been shown to reduce serum cholesterol, and with it, the risk of atherosclerosis (1).

Usually the cholesterol concentration in the serum is divided into two classes on the basis of what type of **lipoprotein** is carrying the cholesterol. **Low-density lipoproteins (LDL)** carry more cholesterol than do the **high-density lipoproteins (HDL).** High levels of **LDL cholesterol** are directly related to cardiovascular risk, while high levels of **HDL cholesterol** offer protection from heart disease (1). The concentration of HDL cholesterol is influenced by heredity, gender, exercise, and diet. Diets high in saturated fats increase LDL cholesterol. A reduction in the sources of saturated fats, including meats, animal fat, palm oil, coconut oil, hydrogenated shortenings, whole milk, cream, butter, ice cream, and cheese would reduce LDL cholesterol. Just substituting unsaturated fats for these saturated fats will lower serum cholesterol. Overall, the recommendation from the American Heart Association is to lower total fat consumption from about 42% to 30% of total caloric intake. Dietary restriction of cholesterol has been shown to be effective in lowering serum cholesterol (1); however, this effect is influenced by the percentage of saturated fat in the diet and the initial level of serum cholesterol (i.e., those with high serum cholesterol levels benefit the most) (40). Based on currently available evidence, it is reasonable and prudent to recommend a decrease in cholesterol in the diet to 300 mg/day or less (1). To achieve these goals, the following suggestions were provided as part of the *Dietary Guidelines for Americans:*

- Choose lean meat, fish, poultry, and dry beans and peas as protein sources.
- Use skim or low-fat milk and milk products.
- Moderate your use of egg yolks and organ meats.
- Limit your intake of fats and oils, especially those high in saturated fat, such as butter, cream, lard, heavily hydrogenated fats (some margarines), shortenings, and foods containing palm and coconut oils.
- Trim fat off meats.
- Broil, bake, or boil rather than fry.
- Moderate your use of foods that contain fat, such as breaded and deep-fried foods.
- Read labels carefully to determine both amount and type of fat present in food.

Protein

Protein, at 4 kcal/gm, is not viewed as a primary energy source, as are fats and carbohydrates. Rather, it is important because it contains the nine essential amino acids, without which the body cannot synthesize all the protein needed for tissues, enzymes, and hormones. The *quality* of protein in a diet is based on how well these essential amino acids are represented. In terms of quality, the *best* sources for protein are eggs, milk, and fish, with *good* sources being meat, poultry, cheese, and soybeans. *Fair* sources of protein include grains, vegetables, seeds and nuts, and other legumes. Given that a meal contains a variety of foods, one food of higher quality protein tends to complement another of lower quality protein to result in an adequate intake of essential amino acids (29).

The adult RDA protein requirement of 0.8 gm/kg is easily met with diets that include a variety of the aforementioned foods. The U.S. RDA is set at 45 gm for high-quality protein and 65 gm for low-quality protein. Nutrition labels list the percent of the U.S. RDA met relative to the quality of protein in the food (29). The protein requirement is also expressed as 10%–12% of total kcal ingested. Overall, most Americans meet either of these recommendations. The protein requirement for athletes is discussed in chapter 23.

Meeting the Guidelines and Achieving the Goals

A good diet would allow an individual to achieve the RDA for protein, minerals, and vitamins, while emphasizing carbohydrates and minimizing fats. This can be accomplished by following one of the *Dietary Guidelines for Americans:* to eat a variety of foods. These guidelines (98) suggested that daily food selections should include:

- Fruits
- Vegetables
- Whole-grain and enriched breads, cereals, and other products made from grains
- Milk, cheese, yogurt, and other products made from milk
- Meats, poultry, fish, eggs, and dry beans and peas

Basic Four Food Group Plan

The Basic Four Food Group Plan is one way to follow these guidelines. Table 18.4 shows the four food groups, meat and meat substitutes, milk and milk products, fruits and vegetables, and grains, their serving size, the

Table 18.4   The Basic Four Food Group Plan

Food Group	Sample Foods and Serving Size	Number of Daily Servings for Adults	Major Nutrients
Meat and meat substitutes	2–3 oz lean meat, fish, or poultry 2 eggs 1 cup nuts ½ cup (2 oz) cottage cheese*	2	Protein, iron, niacin, and riboflavin
Milk and milk products	1 cup (8 fl oz) milk or yogurt 2 cups of cottage cheese* 1.5 cups of ice cream 2 oz cheese food*	2	Protein, calcium, riboflavin, zinc, vitamin D
Fruits and vegetables	Half cup fruit Select from citrus fruits (vitamin C) Dark green or yellow vegetables (vitamin A)	4	Vitamins A and C; Carbohydrates
Grains (breads and cereal products)	1 slice of bread 1 cup (1 oz) ready-to-eat cereal ½–¾ cup cooked cereal, macaroni, rice, or spaghetti	4	Carbohydrates, additional amounts of iron, thiamin, and niacin

*Cottage cheese can count for either the meat or the milk group.

number of servings per day, and the major nutrients supplied. The emphasis is on eating a variety of items within each group in which **nutrient density** is relatively high. Nutrient density describes the nutrient content in 1,000 kcal of a food (96). Selecting foods of high nutrient density keeps the nutrients up and total kcals down. The quantity of each item within a food group in the Basic Four Food Group Plan is based on the quantity of a *specific nutrient* contained therein. For example, the items on the milk list have the calcium content in one cup of milk, and meat portion is based on protein content.

While one can plan daily menus of 1,200–1,400 kcal using the Basic Four Food Group Plan and meet the RDA for all nutrients, it has been shown that those who regularly follow the plan might consume inadequate amounts of vitamin B-6, magnesium, iron, zinc, and vitamin E. In order to deal with these shortcomings, a modification of the Basic Four Food Group Plan has been proposed (55).

- Make the meat serving 3 oz and not 2–3 oz.
- Add two servings of legumes and/or nuts (serving size about 3/4 cup).
- Make the grain servings "whole grain" and not enriched.
- Add one serving of fat or oil for vitamin E.

A problem with this modification is that the caloric content approaches 2,200 kcal, higher than needed for some people, especially women (29, 55). One approach to deal with this is to encourage those people

Table 18.5 The six exchange groups

Group	Serving Size	Similar Foods	Carbohydrate (gm)	Protein (gm)	Fat (gm)	Energy (kcal)
Milk (skim)	1 cup	1 cup skim milk 1 cup yogurt from skim milk	12	8	Trace	90
Vegetable	½ cup	String beans Greens Carrots Beets	5	2	0	25
Fruit	1 serving	½ small banana 1 small apple ½ grapefruit ½ cup orange juice	15	0	0	60
Bread (starch)	1 slice	¾ cup ready-to-eat cereal ½ cup beans ⅓ cup corn 1 small potato	15	3	Trace	80
Meat (lean)	1 oz	1 oz chicken meat, w/o skin 1 oz fish ¼ cup canned tuna, or salmon 1 oz low-fat cheese (<5% butterfat)	0	7	3	55
Fat	1 tsp	1 tsp margarine 1 tsp oil 1 tbsp salad dressing 1 strip crisp bacon	0	0	5	45

who live on 1,900 kcal/day to expend 300 kcal in exercise so they can consume more calories and more easily meet the RDA for nutrients (96).

Exchange System

Another method of planning a diet is the Exchange System. In this system the *caloric content and the percent of carbohydrate, fat, and protein* in each food is the focus of attention, rather than the nutrient density as in the Basic Four Food Group Plan. Foods in each group in the Exchange System would be similar in these characteristics. There are six groups, and table 18.5 shows the breakdown for each. This system is useful in weight control programs since the focus of attention is on calories. By knowing how many "exchanges" from each group are contained in the diet, the caloric content is known. Table 18.6 shows how the Basic Four Food Group Plan and the Exchange System can be used to meet dietary goals (55).

Table 18.6 Using the Basic Four Food Group Plan and an Exchange System to meet dietary goals

Four Food Group Plan	Exchange System	Example	Calories
Milk—2 servings	Milk group—select 2 exchanges	1 cup skim milk 1 cup low-fat yogurt	180
Meat—2 servings	Lean meat Group—select 6 exchanges†	2 oz chicken 2 oz low-fat cheese* 2 oz 95% fat-free luncheon meat	330
Fruits and vegetables—4 servings	Fruits and Vegetables— select 4 exchanges	½ cup cabbage 1 large tomato ½ grapefruit ½ cup orange juice	50 120
Grains (breads and cereal products)—4 servings	Bread Group—select 4 exchanges	2 slices whole wheat bread ½ cup shredded wheat ½ cup cooked pasta	320
		Total	1,000

†In exchange system one serving is equal to 1 oz.
*In exchange system cheese counts as a protein source.

Evaluating the Diet

Independent of your dietary plan, the question arises as to how well you are achieving the guidelines. How do you analyze your diet? The first thing to do is to determine what you are eating, without fooling yourself. The use of the **twenty-four-hour recall** method relies on your ability to remember, from a specific time in one day, what you ate during the previous twenty-four hours. You have to judge the size of the portion you have eaten and make a judgement of whether or not that day was representative of what you normally eat. Other people use **food records,** in which a person records what is eaten throughout the day. It is recommended that a person obtain samples from two weekdays and one weekend day to have a better estimate of usual dietary intake (29, 55). It is important to remember that the RDA standards are to be met over the long run, and variations from those standards

will exist from day to day. When you collect your information you record it on a form used for dietary analysis. Appendix H shows such a form with food items listed, and the nutrients and calories associated with each item. The summary at the bottom of the chart allows you to determine whether or not you are meeting the RDA standards and are achieving the *Dietary Guidelines for Americans.*

Body Composition

Obesity is a major problem in our society, being related to hypertension, elevated serum cholesterol, and adult onset diabetes (67). In addition, there is growing concern that the increase in childhood obesity is going to increase this pool of obese adults. In order to deal with this problem we must be able to monitor changes in body fatness throughout life and evaluate the effectiveness of diet and exercise in dealing with this problem. This section will present a brief overview of the different methods used in body composition analysis, provide detailed explanations of the most common methods, and discuss the role of diet and exercise in weight control.

Methods of Measuring Body Composition

The Metropolitan Life Insurance Company's 1959 height/weight table (89) is one of the most common methods used to make judgements about whether or not a person is overweight (table 18.7). These tables are based on that company's policyholders, and the body weights associated with the lowest rate of mortality are listed by frame size. In 1983 an updated table was published that allowed more weight at each height. While Andres (4) found support for such adjustments, the American Heart Association continues to recommend the 1959 table. It has been suggested that the lower death rates at the higher weights in the 1983 table are a result of better treatment of CHD and diabetes, which allows heavier people to live longer; a reduction in cigarette smoking; and an increase in physical activity (41).

Independent of which table is used, there are some problems associated with their use:

1. persons seeking and receiving insurance are not representative of the general population.
2. some persons are represented more than once in the table, since policies (not people) were tabulated.
3. heights and weights were not measured in every case (some policyholders simply stated these), and
4. body frame size was not measured (4).

In spite of these limitations, one of the most common indices of body composition is calculated from this table. In this procedure the midpoint in the weight range for a medium frame for a given height is used as a standard against which other body weights are compared. Dividing a person's weight by the midpoint in the weight range generates a relative weight (RW) or obesity index. A person with a body weight equal to the midpoint value would have a RW = 1.00. In contrast, if we look at the 1959 table (table 18.7), a man who is six feet tall and weighs 200 lbs, has a RW = 1.23 (200 lb ÷ 163.5 lb). A person who is 10% above normal (RW = 1.10) is classified as overweight, and if 20% above normal (RW = 1.20), is classified as obese. Our male subject at 23% above normal would be classified as obese.

The problem, of course, is that with height/weight tables there is no way to know if the person is heavily muscled or simply overfat. One of the earliest uses of body composition analysis showed that with height/weight tables "All American" football players weighing 200 lbs would have been found unfit for military service and would not have received life insurance (136). Clearly there is a need to distinguish overweight from overfat, and that will be the purpose of the next section of this chapter.

The most direct way to measure body composition is to do a chemical analysis of the whole body to determine the amount of water, fat, protein, and minerals. This is a common method used in nutritional studies on rats, but is useless in providing information for the average person. The following is a brief summary of techniques providing information about (1) the composition of the whole body and (2) the development or change in specific tissues of the body.

Isotope Dilution:
Total body water (TBW) is determined by the isotope dilution method. In this method a subject drinks an isotope of water (tritiate water—^3H_2O), deuterated water (^2H_2O), or ^{18}O-labeled water ($H_2^{18}O$) that is distributed throughout the body water. After three to four hours to allow for distribution of the isotope, a sample of body fluid (serum or saliva) is obtained and the concentration of the isotope is determined. The volume of TBW is obtained by calculating how much body water would be needed to achieve that concentration. A person with a large amount of body water will dilute the isotope to a greater extent. People with large TBW volumes possess more lean tissue and less fat tissue, so TBW can be used to determine body fatness (42, 112).

Table 18.7 Desirable weights for men and women, twenty-five years of age and over

Height* Feet	Inches	Small Frame	Medium Frame	Large Frame
Men				
5	2	112–120	118–129	126–141
5	3	115–123	121–133	129–144
5	4	118–126	124–136	132–148
5	5	121–129	127–139	135–152
5	6	124–133	130–143	138–156
5	7	128–137	134–147	142–161
5	8	132–141	138–152	147–166
5	9	136–145	142–156	151–170
5	10	140–150	146–160	155–174
5	11	144–154	150–165	159–179
6	0	148–158	154–170	164–184
6	1	152–162	158–175	168–189
6	2	156–167	162–180	173–194
6	3	160–171	167–185	178–199
6	4	164–175	172–190	182–204

Height** Feet	Inches	Small Frame	Medium Frame	Large Frame
Women				
4	10	92–98	96–107	104–119
4	11	94–101	98–110	106–122
5	0	96–104	101–113	109–125
5	1	99–107	104–116	112–128
5	2	102–110	107–119	115–131
5	3	105–113	110–122	118–134
5	4	108–116	113–126	121–138
5	5	111–119	116–130	125–142
5	6	114–123	120–135	129–146
5	7	118–127	124–139	133–150
5	8	122–131	128–143	137–154
5	9	126–135	132–147	141–158
5	10	130–140	136–151	145–163
5	11	134–144	140–155	149–168
6	0	138–148	144–159	153–173

*With shoes with one-inch heels.
**With shoes with two-inch heels.
Metropolitan Insurance Companies, New York, N.Y.

Photon Absorptiometry:
A method in which the density of bones is determined. A beam of photons from iodine-125 is passed over a bone or bones, and the transmission of the photon beam through bone and soft tissue is obtained. There is a very strong positive relationship between the absorption of the photons and the density of the bones (27).

Potassium-40:
Potassium is located primarily within the cells, along with a naturally occurring radioactive isotope of potassium: ^{40}K. The ^{40}K can be measured in a whole-body "counter," and is proportional to the mass of lean tissue.

Hydrostatic (Underwater) Weighing:
Water has a density of about 1 gm/ml, and body fat, with a density of about 0.900 gm/ml, will float on water. Lean tissue has a density of about 1.100 in adults and will sink in water. Whole body density provides information about the portion of the body that is lean and fat. Underwater weighing methods are commonly used to determine body density (141), and will be discussed in more detail.

Radiography:
An x-ray of a limb allows one to measure the widths of fat, muscle, and bone, and has been used extensively in tracing the growth of these tissues over time (65). Fat-width measurements can also be used to estimate total body fat (44, 68).

Ultrasound:
Sound waves are transmitted through tissues and the echoes are received and analyzed. This technique has been used to measure the thickness of subcutaneous fat. Present technology allows for whole body scans and the determination of the volumes of various organs (57).

Nuclear Magnetic Resonance (NMR):
In this method electromagnetic waves are transmitted through tissues. Select nuclei absorb and then release energy at a particular frequency (resonance). The resonant-frequency characteristics are related to the type of tissue, and computer analysis of the signal can provide detailed images and calculate the volumes of specific tissues (57).

Total Body Electrical Conductivity (TOBEC):
Body composition is analyzed by TOBEC on the basis that lean tissue and water conduct electricity better than does fat. In this method the subject lies in a large cylindrical coil while an electric current is injected into the coil. The electromagnetic field developed in the space enclosed by the cylindrical coil is affected by the subject's body composition (108, 115, 131).

Bioelectrical Impedance Analysis (BIA):
The basis for BIA is similar to that of TOBEC, but uses a small portable instrument. An electrical current is applied to an extremity and resistance to that current (primarily due to fat content) is measured (115, 131).

Skinfold Thickness:
An estimate of total body fatness is made from a measure of the subcutaneous fat. A number of skinfold measurements are obtained and the values used in equations to calculate body density (81).

Some of these procedures are expensive in terms of personnel and equipment (e.g., potassium-40, TOBEC, radiography, ultrasound, NMR, TBW), and are not used on a routine basis for body composition analysis. BIA shows some promise (82), but there is a need to develop and validate equations on different populations before recommending its widespread use. Two approaches that are used extensively include the **underwater weighing** and skinfold methods. In both of these methods the investigator obtains a measure of **whole body density,** and from this calculates the percentage of the body that is fat and the percentage that is fat free. This is the two-component body composition system described by Behnke that is commonly used to describe changes in body composition. The underwater weighing and skinfold techniques will be described in detail, after a brief discussion of how density values are converted to percent body fat and percent fat-free values.

Two-Component System of Body Composition

The conversion of whole body density values to fat and fat-free tissue components relies on "constants" used for each of those tissue components. Human fat tissue is believed to have a density of 0.900 gm/ml, and fat-free tissue, a density of 1.100 gm/ml. Using these density values, Siri (120) derived an equation to calculate percent body fat from whole body density:

$$\% \text{ body fat} = \frac{495}{\text{Density}} - 450$$

This equation is correct only if the density values for fat tissue and fat-free tissue are 0.900 and 1.100 gm/ml, respectively. Investigators sensed that certain populations might have fat-free tissue densities different from that of 1.100 gm/ml when they observed high values for body fatness for children and the elderly, and extremely low values (<0% body fat) in professional football players (141). Children have lower bone mineral contents, less potassium, and more water per unit fat-free mass, yielding a lower density for fat-free mass (83). Lohman (78) reports density values (gm/ml) of 1.080 at age six, 1.084 at age ten, and 1.097 for boys aged fifteen and one half. The lower values in the prepubescent child would overestimate percent body fat by 5%. Lohman recommends the following modification of Siri's equation for prepubescent children nine to eleven years of age (78, 80).

$$\% \text{ fat} = \frac{530}{\text{Density}} - 489$$

Recommendations were also made relative to other populations having different density values for fat-free tissue. Women have less bone mineral content per unit fat-free mass, even as adults. Lohman (78, 80) recommends the following equation for young adult females:

$$\% \text{ body fat} = \frac{509}{\text{Density}} - 465$$

In contrast to the children and women who had density values below 1.100 for the fat-free mass, Blacks were shown to have a density of 1.113 gm/cc (114). The Siri equation would have to be modified as follows:

$$\% \text{ body fat} = \frac{437}{\text{Density}} - 393$$

While this may appear to be quite complicated, there is good reason to have the correct equation for a specific population. If judgements are to be made about the distribution of obesity in our society, it is nice to not be off by 5% in estimating body fatness. The following sections will discuss how whole body density values are determined by underwater weighing and skinfold procedures.

Underwater Weighing

Density is equal to mass divided by volume (D = M/V). Since we already know body mass (body weight), we only have to determine body volume in order to calculate whole body density (49). The underwater weighing method applies Archimedes' principle, which states that when an object is placed in water it is bouyed up by a counterforce equal to the water it displaces (106). The volume of water displaced (spilled over) would equal the *loss of weight* while the object is completely submerged. Some investigators determine body volume by measuring the actual volume of water displaced; others measure weight while the subject is underwater, and obtain body volume by subtracting the weight measured in water (M_W) from that measured in air (M_A) or ($M_A - M_W$). Both methods of determining volume are reproducible, but percent body fat values are slightly but significantly (0.7%) lower with the volume displacement method (134). The weight of water displaced is converted to a volume by dividing by the density of the water (D_W) at the time of measurement.

$$D = \frac{M}{V} = \frac{M_A}{\dfrac{(M_A - M_W)}{D_W}}$$

This denominator must now be corrected for two other volumes: the volume of air in the lungs at the time of measurement (usually residual volume (V_R)), and the volume of gas in the gastrointestinal tract (V_{GI}). It is recommended that V_R be measured at the time that underwater weight is measured, but measurement on land with the subject in the same position is a suitable alternative (78). Residual volume can also be estimated with gender-specific regression equations, or by taking 24% (males) or 28% (females) of vital capacity. However, the latter two procedures introduce measurement errors of 2%–3% for a given individual (94). V_{GI} can be quite variable, and while some investigators ignore this measure, others assume a 100 ml volume for all subjects.

The density equation can now be rewritten (24).

$$D = \frac{M}{V} = \frac{M_A}{\dfrac{(M_A - M_W)}{D_W} - V_R - V_{GI}}$$

Figure 18.2 shows the equipment used to measure underwater weight. Water temperature is measured to obtain the correct water density. The subject is weighed on land on a scale accurate to within 100 gms. The subject puts on a diver's belt with sufficient weight to prevent floating during the weighing procedure, and sits on the chair suspended from the precision scale. The scale can be read to 10 gms, and has 50 gms major divisions. The subject sits on the chair with the water at chin level and as a maximal exhalation is just about completed, the subject bends over and pulls the head under. When a maximal expiration is achieved, the subject holds that position for about five to ten seconds while the investigator reads the scale. This procedure is repeated six to ten times until the values stabilize. The weight of the diver's belt and chair are subtracted from this weight to obtain the true value for M_W. If V_R were to be measured at the time underwater weight is measured, the subject would have to be breathing through a mouthpiece and valve assembly that could be activated at the correct time (106).

The following data were obtained on a white male, aged thirty-six: $M_A = 75.20$ kg, $M_W = 3.52$ kg, $V_R = 1.43$ liters, $D_W = 0.9944$ at 34° C, $V_{GI} = 0.1$ liters.

$$D = \frac{75.20}{\dfrac{(75.20 - 3.52)}{.9944} - 1.43 - 0.1}$$

$$= \frac{75.20}{70.55} = 1.066$$

This density value is now used in Siri's equation to calculate percent body fat.

$$\% \text{ body fat} = \frac{495}{D} - 450$$

$$14.3\% = \frac{495}{1.066} - 450$$

The underwater weighing procedure in which RV is measured (and not estimated) is the "standard" against which other methods are compared. However, remember that due to the normal biological variability in the fat-free mass in a given population the percent body fat value is estimated to be within ±2.5% of the "true" value (81).

Sum of Skinfolds

Underwater weighing, although a good way to obtain a measurement of body density, is time consuming and requires special equipment and personnel. Paralleling the development of the advanced technologies used in body composition analysis, scientists developed equations that predicted body density from a collection of skinfold measurements. The skinfold method relies on the observation that within any population a certain fraction of the total body fat lies just under the skin (subcutaneous fat), and if one could obtain a representative sample of that fat, overall body fatness (density) could be predicted. Generally, these prediction equations were developed with the underwater weighing method used as the standard. For example, a group of college males and females would have body density measured by underwater weighing, and a variety of skinfold measures would also be obtained. The

Figure 18.2 The underwater weighing technique illustrating two individuals with the same weight and height, but different body composition.

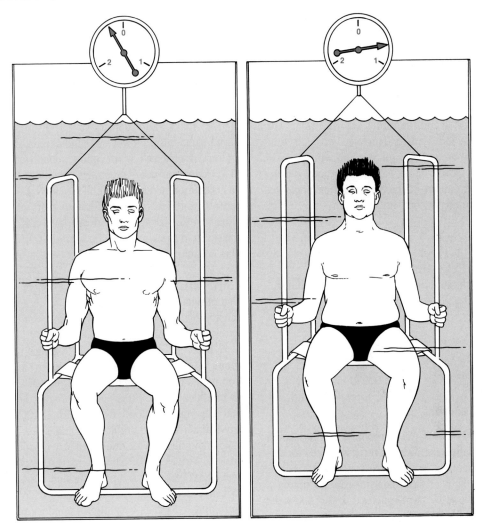

investigator would then determine what collection of skinfolds would most accurately predict the body density determined by underwater weighing.

Investigators found that the subcutaneous fat represented a variable fraction of total fat (20%–70%), depending on age, sex, overall fatness, and the measurement technique used. At a specific body fatness women have less subcutaneous fat than men, and older

subjects of the same sex have less than younger subjects (81). Given that these variables could influence an estimate of body density, it is no surprise that of the more than 100 equations developed, most were found to be "population specific" and could not be used for groups of different ages or sex. This obviously creates problems for exercise leaders in adult fitness programs or elementary or high school physical education teachers when they try to find the equation that works best for their particular group. Fortunately, a good deal of progress has been made to reduce these problems.

Jackson and Pollock (63) and Jackson, Pollock, and Ward (62) have provided "generalized equations" for men and women, that is, equations that could be used across various age groups. In addition, these equations have been validated for athletic and nonathletic populations, including postpubescent athletes (78, 118, 119). In these equations specific skinfold measurements are obtained and the values are used along with age to calculate body density. Here are two such equations, one for men and one for women, which can be used to predict body density (63). The body density value obtained is used in the Siri equation presented earlier to calculate % body fat.

Men

$$Density = 1.1125025 - 0.0013125 (X_1)$$
$$+ 0.0000055 (X_1)^2 - 0.0002440 (X_2)$$

Where X_1 = sum of chest, triceps, subscapular skinfolds, and X_2 = age in years.

Women

$$Density = 1.089733 - 0.0009245 (X_1)$$
$$+ 0.0000025 (X_1)^2 - 0.0000979 (X_2)$$

Where X_1 = sum of triceps, suprailium, and abdominal skinfolds, and X_2 = age in years.

Jackson and Pollock (63) simplified this procedure by providing tabulated % body fatness values for different skinfold thicknesses across age. All that is needed is the sum of skinfolds in order to obtain a % body fatness value. Appendixes I and J show the % body fat tables for men and women, respectively, using the sum of three skinfolds. For example, a woman, aged twenty-five, with a sum of skinfolds equal to 50 mm has % body fat equal to 22.9% (look to the right of the sum of skinfold column where 48–52 is shown, over to the second column—ages 23–27). Estimates of % body fatness from skinfold measures has an error of about ± 3.7% (79).

The use of skinfold measurements was extended to children in the schools for early identification of obesity. The American Alliance for Health, Physical Education, Recreation and Dance (3) developed the Health-Related Fitness Test to evaluate cardiorespiratory function, low back function, and body fatness. The body fatness assessment relied on a tricep and/or subscapular skinfold(s), and percentile norms were developed. The scientists who designed this test could not provide % body fatness values because the assumption that the fat-free mass had a density of 1.100 gm/cc was believed to be false. However, as indicated earlier, based on recent research with young populations the Siri (121) equation used to convert density to % body fat has been modified for these children (78). Lohman (82) recently published charts for two pairs of skinfolds, triceps plus subscapular or triceps plus calf, that relate the skinfold thickness to % fat for children. The triceps plus subscapular standards are shown in figure 18.3.

Body Fatness for Health and Fitness

The previous sections showed how to determine body density by underwater weighing and skinfold procedures. This information on body density is converted to % body fat and can be used to make judgements about one's status relative to health and fitness. Lohman (82) recommends a range of 10%–20% as an optimal health and fitness goal for males. He indicates that this range allows for individual differences in physical activity and preferences, and is associated with little or no health risk due to diseases associated with fatness. Values above 20% increase the risks of diabetes, heart disease, and hypertension. Values of 20%–25% are considered moderately high, 25%–31% as high, and >31% as very high. Females are generally about 3% fatter than males prior to puberty and 11% fatter after puberty. The optimal range of body fat for adult females is 15%–25%, with 25%–30% listed as moderately high, 30%–35% as high, and >35% as very high (82).

Now that we know how to obtain a % body fatness measure, and what the optimal % body fat values are, how can we determine what the optimal body weight

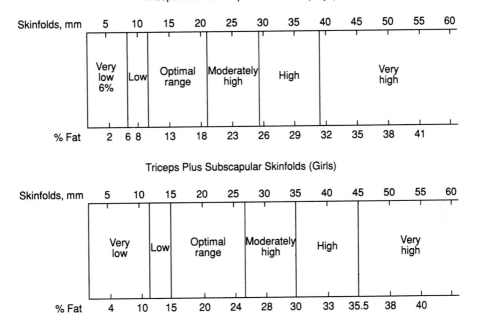

Figure 18.3 Estimation of percent body fat in boys and girls on the basis of the sum of the triceps and subscapular skinfolds. This figure shows fatness values that are too low, as well as those that are too high.

range is? In the following example a female college student has 30% body fat and weighs 142 lbs. Her optimal % fat range is 15%–25%.

Step 1. Calculate fat-free weight:

100% − 30% fat = 70% fat free
70% × 142 lb = 99.4 lb fat-free weight

Step 2. Optimal weight = fat-free weight/(1 − optimal % fat), with optimal % fat expressed as a fraction:

For 15% = 99.4 lb/(1 − .15) = 117 lb;
for 25% = 99.4 lb/(1 − .25) = 132.5 lb
Her optimal weight range is 117–133 lb

Lohman (82) also indicates on his charts (figure 18.3) values for % body fat that are below the optimal range. There is a great pressure in our society to be thin, and this can be carried to an extreme. A far too common problem in our high schools and colleges is **anorexia nervosa,** in which young females (usually) have an exaggerated fear of getting fat. This fear leads to food restriction, increased exercise, and use of laxatives in an attempt to stay thin. Some practice **bulimia** in which large quantities of food are taken in, only to be vomited. These practices lead to such an emaciated state that amenorrhea may occur, and have resulted in death in 5% of the cases (31, 43). The low and very low % body fat values on Lohman's charts are consistent with a way to monitor the movements of people toward these dangerous conditions.

It is clear that to stay in the optimal % body fat range an individual must balance the dietary consumption of calories with energy expenditure. We will now consider that topic.

Obesity and Weight Control

In chapter 14 we discussed the major risk factors associated with degenerative diseases. While high blood pressure, cigarette smoking, and elevated serum cholesterol are the three primary risk factors (107), more and more evidence points to obesity as being a separate independent factor, or one directly tied to two of the above primary risk factors. Two separate epidemiological studies found that increases in relative weight or body mass index (MBI = wt [kg] ÷ ht [m²]) were related to an increase in the risk of heart disease (67, 109). Data from the Framingham Heart Study showed that relative weight was positively related to high serum triglycerides, total cholesterol (with lower HDL), and uric acid, elevated blood pressure, and a greater degree of glucose intolerance (67). The following is a summary of the diseases that are believed to be caused by or associated with obesity (110).

Causal

1. Diseases or conditions in which obesity is a *primary contributing factor:* adult-onset diabetes, menstrual abnormalities, reproductive problems, heart size and function, arthritis, gout, and hypertension.
2. Diseases or conditions in which obesity is a *secondary contributing factor:* endometrial carcinoma.

Assocation

1. Diseases or conditions that are correlated with obesity, but not caused by obesity: atherosclerotic disease, gallbladder disease, and death.

As mentioned earlier, in spite of this information, the 1983 height/weight table of the Metropolitan Life Insurance Company listed higher weights at each height as being associated with lower death rates. In response, a twenty-six-year follow-up study of participants in the Framingham Heart Study recommended against this revision of the height/weight table with data indicating that higher relative weight was associated with increases in cardiovascular diseases (CVD)

and death from CVD (60). The reason for the confusion was that the death rate was actually decreasing while the relative weight was increasing. The decrease in the death rate was believed to be due to decreases in cigarette smoking and improved health care and not the fact that people were fatter (41). It has been suggested that the better treatments available for those with diabetes and heart disease allows them to live longer at the higher body weights. It is a case of where the *average* body weight of a group is not the *optimal* weight for low risk of disease. In fact, Kannel and Gordon (67) have stated that ". . . if everyone were at optimal weight we would have 25% less coronary heart disease and 35% less congestive heart failure and brain infarctions" (67).

Obesity

Obesity refers to the percent of the body weight that is fat, usually >25% for men and >30% for women. However, all obesity is not the same. Recent studies suggest that it is not only the relative body fatness that is related to an increased risk of CVD, but that the distribution of that fatness must also be considered. Individuals with a large waist circumference compared to hip circumference had higher risk of CVD. These data suggest that in addition to skinfold or underwater weighing estimates of body density, measurements of waist and hip circumferences should also be obtained (76, 77). Ratios of waist to hip circumference >1.0 for men and >0.8 for women are associated with an increased risk of CVD, and such individuals are treated even if only borderline obese (10).

In addition to fat tissue distribution, there is a need to determine whether the obesity is due to an increase in the amount of fat in each fat cell (hypertrophic obesity), or an increase in the number of fat cells (hyperplastic obesity), or both. In moderate obesity where the mass of adipose tissue is less than 30 kg, the increase in fat cell size appears to be the primary means of storing the additional fat. Beyond that the cell number is the variable most strongly related to the mass of adipose tissue (12, 58). This is shown in figure 18.4

Figure 18.4 Relationship of fat cell size and fat cell number to total kilograms of body fat. Fat cell size is given in μg of fat, and fat cell number in billions of cells. The increase in body fatness beyond about 30 kg of fat is directly related to an increasing fat cell number; fat cell size remains relatively constant.

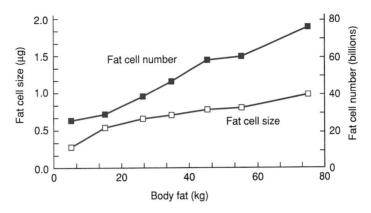

where cell size increases up to about 30-kg body fat, and does not significantly change thereafter. In contrast, fat cell number is strongly related to the mass of adipose tissue (122).

There are about 25 billion fat cells in a normal-weight individual versus 60–80 billion in the extremely obese (12, 58, 122). When a person undergoes dietary restriction, the size of the fat cells decrease but the number does not (12, 58). This high fat cell number is believed to be related to the difficulty obese patients have in maintaining body weight once it has been lost. Figure 18.5 shows the pattern of weight loss, maintenance, and gain of groups classified as having obesity that is hyperplastic, hypertrophic, or both. A "borderline" obese group is also represented. Those with hyperplastic obesity or combined hyperplastic and hypertropic obesity lost weight quickly, kept it off for only a short period of time, and regained it at a high rate. At this point we have seen that dieting does not change fat cell number, and that those who possess a high number of fat cells have difficulty maintaining a reduced body weight. The next question to consider is, when does the fat cell number increase?

In a longitudinal study of children during the first eighteen months of life, the fat cell number did not increase during the first twelve months, the increase in cell size being entirely responsible for the increase in body fat. In contrast, the gain in body fat from twelve to eighteen months was due entirely to an increase in fat cell number with cell size remaining stable (53). When these data were plotted along with data from other studies, the results indicated that cell number increases throughout growth (53, 58). Given that physical activity and dietary intervention in grossly obese young children (eight years old) can slow the rate of growth in fat cell number (52), and that the fat cell number is tied to the inability of obese children to lose their obesity as adults, the emphasis on treatment during childhood is obvious. Unfortunately, in spite of our understanding of the problem, the prevalence of pediatric obesity has increased by 54% among six- to eleven-year-olds and by 39% among twelve- to seventeen-year-olds over the past fifteen to twenty years (72). What causes obesity?

There is clearly no single cause of obesity. Obesity is related to both genetic and environmental variables. In 1965 Mayer (85) commented on the numerous studies showing that 70%–80% of obese children had at least one obese parent, but concluded that it was difficult to interpret those data given the way cultural background interacts with genetics. In effect, the need to do hard physical work in some countries, or extreme social pressure against obesity (discussed later), might not allow a genetic predisposition to express itself. Garn

Figure 18.5 Patterns of weight loss and gain for obese individuals classified as being borderline obese, or having hypertropic, or hyperplastic obesity or both. Those with combined or hyperplastic obesity regained their weight sooner, and at a higher rate than those with hypertropic obesity.

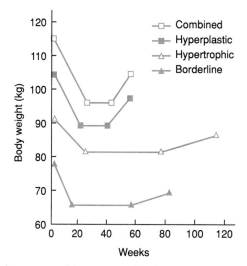

Schematic summary of the mean results of treatment for the four obese groups

and Clark (45) found a strong relationship between parental fatness and the fatness of children. They identified three categories of fatness on the basis of triceps skinfold: lean = <15th percentile; medium = 15th–85th percentile, and obese = >85th percentile. Figure 18.6 shows that parental fatness was related to the fatness of the child. While this might imply that a genetic link exists, when the investigators compared husbands to wives (usually no genetic tie), the relationship was similar to that for their children, suggesting either that there was a tendency of like to mate like, or that communal living exerts a major influence.

A powerful set of data bearing on the topic of genetics and obesity was provided when adopted children (90% placed in first year) were compared, as adults, to their biological and adopted parents (127). On the basis of a completed health questionnaire they were classified as thin (≤4th percentile), median (50th percentile), overweight (92nd–96th percentile), and obese (>96th percentile) using the body mass index (wt. (kg) ÷ ht(m²)). Figure 18.7 shows a strong relationship between the adoptee's weight class and the biological parents' body mass index. There was no relationship between the weight class of the adoptees and the body mass index of the adoptive parents (127). These data suggest a strong genetic component in the determination of adult body mass.

These data would appear to minimize the role of the environment, but the senior author of that study, Stunkard, believed that if the same measurements were

Figure 18.6 Fatness of boys and girls compared to parental fatness combinations. Childhood fatness increases from the lean X lean parent pair, to the obese X obese parent pair.

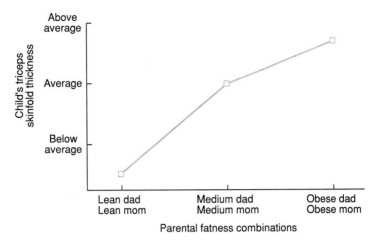

Figure 18.7 Comparison of body mass index of biological and adoptive parents with the adoptee's weight class. In the figure on the left, there is a strong relationship between the weight class of the adoptees and their biological parents. This relationship was not shown for the adoptive parents.

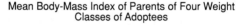

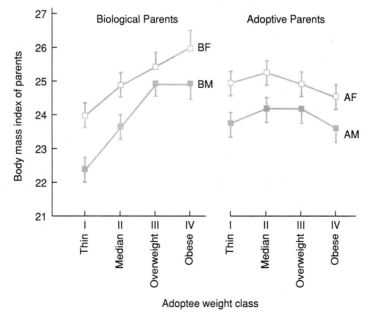

Note the increase in mean body-mass index of biological parents with the increase in weight class of the adoptees. No such increase was found with adoptive parents. Bars represent 1 SEM. BF denotes biological fathers, BM biological mothers, AF adoptive fathers, and AM adoptive mothers.

Figure 18.8 Physiological set point for control of body weight by altering feeding behavior showing the glucostatic (blood glucose), lipostatic (adipose tissue), and ponderostatic (weight) input to the hypothalamus. The signals from these latter mechanisms are compared against a "set-point," and an appropriate increase or decrease in feeding behavior occurs. In this model, exercise can modify the input, and the type of diet can modify feeding behavior.

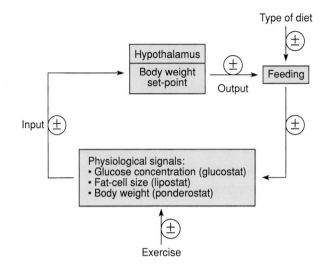

taken on the adoptees when they were with the adoptive parents, a relationship would have been found (72). Further, a co-author, Sorensen, observed an eight-fold increase in obesity in army inductees over a fifteen-year period, too short a time for a change in the gene pool (72). Lastly, observations supporting Mayer's comment that culture might not allow expression of a genetic trait for obesity is found in the relationship of obesity with socioeconomic class. In American women, obesity is inversely related to socioeconomic class: 30% for lower, 18% for middle, and 5% for the upper class (48). Further, women and adolescent girls have been shown to suffer the most direct discrimination because of this obesity (133). Clearly, while we may possess a genetic predisposition for obesity, there are a variety of social factors that influence its appearance.

Set Point and Obesity

Obese individuals, as previously mentioned, have a great deal of difficulty maintaining a reduced weight. In fact, the tendency of a person to return to a certain weight suggests that there is a biological set point for body weight much like the set points for any negative feedback biological control system. While the hypothalamus contains centers associated with satiety and feeding behavior, please understand that the *body weight set point is a concept, rather than a reality* (13). Figure 18.8 shows a physiological model of a body weight set point in which biological signals with regard to blood glucose (glucostatic signal), lipid stores (lipostatic signal), or weight on feet (ponderostatic signal) provide input to the hypothalamus (13). If the collective signals indicate low energy stores, food intake is stimulated until the source of the signal is diminished and the energy stores now equal the set point. Like any biological control system, if the set point were to be increased, body weight would increase to meet this new value. Exercise can modify the signals going to the hypothalamus, and the type of diet can also influence feeding behavior.

In contrast to this physiological model, Booth's cognitive set-point model (13) deals with the role the environment (culture, socioeconomic class, etc.) has on body weight. Figure 18.9 shows that relative to a personally selected "ideal" body weight set point we are constantly receiving a variety of cognitive signals about

Figure 18.9 Cognitive set point for control of body weight by altering feeding behavior. A person's perception of "ideal" body weight is balanced against signals about how one looks, body weight, clothing, size, etc. Exercise can modify the input, and the type of diet can modify feeding behavior.

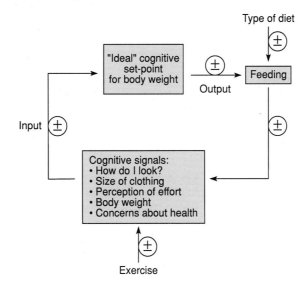

how we look, body weight, clothing size, perception of effort, and concerns about health. A mismatch between the "ideal" set point and these perceptions leads to appropriate eating behavior. Exercise can modify the signals, and the type of diet can influence the feeding behavior. This set-point model is closely related to the behavior modification approach to diet, exercise, and weight control.

Diet, Exercise, and Weight Control

The energy balance equation is a very simple one. Energy balance is achieved when caloric intake equals caloric expenditure. If intake is greater than expenditure a weight gain occurs, and vice versa. The Framingham Heart Study showed that body weight increases as we age. A reasonable question to ask is whether this gain in weight was due to an increase in caloric intake. Interestingly, caloric intake decreased over the same age span (16). We are forced to conclude that energy expenditure has decreased faster than the decrease in caloric intake, and as a result, weight gain has occurred. This weight gain problem can be corrected by understanding and dealing with one or both sides of the energy balance equation. We will first deal with how modifications in energy intake can affect weight loss, and then we will explore the variables on the energy expenditure side of the equation.

Energy Intake

Dieting has become an American cultural phenomenon as people try to deal with the energy intake side of the energy balance equation. The caloric value of 1 lb (454 gm) of adipose tissue is about 3,500 kcal, so a negative energy balance of 500 kcal per day should result in the loss of 1 lb per week. Before we describe the various classes of diets, there are a few general points that must be considered. The rate of weight loss in the first days of a diet will be greater than later in the dietary period. This is because there is a reduction in the carbohydrate store and lean tissue mass at the onset of a diet. As mentioned earlier in this chapter, 1 gm of carbohydrate requires 2.7 gms of water for storage. When this carbohydrate store is decreased at the onset of a diet, the water is lost with it, giving the appearance of a large fat loss. In addition, lean tissue will be lost during a diet and the caloric value of that tissue is only about one-third that of fat tissue. Consequently, in the first 3,500 kcal deficit more than 1 lb will be lost. As the diet continues, the rate of weight loss will slow down. This is because adipose tissue (at 7,700 kcal/kg) represents more of the tissue loss, and the low caloric diet has an effect on the energy expenditure side of the equation (see later discussion). The lean tissue loss could equal as much as 50% of the total weight loss during starvation (6), and about 35% during simple dietary restriction (21). In the starvation study, the parallel loss of lean and fat tissue left some subjects with the same % body fat at the end of weeks of starvation! When refeeding took place there was a rapid gain in body weight related to the replacement of lean tissue.

Diets

Table 18.8 presents a brief summary of the types of diets used in weight-loss programs and their characteristics. These diets may be balanced with regard to the major nutrients, and some may be taken in liquid form. This latter characteristic reduces the need to count calories, is easier to follow, but is monotonous (130). The unbalanced diets vary the proportion of carbohydrate and protein, or may include some exotic food items. Low-carbohydrate, low-calorie diets promote **ketosis,** the production of short-chain fatty acids, which may depress appetite. These diets cause a rapid weight loss due to carbohydrate depletion and a diuresis associated with the need to excrete the ketones. In addition, the low carbohydrate diets do not maintain the body's lean body mass as well as balanced diets of the same caloric content. In general, while low-calorie balanced diets containing more than 800 kcal/day can be used safely, the low-carbohydrate ketogenic diets can cause weakness, apathy, fatigue, vomiting, dehydration, and postural hypotension (130).

The low-calorie diet may be the result of the addition of fiber-rich foods to increase the bulk, which gives one the feeling of fullness without the calorie load. These diets would include the substitution of diet drinks for regular drinks, and skim milk for whole milk.

The last category, fasting, includes both total fasting and supplemental fasting. In supplemental fasting the patient receives about 30–45 gm protein and 20–30 gm carbohydrate per day, along with vitamins and minerals. These approaches are used with the very obese and require direct medical supervision. It must also be remembered that considerable lean body mass is lost with such approaches (130).

There is a clear need to choose a diet that is balanced and causes a small but systematic negative energy balance. One of the *Dietary Guidelines for Americans* was to maintain desirable weight. The recommendations to avoid overeating included: eating slowly, taking smaller portions, and avoiding "seconds." Further, to lose weight the following suggestions were made:

- Eat a variety of foods that are low in calories and high in nutrients.
- Eat more fruits, vegetables, and whole grains.
- Eat less fat, and fatty foods.
- Eat less sugar and sweets.
- Drink less alcoholic beverages.
- Increase your physical activity.

Remember that an energy deficit of about 500 kcal/day will result in the loss of one pound per week, a reasonable rate that will allow one to gradually control what and how one eats. Both of these elements are needed for long term weight control.

Behavior Modification

Behavior modification programs related to weight loss focus on *how* to eat rather than simply on *what* to eat (20). These programs have been shown to be as effective as traditional weight-loss programs (126), and there are no adverse side effects since inappropriate ketogenic diets are avoided.

The behavior modification process begins when an individual has a desire to reduce weight and follows through by recording current food consumption patterns for two to three weeks on a form listing not only what was eaten and the caloric value of the food stuff, but also an identification of the circumstances around which the food was eaten (e.g., time, place, persons,

Table 18.8 Categories of weight-loss diets

Type of Diet	Description	Characteristic(s)
I. Nutritionally Balanced		
Unrestricted calories	Liquid homogenate	Monotonous
Restricted calories: Varied items	Mixed low-calorie diet (800–1,200 kcal)	Carefully controlled caloric intake; palatable (satisfying)?
Formula	Liquid homogenate	Carefully controlled caloric intake; monotonous
II. Nutritionally Unbalanced (may also be calorically restricted)		
Altered proportion of macronutrients	High protein, or carbohydrate, low fat	Reduced efficiency of calorie utilization; reduced fat deposition; difficult to compensate for excluded foods
Altered proportion of macronutrients	Low carbohydrate, high fat or protein	Ketosis, decreased appetite; small excretory loss of calories; difficult to compensate for excluded foods
Specific food item focus	Grapefruit, kelp, vitamin B-6, etc.	Promote lipolysis; reduced efficiency of calorie utilization; monotonous
III. Calorically Dilute	High fiber, low fat	Slowed ingestion rate (more chewing required); impaired digestion/absorption of nutrients; satiety-inducing
IV. Fasting		
Very low-calorie diets	Protein or protein/carbohydrate mixtures, 300–600 kcal per day	Reduce body fat, spare body protein; ketosis
Total fasting		Reduce body fat and protein; highly ketogenic

From J. R. Vassel et al. "Obesity." In *Nutrition Reviews' Present Knowledge in Nutrition.* Copyright © 1984 International Life Sciences Institute-Nutrition Foundation, Washington, D.C. Reprinted by permission.

and mood) (125, 139). This record is taken as a "baseline," and is analyzed both in terms of the adequacy of the diet as well as the patterns of eating. The individual might now set both long- ("I want to lose 20 pounds.") and short-term ("I want to lose 1 pound per week.") goals, and on the basis of these goals an appropriate daily kcal reduction is chosen (500 kcal/day). The manner in which the 500 kcal deficit is achieved is dependent on what is recorded at baseline. For example, a person might consume high-calorie snacks while watching TV. Life-style changes to deal with that pattern might include (1) substituting a low-calorie snack, (2) only eating snacks in other rooms, or (3) not buying the high-calorie snack. The attempt is to change environmental cues (food and space) that trigger the eating of high-calorie snacks (125, 14).

Behavioral change depends on reinforcement to help maintain the appropriate behavior. The individual might reward himself or herself upon meeting each 5-lb goal along the way to the 20-lb target, or contract with someone who would provide positive feedback along the way to achieving the goal. Behavior modification programs are consistent with the concept of personal responsibility associated with fitness and wellness programs. Commercial weight-loss programs such as Weight Watchers® use these behavior modification principles.

Energy Expenditure

The other half of the energy balance equation involves the expenditure of energy and includes the basal metabolic rate, thermogenesis (shivering and nonshivering), and exercise. We will examine each of these relative to its role in energy balance.

Basal Metabolic Rate

Basal metabolic rate (BMR) is the rate of energy expenditure measured under standardized conditions (e.g., supine rest, twelve to eighteen hours after a meal, in a thermoneutral environment). Because of the difficulty of achieving these conditions during routine measurements investigators have measured **resting metabolic rate (RMR)** instead. In this latter procedure the subject simply reports to the lab two to four hours after eating, and after a period of time (thirty to sixty minutes) the metabolic rate is measured. Given the low level of oxygen uptake measured for BMR or RMR (200–400 ml · min^{-1}), a variation of only ± 20 to 40 ml · min^{-1} represents a potential $\pm 10\%$ error. In the following discussion both BMR and RMR will be discussed interchangeably.

The BMR is important in the energy balance equation because it represents the largest fraction of total energy expenditure in the average sedentary person, and it cannot be voluntarily changed (71). The BMR is proportional to body surface area, and after age twenty it decreases approximately 2% and 3% per decade in women and men, respectively. Women have a significantly lower BMR at all ages, due primarily

Weight Watchers® is a registered trademark of Weight Watchers International.

to their higher body fatness (36, 104). Consistent with this, when RMR is expressed per unit of lean tissue mass there is no gender difference. At any body weight the RMR decreases about 0.01 kcal/min for each 1% increase in body fatness (104). While this may appear to be insignificant, this small difference can become meaningful in the progressive increase in weight gain over time. For example, a 5% difference in body fatness at the same body weight results in a difference of 0.05 kcal · min^{-1}, or 3 kcal · hour^{-1}, which is equal to 72 kcal · d^{-1}. With 1 lb of adipose tissue gain equal to about 3,500 kcal, a 72 kcal · d^{-1} imbalance could result in a 7-lb gain per year. Part of the decrease in the BMR with age is related to the gain in body fat over the years.

The range (± 3 SD) in normal BMR values is about $\pm 21\%$ from the average value, and such variation helps to explain the observation that some have an easier time at maintaining body weight than others. If an average adult male has a BMR of 1,500 kcal · day^{-1}, those at $+3$ SD can take in about 300 kcal more per day (21% of 1,500 kcal) to maintain weight, while others at the low end of the range (-3 SD) would have to take in 300 fewer kcals (36, 46).

Body fatness is not the only factor influencing the BMR. In 1919 Benedict et al. (8) showed that prolonged dieting (reduction from about 3,100 kcal to 1,950 kcal) was associated with a 20% decrease in the BMR expressed per kilogram of body weight. This observation was confirmed in the famous Minnesota Starvation Experiment (70), and is shown in figure 18.10. In this figure the BMR is expressed as a percent of the value measured before the period of semistarvation. The percent decrease in BMR is larger "per man" because of the loss of lean tissue (as well as fat tissue), however, when the value is expressed per kilogram of body weight or per unit of surface area (m^2) the BMR is still shown to be reduced. A decrease in the concentration of one of the thyroid hormones (T$_3$), and a reduced level of sympathetic nervous system activity have been implicated in this lower BMR due to caloric restriction (15). What these data mean is that during a period of low caloric intake the energy production of the tissues decreases in an attempt to adapt to the lower caloric intake and reduce the rate of weight loss. This is an appropriate adaptation in periods of

Figure 18.10 Decrease in basal metabolic rate during twenty-four weeks of semi-starvation.

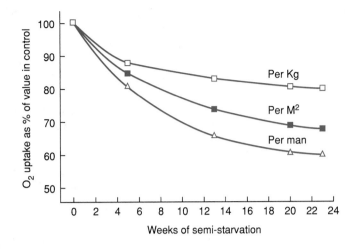

semistarvation, but is counterproductive in weight-reduction programs. This information bears heavily on the use of low-calorie diets as a primary means of weight reduction.

The BMR is also responsive to periods of over-feeding. In the dieting experiment of Benedict et al. (8), mentioned earlier, when the subjects were allowed a day of free eating, the BMR was elevated on the following day. Further, in long-term (fourteen to twenty days) overfeeding to cause obesity, increases in resting and basal metabolic rates have been recorded. In essence, during the dynamic phase of weight gain (going from a lower to a higher weight) more calories are required per kg of body weight to maintain the weight gain than to maintain normal body weight (46, 117). This increased heat production due to caloric intake, called **thermogenesis,** will be discussed in the next section.

In summary, the BMR represents the largest fraction of total energy expenditure in sedentary persons. The BMR decreases with age, and women have lower BMR values than men. Body fatness is related to both the gender difference and to the decline in BMR with age. A reduction in caloric intake by dieting or fasting can reduce the BMR by 20%. It would appear that by maintaining a low percent body fat and a reasonable caloric intake the BMR is maintained as high as possible.

Thermogenesis

Core temperature is maintained at about 37° C by balancing heat production with heat loss. Under thermoneutral conditions the BMR (RMR) provides the necessary heat, but under cold environmental conditions the process of shivering is actuated in which 100% of the energy involved in involuntary muscle contraction appears as heat to maintain core temperature. In addition, some animals (including newborn humans) produce heat by a process called nonshivering thermogenesis, involving brown adipose tissue. This type of adipose tissue is rich in mitochondria and increases heat production in response to norepinephrine (NE). Thyroid hormones, especially T_3, may either directly affect this process, or act in its permissive manner to facilitiate the action of NE (15, 16, 64). Heat production is increased by uncoupling oxidative phosphorylation, that is, oxygen is used without ATP formation, so the energy contained in $NADH_2$ and $FADH_2$ appears directly as heat. Those individuals with large quantities of brown adipose tissue have a greater capacity to "throw off" calories in the form of heat rather than store them in adipose tissue. It has been hypothesized that variations in brown adipose tissue might be related to the ease or difficulty with which one gains weight. In a study to test this hypothesis, norepinephrine, which is known to stimulate

Figure 18.11 Relationship between heat loss following a high-fat diet and the % body fat of the subjects.

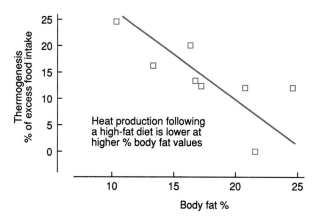

Heat production following a high-fat diet is lower at higher % body fat values

energy production in brown adipose tissue, was infused into lean and obese women. While the obese women had less of a change in heat production than the lean women, it could not be concluded that the lower level of thermogenesis was the cause or the result of the obesity (66). A subsequent study (34) could not confirm these results.

Thermogenesis involves more than brown adipose tissue. There is a "normal" 10%–15% increase in heat production (formally called the specific dynamic effect) with the ingestion of a meal (16). What is interesting is that this response is affected by body fatness in a manner like the BMR. Figure 18.11 shows that the immediate increase in caloric expenditure due to the ingestion of a high-fat meal is higher for those with lower body fatness values (64). This means that fat people conserve the energy intake better than thin people, making weight gain an easier proposition. However, there is more to this story.

In individuals who have been on a diet (underfeeding) just one day of overfeeding leads to an increase in the next day's BMR. The BMR then quickly returns to the level consistent with the low-caloric intake specified in the diet (8). It is as if the body is throwing off extra heat to maintain body weight during this period of relative overfeeding. This phenomenon has also been observed in the chronic overfeeding of human subjects. In Garrow's (47) and Danforth's

(33) reviews of these overfeeding studies the subjects showed an unexplained heat production associated with chronic excess caloric intakes. The elevations of the BMR have been explained on the basis of an increase in the mass of brown adipose tissue (mentioned earlier), and the involvement of other **energy wasteful systems.** These latter systems include a change in the Na^+/K^+ pump activity, or "futile cycles" in which the equivalent of one ATP is lost each in turn of the cycle (15, 16). An example of a futile cycle is when an ATP is used to convert fructose-6-phosphate to fructose-1,6-diphosphate, which, in the next step, is converted back to fructose-6-phosphate. In situations where heat, but no ATP, is produced, the resting oxygen consumption would have to be higher to maintain the normal ATP-consuming systems. Whatever the mechanism by which this dietary thermogenesis is induced, via brown fat or by futile cycles, it must be made clear that, like the BMR, there are marked differences in how individuals respond to an increased dietary intake. Clearly, those who have a normally high BMR and are very responsive to a large caloric excess would have an easier time staying at normal weight than those who do not.

Exercise

Physical activity makes up the most variable part of the energy expenditure side of the energy balance equation. There are those who have sedentary jobs and

Figure 18.12 Pattern of caloric intake for rats versus the durations of exercise. When rats do little or no exercise, caloric intake exceeds what is needed and body weight increases (see top-left part of figure). However, over a broad range of physical activity, caloric intake increases proportional to the activity, and body weight (top line) remains constant.

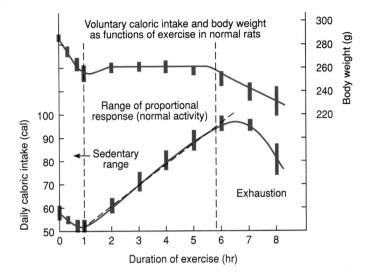

who do little physical activity during their leisure time. Others may have strenuous jobs, or expend 300–1,000 kcal during their leisure time every day or two. Just how important is physical activity in weight control? This section will examine the role of physical activity in the control of appetite, body composition, and weight loss.

Appetite. The classic animal study describing the role of exercise on appetite was conducted by Mayer and colleagues (86). Figure 18.12 shows that when female rats exercised for twenty to sixty minutes per day (sedentary range) the caloric intake actually decreased slightly and the animals lost weight. Over the durations of one to six hours of activity the caloric intake increased proportionately and body weight was maintained, but at a level below that of the sedentary rat. Durations in excess of six hours were associated with a relative decrease in caloric intake and body weight (exhaustion). Twenty-five years after this study, Katch et al. (69) showed that in male rats accomplishing the same amount of work, those exercising at the higher intensity had a greater depression in appetite and weight gain than those at the lower intensity, with both groups being lower than the sedentary animals. In contrast, female rats tend to respond to increasing exercise intensity with an increase in appetite (101).

Data on exercise and appetite in humans are more difficult to obtain. In the aforementioned rat study one can obtain a relatively accurate picture of food consumption, but it is more difficult to do so with a human population. For example, if exercise prevented a "normal" gain of 2 lbs (7,000 kcal) per year in the average adult, that gain could be explained by an excess caloric intake (above expenditure) of only 20 kcal/day (7,000 kcal ÷ 365 days), an amount that is impossible to measure on a day-to-day basis (46). In part, that is what makes this research so difficult to conduct.

Mayer and colleagues (87) studied the relationship of exercise to caloric intake on mill workers in West Bengal, India. Figure 18.13 shows a pattern of response similar to Mayer et al.'s (86) study on rats. In the activity classifications from light to very heavy work, caloric intake increased proportionally so that

Figure 18.13 Pattern of caloric intake versus occupational activity in humans. For occupations ranging from light work to very heavy work there is a balance between caloric intake and physical activity such that body weight remains constant. For sedentary occupations caloric intake (see left side of lower figure) exceeds needs and body weight is higher than expected (see left side of top figure).

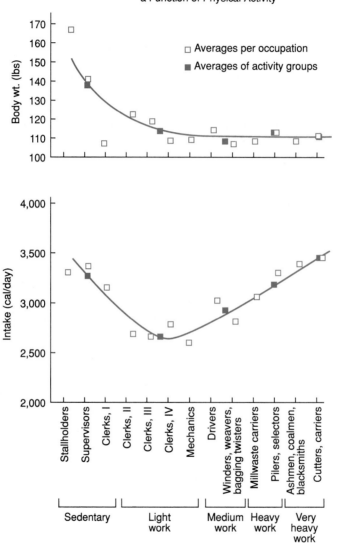

body weight was not different among the various groups. However, in the sedentary classification, caloric intake was as high as for the very heavy work classification, and body weight was higher than the other groups. This suggests that a minimal level of exercise is needed to help regulate appetite. This study has been cited over the years as a primary supporting piece of evidence showing exercise to be important in the regulation of appetite. However, in 1978 Garrow (46) questioned the analysis of the data at the sedentary end of the scale where the group called "Clerks I" had a body weight similar to the more active groups, *but consumed about 400 kcal/day more* than those in the light work category. This analysis of the data would support a conclusion opposite that of Mayer et al. (86).

It should be clear that there would have to be some proportional increase in appetite as subjects increased physical activity, otherwise an athlete would gradually waste away during the course of a competitive season! However, when an exercise program is introduced to obese and/or sedentary individuals, appetite does not appear to increase. In Wilmore's (142) review of such exercise intervention studies, appetite did not increase in proportion to energy expenditure, suggesting a net loss of appetite. In summary, in male animals exercise decreases appetite proportional to exercise intensity, while in female animals exercise stimulates appetite. Generally, in humans, caloric intake is regulated in proportion to energy expenditure over a broad range of exercise intensities and durations to help maintain body weight, but when exercise is introduced to a formally sedentary population, a net decrease in appetite results.

Body Composition. While exercise may help regulate appetite to maintain body weight, exercise has an independent effect on the composition of that weight. This has been shown in both animal as well as human studies. In general, male rats that participate in regular exercise have lower body weights, less lean body mass, and very little body fat compared to their sedentary control litter mates. In contrast, female rats tend to respond to exercise training with an increase in appetite such that they are as heavy as the sedentary group, with a lower fat weight and a higher lean

weight (99). In addition to these general changes in body composition due to exercise, Oscai et al. (100) have shown in rats that exercise or food restriction results in fewer and smaller fat cells. This observation is supported by Hager et al.'s (53) finding that in a group of eight-year-old obese girls a diet/activity program was instrumental in reducing the rate of gain in fat cell number.

The advantage of using exercise compared to caloric restriction alone in weight-loss programs is that the composition of the weight that is lost is more fat tissue than lean tissue. In both animal (99) as well as human (21, 37) studies using dietary restriction alone, lean body mass loss can equal 30%–40% of the weight loss. Exercise plus diet results in less lean body mass loss and a proportionately greater fat loss (99). However, it must be remembered that body composition changes take place slowly in human exercise studies, and the magnitude of the change is small. Wilmore's summary (141) of exercise and body composition studies showed the average decrease in percent body fat to be only 1.6% with fitness programs ranging in duration from 6 to 104 weeks. In summary, moderate exercise conducted on a regular basis appears to be instrumental in regulating appetite and in decreasing percent body fat. When weight loss occurs with an exercise and diet program less lean body mass is lost than when the same weight loss is achieved by diet alone.

Weight Loss. Before we begin our discussion of how physical activity should be used in a weight-loss program, we must emphasize the role that all of the previous factors—dietary intake, BMR, and thermogenesis—can have on energy balance. It is recommended that a person keep a dietary chart for two to three weeks to provide a more accurate estimate of caloric intake. If formulas are used to estimate energy intakes, the value could be off by ±15% (46). The dietary chart would also focus attention on what items could be eliminated or modified to maintain a balanced diet. A point to remember is that any dietary modification should be moderate (e.g., 500 kcal per day) to reduce the chance that the BMR would fall, and to increase the chance that a diet will contain the necessary nutrients needed for optimum health.

Table 18.9 Net caloric cost per mile for walking, jogging, and running

Walking

Mph	2	2.5	3	3.5	4	4.5	5
Meters/min	54	67	80	94	107	121	134
Net cost kcal · kg⁻¹ · mile⁻¹	.77	.77	.77	.77	.96	1.15	1.38

Jogging/Running

Mph	3	4	5	6	7	8	9	10
Meters/min	80	107	134	160	188	215	241	268
Net cost kcal · kg⁻¹ · mile⁻¹	1.53	1.53	1.53	1.53	1.53	1.53	1.53	1.53

Note: Multiply by body weight in kilograms to obtain the number of kilocalories used per mile.
From Edward T. Howley and B. Don Franks, *Health/Fitness Instructor's Handbook.* Copyright © 1986 Human Kinetics Publishers, Champaign, Ill. Reprinted by permission.

It is generally recommended that the negative caloric imbalance be shared between dietary intake and exercise. If an individual wishes to achieve a 500-kcal daily deficit, this can be achieved by increasing energy expenditure 250 kcal and by decreasing caloric intake 250 kcal. While the intensity of activity may play a role in appetite suppression, the primary factor involved in weight loss is the total work accomplished, so low-intensity, long-duration exercise is as good as high-intensity, short-duration exercise in expending calories. For the sedentary, overweight person, low-intensity exercise is the proper choice since it can be done for longer periods of time in each exercise session and can be done each day. In addition, for weight loss considerations, the caloric cost of an activity should be listed as the *net* cost (that above resting) since the *gross* cost of the activity includes energy already associated with resting metabolism. Table 18.9 shows the *net* energy cost per kg for walking and running 1 mile. In chapter 6 the net cost per m · min⁻¹ of horizontal travel was 0.1 ml · kg⁻¹ · min⁻¹ for walking (up to about 3.5 mph), and 0.2 ml · kg⁻¹ · min⁻¹ for jogging or running. This translates to about 0.77 kcal per kg per mile for walking (0.1 ml · kg⁻¹ · meter⁻¹ times 1,609 m · mile⁻¹ times .0048 kcal per ml O_2), and 1.53 kcal per kg per mile for jogging or running. If a 60-kg person wished to expend 250 kcal by walking, a distance of

5.4 miles would have to be covered (250 kcal ÷ [60 kg × 0.77 kcal · kg⁻¹ · mile⁻¹]); the distance would be only 2.7 miles if jogged. If the person walks at relatively high walking speeds, the caloric cost is higher than for the slower walking speeds, and a shorter distance would have to be walked to expend the same number of calories. As mentioned earlier, since it is the total amount of work that is important in weight loss, the total distance walked or jogged does not have to be done at any one time.

In selecting activities to achieve weight loss goals, one must be careful not to overestimate the energy expenditure. If a table of values of the caloric cost of activities lists climbing stairs as requiring 15 kcal · min⁻¹, one must realize that this is an impossible goal to achieve aerobically for those with a maximal oxygen uptake less than 3 l · min⁻¹. Further, while an average value may be stated in such tables, some activities (e.g., swimming) have extreme variations in the energy required for the task. To deal realistically with this problem, Sharkey (115) provides a means of estimating the caloric expenditure associated with exercise for people of different fitness levels. If a person has a $\dot{V}O_2$ max equal to 10 METs, then the appropriate range of exercise intensities to be in the THR zone would be 6–8 METs (60%–80% $\dot{V}O_2$ max). Since 1 MET is 1 kcal · kg⁻¹ · hr⁻¹ (in addition to 3.5 ml · kg⁻¹ · min⁻¹), this subject would be working in the

$\dot{V}O_2$ Max (METs)	*Net* Energy Expenditure	Body Weight (kg)		
(kcal $\cdot$ kg^{-1} $\cdot$ hr^{-1})	at 70% $\dot{V}O_2$ Max	50	70	90
20	13.0	650	910	1,170
18	11.6	580	812	1,044
16	10.2	510	714	918
14	8.8	440	616	792
12	7.4	370	518	666
10	6.0	300	420	540
8	4.6	230	322	414
6	3.2	160	224	288

From Edward T. Howley and B. Don Franks, *Health/Fitness Instructor's Handbook*. Copyright © 1986 Human Kinetics Publishers, Champaign, Ill. Reprinted by permission.

range of 6–8 kcal $\cdot$ kg^{-1} $\cdot$ hr^{-1}. If the person weighs 70 kg and exercises for thirty minutes at 7 kcal $\cdot$ kg^{-1} $\cdot$ hr^{-1}, the person would expend a total of 245 kcal (70 kg $\times$ 7 kcal $\cdot$ kg^{-1} $\cdot$ hr^{-1} $\times$ 0.5 hr). The net caloric expenditure would be about 210 kcal. Table 18.10 summarizes the estimated energy expenditure associated with exercise training for those with different $\dot{V}O_2$ max values. It should be clear that as the person loses weight the number of kcal used per fixed workout decreases, along with a decrease in the BMR. The combined effect of these two elements on the expenditure side of the weight balance equation is that there will be a slowing of the rate of weight loss over time.

Epilogue: Obesity, Diet, and Exercise

At this point in the chapter we have discussed a variety of topics related to energy balance. The question remains, are people obese because they eat too much or expend too little? The answer is not a simple one when comparing obese to normal weight groups. Garrow (47) provides a summary of the research literature showing that you can find both obese and normal weight persons living on the same number of calories per day. The conclusion that is generally drawn from these data is that the obese must be very inactive. Garrow's point is that such a conclusion excludes the influence that a low BMR or low thermogenic response to food has on energy balance. Further, he cites a variety of studies showing either no differences in the physical activity levels of lean and obese subjects, or a difference as small as 100 kcal/day. He indicates that while this difference of 100 kcal/day could explain the obesity *if all other factors are equal,* we know that all other factors are *not* equal. Given the variability in the other factors in the energy balance equation (BMR and thermogenesis), he concludes that it is impossible to show that inactivity is a major factor in causing obesity.

This does not mean that regular physical activity is unimportant in the gradual systematic development of obesity. As mentioned previously, a caloric imbalance of only 20 kcal/day can explain a 2-lb weight gain per year. There is no way to measure such an imbalance, but given the gain in weight with age for the Framingham population, such a small imbalance obviously existed. We believe that it is these small differences in physical activity that occur over time that contribute to the systematic weight gain, while the gain in body fatness may sustain the higher weight due to a lower BMR. For example, when a 70-kg individual who has normally walked one-half mile per day to and from a bus in order to get to work switches to a car pool that has door-to-door service, he or she would have an imbalance of about 27 kcal per day of work. Such normal life-style changes go unnoticed until a person realizes that he or she has gained some weight. Consistent with this is the observation that TV viewing is the strongest predictor of subsequent obesity in children. Not only are the children inactive, but they also eat more while watching TV (72).

The focus on the use of behavior modification in weight control is the identification of current behaviors and then altering those that move us toward a goal. The role of exercise in overall health status transcends weight control, and can be justified for reasons related to the risk factors associated with cardiovascular disease. It is interesting that the quantity of physical activity related to improved cardiovascular function ($\dot{V}O_2$ max) also decreases the risk of cardiovascular disease, and decreases body fatness.

Summary

1. The U.S. government established a set of *Dietary Goals* to improve health status: increase carbohydrates to 55%–60% of total calories, decrease fat intake to 30% of total calories (with saturated fat being only 10%), decrease dietary cholesterol to 300 mg per day, decrease salt consumption to about 3 gm per day.

2. The *Dietary Goals* were regarded as being too specific relative to our knowledge of how nutrition affects health status, so a series of *Dietary Guidelines* were provided that were more general in nature, but consistent with the intent of the *Dietary Goals*.

3. The Recommended Dietary Allowance (RDA) is the quantity of a nutrient that will meet the needs of almost all healthy persons. The U. S. Recommended Daily Allowance is based on the highest RDA for a nutrient and indicates what percent of the RDA is met by the consumption of a product.

4. The classes of nutrients include water, vitamins, minerals, carbohydrate, fat, and protein.

5. The fat-soluble vitamins include A, D, E, and K. These can be stored in the body in large quantities and a toxicity can develop. The water-soluble vitamins include thiamin, riboflavin, niacin, B-6, folacin, B-12, pantothenic acid, biotin, and C. Most of these are involved in energy metabolism. Vitamin C is involed in the maintenance of bone, cartilage, and connective tissue.

6. The major minerals include calcium, phosphorous, potassium, sulfur, sodium, chloride, and magnesium. The trace elements include iron, zinc, copper, iodine, manganese, selenium, chromium, molybdenum, cobalt, arsenic, nickle, fluoride, and vanadium. Inadequate calcium and iron intake have been linked with osteoporosis and anemia, respectively. Those with a genetic predisposition for hypertension due to dietary sodium benefit by a reduction in salt intake.

7. Carbohydrate is a primary source of energy in the American diet, and is divided into two classes: that which can be metabolized (sugars and starches), and dietary fiber. A primary recommendation to improve health status in the American population is to increase the amount of complex carbohydrates to represent about 55%–60% of the calories, and to add more dietary fiber.

8. Fat represents about 42% of the energy intake in the American diet, and the recommended change consistent with good health is to reduce this total to no more than 30%. Saturated fats should not represent more than 10% of the total calories.

9. The Basic Four Food Group Plan for meeting the nutritional requirements include the milk, meat, fruit/vegetable, and grain groups. The emphasis in this plan is to select food high in nutrient density (protein, carbohydrates, vitamins, and minerals).

10. The Exchange System includes six groups organized for their composition of carbohydrate, fat, and protein, with special

consideration for the caloric content. The six groups include milk, vegetable, fruit, bread, meat, and fat.

11. A height/weight table can indicate "overweight" relative to an average weight, but does not provide quantitative information about the compositon of that weight in terms of fat-free mass and fat mass.

12. Body composition can be defined in terms of total body water (isotope dilution), bone density (photon absorptiometry), lean tissue mass (potassium-40), density (underwater weighing), and thickness of various tissues (ultrasound, radiography, skinfolds).

13. In the two-component system the body is divided into fat-free and fat mass, with densities of 1.100 and 0.900, respectively. The estimate of the fat-free densitiy value has been questioned for a number of groups and new values have been substituted.

14. Body density is equal to mass ÷ volume. Underwater weighing is used to determine body volume using the principle of Archimedes: when an object is placed in water it is bouyed up by a counterforce equal to the water it displaces. One can measure the actual volume of water displaced, or the loss of weight while underwater ($M_A - M_W$). The weight of water is divided by the density of water to yield body volume, which must then be corrected for the residual volume and the volume of gas in the GI tract.

15. The percent body fat value has an error of about $\pm 2.5\%$ due the normal biological variation of the fat-free mass.

16. Subcutaneous fat can be "sampled" as skinfold thicknesses, and a sum of skinfolds can be converted to a percent body fat with formulas derived from the relationship of the sum of skinfolds to an underwater weight estimate of body fatness. We now have more generalized formulas based on larger, more representative male and female populations.

17. The recommended body fatness for males is 10%–20%, and for females is 15%–25%. There is concern about obesity and anorexia for those above and below these values, respectively.

18. The weight at any given height has increased over the last two decades, while the death rate has decreased. This lower death rate is believed to be related to better medical care of those with heart disease and diabetes, and not because people are heavier. If everyone were at optimal weight there would be a 25% reduction in CHD, and a 35% reduction in congestive heart failure and stroke.

19. Obesity associated with fat mass in excess of 30 kg is due primarily to an increase in fat cell number, with fat cell hypertrophy being related to smaller degrees of obesity. Those with hyperplasia have a more difficult time losing weight and keeping it off. Fat cell number increases throughout life from about age one, and the focus of attention is on preventing this problem in childhood since those who develop the problem as children carry it into adult life.

20. There is a positive relationship between the fatness of the parents and the fatness of their children. Adopted children resemble their biological parents more than their adoptive parents. However, the rate of increase in obesity in a population whose genetic pool is not dramatically changing suggests a strong environmental influence.

21. Investigators have proposed a set-point theory to explain obesity given the tendency for people who diet to return to their former weight. Theories based on weight sensors (ponderostatic), the blood glucose concentration (glucostatic), and the mass of lipid (lipostatic) have been proposed. A behavioral set-point theory has been proposed that relies on the person making appropriate activity and dietary judgements when body weight, size, or shape does not match up with that person's ideal.

22. Body weight increases with age, while dietary energy intake decreases, indicating that the rate at which we expend calories decreases faster than the decrease in caloric intake.

23. Low-calorie, low-carbohydrate diets cause a faster rate of weight loss at the start of a diet due to the decrease in the carbohydrate store in which 2.7 g water are bound to each gram of carbohydrate. These diets can lead to ketosis, which can cause a variety of problems.

24. The basal metabolic rate (BMR) decreases with age and is related to a higher percent body fat. In addition, the BMR is lower for women at any age due to the natural difference in fatness between men and women. A low-calorie diet causes a decrease in the BMR, which will slow the rate of weight loss over time.

25. The thermogenesis may be associated with brown adipose tissue or with "futile cycles" that use an ATP to generate a reaction, only to lose it as heat in the next step when the product is converted back to the reactant. Both short-term and long-term increases in dietary intake can increase heat production, suggesting that during the dynamic phase of weight gain the body may be trying to throw off excess calories.

26. Given the normal large variation among people in BMR and the ability to develop a thermogenic response, it is difficult to show that lack of exercise (which may amount to only 200 kcal per day) is related to obesity.

27. Male rats experience a decrease in appetite with exercise, while female rats experience an increase. Humans increase appetite over a broad range of energy expenditure to maintain body weight; however, formally sedentary individuals show a net loss of appetite when they undertake an exercise program. Exercise decreases fat mass and the percent body fat in animals and humans.

28. The use of exercise to cause weight loss is related to the net caloric cost of the activity, not the gross cost.

29. Subtle changes in physical activity amounting to no more than the caloric equivalent of walking one-half mile each work day would decrease body weight about 2 lbs a year. It is clear that participation in regular physical activity achieves not only the other health-related goals (e.g., increased CRF, HDL-cholesterol, and fibrinolysis) but also increases the chance that the person will stay in energy balance.

Study Questions

1. Summarize the *Dietary Goals for the U.S.* and contrast them with the current dietary intake.

2. What is the difference between a RDA standard and a U.S. RDA standard?

3. Is there any risk in taking fat-soluble vitamins in large quantities? Explain.

4. Which two minerals are believed to be inadequate in women's diets?

5. Relative to coronary heart disease, why is there a major focus on dietary fat?

6. Compared to the Basic Four Food Groups, what is the rationale for including foods in specific groupings in the Exchange System?

7. Using a height/weight table, how fat is a 6' 2" football player who weighs 235 lb?

8. Identify and describe the following methods of body composition: isotope dilution, potassium-40, ultrasound, bioelectrical impedence analysis, skinfold thickness, and underwater weighing.

9. What is the two-component system for body composition?

10. What is the principle of underwater weighing? Why should a different body density equation be used for children and young women, in contrast to adults?

11. Given: a twenty-year-old college male, 180 lb, 28% fat. What is his target body weight to achieve 17% fat?

12. In terms of the resistance to weight reduction, contrast obesity due to hypertrophy versus hyperplasia of fat cells.

13. Is obesity more related to genetics or the environment? Take a position, and defend it.
14. Contrast a physiological set point with a behavioral set point related to obesity.
15. What causes the average individual to gain weight over the adult years?
16. What happens to the BMR when a person goes on a low-calorie diet?
17. What recommendations would you give about the use of diet alone, versus a combination of diet and exercise?
18. What is thermogenesis and how might it be related to a weight gain in the obese?
19. What is the effect of exercise on appetite and body composition?
20. Explain why small amounts of exercise done on a regular basis may ward off weight gain over the years.

Suggested Readings

Christian, J. L., and J. L. Greger. 1985. *Nutrition for Living.* Menlo Park, Calif.: The Benjamin-Cummings Publishing Company, Inc.

Hamilton, E. M. N., and E. N. Whitney. 1982. *Nutrition: Concepts and Controversies.* 2nd ed. St. Paul, Minn.: West Publishing Company.

Lohman, T. G., A. F. Roche, and R. Martorell, eds. 1988. *Anthropometric Standardization Reference Manual.* Champagne, Ill.: Human Kinetics Publishers.

References

1. AHA Committee Report. 1982. Rationale of the diet-heart statement of the American Heart Association. *Nutrition Today* (Sept./Oct.):16–20, (Nov./Dec.):15–19.
2. Aloia, J. R. 1981. Exercise and skeletal health. *Journal of the American Geriatrics Society* XXIX:104–7.
3. American Alliance for Health, Physical Education, Recreation, and Dance. 1980. *Heart-Related Fitness Test Manual.* Reston, Va.: Author.
4. Andres, R. 1985. Mortality and obesity: The rationale for age-specific height-weight tables. In (E. L. Bierman and W. R. Hazzard, eds.) *Principles of Geriatric Medicine,* Chapter 29, 311–18. New York: McGraw-Hill Book Company.
5. Åstrand, P. O., and K. Radahl. 1986. *Textbook of Work Physiology.* 3d ed. New York: McGraw-Hill Book Company.
6. Barnard, D. L. et al. 1969. Changes in body composition produced by prolonged total starvation and refeeding. *Metabolism* 18:564–69.
7. Behnke, A. R., B. G. Feen, and W. C. Welham. 1942. The specific gravity of healthy men: Body weight ÷ volume as an index of obesity. *Journal of the American Medical Association* 118:495–98.
8. Benedict, F. G. et al. 1919. *Human Vitality and Efficiency Under Prolonged Restricted Diet.* Washington, D.C.: The Carnegie Institution of Washington.
9. Björntrop, P. 1978. The fat cell: A clinical view. In (George Bray, ed.) *Recent Advances in Obesity Research: II:* 153–68. Westport, Conn.: Technomic Publishing Company.
10. ———. 1985. Regional patterns of fat distribution. *Annals of Internal Medicine* 103:994–95.
11. Björntrop, P. et al. 1971. Adipose tissue fat cell size and number in relation to metabolism in randomly selected middle-aged men and women. *Metabolism* 20:927–35.
12. Björntorp, P., and L. Sjöström. 1971. Number and size of adipose tissue fat cells in relation to metabolism in human obesity. *Metabolism* 20: 703–13.
13. Booth, D. A. 1980. Acquired behavior controlling energy intake and output. In (A. J. Stunkard, ed.) *Obesity,* 101–43. Philadelphia W.B. Saunders Company.
14. Bouchard, C. 1985. Reproducibility of body composition and adipose tissue measurements in humans. In (A. F. Roche, ed.) *Body-composition Assessment in Youths and Adults,* 9–13. Columbus, Ohio: Ross Laboratories.
15. Bray, G. A. 1969. Effect of caloric restriction on energy expenditure in obese patients. *The Lancet* 2:397–98.
16. ———. 1983. The energetics of obesity. *Medicine and Science in Sports and Exercise* 15:32–40.
17. Brewer, V. 1983. Role of exercise in prevention of involutional bone loss. *Medicine and Science in Sports and Exercise* 15:445–49.
18. Brody, J. 1981. *Jane Brody's Nutrition Book.* New York: Bantham Books.

19. Brook, C. G. D., J. K. Lloyd, and O. H. Wolf. 1972. Relation between age of onset of obesity and size and number of adipose cells. *British Journal of Nutrition* 2:25–27.

20. Brownell, K. D., and A. J. Stunkard. 1980. Behavioral treatment for obese children and adolescents. In (A. J. Stunkard, ed.) *Obesity,* 415–37. Philadelphia: W.B. Saunders Company.

21. Brozek, J. et al. 1963. Densitometric analysis of body composition: Revision of some quantitative assumptions. *Annals of New York Academy of Science* 110:113–40.

22. Bunt, J. C. 1986. Hormonal alterations due to exercise. *Sports Medicine* 3:331–45.

23. Bureau of Nutrition. *The Prudent Diet.* New York City Department of Health, 93 Worth Street, New York, N.Y. 10013.

24. Buskirk, E. R. 1961. Underwater weighing and body density: A review of procedures. In (J. Brozek and A. Henschel, eds.) *Techniques for Measuring Body Composition.* Washington, D.C.: National Academy of Sciences—National Research Council.

25. Buskirk, E. R., and J. Mendez. 1980. Energy: Caloric requirements. In (R. B. Alfin-Slater and D. Kritchevsky, eds.) *Nutrition and the Adult: Macronutrients,* 49–95. New York: Plenum Press.

26. Buskirk, E. R. et al. 1963. Energy balance of obese patients during weight reduction: Influence of diet restriction and exercise. *Annals of New York Academy of Science* 110 (part II):918–40.

27. Cameron, J. R., and J. Sorenson. 1963. Measurement of bone mineral in-vivo: An improved method. *Science* 142:230–32.

28. Cann, C. E. et al. 1984. Decreased spinal mineral content in amenorrheic women. *Journal of the American Medical Association* 251:626–29.

29. Christian, J. L., and J. L. Greger. 1985. *Nutrition for living.* Menlo Park, Calif.: The Benjamin-Cummings Publishing Company, Inc.

30. Coniglio, J. G. 1984. Fat. In *Nutrition Reviews' Present Knowledge in Nutrition.* 5th ed., Chapter 7, 79–89. Washington, D.C.: The Nutrition Foundation.

31. Crisp, A. H. 1980. *Anorexia nervosa: Let me be.* New York: Grune and Stratton, Inc.

32. Dahlquist, A. 1984. Carbohydrates. In *Nutrition Reviews' Present Knowledge in Nutrition,* 5th ed., Chapter 9, 116–30. Washington, D.C.: The Nutrition Foundation.

33. Danforth, E. et al. 1978. Undernutrition contrasted to overnutrition. In (G. Bray, ed.) *Recent Advances in Obesity Research: II,* 229–36. Westport, Conn.: Technomic Publishing Company, Inc.

34. Daniels, R. J. et al. 1982. Obesity in the Pima Indians: Is there a thrifty gene? *American Journal of Clinical Nutrition* 35:835.

35. DeBakey, M. E. et al. 1984. *The Living Heart Diet.* New York: Raven Press.

36. DuBois, E. F. 1968. Basal energy, metabolism at various ages: Man. In (P. L. Altman and D. S. Dittmer, eds.) *Metabolism,* 345. Bethesda, Md.: Federation of American Societies for Experimental Biology.

37. Durnin, J. V. G. A. 1978. Possible interaction between physical activity, body composition, and obesity in man. In (G. Bray, ed.) *Recent Advances in Obesity Research: II,* 237–41. Westport, Conn.: Technomic Publishing Company, Inc.

38. Eastwood, M. 1984. Dietary fiber. In *Nutrition Reviews' Present Knowledge in Nutrition,* 5th ed, Chapter 12, 156–75. Washington, D.C.: The Nutrition Foundation, Inc.

39. Edholm, O. G. 1977. Energy balance in man. *Journal of Human Nutrition* 31:413–31.

40. Ernst, N. D., and R. I. Levy. 1984. Diet and cardiovascular disease. In *Nutrition Reviews' Present Knowledge in Nutrition,* 5th ed., Chapter 50, 724–39. Washington, D.C.: Nutrition Foundation, Inc.

41. Feinleib, M. 1985. Epidemiology of obesity in relation to health hazards. *Annals of Internal Medicine* 103:1019–24.

42. Finberg, L. 1985. Clinical assessment of total body water. In: (A. F. Roche, ed.) *Body-Composition Assessments in Youth and Adults,* 22–23. Columbus, Ohio: Ross Laboratories.

43. Garfinkle, P. E., and D. M. Garner. 1982. *Anorexia Nervosa.* New York: Brunner/Mazel.

44. Garn, S. M. 1961. Radiographic analysis of body composition. In (J. Brozek and A. Henschel, eds.) *Techniques for Measuring Body Composition,* 36–58. Washington, D.C.: National Academy of Sciences—National Research Council.

45. Garn, S., and D. C. Clark. 1976. Trends in fatness and the origins of obesity. *Pediatrics* 57:443–56.

46. Garrow, J. S. 1978. *Energy Balance and Obesity in Man.* New York: Elsevier North-Holland, Inc.

47. Garrow, J. S. 1978. The regulation of energy expenditure in man. In (G. Bray, ed.) *Recent Advances in Obesity Research: II,* 200–10. Westport, Conn.: Technomic Publishing Company, Inc.

48. Goldblatt, P. B., M. E. Moore, and A. J. Stunkard. 1965. Social factors in obesity. *Journal of the American Medical Association* 192:1039–44.

49. Goldman, R. F., and E. R. Buskirk. 1961. Body volume measurement by underwater weighing: Description of a method. In (J. Brozek and A. Henschel, eds.) *Techniques for measuring body composition,* 78–89. Washington, D.C.: National Academy of Sciences—National Research Council.

50. Gortmaker, J. L. et al. 1987. Increasing pediatric obesity in the United States. *American Journal of Diseases of Children* 141:535–40.

51. Guyton, A. G. 1981. *Textbook of Medical Physiology.* 6th ed. Philadelphia: W. B. Saunders Company.

52. Hager, A., L. Sjöström, and B. Arvidsson. 1978. Adipose tissue cellularity in obese school girls before and after dietary treatment. *American Journal of Clinical Nutrition* 31:68–75.

53. ———. 1977. Body fat and adipose tissue cellularity in infants: A longitudinal study. *Metabolism* 26:607–14.

54. Hallberg, L. 1984. Iron. In *Nutrition Reviews' Present Knowledge in Nutrition.* 5th ed., Chapter 32, 459–78.

55. Hamilton, E. M. N., and E. N. Whitney. 1982. *Nutrition: Concepts and Controversies.* 2d ed. St. Paul: West Publishing Company.

56. Heaney, R. P. 1987. The role of calcium in prevention and treatment of osteoporosis. *The Physician and Sportsmedicine* 15(11):83–88.

57. Heymsfield, S. B. 1985. Clinical assessment of lean tissues: Future directions. In (A. F. Roche, ed.) *Body-Composition Assessment in Youths and Adults.* 53–58. Columbus, Ohio: Ross Laboratories.

58. Hirsch, J., and J. L. Knittle. 1970. Cellularity of obese and nonobese human adipose tissue. *Federation Proceedings* 29:1516–21.

59. Howley, E. T., and B. Don Franks. 1986. *Health/ Fitness Instructor's Handbook.* Champaign, Ill.: Human Kinetics Publishers.

60. Hubert, H. B. et al. 1983. Obesity as an independent risk factor for cardiovascular disease: A 26-year follow-up of participants in the Framingham Heart Study. *Circulation* 67:968–77.

61. Jackson, A. S., and M. L. Pollock. 1978. Generalized equations for predicting body density of men. *British Journal of Nutrition* 40:497–504.

62. Jackson, A. S., M. L. Pollock, and A. Ward. 1980. Generalized equations for predicting body density of women. *Medicine and Science in Sports and Exercise* 12:175–82.

63. ———. 1985. Practical assessment of body composition. *The Physician and Sportsmedicine* 13:76–90.

64. James, W. P. T., and P. Trayhurn. 1981. Thermogenesis and obesity. *British Medical Bulletin* 37:43–48.

65. Johnston, F. E., and R. Malina. 1966. Age changes in the composition of the upper arm in Philadelphia children. *Human Biology* 38:1–21.

66. Jung, R. T. et al. 1979. Reduced thermogenesis in obesity. *Nature* (London) 279: 322–23.

67. Kannel, W. B., and T. Gordon. 1979. Physiological and medical concomitants of obesity: The Framingham study. In *Obesity in America,* 125–43. U.S. Department of Health, Education, and Welfare. NIH Publication No. 79–359.

68. Katch, F. I. 1985. Assessment of lean body tissues by radiography and bioelectrical impedance. In (A. F. Roche, ed.) *Body-Composition Assessment in Youths and Adults,* 46–51. Columbus, Ohio: Ross Laboratories.

69. Katch, V. L., R. Martin, and J. Martin. 1979. Effects of exercise intensity on food consumption in the male rat. *American Journal of Clinical Nutrition.* 32:1401–7.

70. Keys, A. et al. 1950. *The Biology of Human Starvation* (Volume 1). Minneapolis: The University of Minnesota Press.

71. Knittle, J. L. 1972. Obesity in childhood: A problem in adipose tissue cellular development. *Journal of Pediatrics* 81:1048–59.

72. Kolata, G. 1986. Obese children: A growing problem. *Science* 233:20–21.

73. Kral, J. G. 1985. Morbid obesity and related health risks. *Annals of Internal Medicine* 103:1043–47.

74. Krotkiewski, M. et al. 1977. Adipose tissue cellularity in relation to prognosis for weight reduction. *International Journal of Obesity* 1: 395–416.

75. Kushner, R. F., D. A. Schoeller, and B. B. Bowman. 1976. Comparison of total body water (TBW) determination by bioelectrical impedance analysis

(BIA), anthropometry, and D_2O dilution (abstract). *American Journal of Clinical Nutrition* 39:658.

76. Lapidus, L. et al. 1984. Distribution of adipose tissue and risk of cardiovascular disease and death: A 12-year follow-up of participants in the population study of women in Gothenburg, Sweden. *British Medical Journal* 289:1257–61.

77. Larsson, B. et al. 1984. Abdominal adipose tissue distribution, obesity, and risk of cardiovascular disease and death: 13-year follow-up of participants in the study of men born in 1913. *British Medical Journal* 288:1401–4.

78. Lohman, T. G. 1986. Applicability of body composition techniques and constants for children and youths. In (K. B. Pandolf, ed.) *Exercise and Sport Sciences Reviews,* Volume 14, Chapter 11, 325–57. New York: Macmillan Publishing Company.

79. ———. 1982. Body composition methodology in sports medicine. *The Physician and Sportsmedicine* 10(12):47–58.

80. ———. 1985. Research relating to assessment of skeletal status. In (A. F. Roche, ed.) *Body-Composition Assessments in Youth and Adults,* 38–41. Columbus, Ohio: Ross Laboratories.

81. ———. 1981. Skinfolds and body density and their relation to body fatness: A review. *Human Biology* 53:181–225.

82. ———. 1987. The use of skinfold to estimate body fatness in children and youth. *Journal of Alliance for Health, Physical Education, Recreation and Dance* 58 (Nov.–Dec.): 98–102.

83. Lohman, T. G. et al. 1984. Bone mineral measurements and their relation to body density in children, youth and adults. *Human Biology* 56:667–79.

84. Lukaski, H. C. et al. 1984. Assessment of fat-free mass using bioelectrical impedance measurements of the human body (abstract). *American Journal of Clinical Nutrition* 39:657.

85. Mayer, J. 1965. Genetic factors in human obesity. *Annals of New York Academy of Science* 131: 412–21.

86. Mayer, J. et al. 1954. Exercise, food intake, and body weight in normal rats and genetically obese mice. *American Journal of Physiology* 177:544–48.

87. Mayer, J., P. Roy, and K. P. Mitra. 1956. Relation between caloric intake, body weight and physical work: Studies in an industrial male population in West Bengal. *American Journal of Clinical Nutrition* 4:169–75.

88. McArdle, W. D., F. I. Katch, and V. L. Katch. 1981. *Exercise physiology: Energy, nutrition, and human performance.* 2d ed. Philadelphia: Lea & Febiger.

89. Metropolitan Life Insurance Company. 1959. New weight standards for men and women. *Statistical Bulletin Metropolitan Life Insurance Company* 40:1–4.

90. Montoye, H. J. 1975. *Physical Activity and Health: An Epidemiological Study of an Entire Community.* Englewood Cliffs, N.J.: Prentice-Hall, Inc.

91. Montoye, H. J. et al. 1980. Bone mineral in senior tennis players. *Scandanavian Journal of Sport Science* 2:26–32.

92. Montoye, H. J. et al. 1976. Habitual activity and serum lipids: Males age 16–64, in a total community. *Journal of Chronic Diseases* 29: 697–709.

93. Moore, R., and E. R. Buskirk. 1974. Exercise and body fluids. In *Science and Medicine of Exercise and Sport.* 2d ed. (W. R. Johnson and E. R. Buskirk, eds.) New York: Harper & Row Publishers.

94. Morrow, J. R. et al. 1986. Accuracy of measured and predicted residual lung volume on body density measurement. *Medicine and Science in Sports and Exercise* 18: 647–52.

95. Nachtigall, L. E. et al. 1979. Estrogen replacement therapy I: A 10-year prospective study in the relationship to osteoporosis. *Obstetrics and Gynecology* 53:277–81.

96. National Research Council, National Academy of Sciences. 1980. *Recommended Dietary Allowances.* Washington, D.C.: National Academy Press.

97. Nutrition and your health: Dietary guidelines for Americans. 1980. U.S. Department of Agriculture and U.S. Department of Health and Human Services, Washington, D.C.

98. Nutrition and your health: Dietary guidelines for Americans. 1985. 2d ed. U.S. Department of Agriculture and U.S. Department of Health and Human Services, Washington, D.C.

99. Oscai, L. B. 1973. The role of exercise in weight control. In (J. H. Wilmore, ed.) *Exercise and Sport Sciences Reviews* (volume 1), 103–20. New York: Academic Press.

100. Oscai, L. B. et al. 1972. Effects of exercise and food restriction on adipose tissue cellularity. *Journal of Lipid Research* 13:588–92.

101. Oscai, L. B., P. A. Mole, and J. O. Holloszy. 1971. Effects of exercise on cardiac weight and mitochondria in male and female rats. *American Journal of Physiology* 220:1944–48.

102. Owen, R. A. et al. 1980. The national cost of acute care of hip fractures associated with osteoporosis. *Clinical Orthopedics and Related Research* 150:172–76.

103. Oyster, N., M. Morton, and S. Linnell. 1984. Physical activity and osteoporosis in post-menopausal women. *Medicine and Science in Sports and Exercise* 16:44–55.

104. Passmore, R. 1968. Energy metabolism at various weights: Man. Part II. Resing: Adults. In (P. L. Altman and D. S. Dittmer, eds.) *Metabolism* 344–45. Bethesda, Md.: Federation of American Societies for Experimental Biology.

105. Pollock, M. L. 1985. General discussion of sports medicine. In (A. F. Roche, ed.) *Body-Composition Assessment in Youths and Adults,* 83–86. Columbus, Ohio: Ross Laboratories.

106. Pollock, M. L., J. H. Wilmore, and S. M. Fox. 1984. *Exercise in Health and Disease.* Philadelphia: W.B. Saunders Company.

107. Pooling Project Research Group. 1978. Relationship of blood pressure, serum cholesterol, smoking habit, relative weight and ECG abnormalities to incidence of major coronary events: Final report of the pooling project. *Journal of Chronic Diseases* 31:201–306.

108. Presta, E. et al. 1987. Body composition in adolescents: Estimation by total body electrical conductivity. *Journal of Applied Physiology* 63:937–41.

109. Rabkin, S. W., F. A. L. Mathewson, and Ping-hwa Hsu. 1977. Relation of body weight to development of ischemic heart disease in a cohort of young North American men after a 26-year observation period: The Manitoba study. *The American Journal of Cardiology* 39:452–58.

110. Rimm, A. A., and P. L. White. 1979. Obesity: Its risks and hazards. In *Obesity in America.* U.S. Department of Health, Education and Welfare. NIH Publication No. 79–359.

111. Roche, A. F., A. K. Abdel-Malek, and D. Mukherjee. 1985. New approaches to clinical assessment of adipose tissue. In (A. F. Roche, ed.) *Body-Composition Assessments in Youths and Adults,* 14–18. Columbus, Ohio: Ross Laboratories.

112. Schoeller, D. A. et al. 1985. Measurement of total body water: Isotope dilution techniques. In (A. F. Roche, ed.) *Body-Composition Assessment in Youths and Adults,* 24–29. Columbus, Ohio: Ross Laboratories.

113. Schuette, S. A., and H. M. Linkswiler. 1984. Calcium. In *Nutrition Reviews' Present Knowledge in Nutrition.* 5th ed., Chapter 28, 400–12. Washington, D.C.: The Nutrition Foundation.

114. Schutte, J. E. et al. 1984. Density of lean body mass is greater in blacks than in whites. *Journal of Applied Physiology: Respiratory, Environmental, and Exercise Physiology* 56:1647–49.

115. Segal, K. R. et al. 1985. Estimation of human body composition by electrical impedance methods: A comparative study. *Journal of Applied Physiology* 58:1565–71.

116. Sharkey, B. 1984. *The Physiology of Fitness.* 2d ed. Champaign, Ill: Human Kinetics Publishers.

117. Sims, E. A. H. et al. 1973. Endocrine and metabolic effects of experimental obesity in man. *Recent Progress in Hormonal Research* 29:457–87.

118. Sinning, W. E. et al. 1985. Validity of "generalized" equations for body composition analysis in male athletes. *Medicine and Science in Sports and Exercise* 17:124–30.

119. Sinning, W. E., and J. R. Wilson. 1984. Validity of "generalized" equations for body composition analysis in women athletes. *Research Quarterly for Exercise Sport* 55:153–60.

120. Siri, W. E. 1961. Body composition from fluid spaces and density: Analysis of methods. In (J. Brozek and A. Henschel, eds.) *Techniques for Measuring Body Composition,* 223–44. Washington, D.C.: National Academy of Sciences—National Research Council.

121. Sjöström, L. 1980. Fat cells and body weight. In (A. J. Stunkard, ed.) *Obesity,* 72–100. Philadelphia: W. B. Saunders Company.

122. Sjöström, L., and P. Björntorp. 1974. Body composition and adipose tissue cellularity in human obesity. *Acta Media Scandinavica* 195:201–11.

123. Stallones, R. A. 1985. Epidemiologic studies of obesity. *Annals of Internal Medicine* 103:1003–5.

124. Stare, F. J., and M. McWilliams. 1984. *Living Nutrition.* 4th ed. New York: John Wiley & Sons.

125. Stuart, R. B., and B. Davis. 1972. *Slim Chance in a Fat World.* Champaign, Ill.: Research Press.

126. Stunkard, A. J. 1979. Obesity and the social environment: Current status, future prospects. In *Obesity in America,* 206–40. U.S. Department of Health, Education, and Welfare. NIH Publication No. 79–359.

127. Stunkard, A. J. et al. 1986. An adoption study of human obesity. *The New England Journal of Medicine* 314:193–98.

128. U.S. Senate Select Committee on Nutrition and Human Needs. 1977. *Dietary Goals for the U.S.—Supplemental Views.* Washington, D.C.: U.S. Government Printing Office.

129. U.S. Senate Select Committee on Nutrition and Human Needs. 1977. *Eating in America: Dietary Goals for the U.S.* Cambridge, Mass.: The MIT Press.

130. Van Itallie, T. B. 1979. Conservative approaches to treatment. In (G. A. Bray, ed.) *Obesity in America.* Department of Health, Education, and Welfare. NIH Publication No. 79–359.

131. Van Itallie, T. B. et al. 1985. Clinical assessment of body fat content in adults: Potential role of electrical impedance methods: In (A. F. Roche, ed.) *Body-Composition Assessments in Youth and Adults,* 5–8. Columbus, Ohio: Ross Laboratories.

132. Vasselli, J. R., M. P. Cleary, and T. B. Van Itallie. 1984. Obesity. In *Nutrition Reviews' Present Knowledge in Nutrition.* 5th ed., Chapter 4, 35–36. Washington, D.C.: The Nutrition Foundation, Inc.

133. Wadden, T. A., and A. J. Stunkard. 1985. Social and psychological consequences of obesity. *Annals of Internal Medicine* 103:1062–67.

134. Ward, A. et al. 1978. A comparison of body fat determined by underwater weighing and volume displacement. *American Journal of Physiology* 234:E94–E96.

135. Waxman, M., and A. J. Stunkard. 1980. Caloric intake and expenditure in obese boys. *The Journal of Pediatrics* 96:187–93.

136. Welham, W. C., and A. R. Behnke. 1942. The specific gravity of healthy men: Body weight ÷ volume and other physical characteristics of exceptional athletes and of naval personnel. *Journal of the American Medicine Association* 118:498–501.

137. Williams, M. H. 1985. *Nutritional Aspects of Human Physical and Athletic Performance,* 2d ed. Springfield, Ill.: Charles C. Thomas, Publisher.

138. ———. 1985. *The Nutrition for Fitness Answer Book.* Dubuque, Ia.: Wm. C. Brown Publishers.

139. Williams, R. L., and J. D. Long. 1983. *Toward a Self-Managed Lifestyle.* 3d ed. Boston, Mass.: Houghton Mifflin Company.

140. Wilmore, J. H. 1985. Body composition and sports medicine: Research considerations. In (A. F. Roche, ed.) *Body-Composition Assessment in Youths and Adults,* 78–82. Columbus, Ohio: Ross Laboratories.

141. ———. 1983. Body composition in sport and exercise: directions for future research. *Medicine and Science in Sport and Exercise* 15:21–31.

142. ———. 1983. The 1983 C. H. McCloy Research Lecture. Appetite and body composition consequent to physical activity. *Research Quarterly for Exercise and Sport* 54:415–25.

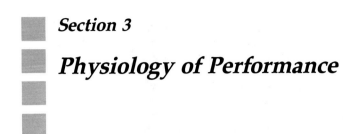

Section 3

Physiology of Performance

19 *Factors Affecting Performance*

Objectives

*B*y studying this chapter, the student will be able to do the following:

1. Identify factors affecting maximal performance.
2. Provide evidence for and against the central nervous system being a site of fatigue.
3. Identify potential neural factors in the periphery that may be linked to fatigue.
4. Explain the role of cross-bridge cycling on fatigue.
5. Summarize the evidence on the order of recruitment of muscle fibers with increasing intensities of activity, and the type of metabolism upon which each is dependent.
6. Describe the factors limiting performance in all-out activities lasting less than ten seconds.
7. Describe the factors limiting performance in all-out activities lasting 10–180 seconds.
8. Discuss the subtle changes in the factors affecting optimal performance as the duration of a maximal performance increases from three minutes to four hours.

Outline

In the last few chapters we have focused on proper exercise and nutrition for health and fitness. The emphasis was on *moderation* for both in order to reduce the risk factors associated with a variety of diseases. We must now change that focus in order to discuss the factors limiting physical performance.

Performance goals require much more time, effort, and risk of injury than fitness goals. What are the requirements for optimal performance? In order to answer this question we must ask another: What kind of performance? It is clear that the requirements for the best performance in the shot put are different from those associated with the marathon. Figure 19.1 shows a diagram of factors influencing performance (3). Every performance requires a certain amount of strength, as well as the "skill" to apply that strength in the best way. Further, energy must be supplied in the manner needed or performance will suffer. Different activities require differing amounts of energy from aerobic and anaerobic processes. Both the environment (altitude and heat) and diet (carbohydrate and water intake) play a role in endurance performance. Lastly, best performances require a psychological commitment to "go for the gold." The purpose of this chapter is to expand on this diagram and discuss factors limiting performance in a variety of activities, which will point the way to the remaining chapters. However, before we do, we will summarize the potential sites for fatigue that would clearly affect performance.

Sites of Fatigue

Fatigue is simply defined as an inability to maintain a power output or force during repeated muscle contractions (6). As the two examples of the shot put and the marathon suggest, the causes of fatigue are varied, and are usually specific to the type of physical activity. Figure 19.2 provides a summary of potential sites of fatigue (7). The discussion of mechanisms starts at the top, i.e., the brain, where a variety of factors can influence the "will to win," and continues to the cross-bridges of the muscles themselves. There is evidence to support most of the sites listed in figure 19.2 as a "weak link" in the development of muscle tension needed for optimal performance. We will provide a summary of the evidence about each weak link, and then apply the information to specific types of performances.

Central Fatigue

The central nervous system (CNS) would be implicated in fatigue if there was (a) a reduction in the number of functioning motor units involved in the activity or (b) a reduction in motor unit firing frequency (5). There is evidence both for and against the concept of "central fatigue"; that is, that fatigue originates in the CNS.

Merton's classic experiments showed no difference in tension development when a *voluntary* contraction was compared to an *electrically induced* maximal contraction. In addition, when the muscle was fatigued by voluntary contractions, electrical stimulation could not restore tension (11). This suggested that the CNS was not limiting performance, and that the "periphery" was the site of fatigue.

Figure 19.1 Factors affecting performance.

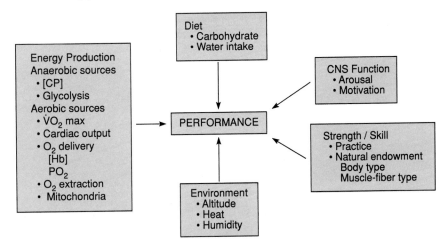

In contrast, the early work of Ikai and Steinhaus (8) showed that a simple shout during exertion could increase what was formerly believed to be "maximal" strength. In addition, later work showed that electrical stimulation of a muscle fatigued by voluntary contractions resulted in an increase in tension development (9). These studies suggest that the upper limit of voluntary strength is "psychologically" set, given that certain motivational or arousal factors are needed to achieve a physiological limit (9). In agreement with these results (that the CNS can limit performance) are two studies by Asmussen and Mazin (1, 2). Their subjects lifted weights thirty times a minute, causing fatigue in 2 to 3 minutes. Following a two-minute pause, the lifting continued. These investigators showed that when either a physical diversion, consisting of the contraction of nonfatigued muscles, or mental diversion, consisting of doing mental arithmetic, was used between fatiguing bouts of exercise, work output was greater than when nothing was done during the pause. In addition, they found that if a person did a series of muscle contractions to the point of fatigue with the eyes closed, simply opening the eyes restored tension (2). These studies suggest that alterations in central nervous system "arousal" can facilitate motor unit recruitment to increase strength, and alter the state of fatigue.

Peripheral Fatigue

While there is evidence both for and against the CNS being a site of fatigue, the vast majority of evidence points to the periphery, where neural, mechanical, or energetic events could hamper tension development.

Neural Factors

Fatigue due to neural factors could be associated with failure at the neuromuscular junction, the sarcolemma, or the transverse tubules (see figure 19.2).

Neuromuscular Junction   The action potential appears to reach the neuromuscular junction even when fatigue occurs, suggesting that the potential "weak link" is a depletion of acetylcholine or a reduced excitability of the motor end plate (11). However, evidence based on simultaneous measurements of electrical activity at the neuromuscular junction and in the individual muscle fibers suggests that the neuromuscular junction is not the site of fatigue (4).

Sarcolemma and Transverse Tubules   There is evidence that stimulating the muscle at a high rate (high frequency) can lead to a slowing of the action potential waveform along the sarcolemma and the transverse tubules. This might be related to an accumulation of K^+, which would increase the excitation threshold of the membranes (10).

Figure 19.2 Possible sites of fatigue.

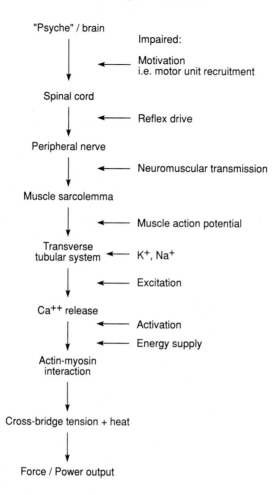

Possible Fatigue Mechanisms

"Psyche" / brain

Impaired:

Motivation
i.e. motor unit recruitment

Spinal cord

Reflex drive

Peripheral nerve

Neuromuscular transmission

Muscle sarcolemma

Muscle action potential

Transverse tubular system ← K^+, Na^+

Excitation

Ca^{++} release

Activation

Energy supply

Actin-myosin interaction

Cross-bridge tension + heat

Force / Power output

Mechanical Factors

The primary mechanical factor that may be related to fatigue is the cross-bridge. The action of the cross-bridge depends on (1) Ca^{++} being available to bind with troponin to allow the cross-bridge to bind with the active site on actin, and (2) ATP, which is needed for both the activation of the cross-bridge to cause movement, and the dissociation of the cross-bridge from actin. A high H^+ concentration, due to a high rate of lactate formation, may interfere with Ca^{++} binding to troponin and reduce tension development (6). One sign of fatigue in isometric contractions is a longer "relaxation time"—the time from peak tension development to baseline tension. This longer relaxation time could be due to a slower cycling of the crossbridge due to (1) Ca^{++} not being pumped back to the sarcoplasmic reticulum fast enough, and/or (2) inadequate ATP, which is needed for dissociation of the cross-bridge as well as for Ca^{++} pumping (10). It is this last factor, the availability of ATP, that has received the greatest attention.

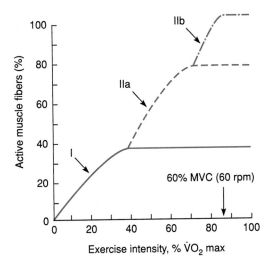

Figure 19.3 Order of muscle fiber type recruitment in exercise of increasing intensity.

Energetics of Contraction

It is no surprise that in order to maintain a certain rate of muscular work ATP must be supplied as fast as it is used. Any factor compromising this delivery of ATP would be linked to fatigue. Chapters 3 and 4 provided extensive detail related to the mechanisms of ATP production, and the roles of creatine phosphate, anaerobic glycolysis, and the oxidative metabolism of carbohydrates and fat during different intensities of exercise. In addition, chapter 8 linked these different methods of ATP production to the different muscle fiber types that are recruited during activity. We will briefly summarize this information.

Figure 19.3 shows the pattern of recruitment of muscle fiber types with increasing intensities of exercise. Up to about 40% of $\dot{V}O_2$ max, the Type I slow-twitch oxidative muscle fiber is recruited to provide tension development (12). This fiber type is dependent on a continuous supply of blood to provide the oxygen needed for the generation of ATP from carbohydrates and fats. Any factor limiting the oxygen supply to this fiber type (e.g., altitude, dehydration, blood loss, or anemia) would cause a reduction in tension development in these fibers and necessitate the recruitment of Type IIa fibers to generate the needed tension.

Type IIa fast-twitch, fatigue-resistant muscle fibers are recruited between 40%–75% $\dot{V}O_2$ max (12). These fast-twitch fibers are rich in mitochondria, as are the Type I fibers, making them somewhat dependent on oxygen delivery for tension development. However, they also have a great capacity to produce ATP via anaerobic glycolysis. The mitochondrial content of Type IIa fibers is sensitive to endurance training, so that with detraining more of the ATP supply would be provided by glycolysis, leading to lactate production (see chapter 13). If oxygen delivery to this fiber type is decreased, or the ability of the fiber to use oxygen is decreased (due to low mitochondrial number), tension development will fall, requiring Type IIb fibers to come into play to maintain tension.

Type IIb is the fast-twitch muscle fiber with a low mitochondrial content. This fiber can generate great tension via anaerobic sources of energy, but fatigues quickly. It comes into play at about 75% $\dot{V}O_2$ max, making heavy exercise dependent upon its ability to develop tension (12).

Factors Limiting All-Out Anaerobic Performances

As the intensity of exercise increases, the recruitment of muscle fibers progresses from Type I → Type IIa → Type IIb. This means that the ATP supply needed for tension development is becoming more and more dependent upon anaerobic sources of ATP (12). In this way, fatigue is specific to the type of task undertaken. If a task requires that only Type I fibers be recruited then the factors limiting performance will be very different from those associated with tasks requiring Type IIb fibers. With this review and summary in mind, let's now examine the factors limiting performance.

Ultra Short-Term Performances (Less than Ten Seconds)

The events that fit into this category include the shot put, high jump, long jump, and 50–100-meter sprints. These events require that tremendous amounts of energy be produced in a short period of time (high-power events), and it should be no surprise that all muscle fibers would be involved. Figure 19.4 shows that

Figure 19.4 Factors affecting fatigue in ultra short-term events.

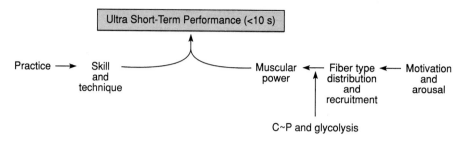

maximal performance is limited by the fiber type distribution (Type I versus Type II), which is genetically determined (see chapter 8), the number of muscle fibers recruited, which is influenced by the level of motivation (8), and the skill and technique of the athlete, which is due to practice. It should be no surprise that the anaerobic sources of ATP—the ATP-PC system and glycolysis—provide the energy. Chapter 20 provides tests for anaerobic power and chapter 21 provides a detailed list of the activities dependent upon such power.

Short-Term Performances (10 to 180 Seconds)

Maximal performances in the ten to sixty second range are still predominantly (>70%) anaerobic, using the high force fast-twitch fiber, but when a maximal performance is extended to three minutes, about 60% of the energy is coming from the slower aerobic ATP-generating processes. As a result of this transition from anaerobic to aerobic energy production, maximal running speeds slow as the length of the race increases. Given that the ATP-PC system can only supply ATP for several seconds, the vast majority of the anaerobically supplied ATP will be derived from anaerobic glycolysis (see chapter 3). Figure 19.5 shows that this will cause an accumulation of H^+ in muscle as well as blood. The elevated H^+ concentration may actually interfere with the continued production of ATP via glycolysis (13), or the contractile machinery itself, by interfering with troponin's ability to bind with Ca^{++}

(6). In an effort to slow H^+ accumulation, some athletes have attempted to ingest buffers prior to a race. This procedure is discussed in detail in chapter 25, dealing with ergogenic aids and performance.

Factors Limiting All-Out Aerobic Performances

As the duration of a performance increases, more demand is placed on the aerobic sources of energy. In addition, environmental factors such as heat, humidity, and water and carbohydrate ingestion play a role in fatigue.

Moderate-Length Performances (Three to Twenty Minutes)

While 60% of ATP production is derived from aerobic processes in a three-minute maximal effort, the value jumps to 90% in a twenty-minute all-out performance. Given this dependence on oxidative energy production, the factors limiting performance would include both the cardiovascular system, which delivers oxygen rich blood to the muscles, and the mitochondrial content of the muscles involved in the activity. Since speed is a prerequisite in races lasting less than twenty minutes, Type IIa fibers, which are rich in mitochondria, are very much involved in supplying the ATP aerobically. Races lasting less than twenty minutes would be run at 90%–100% of maximal aerobic power, so the athlete with the highest $\dot{V}O_2$ max would have a distinct advantage. However, due to the fact that Type IIb fibers would also be recruited, high levels of blood

Figure 19.5 Factors affecting fatigue in short-term events.

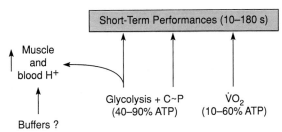

Figure 19.6 Factors affecting fatigue in aerobic performances lasting three to twenty minutes.

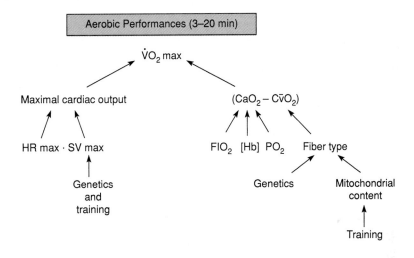

lactic acid are also experienced, and H^+ accumulation would affect tension development as previously described (6, 13). Figure 19.6 summarizes the factors affecting performances requiring a high maximal oxygen uptake. The maximal stroke volume is the crucial key to a high cardiac output (see chapter 13), and is influenced by both genetics and training. The arterial oxygen content (CaO_2) is influenced by the arterial hemoglobin content [Hb], the fraction of inspired oxygen (FIO_2), and PO_2 of the inspired air. Chapter 24 discusses the effect of altitude (low PO_2) on $\dot{V}O_2$ max and chapter 25 discusses the use of blood doping (to raise the [Hb]) and oxygen breathing on aerobic performance. Training programs are discussed in chapter 21.

Intermediate-Length Performances (Twenty-One to Sixty Minutes)

In all-out performances lasting twenty-one to sixty minutes, the athlete will generally work at <90% $\dot{V}O_2$ max. A high $\dot{V}O_2$ max is certainly a prerequisite for success, but now other factors come into play. For example, an individual who is an "economical" runner can move at a slightly higher speed for the same amount of oxygen compared to a runner who is not economical. Differences in running economy are due to biomechanical and/or bioenergetic factors. In this case measurements of both $\dot{V}O_2$ max and running economy would be needed to predict performance (see chapter 20). However, there is another variable that

Figure 19.7 Factors affecting fatigue in aerobic performances lasting twenty-one to sixty minutes.

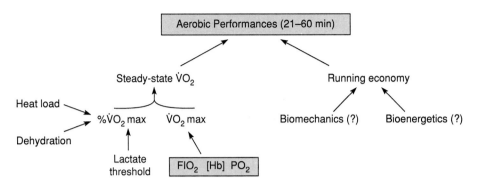

must be considered. Since races of this duration are not run at $\dot{V}O_2$ max, a person who can run at a high percentage of $\dot{V}O_2$ max would have an advantage. The ability to run at a high percentage of $\dot{V}O_2$ max is related to the concentration of lactate in the blood. One of the best predictors of race pace is the lactate threshold; the procedures to follow in estimating the maximal running speed for long distance races are presented in chapter 20. Factors limiting performance in runs of twenty-one to sixty minutes are summarized in figure 19.7. Please note that we must now consider the environmental factors of heat and humidity, as well as the state of hydration of the runner. The heat load will require that a portion of the cardiac output be directed to the skin, pushing the cardiovascular system closer to maximum at any running speed. See chapters 23 and 24 for information on how to deal with dehydration and environmental heat loads.

Long-Term Performances (One to Four Hours)

These are clearly aerobic performances involving little anaerobic energy production. Using the shorter aerobic performances (<sixty minutes) as a lead in, the longer the performance the greater the chance that environmental factors will play a role in the outcome. In addition, for performances greater than one hour the ability of the muscle and liver carbohydrate stores to supply glucose may be exceeded. As pointed out in chapter 4, fatty acids provide more fuel for oxidative

metabolism as exercise continues. However, it is clear that some muscle fibers (Type IIa) must have intramuscular glycogen available, or muscle tension and performance will decline. Chapter 23 provides information about the optimal diet for performance in long-term events. Figure 19.8 summarizes the factors limiting performance in long distance events.

In conclusion, the factors limiting performance are specific to the type of performance. Short-term explosive performances are dependent on Type IIb fibers that can generate great power through anaerobic processes. In contrast, longer duration aerobic events require a cardiovascular system that can deliver oxygen at a high rate to muscle fibers with many mitochondria. It is clear that the testing and training of athletes must focus on the factors limiting performance for the specific event. For example, dietary carbohydrate and fluid ingestion are much more crucial for the long distance runner than the high jumper. The following chapters will explore how to appropriately test, train, and feed athletes for optimal performance.

Summary

1. Optimal performance depends on strength, skill, an appropriate energy supply, and motivation.
2. Increases in CNS arousal facilitates motor unit recruitment to increase strength and alter the state of fatigue.

Figure 19.8 Factors affecting fatigue in aerobic performances lasting one to four hours.

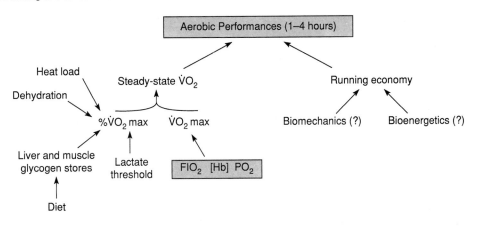

3. The ability of the muscle membrane to conduct an action potential may be related to fatigue in activities demanding a high frequency of stimulation.

4. The cross-bridge's ability to "cycle" is important in continued tension development. The effect of a high H^+ concentration on the ability of Ca^{++} to bind troponin, the inability of the lateral sac to take up Ca^{++}, or the lack of ATP needed to dissociate the cross-bridge from actin may be related to fatigue.

5. Muscle fibers are recruited in the following order with increasing intensities of exercise: Type I $\rightarrow$ Type IIa $\rightarrow$ Type IIb. The progression moves from the most to the least oxidative muscle fiber type. Intense exercise demands that Type IIb fibers be recruited, resulting in an increase in lactate production.

6. In events lasting less than ten seconds, optimal performance is dependent on the recruitment of appropriate Type II fibers to generate the great forces that are needed. Motivation or arousal is required, as well as the skill needed to direct the force. The primary energy sources are anaerobic, with the focus on creatine phosphate.

7. In short-term performances lasting 10–180 seconds, there is a shift from 70% of the energy supplied anaerobically at ten seconds to 60% being supplied aerobically at 180 seconds. Anaerobic glycolysis provides a substantial portion of the energy, resulting in elevated lactate levels.

8. In moderate-length performances lasting three to twenty minutes, aerobic metabolism provides 60%–90% of the ATP, respectively. These activities require an energy expenditure near $\dot{V}O_2$ max, with Type II fibers being recruited. Any factor interfering with oxygen delivery (e.g., altitude or anemia) would decrease performance since it is so dependent on aerobic energy production. High levels of lactate accompany these types of activities.

9. Intermediate-length activities lasting twenty-one to sixty minutes are usually conducted at less than 90% $\dot{V}O_2$ max, and are predominately aerobic. Given the length of the activity, environmental factors such as heat, humidity, and the state of hydration of the subject play a role in the outcome.

10. In long-term performances of one to four hours duration, environmental factors play a more important role as the muscle and liver glycogen stores try to keep up with the rate at

which carbohydrate is used. Diet, fluid ingestion, and the ability of the athlete to deal with heat and humidity all influence the final outcome.

Study Questions

1. List the factors influencing performance.
2. Is the limiting factor for strength development located in the CNS or out in the periphery? Support your position.
3. What points along the peripheral nervous system could be potential sites of fatigue?
4. Describe the pattern of recruitment of muscle fiber types during activities of progressively greater intensity, and explain them.
5. As the duration of a maximal effort increases from less than ten seconds to those lasting 10–180 seconds, what factor becomes limiting in terms of energy production?
6. Draw a diagram of the factors limiting maximal running performances of 1,500 m to 5 km.
7. While a high $\dot{V}O_2$ max is essential to world class performance, what role does running economy play in a winning performance?
8. Given that lactate accumulation will adversely affect endurance performance, what test might be an indicator of maximal sustained running (swimming, cycling) speed?
9. What effect do environmental factors, such as altitude and heat, play in very long distance performances of one to four hours duration?

Suggested Readings

Jones, N. L., N. McCarney, and A. J. McComas, eds. 1986. *Human Muscle Power.* Champaign, Ill.: Human Kinetics Publishers.
Porter, Ruth, ed. 1981. *Human Muscle Fatigue: Physiological Mechanisms.* London: Pitman Medical.
Simonson, E. 1971. *Physiology of Work Capacity and Fatigue.* Springfield, Ill.: Charles C. Thomas.

References

1. Asmussen, E., and B. Mazin. 1978. Recuperation after muscular fatigue by "diverting activities." *European Journal of Applied Physiology* 38:1–7.
2. ———. 1978. A central nervous component in local muscle fatigue. *European Journal of Applied Physiology* 38:9–15.
3. Åstrand, P. O., and K. Rodahl. 1977. *Textbook of Work Physiology.* 2d ed. New York: McGraw-Hill Book Company.
4. Bigland-Ritchie, B. 1981. EMG and fatigue of human voluntary and stimulated contractions. In *Human Muscle Fatigue: Physiological Mechanisms,* 130–56. London: Pitman Medical.
5. Edwards, R. H. T. 1981. Human muscle function and fatigue. In *Human Muscle Fatigue: Physiological Mechanisms,* 1–18. London: Pitman Medical.
6. Fuchs, F., V. Reddy, and F. N. Briggs. 1970. The interaction of cations with the calcium-binding site of troponin. *Biochim. Biophys. Acta.* 221:407–9.
7. Gibson, H., and R. H. T. Edwards. 1985. Muscular exercise and fatigue. *Sports Medicine* 2:120–32.
8. Ikai, M., and A. H. Steinhaus. 1961. Some factors modifying the expression of human strength. *Journal of Applied Physiology* 16:157–63.
9. Ikai, M., and K. Yabe. 1969. Training effect of muscular endurance by means of voluntary and electrical stimulation. *European Journal of Applied Physiology* 28:55–60.
10. Jones, D. A. 1981. Muscle fatigue due to changes beyond the neuromuscular junction. In *Human Muscle Fatigue: Physiological Mechanisms,* 178–96. London: Pitman Medical.
11. Merton, P. A. 1954. Voluntary strength and fatigue. *Journal of Physiology* 123:553–64.
12. Sale, D. G. 1987. Influence of exercise and training on motor unit activation. In (K. B. Pandolf, ed.) *Exercise and Sport Sciences Reviews* Volume 15, 95–151. New York: MacMillan Publishing Company.
13. Trevidi, B., and W. H. Danforth. 1966. Effect of pH on the kinetics of frog muscle phosphofructokinase. *Journal of Biological Chemistry* 241:4110–12.

20 *Work Tests to Evaluate Performance*

Objectives

*B*y studying this chapter, you should be able to do the following:
1. Discuss the rationale for the determination of $\dot{V}O_2$ max in the evaluation of exercise performance in athletes competing in endurance events.
2. Explain the concept of "specificity of $\dot{V}O_2$ max."
3. State the rationale for the assessment of the lactate threshold in the endurance athlete.
4. Discuss the purpose and technique(s) involved in the measurement of exercise economy.
5. Provide an overview of how laboratory tests performed on the endurance athlete might be interpreted as an aid in predicting performance.
6. Describe several tests that are useful in assessing anaerobic power.
7. Discuss the techniques used to evaluate strength.

Outline

Key Terms

dynamometer
isokinetic
Margaria power test
maximal oxygen uptake
muscular strength
power tests
Sargent's jump-and-reach test
Wingate test

In general, there have been two principal approaches to the assessment of physical performance: (1) field tests of general physical fitness, which include a variety of measurements requiring basic performance demands and (2) laboratory assessments of physiological capacities such as maximal aerobic power ($\dot{V}O_2$ max), anaerobic power, and exercise economy (1, 25). It can be argued that physical fitness testing may be important for an overall assessment of general conditioning, particularly in terms of evaluating student progress in a physical education conditioning class (1, 31). However, use of these test batteries does not provide the detailed physiological information needed to assess an athlete's potential. Therefore, more specific laboratory tests are required to provide detailed physiological information relative to performance in specific athletic events. It is the purpose of this chapter to discuss laboratory tests designed to measure physical work capacity. Specifically, much of the chapter will center around laboratory tests to evaluate the maximum energy transfer capacities discussed in chapters 3 and 4.

Laboratory Assessment of Physical Performance

Designing laboratory tests to assess physical performance requires an understanding of those factors that contribute to success in a particular sport or athletic event. In general, physical performance is determined by the individual's capacity for maximal energy output (i.e., maximal oxygen transport, aerobic, and anaerobic processes), muscular strength, coordination/economy of movement, and psychological factors (e.g., motivation and tactics) (1, 2). Figure 20.1 illustrates a simple model of the components that interact to determine the quality of physical performance. Many types of athletic events require a combination of several of the above factors for an outstanding performance to occur. However, often one or more of the these factors plays a dominating role in determining athletic success. In golf, there is little need for a high-energy output, but proper coordination is essential. Sprinting 100 meters rquires not only good technique, but a high anaerobic power output as well. In distance running, cycling, or swimming, a high capacity for aerobic energy-yielding processes is essential for success. Again, laboratory evaluation of performance requires an understanding of those factors that are important for optimal performance in a particular athletic event. Thus, a test that stresses the same physiological systems required by a particular sport or athletic event would appear to be a valid means of assessing physical performance. Let's begin our discussion of performance testing by a discussion of tests to assess the maximal aerobic energy output of an athlete.

Direct Testing of Maximal Aerobic Power

Maximal oxygen uptake was first mentioned in chapter 4, and is defined as the highest oxygen uptake that an individual can obtain during exercise (1). By necessity, the type of exercise performed to determine $\dot{V}O_2$ max must use large muscle groups (e.g., legs). Direct measurement of $\dot{V}O_2$ max is generally performed in a laboratory using a motorized treadmill or cycle ergometer, and open-circuit spirometry is used to measure pulmonary gas exchange (chapter 6). However, $\dot{V}O_2$ max

Figure 20.1 Factors that contribute to physical performance. See text for details.

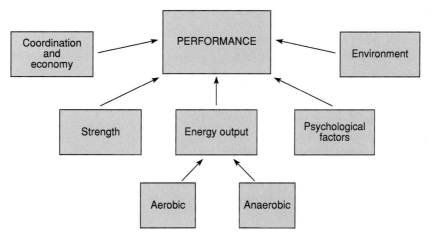

has also been measured during both free and tethered swimming, bench stepping, ice skating, and during rowing (3, 8, 26, 28, 50).

Historically, the measurement of $\dot{V}O_2$ max has been considered the test of choice for predicting success in endurance events such as distance running (7, 10, 16, 17, 19, 21, 24, 30, 51). For example, relative $\dot{V}O_2$ max (i.e., $\dot{V}O_2$ max expressed in ml $\cdot$ kg^{-1} $\cdot$ min^{-1}) has been shown to be the single most important factor in predicting distance running success in a heterogeneous group of athletes (11, 12, 16). The logical explanation for this finding is that since distance running is largely an aerobic event (chapter 4), those individuals with a high $\dot{V}O_2$ max should have an advantage over individuals with lower aerobic capacities. However, as one would expect, the correlation between $\dot{V}O_2$ max and distance running performance is low in a homogeneous group of runners (i.e., similar $\dot{V}O_2$ max) (9, 36). These observations suggest that although a high $\dot{V}O_2$ max is important in determining distance running success, other variables are important as well. Therefore, measurement of $\dot{V}O_2$ max is only one in a battery of tests that should be used in evaluating physical work capacity in endurance athletes.

Specificity of Testing

As stated previously, running on a treadmill or pedaling a cycle ergometer are the two most common forms of exercise used to determine $\dot{V}O_2$ max. However, much evidence exists to suggest that a test to determine $\dot{V}O_2$ max should involve the specific movement used by the athlete in his or her event (3, 4, 32). For example, If the athlete being tested is a runner, it is important that $\dot{V}O_2$ max be assessed during running. Likewise, if the athlete being evaluated is a trained cyclist, then the exercise test should be performed on the cycle ergometer. Further, specific testing procedures have been established for cross-country skiers and swimmers as well (26, 28).

Exercise Test Protocol

A test to determine $\dot{V}O_2$ max generally begins with a submaximal "warm-up" load that may last three to five minutes. After the warm-up period, the power output can be increased in several ways: (1) the work rate may be increased to a load that in preliminary experiments has been shown to represent a load near the predicted maximal load for the subject, (2) the load may be increased stepwise each minute until the subject reaches a point where the power output cannot be maintained, or (3) the load may be increased stepwise every two to four minutes until the subject cannot maintain the desired work rate. When any one of these procedures is carefully followed, they yield approximately the same $\dot{V}O_2$ max (1, 23, 35), although an exercise protocol that does not exceed ten to twelve minutes seems preferable (6, 23).

The criteria to determine if $\dot{V}O_2$ max has been obtained was discussed in chapter 15. However, because of the importance of this measure, some important issues will be reviewed here. The primary criterion to determine if $\dot{V}O_2$ max has been reached during an incremental exercise test is a plateau in oxygen uptake with a further increase in work rate (46). This concept is illustrated in figure 20.2. Unfortunately, when testing untrained subjects, a plateau in $\dot{V}O_2$ is rarely observed during an incremental exercise test. Does this mean that the subject did not reach his or her $\dot{V}O_2$ max? This possiblilty exists, but it is also possible that the subject reached his or her $\dot{V}O_2$ max at the last work rate, but could not complete another exercise stage and therefore a plateau in $\dot{V}O_2$ was not observed. In light of this possibility, several investigators have suggested that the validity of a $\dot{V}O_2$ max test be determined from not one but several criteria. For example, Williams et al. (49) and McMiken and Daniels (29) have proposed that a $\dot{V}O_2$ max test be judged as valid if any two of the following criteria are met: (1) a respiratory exchange ratio > 1.15, (2) a heart rate during the last exercise stage that is ± 10 beats $\cdot$ min^{-1} within the subject's predicted max heart rate, or (3) a plateau in $\dot{V}O_2$ with an increase in work rate.

Determination of Peak $\dot{V}O_2$ in Paraplegic Athletes

Again, by definition, $\dot{V}O_2$ max is the highest $\dot{V}O_2$ that can be attained during exercise using large muscle groups (1). However, subjects with injuries to or paralysis of their lower limbs can have their aerobic fitness evaluated through arm ergometry, which substitutes arm cranking for cycling or running. Given the aforementioned defintion of $\dot{V}O_2$ max, the highest $\dot{V}O_2$ obtained during an incremental arm ergometry test is not referred to as $\dot{V}O_2$ max, but is called the "peak $\dot{V}O_2$" for arm exercise.

Figure 20.2 Changes in oxygen uptake during an incremental cycle ergometer test designed to determine $\dot{V}O_2$ max. The observed plateau in $\dot{V}O_2$ with an increase in work rate is considered to be the "gold standard" for validation of $\dot{V}O_2$ max.

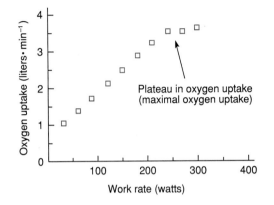

The protocols used to determine peak $\dot{V}O_2$ during arm ergometry are similar in design to the previously mentioned treadmill and cycle ergometer protocols (40, 41). However, recent evidence suggests that in subjects who are not specifically arm trained, a higher peak $\dot{V}O_2$ is obtained during arm ergometry if the test begins at some predetermined load that represents approximately 50%–60% of peak $\dot{V}O_2$ during arm work (47). A logical explanation for these findings is that an "accelerated" incremental arm testing protocol that rapidly reaches a high power output might limit local fatigue early in the test and therefore allow the subject to reach a higher power output and therefore obtain a higher peak $\dot{V}O_2$.

In an effort to provide a more specific form of testing for paraplegics who are wheelchair racing athletes, some laboratories have modified a wheelchair by connecting the wheels to a cycle ergometer in such a way that the resistance to turn the wheels can be adjusted in the same manner as the load is altered on the cycle ergometer (38). This allows wheelchair athletes to be tested using the exact movement that they use during a race, and is therefore superior to using arm ergometry to evaluate peak $\dot{V}O_2$ in this population.

Use of the Lactate Threshold to Evaluate Performance

Numerous investigators have provided evidence that some measure of the maximal steady state running speed is useful in predicting success in distance running events from 2 miles to the marathon (13, 14, 23, 36, 43, 44). The most common laboratory measurement to estimate this maximal steady state speed is the determination of the lactate threshold. Recall that the lactate threshold represents an exercise intensity where blood lactic acid levels begin to systematically increase. Since fatigue is associated with high levels of blood and muscle lactic acid, it is logical that the lactate threshold would be related to endurance performance in events lasting longer than twelve to fifteen minutes (25). Although much of the research examining the role of the lactate threshold in predicting endurance performance has centered around distance running, the same principles apply to predicting performance in endurance cycling, swimming, and cross-country skiing.

Direct Determination of Lactate Threshold

Similar to the assessment of $\dot{V}O_2$ max, the determination of the lactate threshold requires athletes to be tested in a manner that simulates their competitive movements (i.e., specificity of testing). Testing protocols to determine the lactate threshold generally begin with a two to five minute warm-up at a low work rate followed by a stepwise increase in the power output every one to three minutes (37, 44, 48). In general, the stepwise increases in work rate are small in order to provide better resolution in the determination of the lactate threshold.

To determine the blood concentration of lactic acid, blood samples are obtained at each work rate from a catheter (an indwelling tube) placed in an artery or vein in the subject's arm. After the test, these blood samples are chemically analyzed and the lactic acid concentration at each exercise stage is then graphed against the oxygen consumption at the time the sample is removed. This idea is illustrated in figure 20.3. How

Figure 20.3 Typical graph of the changes in blood lactic concentrations during an incremental exercise test. The sudden rise in blood lactic acid is called the "lactate threshold."

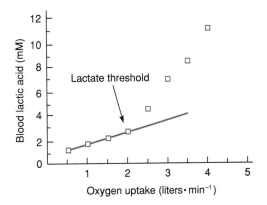

does one determine the lactate threshold? Recall that the formal definition of the lactate threshold is the point after which there is a systematic and continuous rise in blood lactate concentration. Although several techniques are available, the simplest and most common procedure is to allow two independent investigators to subjectively pick the lactate "breakpoint" by visual inspection of the lactate/$\dot{V}O_2$ plot (37, 48). If the two investigators disagree as to where the threshold occurs, a third investigator is used to arbitrate.

In practice, the lactate "break point" can often be chosen by using a ruler and drawing a straight line through the lactate concentrations at the first several work rates. The last point on the line is considered the lactate threshold (figure 20.3). The obvious advantage of this technique is its simplicity . The disadvantage of this procedure is that not all investigators agree that this procedure yields valid and reliable results (37). In light of this concern, several researchers have proposed that complex computer programs be used to more accurately predict the lactate threshold, or that an arbitrary lactate value (e.g., 4 mM) be used as an indication of the lactate threshold (25).

Figure 20.4 Example of the ventilatory threshold determination. Note the linear rise in ventilation up to an oxygen uptake of 2.0 liters/minute—above which ventilation begins to increase in an alinear fashion. This break in linearity of ventilation is termed the "ventilatory threshold" and can be used as an estimate of the lactate threshold.

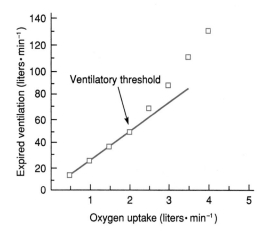

Prediction of the Lactate Threshold by Ventilatory Alterations

A technique to estimate the lactate threshold that does not require blood withdrawal has obvious appeal to both investigators and experimental subjects. This need for a noninvasive methodology to determine the lactate threshold has led to the widespread use of ventilatory and gas exchange measures to estimate the lactate threshold. Recall from chapter 10 that the rationale for the use of the "ventilatory threshold" as a "marker" of the lactate threshold is linked to the belief that the increase in blood lactic acid concentration at the lactate threshold stimulates ventilation via hydrogen ion influence on the carotid bodies. Although there are several noninvasive techniques in use today, the least complex procedure to estimate the lactate threshold by gas exchange is to perform an incremental exercise similar to the previously discussed test used to determine the lactate thesehold. Upon completion of the test, the minute ventilation at each work rate during the test is graphed as a function of the oxygen uptake. Figure 20.4 illustrates this procedure. Similar to the determination of the lactate threshold,

the usual procedure is to allow two independent researchers to visually inspect the graph and subjectively determine the point where there is a sudden increase in ventilation (figure 20.4). The point where ventilation increases rapidly is considered the ventilatory threshold and is used as an estimate of the lactate threshold. Although some authors have criticized this technique for a lack of precision (37), it seems clear that this procedure is useful in predicting success in endurance events (36).

Tests to Determine Exercise Economy

The topic of exercise economy was first introduced in chapter 6. The economy of a particular sport movement (e.g., running or cycling) has a major influence on the energy cost of the sport and consequently interacts with $\dot{V}O_2$ max in determining endurance performance (9, 25). For example, a runner who is uneconomical will expend a greater amount of energy to run at a given speed when compared to an efficient runner. With all other variables being equal, the more economical runner would likely defeat the less economical runner in head-to-head competition. Therefore, the measurement of exercise economy would seem appropriate when performing a battery of laboratory tests to evaluate an athlete's performance potential.

How is exercise economy evaluated? Conceptually, the exercise economy is assessed by graphing energy expenditure during the particular activity (e.g., running, cycling, etc.) at several speeds. In general, the energy costs of running, cycling, or swimming can be determined using similar methods. Let's use running as an example to illustrate this procedure. The economy of running is quantified by measuring the oxygen cost of steady state running on a horizontal treadmill at several speeds. The oxygen requirement of running is then graphed as a function of running speed (5, 18). Figure 20.5 illustrates the change in $\dot{V}O_2$ in two runners at a variety of running speeds. Notice that at any given speed, runner B requires less oxygen and therefore expends less energy than runner A (i.e., runner B is more economical than runner A). Again, a marked difference in running economy between athletes can have an important impact on performance.

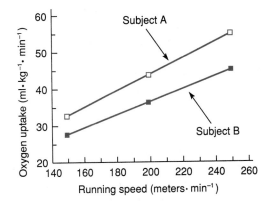

Figure 20.5 An oxygen cost-of-running curve for two subjects. Note the higher $\dot{V}O_2$ cost of running at any given running speed for subject A when compared to subject B. See text for details.

Estimating Success in Distance Running

Over the past fifteen to twenty years, numerous investigators have attempted to apply laboratory tests to predict performance in a variety of sports (cross-country skiing, distance running, swimming, etc.). In general, the sport that has received the most attention is distance running. Conceptually, prediction of potential performance in any endurance sport involves use of similar laboratory measurements ($\dot{V}O_2$ max, economy of movement, etc.). We will use distance running as an example of how a sport scientist or coach might use laboratory measurements to estimate an athletes's performance in a particular event. Let's begin our discussion with a brief overview of the physiological factors that contribute to distance running success. As previously mentioned, the best test for determining an endurance runner's potential is $\dot{V}O_2$ max. However, other factors modify the pace that can be maintained for races of different lengths. For example, anaerobic energy contributes significantly to the ability to maintain a specified pace during shorter distance runs (e.g., 1,500 meters) (7, 25). In longer runs (5,000 to 10,000 meters), running economy and the anaerobic threshold may play important roles in determining success (14, 36, 44). In short, in order to

predict endurance performance, the coach or sport scientist must determine the athlete's maximal race pace that can be maintained for a particular racing distance.

To illustrate how performance in distance running might be estimated, consider an example of predicting performance in a 10,000-meter race. We begin with an assessment of the athlete's running economy and then perform an incremental treadmill test to determine $\dot{V}O_2$ max and the lactate threshold. The test results for our runner (Johnny Runfast) are graphed in figure 20.6. How do we determine the maximal race pace from the laboratory data? Numerous studies have shown that a close relationship exists between the lactate or ventilatory threshold and the maximal pace that can be maintained during a 10,000-meter race (14, 36, 44). For instance, it appears that well-trained runners can run 10,000 meters at a pace that exceeds their lactate threshold by approximately 5 m · min⁻¹ (33, 34). With this information and the data from figure 20.6, we can now predict a finish time for Johnny. First, we examine figure B to determine the $\dot{V}O_2$ at the lactate threshold. The lactate threshold occurred at a $\dot{V}O_2$ of 40 ml · kg⁻¹ · min⁻¹, which corresponds to a running speed of 200 m · min⁻¹ (part A of figure 20.6). Assuming that Johnny can exceed this speed by 5 m · min⁻¹, the projected average race pace for a 10,000-meter run would be 205 m · min⁻¹. Therefore, an estimate of Johnny's finish time could be obtained by dividing 10,000 meters by his predicted running speed (m · min⁻¹):

Estimated finish time = 10,000 m ÷ 205 m · min⁻¹
= 48.78 min

Although theoretical predictions of performance such as the example above can generally estimate performance with a reasonable degree of precision, a number of outside factors can influence racing performance. For example, motivation and race tactics play an important role in distance running success. Further, environmental conditions (heat/humidity, altitude, etc.) also influence an althlete's utimate performance.

Figure 20.6 Incremental exercise test results for a hypothetical runner. These test results can be used to predict performance in an endurance race. See text for details.

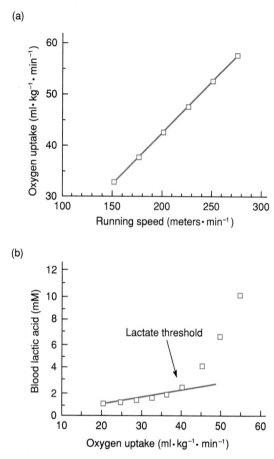

(a)

(b)

Figure 20.7 The percent contribution of the ATP-PC system, anaerobic glycolysis, and aerobic metabolism as a function of time during a maximal effort.

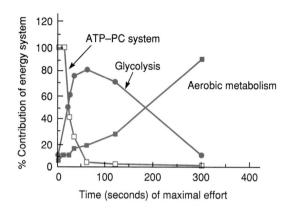

less than ten seconds are considered to principally use the ATP-PC system to produce ATP, while events lasting thirty to sixty seconds utilize anaerobic glycolysis as the major bioenergetic pathway to synthesize ATP. This principle is illustrated in figure 20.7 and should be remembered when designing tests to evaluate an athlete's anaerobic power for a specific sport.

Tests of Short-Term Maximal Anaerobic Power

Several practical "field tests" have been developed to assess the maximal capacity of the ATP-PC system to produce ATP over a very short time period (e.g., one to six seconds) (27). These tests are generally referred to as "**power tests.**" Recall from chapter 6 that power is defined as:

$$\text{Power} = [F \times D] \div T$$

where F is the force generated, D is the distance over which the force is applied, and T is the time required to perform the work.

Margaria Power Test

One of the most commonly used power tests is the **Margaria power test** (27). This popular test requires the subject to run up a flight of steps as quickly as possible, and is conducted in the following manner.

Determination of Anaerobic Power

For the assessment of anaerobic power, it is essential that the test employed use the muscle groups involved in the sport (i.e., specificity) and involve the energy pathways utilized in the performance of the event. In general, tests to assess maximal anaerobic power can be classified into (1) short-term tests designed to test the maximal capacity of the "ATP-PC system," and (2) medium-term tests to evaluate the maximal capacity for anaerobic glycolysis (sometimes referred to as anaerobic endurance). Remember that events lasting

Figure 20.8 Illustration of the performance of a Margaria power test. The subject begins with a running start and leaps three steps at a time up a stairs. The time required to leap up a total of six steps is recorded and the power output computed. See text for details.

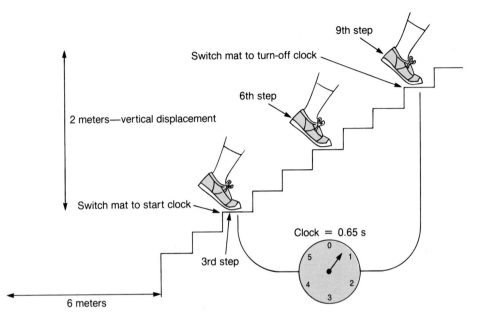

After several practice opportunities, the subject bounds up nine steps, taking three steps at a time. A timing "switch" mat starts a clock at step three and a second "switch" mat stops the clock at step nine which ends the test (see figure 20.8). The power output is calculated by mutliplying the subject's body weight (i.e., the force) times the vertical distance traveled (usually 1–2 meters), and dividing by the time required to perform the test. Consider an example of an athlete (75 kg) who transverses six steps (vertical displacement = 2 meters) in 0.65 seconds. The power output is calculated as:

$$F = 75 \text{ kg}$$
$$D = 2 \text{ m}$$
$$T = 0.65 \text{ sec}$$
$$\text{power} = (75 \text{ kg} \times 2 \text{ m}) \div 0.65 \text{ sec}$$
$$= 230.8 \text{ kg-m} \cdot \text{sec}^{-1}$$

The Margaria power test has been shown to predict success in a 40-yard dash with a fair degree of accuracy (28). However, the absolute score or power output of the Margaria test needs to be interpreted with some caution. For example, if two athletes who differ in body weight perform a Margaria test in the same time, the heavier athlete will have a higher power output. This means that the larger athlete can generate a higher power output than the smaller athlete. However, in a weight-bearing acitivity like running the 100-meter dash, a higher Margaria score does not necessarily mean that the heavier athlete will complete the race in a faster time than the lighter athlete, since body weight is carried along.

Jumping Power Tests

For many years, tests such as the standing long jump or **Sargent's jump-and-reach test** have been used as field tests to evaluate an individual's explosive anaerobic power. The standing long jump is the distance covered in a horizontal leap from a crouched position, while the Sargent's jump-and-reach test is the difference between the standing reach height and the maximum jump-and-touch height. In general, both tests probably fail to adequately assess an individual's maximal

ATP-PC system capacity because of the brief duration of each test. Neither test is considered a good predictor of success in running a short dash (28).

Running Power Tests

The 40-yard dash has been a popular test to evaluate power output in football players for many years. The athlete generally performs two to three timed 40-yard dashes with full recovery between efforts. The fastest time recorded is considered an indication of the individual's power output. Although a 40-yard dash is a rather specific test of power output for football players, there is little evidence that a 40-yard run in a straight line is a reliable predictor of an athlete's success at a particular position. Perhaps a shorter run (e.g., 10–20 yards), with several changes in direction, might provide a more specific test of power output in football players (28).

Recently, Stuart and colleagues (42) have proposed a fitness test for football players that is designed to evaluate the athlete's ability to perform repeated short bursts of power. The test is conducted in the following way. After a brief warm-up, the athlete performs a series of ten timed 40-yard dashes (maximum effort), with a twenty-five second recovery between dashes. The twenty-five second recovery period is designed to simulate the elapsed time between plays in a football game. The athletes' time for each 40-yard dash is graphed as a function of the trial number. This procedure is illustrated in figure 20.9 where line A represents data from a well-conditioned athlete and line B is data from a less fit athlete. Notice that both lines A and B have negative slopes (fatigue slope). This demonstrates that each of the two athletes is slowing down with each sequential 40-yard trial. Athletes who are highly conditioned will be able to maintain faster 40-yard dash times over the ten trials when compared to less conditioned athletes, and therefore will have a less negative fatigue slope. In an effort to establish a set of standards for this test, Stuart and co-workers have proposed that athletes be classified into one of four classifications on the basis of the maximal running velocity percentage that can be maintained over the final three 40-yard dash trials (see table 20.1). At present,

Figure 20.9 Illustration of the use of a series of timed 40 yard dashes to determine the anaerobic fitness of football players. In this illustration, subject A shows a small but constant decline in running speed with each additional dash. In contrast, subject B shows a large systematic decline in speed across dash trials. Therefore, subject A is considered to be in better condition than subject B. See text for details.

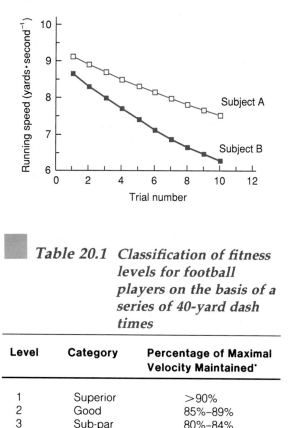

Table 20.1 *Classification of fitness levels for football players on the basis of a series of 40-yard dash times*

Level	Category	Percentage of Maximal Velocity Maintained*
1	Superior	>90%
2	Good	85%–89%
3	Sub-par	80%–84%
4	Poor	<79%

The "percentage of the maximal velocity maintained" is calculated by averaging the velocity of the last three trials and dividing by the average velocity over the first three trials. This ratio is then expressed as a percentage. See text for further details.

levels 1 and 2 are considered acceptable levels of fitness for football players of any position, while levels 3 and 4 are labeled as sub-par fitness standards.

Tests of Medium-Term Anaerobic Power

As illustrated in figure 20.7, the ATP-PC system for production of ATP during intense exercise is important for short bursts of exercise (one to ten seconds), whereas glycolysis becomes an important metabolic pathway for energy production in events lasting longer than fifteen seconds. In an effort to evaluate the maximal capacity for anaerobic glycolysis to produce ATP during exercise, several medium-term anaerobic power tests have been developed. Like other performance tests, anaerobic power tests should involve the specific muscles used in a particular sport.

Cycling Anaerobic Power Tests

Researchers at the Wingate Institute in Israel have developed a thirty-second, maximal effort cycling test (**Wingate test**) designed to determine both peak anaerobic power and mean power output over the thirty-second test. This test has been shown to be highly reproducible (20) and offers an excellent means of evaluating anaerobic power output in cyclists. The test is adminstered in the following manner. The subject performs a short, two- to four-minute warm-up on the cycle ergometer at an exercise intensity sufficient to elevate heart rate to 150–160 beats · min^{-1}. After a three- to five-minute rest interval, the test begins with the subject pedaling the cycle ergometer as fast as possible without resistance on the flywheel. After the subject reaches full pedaling speed (e.g., two to three seconds), the test adminstrator quickly increases the flywheel resistance to a predetermined load. This predetermined load is an estimate (based on body weight) of a work load that would exceed the subject's $\dot{V}O_2$ max by 20%–60% (see table 20.2). The subject continues to pedal as rapidly as possible, and the pedal rate is recorded every five seconds during the test. The highest power output over the first few seconds is considered the peak power output and is indicative of the maximum rate of the ATP-PC system to produce ATP during this type of exercise. The decline in power output during the test is used as an index of fatigue and presumably represents the maximal capacity to produce ATP via a combination of the ATP-PC system

and glycolysis. The decrease in power output is expressed as the percentage of peak power decline. In practice, the peak power output obtained during a Wingate test occurs near the beginning of the test, and the lowest power output is recorded during the last five seconds of the test. The difference in these two power outputs (i.e., highest power output − lowest power output) is then divided by the peak power output and expressed as a percentage. For instance, if the peak power output was 600 watts and the lowest power output during the test was 200 watts, then the decline in power output would be computed as:

$$(600 - 200) \div 600 = .666 \times 100 = 67\%$$

The 67% decline in power output means that the athlete decreases his or her peak power output by 67% over the thirty-second exercise period.

Table 20.2 *The resistance setting for the Wingate test is based on the subject's body weight*

Subject's Body Weight (kg)	Resistance Setting on the Flywheel (kg)
20–24.9	1.75
25–29.9	2.0
30–34.9	2.5
35–39.9	3.0
40–44.9	3.25
45–49.9	3.5
50–54.9	4.0
55–59.9	4.25
60–64.9	4.75
65–69.9	5.0
70–74.9	5.5
75–79.9	5.75
80–84.9	6.25
> 85	6.5

From B. Noble, *Physiology of Exercise and Sport.* Copyright © 1986. C. V. Mosby College Publishing. St. Louis.

Running Anaerobic Power Tests

Maximal runs of distances from 200–800 meters have been used to evaluate anaerobic power output in runners (39, 45). Because such factors as running technique, motivation, etc. influence the performance of these types of power tests, the development of appropriate norms has been difficult. However, this type of test can be used effectively to determine improvement within individuals as a result of a training regime.

Evaluation of Muscular Strength

Muscular strength is defined as the maximum force that can be generated by a muscle or muscle group (1). Measurement of muscular strength is a common practice in the evaluation of training programs for football players, shot putters, weight lifters, and other power athletes. Historically, muscular strength has been assessed by using one of four methods (28): (1) one-repetition maximum, (2) dynamometry, (3) tensiometry, and (4) isokinetic dynamometers interfaced with a microcomputer.

One-Repetition Maximum

The one-repetition maximum (1-RM) method of evaluating muscular strength involves the performance of a single, maximal lift. This refers to the maximal amount of weight that can be lifted during one complete dynamic repetition of a particular movement (e.g., bench press). To test the 1-RM for any given muscle group, the subject selects a beginning weight that is close to the anticipated 1-RM weight. If one repetition is completed, the weight is increased by a small increment and the trial repeated. This process is continued until the maximum lifting capacity is obtained. The highest weight moved during one repetition is considered the 1-RM. The 1-RM test can be performed using free weights (barbells) or an adjustable resistance exercise machine.

Figure 20.10 Use of the typical hand-grip and back-lift dynamometer.

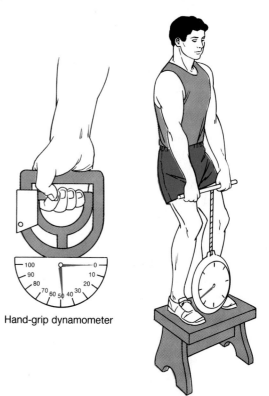

Hand-grip dynamometer

Back-lift
dynamometer

Dynamometry

A **dynamometer** is a device capable of measuring force. Hand-grip and back-lift dynamometers have been used to evaluate grip strength and back strength, respectively, for many years. Dynamometers operate in the following way. When force is applied to the dynamometer, a steel spring is compressed and moves a pointer along a scale. By calibrating the dynamometer with known weights, one can determine how much force is required to move the pointer a specified distance on the scale. Figure 20.10 illustrates the use of a hand-grip and back-lift dynamometer to assess grip and back strength.

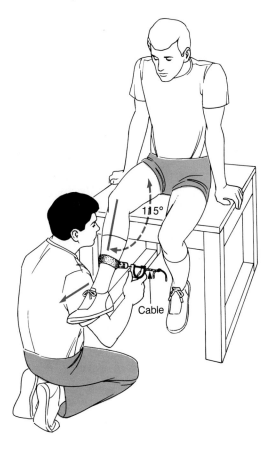

Figure 20.11 Use of the cable tensiometer to measure static force during a knee extension.

115°

Cable

Cable Tensiometry

The cable tensiometer is a tension-measuring device, and was one of the first techniques used to measure isometric force in a variety of muscle groups. Figure 20.11 illustrates the use of the cable tensiometer to measure leg strength during a knee extension. As the subject applies force over the cable, the cable tightens and the tensiometer pointer is deflected to indicate the amount of force applied during the movement.

The fact that the tensiometer is lightweight and portable, makes it an attractive device for making strength measurements in the field. The cable tensiometer has been used in physical therapy to evaluate training progress to injured limbs. It has been argued that since the cable tensiometer can be applied to measure static strength at many different joint angles, this technique might be more effective in evaluating strength gains during therapeutic training than conventional weight-lifting tests (28).

Computerized Assessment of Strength

Over the past several years, several commercial computer-assisted devices to assess dynamic muscular force have been developed. In general, the most common type of computerized strength measurement device on the market is an isokinetic dynamometer, which provides variable resistance. The term **isokinetic** means moving at a constant rate of speed. A variable resistance isokinetic dynamometer is an electronic-mechanical instrument that maintains a constant speed of movement while varying the resistance during a particular movement. The resistance offered by the instrument is an accommodating resistance, which is designed to match the force generated by the muscle. A force transducer inside the instrument constantly monitors the muscular force generated at a constant speed and relays this information to a computer, which calculates the average force generated over each time period and joint angle during the movement. An example of this type of instrument is pictured in figure 20.12.

A typical computer printout of data obtained during a maximum effort leg extension on a computerized isokinetic dynamometer is illustrated in figure 20.13. This type of strength assessment provides a great deal more information than that supplied by a 1-RM test. For instance, the force curve pictured in figure 20.13 illustrates that the subject generates the smallest amount of force early in the movement pattern, and the greatest amount of force is generated during the middle portion of the movement. The 1-RM test provides only the final outcome, which is the maximum amount of weight lifted during this particular movement. That is, a 1-RM test does not provide information concerning the differences in force generation over the full range of movement. Therefore, a computer-assisted isokinetic instrument appears to offer advantages over the more traditional 1-RM test.

Figure 20.12 Use of a commerically available computer-assisted isokinetic dynamometer to measure strength during a knee extension. (Franz Edson)

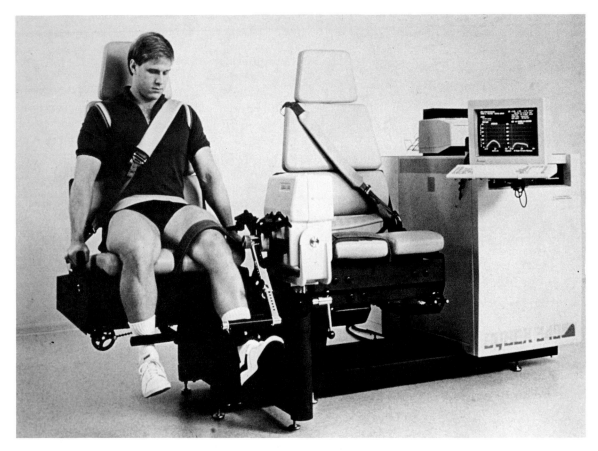

Summary

1. Designing laboratory tests to assess physical performance requires an understanding of those factors that contribute to success in a particular sport. In general, physical performance is determined by the interaction of the following factors:
   a. maximal energy output
   b. muscular strength
   c. coordination/economy of movement
   d. psychological factors such as motivation and tactics

2. Measurement of $\dot{V}O_2$ max requires the use of large muscle groups and should be specific to the movement required by the athlete in his or her event or sport.

3. A $\dot{V}O_2$ max test can be judged to be valid if two of the following criteria are met:
   a. a respiratory exchange ratio $> 1:15$
   b. a HR during the last test stage that is $\pm$ 10 beats $\cdot$ min^{-1} within the predicted HR max.
   c. a plateau in $\dot{V}O_2$ with an increase in work rate

Figure 20.13 Example of a "computer printout" from a computer-assisted isokinetic dynamometer during a maximal effort knee extension.

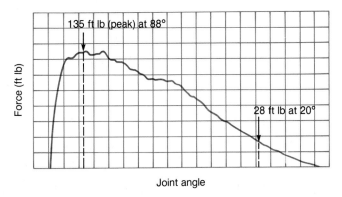

4. Arm crank ergometry and wheelchair ergometry have been used to determine the peak $\dot{V}O_2$ in paraplegic athletes.

5. Prediction of success in an endurance event can be made by a laboratory assessment of the athlete's movement economy, $\dot{V}O_2$ max, and lactate threshold. These parameters can be used to estimate the athlete's maximal pace during the event in question.

6. Anaerobic power tests are classified as: (1) short-term tests to determine the maximal capacity of the ATP-PC system, and (2) medium-term tests to evaluate the maximal capacity for anaerobic glycolysis. Tests of short-term maximal aerobic power include the Margaria power test, jumping power tests, and running power tests. Medium-term power tests can be performed on the cycle ergometer during a maximal run of over 200–800 meters.

7. Evaluation of muscular strength is useful in assessing training programs for athletes involved in power sports or events. Muscular strength can be evaluated using any one of the following techniques: (1) one-repetition maximum, (2) dynamometry, (3) cable tensiometry, or (4) a computerized dynamometer.

Study Questions

1. Discuss the rationale behind laboratory tests designed to assess physical performance in athletes. How do these tests differ from general physical fitness tests?

2. Define maximal oxygen uptake. Why might relative $\dot{V}O_2$ max be the single most important factor in predicting distance running success in a heterogeneous group of runners?

3. Discuss the concept of "specificity of testing" for the determination of $\dot{V}O_2$ max. Give a brief overview of the design of an incremental test to determine $\dot{V}O_2$ max. What criteria can be used to determine the validity of a $\dot{V}O_2$ max test?

4. Briefly, explain the technique employed to determine the lactate threshold and the ventilatory threshold.

5. Describe how the economy of running might be evaluated in the laboratory.

6. Discuss the theory and procedures involved in predicting success in distance running.

7. Explain how short-term maximal anaerobic power can be evaluated by field tests.

8. Describe how the Wingate test is used to assess medium-term anaerobic power.

9. Provide an overview of the 1-RM technique to evaluate muscular strength. Why might a computer-assisted dynamometer be superior to the 1-RM technique in assessing strength changes?

Suggested Readings

Bar-Or, O. 1987. The Wingate test: An update on methodology, reliability and validity. *Sports Medicine* 4:268–89.

Kenney, W., and J. Hodgson. 1985. Variables predictive of performance in elite middle-distance runners. *British Journal of Sports Medicine* 19:207–9.

Londeree, B. 1986. The use of laboratory test results with long distance runners. *Sports Medicine* 3:201–13.

Vandewalle, H., G. Peres, and H. Monod. 1987. Standard anaerobic exercise tests. *Sports Medicine* 4:268–89.

References

1. Åstrand, P. O., and K. Rodahl. 1986. *Textbook of Work Physiology.* New York: McGraw-Hill.

2. Berger, R. 1982. *Applied Exercise Physiology.* Philadelphia: Lea & Febiger.

3. Bouckaert, J., J. Pannier, and J. Vrijens. 1983. Cardiorespiratory response to bicycle and rowing ergometer exercise in oarsmen. *European Journal of Applied Physiology* 51:51–59.

4. Bouckaert, J. and J. Pannier. 1984. Specificity of $\dot{V}O_2$ max and blood lactate determinations in runners and cyclists. *International Archives of Physiology and Biochemistry* 93:30–31.

5. Bransford, D., and E. Howley. 1977. Oxygen cost of running in trained and untrained men and women. *Medicine and Science in Sports and Exercise* 9:41–44.

6. Buchfuhrer, M. et al. 1983. Optimizing the exercise protocol for cardiopulmonary assessment. *Journal of Applied Physiology* 55:1558–64.

7. Bulbulian, R., A. Wilcox, and B. Darabos. 1986. Anaerobic contribution to distance running performance of trained cross-country athletes. *Medicine and Science in Sports and Exercise* 18:107–13.

8. Burke, E. 1976. Validity of selected laboratory and field tests of physical working capacity. *Research Quarterly* 47:95–104.

9. Conley, D., and G. Krahenbuhl. 1980. Running economy and distance running performance of highly trained athletes. *Medicine and Science in Sports and Exercise* 12:357–60.

10. Costill, D. 1979. *A Scientific Approach to Distance Running.* Los Altos: Track and Field News Press.

11. Costill, D. 1970. Metabolic responses to distance running. *Journal of Applied Physiology* 28:251–55.

12. Costill, D. 1967. The relationship between selected physiological variables and distance running performance. *Journal of Sports Medicine and Physical Fitness* 7:61–66.

13. Costill, D., H. Thompson, and E. Roberts. 1973. Fractional utilization of the aerobic capacity during distance running. *Medicine and Science in Sports* 5:248–52.

14. Farrell, P. et al. 1979. Plasma lactate accumulation and distance running performance. *Medicine and Science in Sports* 11:338–44.

15. Foster, C. 1983. $\dot{V}O_2$ max and training indices as determinants of competitive running performance. *Journal of Sports Sciences* 1:13–27.

16. Foster, C., J. Daniels, and R. Yarbough. 1977. Physiological correlates of marathon running and performance. *Australian Journal of Sports Medicine* 9:58–61.

17. Hagan, R., M. Smith, and L. Gettman. 1981. Marathon performance in relation to maximal aerobic power and training indices. *Medicine and Science in Sports and Exercise* 13:185–89.

18. Hopkins, P., and S. Powers. 1982. Oxygen uptake during submaximal running in highly trained men and women. *American Corrective Therapy Journal* 36:130–32.

19. Hughson, R., C. Orok, and L. Staudt. 1984. A high-velocity treadmill running test to assess endurance running potential. *International Journal of Sports Medicine* 5:23–25.

20. Jacobs, I. 1980. The effects of thermal dehydration on performance of the Wingate anaerobic test. *International Journal of Sports Medicine* 1:21–24.

21. Kenney, W., and J. Hodgson. 1985. Variables predictive of performance in elite middle-distance runners. *British Journal of Sports Medicine* 19:207–9.

22. LaFontaine, T., B. Londeree, and W. Spath. 1981. The maximal steady state versus selected running events. *Medicine and Science in Sports and Exercise* 13:190–92.

23. Lawler, J., S. Powers, and S. Dodd. 1987. A time saving incremental cycle ergometer protocol to determine peak oxygen consumption. *British Journal of Sports Medicine* 21:171–73.

24. Lehmann, M. et al. 1983. Correlations between laboratory testing and distance running performance in marathoners of similar ability. *International Journal of Sports Medicine* 4:226–30.

25. Londeree, B. 1986. The use of laboratory test results with long distance runners. *Sports Medicine* 3:201–13.

26. Magel, J., and J. Faulker. 1967. Maximum oxygen uptake of college swimmers. *Journal of Applied Physiology* 22:929.

27. Margaria, R. 1966. Measurement of muscular power in man. *Journal of Applied Physiology* 21:1662.

28. McArdle, W., F. Katch, and V. Katch. 1986. *Exercise Physiology: Energy, Nutrition, and Human Performance.* Philadelphia: Lea & Febiger.

29. McMiken, D., and J. Daniels. 1976. Aerobic requirements of maximal aerobic power in treadmill and track running. *Medicine and Science in Sports and Exercise* 8:14–17.

30. Murase, Y. et al. 1981. Longitudinal study of aerobic power in superior junior athletes. *Medicine and Science in Sports and Exercise* 13:180–84.

31. Noble, B. 1986. *Physiology of Exercise and Sport.* St. Louis: Mosby College Publishing.

32. Pannier, J., J. Vrijens, and C. Van Cauter. 1980. Cardiorespiratory response to treadmill and bicycle exercise in runners. *European Journal of Applied Physiology* 43:243–51.

33. Pollock, M. 1977. Submaximal and maximal working capacity of elite distance runners: cardiorespiratory aspects. *Annuals of the New York Academy of Sciences* 301:310–22.

34. Pollock, M., A. Jackson, and R. Pate. 1980. Discriminant analysis of physiological differences between good and elite runners. *Research Quarterly* 51:521–32.

35. Pollock, M. et al. 1976. A comparative analysis of four protocols for maximal treadmill stress testing. *American Heart Journal* 92:39–46.

36. Powers, S. et al. 1983. Ventilatory threshold, running economy, and distance running performance of trained athletes. *Research Quarterly for Exercise and Sport* 54:179–82.

37. Powers, S., S. Dodd, and R. Garner. 1984. Precision of ventilatory and gas exchange alterations as a predictor of the anaerobic threshold. *European Journal of Applied Physiology* 52:173–77.

38. Sawka, M. et al. 1983. Determination of maximal aerobic power during upper body exercise. *Journal of Applied Physiology* 54:113–17.

39. Schnabel, A., and W. Kinderman. 1983. Assessment of anaerobic capacity in runners. *European Journal of Applied Physiology* 52:42–46.

40. Schwade, J., G. Blomquist, and W. Shapiro. 1977. A comparsion of the response to arm and leg work in patients with ischemic heart disease. *American Heart Journal* 94:203–8.

41. Shaw, D. et al. 1974. Arm crank ergometer: A new method for the evaluation of coronary heart disease. *American Journal of Cardiology* 33:801–5.

42. Stuart, M. K., S. Powers, and J. Nelson. Development of an anaerobic fitness test for football players. Unpublished observations.

43. Tanaka, K., and Y. Matsuura. 1984. Marathon performance, anaerobic threshold, and onset of blood lactate accumulation. *Journal of Applied Physiology* 57:640–43.

44. Tanaka, K. et al. 1983. Relationships of anaerobic threshold and onset of blood lactate accumulation with endurance performance. *European Journal of Applied Physiology* 52:51–56.

45. Taunton, J. H. Maron, and J. Wilkinson. 1981. Anaerobic performance in middle and long distance runners. *Canadian Journal of Applied Sports Sciences* 6:109–13.

46. Taylor, H., E. Buskirk, and A. Henschel. 1955. Maximal oxygen uptake as an objective measure of cardiorespiratory performance. *Journal of Applied Physiology* 8:73–80.

47. Walker, R., S. Powers, and M. Stuart. 1986. Peak oxygen uptake in arm ergometry: Effects of testing protocol. *British Journal of Sports Medicine* 20:25–26.

48. Wasserman, K. et al. 1973. Anaerobic threshold and respiratory gas exchange during exercise. *Journal of Applied Physiology* 35:236–43.

49. Williams, J., S. Powers, and S. Stuart. 1986. Hemoglobin desaturation in highly trained athletes during heavy exercise. *Medicine and Science in Sports and Exercise* 18:168–73.

50. Williams, L. 1978. Prediction of high-level rowing ability. *Journal of Sports Medicine and Physical Fitness* 18:11–15.

51. Wyndham, C. et al. 1969. Physiological requirements for world-class performances in distance running. *South African Medical Journal* 43:996–1002.

21 *Training for Performance*

Objectives

*B*y studying this chapter, you should be able to do the following:
1. Discuss the concept of designing a sport-specific training program based on an analysis of the energy systems utilized by the activity.
2. List and discuss the general principles of physical conditioning for improved sport performance.
3. Define the terms overload, specificity, and reversibility.
4. Outline the use of interval training and continuous training in the improvement of the maximal aerobic power in athletes.
5. Discuss the guidelines associated with planning a training program designed to improve the anaerobic power of athletes.
6. Outline the principles of training for the improvement of strength.
7. Discuss the role of gender differences in the development of strength.
8. List the factors that contribute to delayed onset muscle soreness.
9. Discuss the use of static and ballistic stretching to improve flexibility.
10. Outline the goals of: (1) off-season conditioning, (2) preseason conditioning, and (3) in-season conditioning.
11. List and discuss several common training errors.

Outline

Key Terms

ballistic stretching

delayed onset muscle soreness (DOMS)

hyperplasia

hypertrophy

progressive resistance exercise (PRE)

repetition

rest interval

set

static stretching

variable resistance exercise

work interval

Traditionally, coaches and trainers have planned conditioning programs for their team by following regimens used by teams that have successful win-loss records. This type of reasoning is not sound, since win-loss records alone do not scientifically validate the specific conditioning program used by the successful team. In fact, the successful team might be victorious by virtue of having superior athletes and not as a result of an outstanding conditioning program. It seems clear that the planning of an effective athletic conditioning program can best be achieved by the application of proven physiological training principles. Optimizing training programs for athletes is important, since failure to properly condition an athletic team results in a poor performance and often, defeat. It is the purpose of this chapter to present an overview of how to apply scientific principles to the development of an athletic conditioning program.

Training Principles

The overall objective of a sport conditioning program is to improve performance by increasing the energy output during a particular movement (2, 39, 46). Recall that throughout this book (e.g., chapters 3, 4, and 20), emphasis has been placed on the fact that dissimilar sport activities utilize different metabolic pathways or "energy systems" to produce the ATP needed for movement. An understanding of exercise metabolism is important to the coach or trainer since the design of a conditioning program to optimize athletic performance requires knowledge of the principal energy systems utilized by the sport. Consider a few examples. The performance of a 60-meter dash uses the ATP-CP system almost exclusively to produce the

needed ATP. In contrast, a marathon runner depends on aerobic metabolism to provide the needed energy to complete the race. Unfortunately, few sport activities use one energy pathway exclusively. For instance, soccer uses a combination of metabolic pathways to provide the needed ATP. Knowledge of the relative anaerobic-aerobic contributions to ATP production during an activity is the cornerstone of planning a conditioning program. A well-designed conditioning program allocates the appropriate amount of aerobic and anaerobic conditioning time to match the energy demand of the sport. For instance, if an activity derives 40% of its ATP from anaerobic pathways and 60% from aerobic pathways (e.g., 1,500-meter run), the training program should be divided 40%/60% between anaerobic/aerobic training (2, 39). Table 21.1 contains a list of various sports and an estimation of their predominant energy systems. This information can be used by the coach or trainer to allocate the appropriate amount of time to training each energy system.

The above discussion does not necessarily imply that power athletes (e.g., sprinters) should not perform aerobic training. On the contrary, aerobic activity during the preseason to strengthen tendons and ligaments is generally recommended for all athletes.

Overload, Specificity, and Reversibility

The terms overload, specificity, and reversibility were introduced in chapters 13 and 15, and will be repeated here only briefly. Recall that an organ system (e.g., cardiovascular, skeletal muscle, etc.) increases its capacity in response to a training overload. That is, the training program must stress the system above the level to which it is accustomed. Conversely, when an athlete

Table 21.1 *The predominant energy systems for selected sports*

Sport/Activity	%ATP Contribution by Energy System		
	ATP-PC	Lactic Acid	Aerobic
Baseball	80	15	5
Basketball	80	10	10
Field hockey	60	20	20
Football	90	10	—
Golf(swing)	100	—	—
Gymnastics	90	10	—
Ice hockey:			
Forwards/defense	80	20	—
Goalie	95	5	—
Rowing	20	30	50
Soccer:			
Goalie/wings/strikers	80	20	—
Halfbacks	60	20	20
Swimming:			
Diving	98	2	—
50 meters	95	5	—
100 meters	80	15	—
200 meters	30	65	5
400 meters	20	40	40
1,500 meters	10	20	70
Tennis	70	20	10
Track and field:			
100/200 meters	98	2	—
Field events	90	10	—
400 meters	40	55	5
800 meters	10	60	30
1,500 meters	5	35	60
5,000 meters	2	28	70
Marathon	—	2	98
Volleyball	90	10	—
Wrestling	45	55	—

From E. L. Fox and D. Mathews, *Interval Training: Conditioning for Sports and General Fitness.* Copyright 1974. Saunders College/Harcourt Brace Jovanovich, Orlando.

stops training, the training effect is quickly lost (reversibility). Studies have demonstrated that within two weeks after the cessation of training, significant reductions in $\dot{V}O_2$ max can occur (12, 13). A classic study of Saltin and colleagues (44) demonstrated that after twenty days of bed rest, a group of subjects showed a 25% reduction is $\dot{V}O_2$ max and maximal cardiac output. These rather dramatic decrements in working capacity as a result of inactivity clearly demonstrate the rapid reversibility of training.

The concept of specificity refers to not only the specific muscles involved in a particular movement, but also to the energy systems that provide the necessary ATP required to complete the movement under competitive conditions. Therefore, training programs need to deal with specificity by using not only those muscle groups engaged during competition, but also the energy systems that will be providing the ATP. For instance, "specific training" for a sprinter would involve running high-intensity dashes. Similarly, specific training for a marathoner would involve long, slow-paced runs in which virtually all of the ATP needed by the working muscles would be derived from aerobic metabolism.

Influence of Gender, Initial Fitness Level, and Genetics

At one time, it was believed that conditioning programs for women had special requirements that differed from those used to train men. Today, however, ample evidence exists to demonstrate that men and women respond to training programs in a similar fashion (6, 8, 41, 42). Therefore, the same general approach to physiological conditioning can be used in planning programs for men and women.

It is a common observation that individuals differ greatly in the degree of improvement resulting from training programs. Many factors contribute to the observed individual variations in the training response. One of the most important influences is the athlete's beginning level of fitness. In general, the amount of training improvement is always greater in those individuals who are less conditioned at the beginning of the training program (45). It has been demonstrated that sedentary middle-aged men with heart disease may improve their $\dot{V}O_2$ max by as much as 50%, whereas the same training program in normal active adults improves $\dot{V}O_2$ max by only 10%–15% (34, 39). Similarly, conditioned athletes may only improve their level of conditioning by 3%–5% following an increase in training intensity. However, it needs to be emphasized that this 3%–5% improvement in the trained athlete may be the difference in winning an Olympic gold medal versus failing to place in the event.

Additionally, it seems likely that genetics plays an important role in how an individual responds to a training program (2). For instance, an individual with a high genetic endowment for endurance sports is likely to respond differently to endurance training when compared to an individual with a markedly different genetic profile. It is for this reason, and the fact that athletes begin conditioning programs at different levels of fitness, that training programs should be individualized. It is unrealistic to expect each athlete on the team to perform the same amount of work or to exercise at the same work rate during training sessions.

Note that while training can greatly improve performance, there is an absolute need for a genetic predisposition for athletic talent if the individual is to compete at a world-class level. For example, there is a limit to how much training can improve aerobic power. Therefore, those individuals with a low genetic endowment for aerobic power cannot, under any training program, increase their $\dot{V}O_2$ max to world-class levels. Åstrand and Rodahl (2) have commented that although this seems to be unfair, it is nonetheless a fact that our parents' genetic makeup is important in determining our failure or success in athletics.

Components of a Training Session: Warm-Up, Workout, and Cool Down

Every training session should consist of three components: (1) warm-up, (2) workout, and (3) cool down. This idea was first introduced in chapter 16 and will be mentioned only briefly here. The warm-up or preliminary exercise prior to a training workout has several important objectives. First, warm-up exercises increase cardiac output and blood flow to the skeletal muscles to be used during the training session. Secondly, the warm-up activity results in an increase in muscle temperature, which elevates muscle enzyme activity (38). Finally, preliminary exercise affords the athlete an opportunity to perform stretching exercises. The duration of the warm-up may be from ten to twenty minutes, depending on environmental conditions and the nature of the training acitivity (14, 52). Although some disagreement exists, it is commonly believed that a proper warm-up may reduce the possibility of muscle injury due to pulls or strains (5, 24). Additional research is needed to definitively answer this question.

Immediately following the training session, a period of light, "cool down" exercises should be performed. The principal objective of a cool down is to return "pooled" blood from the exercised skeletal muscles back to the central circulation. Similar to the warm-up, the length of the cool down may vary from ten to thrity minutes, depending on environmental conditions, the age and fitness level of the individual, and the nature of the training session.

Training to Improve Aerobic Power

Recall from chapter 13 that endurance training improves $\dot{V}O_2$ max by increasing both maximal cardiac output and increasing the a-$\bar{v}O_2$ difference (i.e., increasing the muscle's ability to extract O_2). Therefore, a training program designed to improve maximal aerobic power must overload both the circulatory system and stress the oxidative capacities of skeletal muscles as well (2, 10, 14). As in all training regimens, specificity is critical. The athlete should stress the specific muscles to be used in his or her sport. In other words, runners should train by running, cyclists should train on the bicycle, swimmers should swim, and so forth.

There are three principal aerobic training methods used by athletes: (1) interval training, (2) long, slow distance (low intensity), and (3) high-intensity, continuous exercise. Although controversy exists as to which of these training methods results in the greatest improvement in $\dot{V}O_2$ max, there is growing evidence that it is training intensity and not duration that is the most important factor in improving $\dot{V}O_2$ max (7, 15, 18, 21, 26, 33, 43). However, from a psychological standpoint, it would appear that a mixing of all three methods would provide the needed variety to prevent the athlete from becoming bored with a rather singular and monotonous training program.

Note that improvement of $\dot{V}O_2$ max is only one variable related to endurance. Recall from chapter 20 that although a high $\dot{V}O_2$ max is important for success in endurance events, both movement economy and the lactate threshold are also important variables. Therefore, training to improve endurance performance should not only be geared toward the improvement of $\dot{V}O_2$ max, but should also increase the lactate threshold and improve running economy as well. A brief discussion of various training methods used to improve endurance performance follows.

Interval Training

Interval training involves the performance of repeated exercise bouts, with brief recovery periods in between. The length and intensity of the work interval depends on what the athlete is trying to accomplish. For instance, a longer work interval has a greater involvement of aerobic energy production, while a shorter, more intense interval provides greater participation of anaerobic metabolism. Therefore, interval training that is designed to improve $\dot{V}O_2$ max should generally utilize intervals > 60 sec to maximize the involvement of aerobic ATP production. Further, it is generally believed that high-intensity intervals are more effective in improving aerobic power, and perhaps the lactate threshold, than low-intensity intervals (20, 22, 37).

One obvious advantage of interval training over continuous running is that this method of training provides a means of performing large amounts of high-intensity exercise in a short time. Further, this training method offers two ways of providing a training overload. For example, the interval training prescription can be modified to provide "overload" in terms of either increasing the total number of exercise intervals performed, or the intensity of the work interval. Adjustments to either of these factors allow the coach or athlete to alter the workout plan to accomplish specific training goals.

How does one design an interval workout? A complete discussion of the theory and rationale of designing an interval training program to improve athletic performance is beyond the scope of this chapter. For a detailed discussion of interval training, the reader is referred to Fox and Mathews (20). Additionally, table 21.2 provides some general guidelines for determining the intensity for running or swimming intervals.

In planning an interval training session, the following variables need to be considered: (1) length of the work interval, (2) intensity of the effort, (3) duration of the rest interval, (4) number of interval sets, and (5) the number of work repetitions. The length of the **work interval** refers to the distance to be covered during the work effort. In training to improve aerobic power, the work interval should generally last longer than sixty seconds. The intensity of the work effort during interval training can be monitored from a ten-second HR count upon completion of the interval (i.e., 10 sec HR count $\times$ 6 = HR per min). In general, exercise HR's should reach 85%–100% of the maximal HR during interval training. The time between work efforts is termed the **rest interval,** and consists of light activity such as walking. The length of the rest

Table 21.2 *Guidelines for determining the intensity or work rate during interval training for running and swimming different distances.*

Interval Training Distances (Yards)		Work Rate for Each Interval
Run	Swim	
100	25	One to five seconds slower than best time
220	50	Three seconds slower than best time
440	100	One to four seconds faster than average 440-yard run or 100-yard swim times recorded during a mile run or 440-yard swim
880–1,320	165–320	Three to four seconds slower than the average 440-yard run or 100-yard swim times recorded during a mile run or 440-yard swim

Modified from reference 20.

interval is generally expressed as a ratio of the duration of the work interval. For example, if the work interval for running 400 meters was seventy-five seconds, a rest interval of seventy-five seconds would result in a 1:1 ratio of work to rest. Generally, the rest interval should be at least as long as the work interval (2). In planning an interval training program for athletes who are not already highly trained, a work:rest ratio of 1:3 or 1:2 seems preferable. As a rule of thumb, the HR should drop to approximately 120 beats · min⁻¹ near the end of the recovery interval (2).

A **set** is a specified number of work efforts performed as a unit. For instance, a set may consist of 8 × 400-meter runs with a prescribed rest interval between each run. The term **repetition** is the number of work efforts within one set. In the example just given, 8 × 400-meter run repetitions constituted one set. The number of repetitions and sets performed per workout depends on the purpose of the particular training session and the fitness levels of the athletes involved.

Long, Slow Distance
The use of long, slow distance (LSD) runs (or cycle rides, long swims, etc.) became a popular means of training for endurance events in the 1970s. In general, this method of training involves performing exercise at a low intensity (i.e., 57% $\dot{V}O_2$ max or approximately 70% of max HR) for durations that are generally greater in length than the normal competition distance. Although it seems reasonable that this type of training is a useful means of preparing an athlete to compete in long endurance competitions (marathon running), recent evidence suggests that short-term, high-intensity exercise is superior to long-term, low-intensity exercise in improving $\dot{V}O_2$ max (33, 34).

High-Intensity, Continuous Exercise
Again, there is a growing volume of evidence to suggest that continuous high intensity exercise is an outstanding means of improving $\dot{V}O_2$ max and the lactate threshold in athletes (15, 18, 21, 26, 33). At present, the exact exercise intensity that elicits maximal improvement in $\dot{V}O_2$ max is unknown. However, it seems likely that a work rate that is equal to or slightly above the lactate threshold provides excellent improvement in maximum aerobic power and thus is a useful guideline for planning training programs (43). Recall from chapter 20 that the lactate threshold can be determined in the laboratory during an incremental exercise test. Additionally, the lactate threshold can be estimated noninvasively using the ventilatory threshold

(chapters 10 and 20). In the field, it is not practical to take repeated blood samples to determine the training speed that equals the lactate threshold during each training session, nor is it practical to continuously monitor ventilation during training. Therefore, the athlete needs a simple, noninvasive means of evaluating exercise intensity. Exercise heart rate appears to be the most practical means of evaluating exercise intensity during training. During the laboratory assessment of the lactate threshold or ventilatory threshold, it is standard practice to record heart rate stage-by-stage. The heart rate that corresponds to the metabolic rate at which the lactate threshold occurred can then be used by the athlete during training sessions as a guide to optimize training intensity.

The objective during high-intensity, continuous training is to exercise at a heart rate near the lactate threshold for approximately twenty-five to fifty minutes, with the duration of the training session being dependent on the fitness level of the athlete. As the athlete improves, it may become necessary to repeat the laboratory testing and alter the training intensity accordingly.

Training for Improved Anaerobic Power

Athletic events lasting less than sixty seconds depend largely on anaerobic production of the necessary energy. In general, training to improve anaerobic power centers around the need to enhance either the ATP-CP system or anaerobic glycolysis (lactic acid system). However, some activities require major contributions of both of the above anaerobic metabolic pathways to provide the necessary ATP for competition (see table 21.1). Again, it is critical that the training program use the specific muscle groups that are required by the athlete during competition.

Training to Improve the ATP-CP System
Sports such as football, weight lifting, and short dashes in track (100 meters) depend on the ATP-CP system to provide the bulk of the energy needed for competition. Therefore, optimal performance requires a training program that will maximize ATP production via the ATP-CP pathway.

Training to improve the ATP-CP system involves a special type of interval training. In order to maximally stress the ATP-CP metabolic pathway, short, high-intensity intervals (five to ten seconds duration) using the muscles utilized in competition are ideal. Because of the short durations of this type of interval, little lactic acid is produced and recovery is rapid. The rest interval may range between thirty to sixty seconds depending on the fitness levels of the athletes. For example, a training program for football players might involve repeated 30-yard dashes (with several directional changes), with a thirty-second rest period between efforts (chapter 20). The number of repetitions per set would be determined by the athletes' fitness levels, environmental factors, and perhaps other considerations.

Training to Improve the Glycolytic System
After approximately ten seconds of a maximal effort, there is a growing dependence on energy production from anaerobic glycolysis (2, 19, 23). In order to improve the capacity of this energy pathway, the athlete must overload the "system" via short-term, high-intensity efforts. In general, high-intensity intervals of twenty to sixty seconds duration are useful in overloading this metabolic pathway.

This type of anaerobic training is both physically and psychologically demanding and thus requires a high commitment on the part of the athlete. Further, this type of training may drastically reduce muscle glycogen stores. It is for these reasons that athletes often alternate hard interval training days and light training sessions.

Training to Improve Muscular Strength

The goal of a strength training program is to increase the maximum amount of force that can be generated by a particular muscle group. In general, any muscle that is regularly exercised at a high intensity (i.e., intensity near its maximum force generating capacity) will become stronger (48). Strength training exercises can be classified into three categories: (1) isometric or static, (2) isotonic (includes **variable resistance exercise**), and (3) isokinetic. Recall that isometric exercise is the application of force without joint movement, and that isotonic exercise involves force application with joint movement (chapter 8). Variable resistance exercise is the term used to describe machines such as Nautilus® equipment, which provide a variable amount of resistance during the course of an isotonic contraction. Isokinetic exercise is the exertion of force at a constant speed. Although isometric exercise has been shown to improve strength, either isotonic or isokinetic strength training are generally preferred in the preparation of athletes because isometric training does not increase strength over the full range of motion—only at the specific joint angle maintained during training (19, 48, 52).

What physiological adaptations occur as a result of strength training? One of the obvious and perhaps most important physiological changes that occurs following a strength training program is the increase in muscle mass. Recall from chapter 8 that the amount of force that can be generated by a muscle group is proportional to the cross-sectional area of the muscle (36). Therefore, larger muscles exert greater force than smaller muscles. Many investigators believe that the increase in muscle size via resistance training is due to **hypertrophy** (an increase in muscle fiber diameter due to an increase in the number and size of myofibrils) (11, 27, 28, 29). However, Gonyea and associates argue that muscles also increase their size in response to strength training by **hyperplasia** (increase in the number of muscle fibers) (30, 31, 32, 47). Although this issue remains controversial, it appears that most of the current evidence supports the concept that increases in muscle size due to training occur via hypertrophy (11, 27, 28, 29, 48).

Strength training may also induce central nervous system changes, which can increase the number of motor units recruited, alter motor neuron firing rates, enhance motor unit synchronization during a particular movement pattern, and result in the removal of neural inhibition (40). These four processes result in an improvement in the amount of muscular force generated and appear to occur within the few weeks after starting a strength training program (40).

Progressive Resistance Exercise

The most common form of strength training is weight lifting using free weights or various types of weight machines (i.e., isotonic or isokinetic training). In order to improve strength, weight training must employ the overload principle by periodically increasing the amount of weight (resistance) used in a particular exercise. This method of strength training was first described in 1948 by DeLorme and Watkins (16) and is called **progressive resistance exercise (PRE).** Since this early work, numerous other systems of training to improve muscular strength have been proposed, but the concept of PRE is the basis for most weight-training programs.

General Strength-Training Principles

Again, muscles increase their strength by a systematic overload of being forced to contract at tensions near their maximum. If muscles are not overloaded, then there is no improvement in strength. Perhaps the first application of the overload principle was applied by the famous Olympic wrestler, Milo of Crotona (500 B.C.). Milo incorporated overload in his training routine by carrying a bull calf on his back each day until the animal reached maturity. Since the days of Milo, athletes have applied overload to training by lifting heavy objects.

The perfect training regimen for optimum improvement of strength remains controversial. However, many studies have demonstrated that the ideal number of repetitions is between four to eight repetitions maximum (RM) and practiced in multiple sets of three or more (3, 4, 48). Clearly, strength gains are less when the number of repetitions are greater than fifteen. Rest days between strength workouts seems critical for optimal strength improvement (3, 48). Therefore, a training schedule of three to four days per week is recommended.

Similar to other training methods, strength training should involve those muscles used in competition. Indeed, strength training exercises should stress the muscles in the same movement pattern used during the athletic competition. For example, a shot putter should perform exercises that strengthen the specific muscles of the arm, chest, back, and legs that are involved in "putting the shot."

Table 21.3 *Summary of potential advantages and disadvantages of weight training programs using various types of equipment.*

Program	Equipment	Advantages	Disadvantages
Isometric	Variety of home-designed devices	Minimal cost; less time required	Not directly applicable to most sport activities; may become boring; progress is difficult to monitor
Isotonic	Free weights	Low cost; specialized exercises may be designed to simulate a particular sport movement; progress easy to monitor	Injury potential due to dropping weights; increase workout time due to time required to change weights
Isotonic	Commercial weight machines (i.e., Universal)	Generally safe; progress easy to monitor; small amount of time required to change weight	Does not permit specialized exercise; high cost
Variable resistance	Commercial devices (e.g., Nautilus)	Has a cam system that provides a varible resistance that changes to match the joint's ability to produce force over the range of motion; progress easy to monitor; safety	High cost; limited specialized exercises
Isokinetic	Commerical isokinetic devices (e.g., Cybex)	Allows development of maximal resistance over full range of motion; exercises can be performed at a variety of speeds	High cost; limited specialized exercises

Modified from reference 8.

Free Weights versus Machines

Over the past several years, much controversy has centered around the question of whether training with free weights (barbells) or various types of weight machines (Nautilus®, Universal®, etc.) produces the greatest strength gains in athletes. At present, a definitive answer to this question is not available. However, Stone et al. (48) argues that strength training using free weights is superior to training with commerical weight machines (both isotonic and isokinetic) on the basis of the following reasoning: (1) data exists to support the notion that free weights produce greater strength gains during short-term training periods than many types of weight machines (49, 50), (2) use of free weights provides movement versatility and allows a greater specificity of training than weight machines, (3) training with free weights (unlike many weight machines) involves large muscle mass and multi-segment exercise, which forces the athlete to control both balance and stabilizing factors. This type of training is useful since most sports require the athlete to maintain balance and body stability during competition (48). Table 21.3 summarizes some of the advantages and disadvantages of strength training using isometric, isotonic (free weights, Nautilus®, etc.), and isokinetic machines.

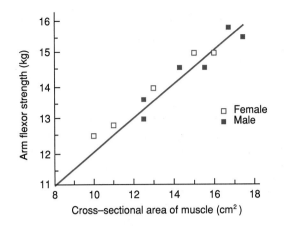

Figure 21.1 Arm flexor strength of men and women graphed as a function of muscle cross-sectional area.

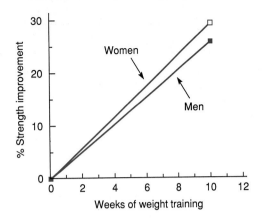

Figure 21.2 Strength changes in men and women as a result of a ten-week strength training program.

Gender Differences in Response to Strength Training

It is well established that when absolute strength (i.e., total amount of force applied) is compared between untrained men and women, men are typically stronger. This difference is greatest in the upper body where men are approximately 50% stronger than women, whereas men are only 30% stronger than women in the lower body (41). This apparent sex difference in strength is eliminated when force production in men and women is compared on the basis of the cross-sectional area of muscle. Figure 21.1 illustrates this point. Notice that as the cross-sectional area of muscle increases (x-axis), the arm flexor strength (y-axis) increases in a linear fashion and is independent of sex. That is, human muscle can generate 3–4 kg of force per cm² of muscle cross-section regardless of whether the muscle belongs to a male or female (36).

An often-asked question is "Do women gain strength as rapidly as men when training with weights?" In an effort to answer this question, Wilmore and colleagues (51) compared the strength change between a group of untrained men and women before and after ten weeks of isotonic weight training. Their findings suggested that no differences existed between sexes in the percent of strength gained during the training period (see figure 21.2). Similar findings

have been reported in other studies, and imply that men and women respond similarly to acute weight training (42). However, the aforementioned studies are considered short-term training periods and may not reflect what occurs over long-term training. For instance, it is generally believed that men exhibit a greater degree of muscular hypertrophy than women as a result of long-term weight training. This gender difference in muscular hypertrophy appears to be related to the fact that men have twenty to thirty times higher blood levels of testosterone. Further research is needed to determine whether men and women differ in strength gains over long-term weight training.

Muscle Soreness

It is a common experience for novice weight trainers and sometimes even veteran strength athletes to notice a **delayed onset muscle soreness (DOMS)** that appears twenty-four to forty-eight hours after strenuous exercise. The search for an answer to the question of "What causes DOMS?" has extended over many years. A number of possible explanations have been proposed, including a buildup of lactic acid in muscle, muscle spasms, and torn muscle and connective tissue. Based on present evidence, it appears that DOMS is due to tissue injury caused by excessive mechanical force exerted upon muscle and connective tissue (1, 9,

25). Perhaps the strongest data to support this viewpoint comes from electron microscropy studies in which electron micrographs taken of muscles suffering from DOMS reveal microscopic tears in these muscle fibers (25).

How does DOMS occur and what is the physiological explanation for DOMS? Armstrong (1) has proposed that DOMS occurs in the following manner: (1) strenuous muscular contractions (especially eccentric contractions) result in structural damage in muscle and perhaps connective tissue as well, (2) calcium leaks out of the sarcoplasmic reticulum and collects in the mitochondria, which inhibits oxidative phosphorylation (i.e., ATP production is halted), (3) the buildup of calcium also activates enzymes (proteases), which degrade cellular proteins including contractile proteins, (4) this breakdown of muscle cells results in an inflammatory process, which includes an increase in prostaglandin and histamine production, and finally (5) the accumulation of histamines, potassium, prostaglandins, and edema surrounding muscle fibers stimulates free nerve endings (pain receptors), which results in the sensation of DOMS (see figure 21.3).

How does one avoid being a victim of DOMS following exercise? It appears that DOMS occurs most frequently following intense exercise using muscles that are unaccustomed to being worked. Further, eccentric exercise appears to cause greater suffering from DOMS than concentric work. Therefore, a general recommendation for the avoidance of DOMS is to begin an exercise training program gradually. That is, avoid intense exercise (particularly eccentric) during the first five to ten training sessions. This pattern of slow progression allows the exercised muscles to "adapt" to the exercise stress and therefore reduces the incidence or severity of DOMS.

Training for Improved Flexibility

The ability to move joints through a full range of motion is important in many sports. Loss of flexibility can result in a reduction of movement efficiency and may increase the chance of injury in some sports (5).

Figure 21.3 Proposed model for the occurrence of delayed muscular soreness.

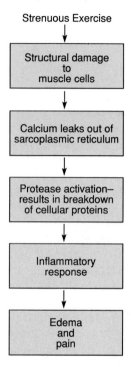

Proposed Model to Explain Delayed Muscular Soreness

Strenuous Exercise

Structural damage to muscle cells

Calcium leaks out of sarcoplasmic reticulum

Protease activation—results in breakdown of cellular proteins

Inflammatory response

Edema and pain

Therefore, many athletic trainers and coaches recommend regular stretching exercises to improve flexibility and thus reduce the chance of injury and perhaps optimize the efficiency of movement.

It should be noted however, that a high degree of flexibility in all joints may not be desirable in all sports. For instance, excessive flexibility is often indicative of proneness to injury in contact sports. For example, the shoulder joint is structurally very weak. This is because the glenoid fossa of the scapula (socket where the head of the humerus fits) is very shallow. Therefore, the main stability of the shoulder joint is provided by the surrounding musculature. Hence, an increase in shoulder muscle mass might reduce flexibility, but would lower the chance of shoulder injury in contact sports by increasing shoulder stability.

There are two general stretching techniques in use today: (1) **static stretching** (continuously holding a stretch position), and (2) **ballistic stretching** (bouncing or bobbing stretching). Although both techniques result in an improvement in flexibility, static stretching is considered to be superior over ballistic stretching because: (1) there is less chance of injury (5), and (2) static stretching causes less muscle spindle activity when compared to ballistic stretching. Stimulation of muscle spindles during ballistic stretching can produce a stretch reflex and therefore result in muscular contraction. This type of muscular contraction counteracts the desired lengthening of the muscle and may increase the chance of injury.

Research has shown that thirty minutes of static stretching exercises performed twice per week will improve flexibility within five weeks (17). It is recommended that the stretch position be held for ten seconds at the beginning of a flexibility program and increased up to sixty seconds after several training sessions. Each stretch position should be repeated three to five times, with the number increased up to ten repetitions. Overload is applied by increasing the range of motion during the stretch position and increasing the amount of time the stretch position is held.

Preceding a static stretch with an isometric contraction of the muscle group to be stretched is an effective means of improving muscle relaxation and may enhance the development of flexibility (5, 17, 52). Muscular relaxation follows an isometric contraction because the contraction stimulates Golgi tendon organs, which inhibit contraction during the subsequent stretching exercise.

Year-Round Conditioning for Athletes

It is common for today's athletes to engage in year-round conditioning exercises. This is necessary to prevent excessive weight gain, particularly in sports such as wrestling, and prevent extreme physical detraining between competitive seasons. By convention, the training periods of athletes are divided into three phases: (1) off-season training, (2) preseason training, and (3) in-season training. A brief description of each training period follows.

Off-Season Conditioning

In general, the objectives of off-season conditioning programs are to: (1) prevent excessive fat weight gain, (2) maintain muscular strength or endurance, (3) maintain ligament and bone integrity, and (4) maintain a reasonable skill level in the athlete's specific sport. Obviously, the exact nature of the off-season conditioning program will vary from sport to sport. For example, a football player would spend considerably more time performing strength-training exercises than a distance runner. Conversely, the runner would incorporate more running into an off-season conditioning program than the football player. Hence, specific exercises should be selected on the basis of the sport's demands (19).

No matter what the sport, it is critical that an off-season conditioning program provide variety for the athlete. Further, off-season conditioning programs generally use a training regimen that is is composed of low-intensity, high-volume work. This combination of low-intensity training and variety may prevent the occurrence of "overtraining syndromes" and the development of psychological staleness. Figure 21.4 contains a list of some recommended training activities for off-season conditioning.

Off-season conditioning allows the athletes to concentrate on fitness areas where they may be weak. Therefore, it is important that off-season programs be designed for the individual. For instance, a basketball player may lack leg strength and power and therefore have a limited vertical jump. An off-season conditioning program allows this athlete to engage in specific strength training acitivites which will improve leg power and enhance vertical jumping capacity.

Preseason Conditioning

The principal objective of preseason conditioning (e.g., eight to twelve weeks prior to competition) is to increase to a maximum the capacities of the predominant energy systems used in a particular athletic event (19). In the transition from off-season conditioning to preseason conditioning there is a gradual shift from low-intensity, high-volume exercise to high-intensity, low-volume exercise. As in all phases of a training cycle, the program should be sport specific.

Figure 21.4 Recommended activities for the various phases of year-round training.

Suggested Activities for the Various Phases of
A Year-Round Training Program

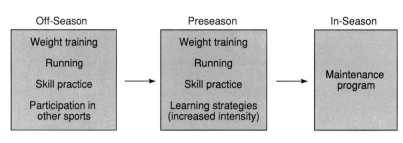

For a detailed preseason conditioning program for specific sports the reader is referred to Fox (19). In general, the types of exercise performed during preseason conditioning are similar to those used during off-season conditioning (figure 21.4). The principal difference between off-season and preseason conditioning is the intensity of the conditioning effort. During preseason conditioning, the athlete applies a progressive overload by increasing the intensity of workouts, whereas off-season conditioning involves high-volume, low-intensity workouts.

In-Season Conditioning

The general goal of in-season conditioning for most sports is to maintain the fitness level achieved during the preseason training program. For instance, in a sport such as football, in which there is a relatively long competitive season, the athlete must be able to maintain strength and endurance during the entire season. A complicating factor in planning an in-season conditioning program for many team sports is that the season may not have a clear-cut ending. That is, at the end of the regular season, play-off games may extend the season an additional several weeks. Therefore, it is difficult in these types of sports to plan a climax in the conditioning program, thus, the need for a maintenance training program.

In planning an in-season conditioning program, the goal is to design a program that is of sufficient volume and intensity to maintain reasonable strength and endurance during the entire playing season. Note that strength can be maintained during the competitive season by as little as one workout every seven to ten days (48). However, maintenance of cardiovascular fitness appears to require a minimum of two to three training days per week (35).

Common Training Mistakes

Some of the most common training errors include: (1) overtraining, (2) undertraining, (3) using exercises and work-rate intensities that are not sport specific, and (4) failure to plan long-term training schedules to achieve specific goals. Let's discuss each of these training errors briefly.

Overtraining may be a more significant problem than undertraining for several reasons. First, overtraining (workouts that are too long or too strenuous) may result in injury or reduce the athlete's resistance to disease. Further, overtraining may result in a psychological staleness, which can be identified by a general lack of enthusiasm on the part of the athlete. The general symptoms of overtraining are: (1) loss in body weight due to a reduction in appetite, (2) chronic fatigue, (3) psychological staleness, (4) multiple colds or sore throats, and/or (5) a decrease in performance.

An overtrained athlete may exhibit one or all of these symptoms (5, 19, 52). Therefore, it is critical that the coach or trainer recognize the classic symptoms of overtraining and be prepared to reduce their athletes' work loads when overtraining symptoms appear. It was stated earlier in this chapter that specific training programs should be planned for athletes when possible to compensate for individual differences in genetic potential and fitness levels. This is an important point to remember when planning training programs for athletic conditioning.

Another common mistake in the training of athletes is the failure to plan sport-specific training exercises. Often coaches or trainers fail to understand the importance of the law of specificity, and develop training exercises that do not enhance the energy capacities of the skeletal muscles used in competition. This error can be avoided by achieving a broad understanding of the training principles discussed earlier in this chapter.

Finally, coaches, trainers, and athletes should plan and record training schedules designed to achieve specific fitness objectives at various times during the year. Failure to plan a training strategy may result in misuse of training time and ultimately result in inferior performance.

Summary

1. The general objective of sport conditioning is to improve performance by increasing the maximum energy output during a particular movement. A conditioning program should allocate the appropriate amount of training time to match the aerobic and anaerobic energy demands of the sport.

2. Muscles respond to training as a result of a progressive overload. When an athlete stops training, there is a rapid decline in fitness due to detraining (reversibility).

3. In general, men and women respond to conditioning in a similar fashion. The amount of training improvement is always greater in those individuals who are less conditioned at the onset of the training program.

4. Every training session should consist of a warm-up period, workout session, and a cool down period.

5. Historically, training to improve maximal aerobic power has used three methods: (1) interval training, (2) long, slow distance, and (3) high-intensity, continuous exercise. Although controversy exists as to which of the above training methods results in the greatest improvement in $\dot{V}O_2$ max, there is growing evidence that it is intensity and not duration that is the most important factor in improving $\dot{V}O_2$ max.

6. Training to improve anaerobic power involves a special type of interval training. In general, the intervals are of short duration and consist of high-intensity exercise (near-maximal effort).

7. Improvement in muscular strength can be achieved via progressive overload by using either isometric, isotonic, or isokinetic exercise. Isotonic or isokinetic training seems preferable to isometric exercise in developing strength gains in athletes, since isometric strength gains occur only at the specific joint angles that are held during isometric training.

8. Although untrained men exhibit greater absolute strength than untrained females, there does not appear to be gender differences in strength gains during a short-term weight-training program.

9. Delayed onset muscle soreness (DOMS) is thought to occur due to microscopic tears in muscle fibers or connective tissue. This results in cellular degradation and an inflamatory response, which results in pain within twenty-four to forty-eight hours after strenuous exercise.

10. Improvement in joint mobility (flexibility) can be achieved via static or ballistic stretching, with static stretching being the preferred technique.

11. Year-round conditioning programs for athletes include an off-season program, preseason program, and an in-season program. The

general objectives of an off-season conditioning program are to prevent excessive fat weight gain, maintain muscular strength and endurance, maintain bone and ligament strength, and preserve a reasonable skill level in the athletes's specific sport.

12. Common mistakes in training include undertraining, overtraining, performing nonspecific exercises during training sessions, and failure to carefully schedule a long-term training plan.

Study Questions

1. Explain how knowledge of the energy systems used in a particular activity or sport might be useful in designing a sport-specific training program.

2. Provide an outline of the general principles of designing a training program for the following sports: (1) football, (2) soccer, (3) basketball, (4) volleyball, (5) distance running (5,000 meters), and (6) 200-meter dash (track).

3. Define the following terms as they relate to interval training: (1) work interval, (2) rest interval, (3) work-to-rest ratio, and (4) set.

4. How can interval training be used to improve both aerobic and anaerobic power?

5. List and discuss the three most common types of training programs used to improve $\dot{V}O_2$ max.

6. Discuss the practical and theoretical differences between an interval training program used to improve the ATP-PC system, and a program designed to improve the lactic acid system.

7. List the general principles of strength development.

8. Define the terms isometric, isotonic, and isokinetic.

9. Outline the model to explain delayed onset muscle soreness proposed by Armstrong.

10. Discuss the use of static and ballistic stretching to improve flexibility. Why is a high degree of flexibility not desired in all sports?

11. List and discuss the objectives of: (1) off-season conditioning, (2) preseason conditioning, and (3) in-season conditioning.

12. What are some of the more common errors made in the training of athletes?

Suggested Readings

Burke, E. J., ed. 1980. *Toward an Understanding of Human Performance*. Ithaca, N.Y.: Movement Publications.

Daniels, J., R. Fitts, and G. Sheehan. 1978. *Conditioning for Distance Running*. New York: John Wiley & Sons.

Fox, E. L. 1984. *Sports Physiology*. Philadelphia: W. B. Saunders Company.

Fox, E. L., T. Kirby, and A. R. Fox. 1987. *Bases of Fitness*. New York: Macmillan Publishing Company.

Stone, M., and H. O'Bryant. 1984. *Weight Training: A Scientific Approach*. Minneapolis: Burgess Publishing Company.

Wilmore, J., and D. Costill. 1988. *Training for Sport and Activity*. Dubuque, Ia.: Wm. C. Brown.

References

1. Armstrong, R. 1984. Mechanisms of exercise-induced delayed onset of muscular soreness: A brief review. *Medicine and Science in Sports and Exercise* 16:529–38.

2. Åstrand, P. O., and K. Rodahl. 1986. *Textbook of Work Physiology*. New York: McGraw-Hill.

3. Berger, R. A. 1982. *Applied Exercise Physiology*. Philadelphia: Lea & Febiger.

4. Berger, R. A. 1962. Optimum repetitions for the development of strength. *Research Quarterly* 33:334–38.

5. Brooks, G. A., and T. Fahey. 1987. *Fundamentals of Human Performance*. New York: Macmillan Publishing Company.

6. Burke, E. 1977. Physiological similar effects of similar training programs in males and females. *Research Quarterly* 48:510–17.

7. Burke, E., and B. D. Franks. 1975. Changes in $\dot{V}O_2$ max resulting from bicycle training at different intensities holding total mechanical work constant. *Research Quarterly* 46:31–37.

8. Burke, E. J. (ed.) 1980. *Toward an Understanding of Human Performance*. Ithaca, N.Y.: Mouvement Publications.

9. Clarkson, P. et al. 1986. Muscle soreness and serum creatine kinase activity following isometric, eccentric, and concentric exercise. *International Journal of Sports Medicine* 7:152–55.

10. Costill, D. 1979. *A Scientific Approach to Distance Running*. Los Altos: Track and Field News.

11. Costill, D. et al. 1979. Adaptations in skeletal muscle following strength training. *Journal of Applied Physiology* 46:96–99.

12. Coyle, E. et al. 1984. Time course of loss of adaptations after stopping prolonged intense endurance training. *Journal of Applied Physiology* 57:1857–64.

13. Coyle, E. et al. 1985. Effects of detraining on responses to submaximal exercise. *Journal of Applied Physiology* 59:853–59.

14. Daniels, J., R. Fitts, and G. Sheehan. 1978. *Conditioning for Distance Running*. New York: John Wiley & Sons.

15. Davies, C. T. M., and A. Knibbs. 1971. The training stimulus: The effects of intensity, duration, and frequency of effort on maximum aerobic power output. *Int. Z. Angew* 20:299–305.

16. Delorme, T., and A. Watkins. 1948. Techniques of progressive resistance exercise. *Archives of Physical and Rehabilitative Medicine* 29:263–66.

17. DeVries, H. 1962. Evaluation of static stretching procedures for improvement of flexibility. *Research Quarterly* 33:222–29.

18. Dudley, G., W. Abraham, and R. Terjung. 1982. Influence of exercise intensity and duration on biochemical adaptations in skeletal muscle. *Journal of Applied Physiology* 53:844–50.

19. Fox, E. L. 1984. *Sports Physiology*. Philadelphia: W. B. Saunders Company.

20. Fox, E. L., and D. Mathews. 1974. *Interval Training: Conditioning for Sports and General Fitness*. Philadelphia: W. B. Saunders Company.

21. Fox, E. et al. 1973. Intensity and distance of interval training programs and changes in maximal aerobic power. *Medicine and Science in Sports* 5:18–22.

22. Fox, E. et al. 1975. Frequency and duration of interval training programs and changes in aerobic power. *Journal of Applied Physiology* 38:481–84.

23. Fox, E., S. Robinson, and D. Wiegman. 1969. Metabolic energy sources during continuous and interval running. *Journal of Applied Physiology* 27:174–78.

24. Franks, B. 1983. In (M. Williams, ed.). *Ergogenic Aids in Sports*. Champaign, Ill.: Human Kinetics, Inc.

25. Friden, J., M. Sjostrom, and B. Ekblom. 1983. Myofibrillar damage following eccentric exercise in man. *International Journal of Sports Medicine* 4:170–76.

26. Gibbons, E. et al. 1983. Effects of various training intensity levels on anaerobic threshold and aerobic capacity in females. *Journal of Sports Medicine and Physical Fitness* 23:315–18.

27. Goldberg, A. 1965. Muscle hypertrophy in hypophysectomized rats. *Physiologist* 8:175–78.

28. Gollnick, P. et al. 1981. Muscular enlargement and number of fibers in skeletal muscles of rats. *Journal of Applied Physiology* 50:936–43.

29. Gollnick, P. et al. 1983. Fiber number and size in overloaded chicken anterior latissimus dorsi muscle. *Journal of Applied Physiology* 54:1292–97.

30. Gonyea, W. 1980. The role of exercise in inducing skeletal muscle fiber splitting. *Journal of Applied Physiology* 48:421–26.

31. Gonyea, W. et al. 1986. Exercise induced increases in muscle fiber number. *European Journal of Applied Physiology* 55:137–41.

32. Gonyea, W., G. Ericson, and F. Bonde-Peterson. 1977. Skeletal muscle fiber splitting induced weight lifting exercise in cats. *Acta Physiologica Scandanavica* 99:105–9.

33. Hickson, R., H. Bomze, and J. Holloszy. 1977. Linear increase in aerobic power induced by a strenuous program of endurance exercise. *Journal of Applied Physiology* 42:372–76.

34. Hickson, R. et al. 1981. Time course of the adaptive responses of aerobic power and heart rate to training. *Medicine and Science in Sports and Exercise* 13:17–20.

35. Hickson, R., and M. Rosenkoetter. 1981. Reduced training frequencies and maintenance of increased aerobic power. *Medicine and Science in Sports and Exercise* 13:13–16.

36. Ikai, M., and T. Fukunaga. 1968. Calculation of muscle strength per unit of cross sectional area of a human muscle by means of ultrasonic measurements *Int. Z. Angew. Physiol.* 26:26–31.

37. Knuttgen, H. et al. 1973. Physical conditioning through interval training with young male adults. *Medicine and Science in Sports* 5:220–26.

38. Martin, B. et al. 1975. Effect of warmup on metabolic responses to strenuous exercise. *Medicine and Science in Sports* 7:146–49.

39. McArdle, W., F. Katch, and V. Katch. 1986. *Exercise Physiology: Energy, Nutrition, and Human Performance.* Philadelphia: Lea & Febiger.

40. Moritani, T., and H. DeVries. 1979. Neural factors versus hypertrophy in the time course of muscle strength gain. *American Journal of Physical Medicine* 58:115–19.

41. Morrow, J., and W. Hosler. 1981. Strength comparsions in untrained men and trained women. *Medicine and Science in Sports and Exercise* 13:194–98.

42. O'Shea, J., and J. Wegner. 1981. Power weight training in the female athlete. *Physician and Sports Medicine* 9:109–14.

43. Priest, J., and R. Hagan. 1987. The effects of maximum steady-state pace on running performance. *British Journal of Sports Medicine* 21:18–21.

44. Saltin, B. et al. 1968. Response to exercise after bed rest and after training. *Circulation* 38(Suppl. 7):1–78.

45. Sharkey, B. 1970. Intensity and duration of training and the development of cardiorespiratory endurance. *Medicine and Science in Sports* 2:197–202.

46. Sharkey, B. 1984. *Physiology of Fitness.* Champaign, Ill.: Human Kinetics.

47. Sola, O., D. Christensen, and A. Martin. 1973. Hypertrophy and hyperplasia of adult chicken anterior latissimus dorsi muscle following stretch with and without denervation. *Experimental Neurology* 41:76–100.

48. Stone, M., and H. O'Bryant. 1984. *Weight Training: A Scientific Approach.* Minneapolis: Burgess Publishing Company.

49. Stone, M., R. Johnson, and D. R. Carter. 1979. A short term comparision of two different methods of resistance training on leg strength and power. *Athletic Training* 14:158–60.

50. Wathen, D. 1980. A comparsion of the effects of selected isotonic and isokinetic exercises, modalities, and programs on the vertical jump in college football players. *National Strength Coaches Association Journal* 2:47–48.

51. Wilmore, J. 1974. Alterations in strength, body composition, and anthrometric measurements consequent to a 10-week weight training program. *Medicine and Science in Sports* 6:133–39.

52. Wilmore, J., and D. Costill. 1988. *Training for Sport and Activity* Dubuque, Ia.: Wm. C. Brown.

22 *Training for Special Populations*

Objectives

*B*y studying this chapter, you should be able to do the following:
1. List those conditions in Type I diabetics that might limit their participation in a vigorous training program.
2. Explain the rationale for the selection of an insulin injection site for Type I diabetics prior to a training session.
3. List the precautions that should be taken by asthmatics during a training session.
4. Discuss the question "Does exercise promote seizures in epileptics?"
5. Discuss the possibility that chronic exercise presents a danger to: (1) the cardiopulmonary system, or (2) the musculoskeletal system of children?
6. Describe the incidence of amenorrhea in female athletes versus the general population.
7. List those factors thought to contribute to "athletic" amenorrhea?
8. Discuss the general recommendations for training during menstruation?
9. List the general guidelines for exercise during pregnancy.

Outline

Key Terms

amenorrhea
apophyses
articular cartilage
dysmenorrhea
epilepsy
epiphyseal plate or growth plate

Certainly the general physiological principles of exercise training to improve performance apply to any individual interested in improving athletic performance (chapter 21). However, there are several special populations that require individual consideration when discussing exercise training for competition. For instance, should diabetics, asthmatics, or epileptics engage in vigorous athletic training? Further, does vigorous exercise have potentially harmful effects on growth and development in children? Finally, are there special concerns for the female athlete engaged in heavy physical training? It is the purpose of this chapter to address each of the above questions. Let's begin our discussion with the topic of exercise training for the diabetic.

Competitive Training for Diabetics

As discussed in chapter 17, there is a beneficial effect of exercise on diabetes, and regular exercise is often recommended by physicians for diabetics as a part of their therapeutic regimen (i.e., to help maintain control of blood glucose levels) (14). We will limit our discussion to Type I diabetics since Type II diabetics are less likely to engage in training for performance purposes. Can Type I diabetics train vigorously and take part in competitive athletics? The answer to this question is a qualified yes. In long-term diabetic patients with microvascular complications (damage to small blood vessels) or neuropathy (nerve damage), exercise should be limited and extensive training is not generally recommended (27). However, in individuals free from complications, diabetes in itself should not limit the type of exercise or sporting event (31).

What precautions should the diabetic athlete take to allow safe participation in training programs? An overview of exercise training for fitness in diabetic populations was presented in chapter 17 and will be reviewed here only briefly. The key to safe participation in sport conditioning for the diabetic athlete is to learn to avoid hypoglycemic episodes during training. Since diabetics vary in their response to insulin, each diabetic athlete, in cooperation with his or her personal physician, must determine the appropriate combination of exercise, diet, and insulin for optimal control of blood glucose concentrations. In general, exercise should take place after a meal and should be part of regular routine. It is often recommended that a reduction in the amount of insulin injected be considered on days in which the athlete is engaged in strenuous training (14, 29, 31). A major concern for the diabetic athlete is the site of the insulin injection prior to exercise. Insulin injected subcutaneously in the leg prior to running (or other forms of leg exercise) results in an increased rate of insulin uptake due to elevated leg blood flow. This may result in an exercise-induced hypoglycemia and can be avoided by using an insulin injection site in the abdomen or the arm (31). Conversely, if the training regimen requires arm exercise (e.g., rowing), the site of insulin injection should be away from the working muscle (e.g., abdomen). Having a glucose solution or carbohydrate snack available during training sessions may help avoid hypoglycemic incidents during workouts.

Can diabetics obtain the same benefits from training as nondiabetics? The consensus answer to this question is yes. Although untrained diabetic children tend to be less fit than normal children, young diabetics respond to a conditioning program in a similar manner to healthy children (27). Empirical observations suggest that when the diabetic athlete's blood glucose is carefully regulated, he or she can compete and excel in a variety of competitive sports.

Training for Asthmatics

It is generally agreed that most children, adolescents, and adults with asthma may safely participate in all sports, provided they are able to control exercise-induced bronchospasms via medication or careful monitoring of activity levels (27). A prerequisite for planning training programs for asthmatics is that the proper therapeutic regimen for managing the athlete's particular type of asthma be worked out prior to commencement of a vigorous training program (chapter 17). Once the asthma is under control, planning the training schedule for asthmatic athletes is identical to that prescribed for athletes without asthma (chapter 21). However, as mentioned in chapter 17, it is often recommended that the asthmatic athlete keep an inhaler (containing a bronchodilator) handy during training sessions, and that workouts be conducted with other athletes in case a major attack occurs.

Epilepsy and Physical Training

The term **epilepsy** refers to a transient disturbance of brain function, which may be characterized by a loss of consciousness, muscle tremor, and sensory disturbances. Since the occurrence of epilepic seizures are not easily predicted, should epileptics engage in vigorous training programs? Unfortunately, there is little information available to answer this question. Before a clear-cut recommendation for the participation of epileptics in athletics can be made, two fundamental questions must be answered. First, does intense physical activity increase the risk of an epileptic seizure? Secondly, does the occurrence of a seizure during a particular sports activity expose the athlete to unnecessary risk? Let's examine the available evidence concerning each of these questions.

Does Exercise Promote Seizures?
There is one rare type of epileptic seizure that has been shown to be induced by exercise per se (6). These are tonic (continous motor activity) seizures and have been reported to occur during a variety of sports activities. Fortunately, this particular type of seizure can be controlled in most instances by anticonvulsant drugs.

In other types of seizure disorders, physicians remain divided in their opinions as to whether exercise increases the risk of seizure occurrence. A report by Gotze et al. (17) suggests that exercise does not increase the risk of seizures in epileptic children or adolescents. In fact, Gotze (17) argues that exercise appears to reduce the incidence of seizures in epileptics by increasing the threshold for seizures. In contrast, Kuijer (23) has suggested that the epileptic is at an increased risk of experiencing a seizure during recovery from exercise. He contends that hyperventilation during recovery from exercise may be the stimulus for the activation of this type of seizure.

Another specific concern for the participation of epileptics in contact sports is whether a blow to the head might mediate a seizure. Again, physicians remain divided in their opinions. Some authors believe the risks are high (20), while Livingston (24) argues that no studies exist to prove that repeated head trauma in epileptics causes a recurrence of seizures. Livingston's argument is based on thirty-six years of personal experience with hundreds of seizure patients who have participated in a variety of contact sports such as football, wrestling, and even boxing. While all of these contact sports predispose the athlete to head trauma, Livingston (24) states that he has not observed a single case where recurrent seizures occurred due to head trauma.

Risk of Injury Due to Seizures
Clearly, there are many competitive sports activities (e.g., football, boxing) during which the occurrence of a seizure would expose the athlete to a risk of harm. However, the occurrence of a seizure during many types of daily routine activities (e.g., climbing stairs) or recreational sports (e.g., SCUBA diving, mountain climbing) could also pose a threat to the epileptic. Whether or not the epileptic should participate in

physical training or sports must be determined on an individual basis by the use of common sense and advice from a sports physician. The benefit-risk ratio of sports participation may vary greatly from case to case and is dependent on the exact nature of the patient's epilepsy and the sport being considered. A child with only a minor seizure problem may, with the aid of medication, experience only a rare seizure with little visible alteration in behavior or consciousness due to the seizure. This type of epileptic could likely participate in almost any training activity without harm (4, 17). In contrast, an epileptic who experiences frequent and major seizures would not be a candidate for many types of sports. For a detailed discussion of epilepsy and exercise, see Strauss in the suggested reading list.

Sports Conditioning for Children

There are many unanswered questions related to the physiologic responses of the healthy child to various types of exercise. This is due to the limited number of investigators studying children and exercise, and because of ethical considerations in studying children. For instance, few investigators would puncture a child's artery, take a muscle biospsy, or expose a child to harsh environments (e.g., heat, cold, high altitudes) to satisfy scientific curiosity. Because of these ethical constraints, current knowledge concerning training for children is limited primarily to the cardiopulmonary system, with a growing body of information concerning the possiblility of musculoskeletal injury as a result of specific types of sports training. The following discussion addresses some of the important issues concerning child participation in vigorous conditioning programs.

Training and the Cardiopulmonary System
As youth sports teams increased in popularity, one of the first questions asked was "Are the hearts of children strong enough for intensive sports conditioning?" In other words, is there a possibility of "overtraining" young athletes, with the end result being permanent damage to the cardiovascular system? The answer to this question is "no." Children involved in endurance sports such as running or swimming improve their

maximal aerobic power comparable to adults and show no indices of damage to the cardiopulmonary system (11, 12). In fact, over the past several years, children have safely trained and completed marathon runs in less than four hours. If proper techniques of physical training are employed, with a progressive increase in cardiopulmonary stress, children appear to adapt to endurance training in a fashion similar to adults (11, 12, 27).

Training and the Musculoskeletal System
Clearly, organized vigorous training in some types of sports (e.g., swimming, basketball, volleyball, track and field) does not appear to adversely affect growth and development in children (27). This is true for both boys (12) and girls (2). In fact, moderate physical training has been shown to augment or optimize growth in children (1, 2, 11, 12). Therefore, many investigators have concluded that a certain amount of physical activity is necessary for normal growth and development (1, 2, 27). However, is there danger of overtraining? Can children perform heavy endurance training or strength training without long-term musculoskeletal problems? This issue remains controversial. There is evidence that the growing bones of a child are more susceptible to certain types of mechanical injury than those of the adult, primarily because of the presence of growth cartilage (27). Growth cartilage is present at the growth plate (**epiphyseal plate**), **articular cartilage** (cartilage at joints), and the sites of major muscle-tendon insertion (**apophyses**) in the child (27). The location of the growth plate, articular cartilage, and the apophyses for the knee joint is illustrated in figure 22.1. The growth plate is the site of bone growth in long bones. The time at which bone growth ceases varies from bone to bone, but is generally complete by eighteen to twenty years of age (27). Upon completion of growth, growth plates ossify (harden with calcium) and disappear, and growth cartilage is replaced by a permanent "adult" cartilage.

Is there an optimal level of training for children, above which musculoskeletal injuries may occur? The apparent answer to this question is yes. Clinical evidence suggests that excessive throwing in organized youth league baseball may result in injury to the elbow

Figure 22.1. Location of the growth plate (epiphyseal plate), articular cartilage, and apophyses associated with the long bones in the leg.

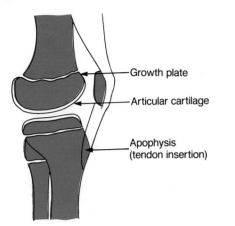

(Little League elbow) (27). This same problem is not observed in free-play situations (27). Another major concern for children participating in endurance training (e.g., running) or strength training (e.g., weight lifting) is that the constant microtrauma of repetitive training can cause premature closure of the growth plate and therefore retard normal long bone growth. Experimental literature on training and specific bone lengths indicates reduced bone lengths in rats and mice exposed to forced swimming and running (27). Unfortunately, corresponding data on humans does not exist. However, given the evidence available on the influence of physical activity on bone growth and development, it appears that the advice of Steinhaus (30) offered over fifty years ago seems to be sound. That is, the pressure effects of regular physical activity may stimulate bone growth to an optimal length, but excessive pressure (overtraining) can retard linear growth. The practical problem in dealing with young athletes is that it is difficult to define excessive pressure. In other words, how much training is optimal to bring about the desired physiological training responses without causing musculoskeletal problems? At present, a simple answer to this question is not available. There is an obvious need for detailed research in this area to produce guidelines for youth coaches and trainers in the development of conditioning programs for children engaged in competitive athletics.

Factors Important to Women Involved in Vigorous Training

Involvement of large numbers of women in competitive athletics has been a fairly recent phenomenon. Over the past two decades, the number of women that are actively engaged in competitive athletics has increased exponentially. Unfortunately, many of the decisions regarding the participation of women in sports and exercise programs have been made on the basis of limited, or absent physiological information. Research concerning women and exercise was scarce until the last few years, and even now is in its infancy. Although many questions concerning the female athlete remain to be answered, current research indicates that there is little reason to limit the healthy female athlete from active participation in endurance or power sports (19). In fact, the general responses of females to exercise and training are basically the same as those described for males. This is logical since the same cellular mechanisms that regulate most physiological and biochemical responses to exercise are the same for both sexes. However, there are several specific concerns related to female participation in vigorous training.

Exercise and Menstrual Disorders

Over the past several years there have been increasing reports concerning the influence of intense exercise training on the length of the menstrual cycle (8, 9, 13, 15, 18, 26). Indeed, there are numerous reports in the literature of female athletes that experience "athletic" amenorrhea. The term **amenorrhea** refers to a cessation of menstruation, and is generally defined as less than four menses per year (25).

How common is athletic amenorrhea? It appears that the incidence of amenorrhea is higher in some sports than in others. For example, the occurrence of irregular menses is rather high in distance running and ballet dancing, while much lower incidences are reported for swimming or cycling (3, 25). Dale (8) reports that the incidence of amenorrhea in the general population is only approximately 3%, while the incidence in distance runners is 24%.

What causes menstrual cycle dysfunction in athletes? At present a definitive answer is not possible, but current belief is that the cause may vary between

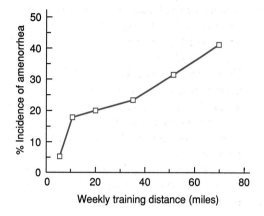

Figure 22.2 The relationship between training distance and the incidence of amenorrhea. Notice that as the training distance increases, there is a direct increase in the incidence of amenorrhea.

Training and Menstruation

The consensus opinion among physicians is that there is little reason for the healthy female athlete to avoid training or competition during menses (19). In fact, data are accumulating to show that world records have been established during all phases of the menstrual cycle. Therefore, it is not recommended that the female athlete alter her training or competitive schedule because of menses.

Dysmenorrhea (painful menstruation) is one of the greatest concerns of the female athlete. Several reports show that the incidence of dysmenorrhea is higher in athletic populations than nonathletic groups (19). The explanation for this observation is unknown. It is believed that prostaglandins (a type of naturally occuring fatty acid) are responsible for dysmenorrhea in both athletes and nonathletes. The release of prostaglandins begins just prior to the onset of menstrual flow, and may last for two to three days after menses begins. These prostaglandins cause the smooth muscle in the uterus to contract, which in turn causes ischemia (reduced blood flow) and pain (19).

Although athletes that experience dysmenorrhea can continue to train, this is often difficult since physical activity may increase the discomfort. Athletes who experience severe dysmenorrhea should see a physician for treatment. Hale (19) reports that athletes often experience a reduction in dysmenorrhea pain with the use of antiprostaglandin drugs. These drugs are considered safe and can be taken without interrupting training schedules.

Training during Pregnancy

Chapter 17 provided a brief overview of what is currently known about exercising for fitness during pregnancy. While it is generally agreed that women who are physically fit prior to becoming pregnant may continue to perform moderate intensity (short duration) exercise during pregnancy (5, 10, 22), controversy exists concerning the wisdom of intense training for pregnant women. Animal studies have demonstrated that long-duration exercise (more than thirty minutes) during pregnancy results in a reduction in both uterine blood flow and fetal weight at term (7, 16, 28, 32). In particular, one study reported that placental diffusion

individual athletes and is probably due to multiple factors. Although early studies linked a low percentage of body fat with athletic amenorrhea (25), recent evidence does not fully support the notion that low body fat is the principal cause of amenorrhea (15, 33). Whatever the cause of amenorrhea in athletes, it appears to be related to training intensity (13). Figure 22.2 illustrates this point. Notice that as the weekly training distances increase, the incidence of athletic amenorrhea increases in proportion to the increase in training stress. This finding can be interpreted to mean that intense training either directly or indirectly influences the incidence of amenorrhea. There are at least two ways in which training might influence normal reproductive function. First, it has been proposed that since exercise alters blood hormone concentrations (21), this change in hormone concentration may result in a modification of feedback to the hypothalamus (chapter 5). This altered feedback, in turn, may influence the release of female reproductive hormones and therefore modify the menstrual cycle (25). A second possibility is that high training mileage may result in increased psychological stress. Psychological stress may disrupt the menstrual cycle by increasing blood levels of catecholamines or endogenous opiates, which have a role in regulating the reproductive system (25).

capacity decreases as a direct function of both the duration and intensity of exercise during pregnancy (16). If these results can be extrapolated to humans, it appears that heavy training may have detrimental effects on fetal development. In light of these animal reports that suggest potential fetal harm if the pregnant mother engages in heavy or long-duration exercise, Hale (19) has recommended that the pregnant female be discouraged from engaging in vigorous exercise. For those athletes wishing to maintain fitness during pregnancy, Hale recommends aquatic programs, since swimming or other forms of aquatic exercise allows cardiovascular training in a medium that offers the body support and accelerated heat transfer. Specific guidelines for exercise during pregnancy were listed in chapter 17 (table 17.4).

Summary

1. Type I diabetics who are free of diabetic complications should not be limited in the type or quantity of exercise. The key for safe sports participation for the Type I diabetic is for the athlete to learn to avoid hypoglycemic episodes.
2. Asthmatics can safely participate in all sports, provided they are able to control exercise-induced bronchospasms via medication or careful monitoring of activity levels.
3. The question of safe participation for epileptics in training programs must be determined on an individual basis. The benefit-risk ratio of sports participation may vary greatly from case to case, and is dependent on the type of epilepsy involved and the sport being considered.
4. Although physical activity has been shown to optimize growth in children, questions remain as to the possibility of overtraining with resultant injuries to the musculoskeletal system. In particular, there is evidence that the growing bones of children are more susceptible to certain types of mechanical injury than adults due to the presence of growth cartilage.
5. The incidence of amenorrhea in female athletes appears to be highest in distance runners when compared to other sports such as swimming or cycling. Although the cause of amenorrhea in female athletes is not clear, it appears likely that multiple factors (e.g., the amount of training and psychological stress) may be involved.
6. There appears to be little reason for female athletes to avoid training during menstruation unless they experience severe discomfort due to dysmenorrhea. Athletes who experience severe dysmenorrhea should see a physician for treatment.
7. Present data suggest that long-duration or intense training should be avoided during pregnancy.

Study Questions

1. What is the recommendation for Type I diabetics with no physical complications for entering a competitive training program?
2. What factors should be considered when advising the diabetic athlete concerning safe participation in athletic conditioning? Include in your discussion suggestions concerning meal timing, injection sites for insulin, and the availability of glucose drinks during training sessions.
3. What is the current opinion concerning the safe participation of asthmatics in competitive athletics?
4. Define the term epilepsy.
5. Discuss the possibility that exercise increases the risk of seizures for epileptics.
6. What factors should be considered in assessing the risk-to-benefit ratio of sports participation for epileptics?
7. Discuss the notion that intense exercise might result in permanent damage to: (a) the cardiovascular system, or (b) musculoskeletal system in children.
8. Outline several possible causes of "athletic" amenorrhea.

9. What is the current recommendation for training and competition during menstruation?
10. Discuss the role of prostaglandins in mediating dysmenorrhea.
11. Based on present information, what are reasonable guidelines for advising the pregnant athlete concerning the intensity and duration of training?

Suggested Readings

Loucks, A., and S. Horvath. 1985. Athletic amenorrhea: A review. *Medicine and Science in Sports and Exercise* 17:56–72.

Micheli, L. 1984. *Pediatric and Adolescent Sports Medicine*. Philadelphia: W.B. Saunders Company.

Powers, S. 1984. Children and exercise. In (J. Thomas, ed.) *Motor Development during Childhood and Adolescence*. Minneapolis: Burgess Publishing Company.

Strauss, R., ed. 1984. *Sports Medicine*. Philadelphia: W.B. Saunders Company.

References

1. Adams, E. 1938. A comparative anthropometric study of hard labor during youth as a stimulator of physical growth of young colored women. *Research Quarterly* 9:102–8.
2. Åstrand, P. O. et al. 1963. Girl Swimmers. *Acta Paediatric Scandanavica* 147(Suppl.):1–75.
3. Baker, E. 1981. Menstrual dysfunction and hormonal status in athletic women: A review. *Fertility and Sterility* 36:691–96.
4. Bennett, D. 1981. Sports and epilepsy: To play or not to play. *Seminars in Neurology* 1:345–57.
5. Bullard, J. 1981. Exercise and pregnancy. *Canadian Family Physician* 27:977–82.
6. Burger, L., R. Lopez, and F. Elliot. 1972. Tonic seizures induced by movement. *Neurology* 22:656–59.
7. Curet, L. et al. 1976. Effect of exercise on cardiac output and distribution of uterine blood flow in pregnant ewes. *Journal of Applied Physiology* 40:725–28.
8. Dale, E., D. Gerlach, and A. Wilhute. 1979. Menstrual dysfunction in distance runners. *Obstetrics and Gynecology* 54:47–53.
9. Dale, E. et al. 1979. Physical fitness profiles and reproductive physiology of the female distance runner. *Physician and Sportsmedicine* 7:83–95.
10. Dressendorfer, R. 1978. Physical training during pregnancy and lactation. *Physician and Sportsmedicine* 6:74–80.
11. Ekblom, B. 1969. Effect of physical training on oxygen transport system in man. *Acta Physiologica Scandanavica* 328(Suppl.):1–45.
12. Eriksson, B. 1972. Physical training, oxygen supply and muscle metabolism in 11–13 year-old boys. *Acta Physiologica Scandanavica* 384(Suppl.):1–48.
13. Feicht, C. et al. 1978. Secondary amenorrhea in athletes. *Lancet* 2:1145–46.
14. Felig, P., and V. Koivisto. 1979. The metabolic response to exercise: Implications for diabetes. In (D. Lowenthal, K. Bharadwaja, and W. Oaks, ed.) *Therapeutics through Exercise*. New York: Grune and Stratton.
15. Galle, P. et al. 1983. Physiologic and psychologic profiles in a survey of women runners. *Fertility and Sterility* 39:633–39.
16. Gilbert, R. et al. 1979. Placental diffusing capacity and fetal development in exercising or hypoxic guinea pigs. *Journal of Applied Physiology* 46:828–34.
17. Gotze, W., S. Kubicki, and M. Munter. 1967. Effect of physical activity on seizure threshold investigated by electroencephalographic telemetry. *Diseases of the Nervous System* 28:664–67.
18. Gray, D., and E. Dale. 1983. Variables associated with secondary amenorrhea in women runners. *Journal of Sports Sciences* 1:55–67.
19. Hale, R. 1984. Factors important to women engaged in vigorous physical activity. In (R. Strauss, ed.) *Sports Medicine*. Philadelphia: W.B. Saunders Company.
20. Jennett, B. 1974. Early traumatic epilepsy: Incidence and significance after non-muscle injuries. *Archives of Neurology* 30:394–98.
21. Jurkowski, J. et al. 1978. Ovarian hormonal responses to exercise. *Journal of Applied Physiology* 44:109–14.
22. Kolata, G. 1983. Exercise during pregnancy reassessed. *Science* 219:832–33.
23. Kuijer, A. 1980. Epilepsy and exercise, electroencephalographical and biochemical studies. In (J. Wada and J. Penry, ed.) *Advances in Epileptology: The X Epilepsy International Symposium*. New York: Raven Press.

24. Livingston, S., and W. Berman. 1973. Participation of epileptic patients in sports. *Journal of American Medical Association* 224:236–38.

25. Loucks, A., and S. Horvath. 1985. Athletic amenorrhea: A review. *Medicine and Science in Sports and Exercise* 17:56–72.

26. Lutter, J., and S. Cushman. 1982. Menstrual patterns in female runners. *Physician and Sportsmedicine* 10:60–72.

27. Micheli, L. 1984. *Pediatric and Adolescent Sports Medicine*. Philadelphia: W.B. Saunders Company.

28. Nelson, P., R. Gilbert, and L. Longo. 1983. Fetal growth and placental diffusing capacity in guinea pigs following long-term maternal exercise. *Journal of Developmental Physiology* 5:1–10.

29. Pruett, E. 1985. Insulin and exercise in the non-diabetic man. In (K. Fotherly and S. Pal, ed.) *Exercise Physiology*. New York: Walter de Gruyter.

30. Steinhaus, A. 1933. Chronic effects of exercise. *Physiological Review* 13:103–147.

31. Sutton, J. 1984. Metabolic responses to exercise in normal and diabetic individuals. In (R. Strauss, ed.) *Sports Medicine*. Philadelphia: W.B. Saunders Company.

32. Terada, J. 1974. Effect of physical activity before pregnancy on fetuses of mice exercised forcibly during pregnancy. *Teratology* 10:141–44.

33. Warren, M. 1980. The effects of exercise on pubertal progression and reproductive function in girls. *Journal of Clinical Endocrinology and Metabolism* 51:1150–57.

23 *Nutrition, Body Composition, and Performance*

Objectives

*B*y studying this chapter, you should be able to do the following:

1. Describe the effect of various carbohydrate diets on muscle glycogen and on endurance during heavy exercise.
2. Contrast the "classic" method of achieving a supercompensation of the muscle glycogen stores with the "modified" method.
3. Describe some of the problems when glucose is ingested immediately prior to exercise.
4. Identify the type of individual who would most benefit from carbohydrate ingestion *during* a prolonged endurance performance.
5. Contrast the evidence that protein is oxidized at a faster rate during exercise with the evidence that the use of labelled amino acids may be an inappropriate methodology to study this issue.
6. Describe the need for protein *during* the adaptation to a new, more strenuous exercise level with the protein need when the adaptation is complete.
7. Defend the recommendation that a protein intake that is 12% of energy intake is sufficient to meet an athlete's need.
8. Describe the "best" way to replace water, citing evidence to support your position.
9. Describe the characteristics of the beverage that should be used to replace water deficits and problems associated with too much glucose in the solution.
10. Describe the salt requirement of the athlete, compared to the sedentary individual, and the recommended means of maintaining sodium balance.
11. List the steps leading to iron deficiency anemia and the special problem that athletes have in maintaining iron balance.
12. Provide a brief summary of the effects of vitamin supplementation on performance.
13. Characterize the role of the pregame meal on performance and the rationale for limiting fats and proteins.
14. Describe the various components of the somatotype and what the following ratings signify: 171, 711, and 117.
15. Describe what the endomorphic and mesomorphic components in the Heath-Carter method of somatotyping represent in conventional body composition analysis.
16. Explain why one must be careful in recommending specific body fatness values for individual athletes.

Outline

Key Terms

ectomorphy
endomorphy
glucose polymer
mesomorphy
somatotype
supercompensation

This chapter on nutrition, body composition, and performance is an extension of chapter 18, since the primary emphasis must be on achieving health-related goals before performance-related goals are examined. In fact, the information presented here must be examined in light of what the average person needs. Does an athlete need additional protein? What percent body fat is a reasonable goal for an athlete? We will address these questions in that order.

Nutrition and Performance

The nutritional goals of the United States were identified in chapter 18 and are restated here:

Average American Diet

Current Diet → **Dietary Goal for Health**
46% Carbohydrate → 58% Carbohydrate
42% Fat → 30% Fat
12% Protein → 12% Protein

The dietary changes required for performance will be discussed relative to these dietary goals needed for health.

Carbohydrate

The dietary goals associated with health recommend that we increase the percent of calories derived from carbohydrate from the current value of about 46% to about 58%. In his analysis of the literature, Brotherhood (9) found the average percent of carbohydrate in the diet of athletes to be 46%, which is surprisingly low given the importance of carbohydrate in prolonged moderate to heavy exercise (see chapter 4). This section will consider the use of carbohydrates in the days prior to a performance and, secondly, during the performance itself.

Carbohydrate Diets and Performance

In 1967, three studies were published from the same Swedish laboratory that set the stage for our understanding of the role of muscle glycogen in performance (1, 6, 48). Hermansen et al. (48) showed muscle glycogen to be systematically depleted during heavy (77% $\dot{V}O_2$ max) exercise and when exhaustion occurred glycogen content was near zero. Ahlborg et al. (1) found that work time to exhaustion was directly related to the initial glycogen store in the working muscles. Bergstrom et al. (6) confirmed and extended this by showing that by manipulating the quantity of carbohydrate in the diet the concentration of glycogen in muscle could be altered and, along with it, the time to exhaustion. In their study subjects consumed 2,800 kcal · d^{-1} using either a low CHO (fat and protein) diet, a mixed diet, or a high-carbohydrate diet where 2,300 kcal came from carbohydrate. Glycogen contents of the quadriceps femoris muscle were, respectively, 0.63 (low), 1.75 (average), and 3.31 (high) g/100 g muscle, and performance time for exercise at 75% $\dot{V}O_2$ max averaged 57, 114, and 167 minutes. Figure 23.1 shows these results. In brief, the muscle glycogen content and performance time could be varied with diet. These laboratory findings were confirmed by Karlsson and Saltin (49), who had trained subjects run a 30-km race twice, once following a high carbohydrate diet and the other time after a mixed diet. The initial muscle glycogen level was 3.5 gm/100 g muscle

Figure 23.1 Effect of different diets on the muscle glycogen concentration and work time to exhaustion.

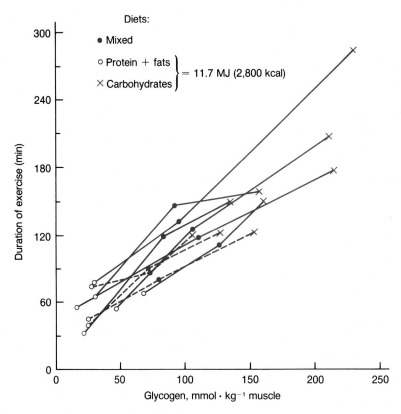

following the CHO diet and 1.7 gm/100 g muscle following the mixed diet. The best performance of all subjects occurred during the high CHO diet. Interestingly, the pace at the start of the race was not faster; instead, they were able to maintain the pace for a longer period of time. An important finding in this study is that compared to the high CHO diet, pace did not fall off for those on the mixed diet until about halfway through the race (about one hour or so). This suggests that the normal mixed diet used in their study would be suitable for athletic events lasting less than one hour.

Given the importance of muscle glycogen in prolonged endurance performance, it is no surprise that investigators have tried to determine what conditions will yield the highest muscle glycogen content. In 1966 Bergstrom and Hultman (6) had subjects do one-legged exercise to exhaust the glycogen store in the exercised leg while not affecting the resting leg's glycogen store. When this procedure was followed with a high-carbohydrate diet, the glycogen content was more than twice as high in the previously exercised leg, compared to the control leg. Further, they found that in subjects who had the high-carbohydrate diet following the protein/fat diet (plus doing exhausting exercise) the muscle glycogen stores were higher than when the mixed diet preceded the high-carbohydrate treatment (6). This combination of information led to the following *classical method* of achieving a muscle glycogen **"supercompensation"**:

1. two sessions of strenuous exercise to exhaust muscle glycogen store

2. a fat/protein diet for three days while continuing to train
3. high-carbohydrate diet (90% CHO) for three days, with inactivity.

There were some practical problems with this approach to achieving a high muscle glycogen content given that it required seven days to prepare for a race. Further, some subjects could not tolerate either the extremely low (high fat and protein) or high (90%) carbohydrate diets. Sherman et al. (62) proposed a *modified plan* that causes supercompensation. The plan requires a tapering of the workout at 70%–75% $\dot{V}O_2$ max from ninety minutes to forty minutes while eating a 50% CHO diet (350 gm/day). This is followed by two days of twenty-minute workouts while eating a 70% CHO diet (500–600 gm · d^{-1}) and, finally, a day of rest prior to the competition with the 70% CHO diet (or 500–600 gm · d^{-1}). This regimen was shown to be effective in increasing the glycogen stores to *high values* consistent with good performance (see figure 23.2).

The point that must be emphasized is that a person who is achieving the dietary goal of 58% of calories from carbohydrate is already close to the high-carbohydrate diets recommended for optimal performance. If an athlete requires 4,000 kcal per day for caloric balance and 58% are derived from carbohydrates, then 2,320 kcal (58% of 4,000 kcal) or 580 gm of carbohydrate will be consumed. This quantity is consistent with what is needed to restore muscle glycogen to normal levels twenty-four hours after strenuous exercise (17). This is important for training considerations, and this "regular" diet would require little or no change to meet the 70% carbohydrate diet (500–600 gm · d^{-1}) described by Sherman et al. (62).

Carbohydrates Immediately Prior to or During a Performance

Muscle glycogen is not the only source of carbohydrate used during exercise. Liver glycogen maintains the blood glucose that is taken up by muscle at an accelerated rate during exercise (see chapter 4). Scientists have tried to determine if the feeding of carbohydrate immediately prior to or during exercise could reduce the rate at which muscle glycogen is

used, as well as preventing a hypoglycemic condition. Hypoglycemia (blood glucose concentration <2.5 mmoles/liter) has been shown to occur during exercise at 58% $\dot{V}O_2$ max for 3.5 hours (3) and at 74% $\dot{V}O_2$ max for 2.5 hours (20). However the number of subjects who demonstrate central nervous system disfunction varied from none (34) to only 25% of the subjects (20). While there is no absolutely clear association between hypoglycemia and fatigue, the maintenance of the plasma glucose concentration by ingesting carbohydrates during exercise increases the time to fatigue in those subjects who tend to become hypoglycemic with exercise (20).

The timing and the type of carbohydrate taken in to slow down the depletion of the body's carbohydrate stores is important. It has been shown that when 75 g of glucose are ingested thirty to forty-five minutes before exercise requiring 70%–75% $\dot{V}O_2$ max, plasma glucose and insulin are elevated at the start of exercise, and muscle glycogen is used at a *faster rate* during the exercise (14, 54). This is counter to the goal of sparing muscle glycogen, and performance has been shown to decrease 19% with such a treatment (36). When 75 g of fructose were substituted for glucose, the elevation in plasma glucose and insulin were not observed and muscle glycogen depletion was less than observed with the glucose treatment (54).

In order to avoid this hyperinsulin response, carbohydrate feedings should be given immediately before or just after exercise starts. In addition, in an attempt to further reduce the chance of a hyperinsulin response, subjects have been fed **glucose polymers** (GP), short chains of glucose molecules. An advantage of the GP is that for the same number of gm of carbohydrate in solution, there is a lower osmolality, which should speed up the rate at which it enters the small intestine and increase the rate of absorption of fluid and electrolytes (45, 52, 59).

Coyle et al. (20) evaluated the effectiveness of GP given during exercise on a subject's ability to maintain a work rate of 74% $\dot{V}O_2$ max. In the control condition, seven of the ten subjects experienced a gradual decline in blood glucose throughout the test, reaching values of 2.5 mM, but only two experienced the CNS symptoms associated with hypolycemia. The GP treatment

Figure 23.2 Modification of the classic glycogen loading technique to achieve high muscle glycogen levels with minimal changes in a training or diet routine. Glycogen levels are in glucose units (gu) per kilogram (kg).

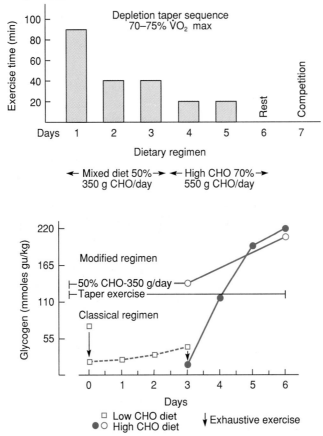

improved endurance performance in these seven subjects (time to fatigue increased from 126 to 159 minutes), and the plasma glucose concentration was maintained throughout the test. The three subjects who did not experience a hypoglycemic condition in the control test did not improve performance with the GP. Given that all subjects experienced fatigue with the GP treatment, it was concluded that while carbohydrate feeding cannot prevent fatigue, in some subjects it may increase the time needed to exhaust the muscle glycogen stores. Consistent with our previous discussion, the focus of attention is on muscle glycogen, which

is needed for work at high intensities. Even though the plasma glucose concentration was maintained with GP ingestion, plasma glucose cannot be taken across the muscle membrane fast enough to meet the muscle's carbohydrate demands at 74% $\dot{V}O_2$ max (18). Work by Ivy et al. (50) supports these observations.

Protein

The adult RDA for protein is 0.8 gm · kg^{-1} · d^{-1} and is easily met by a diet having 12% of its energy (kcal) as protein. For example, the RDA for energy for a nineteen to twenty-two year-old male weighing 70 kg is about 2,900 kcal/day. If 12% of that is protein then 348 kcal are taken in as protein (12% of 2,400 kcal). At 4 kcal $\cdot$ g^{-1}, this person would consume approximately 87 gms protein per day, representing 1.2 g $\cdot$ kg^{-1} $\cdot$ day^{-1} (87 g / 70 kg), or more than the RDA requirement for optimal health. Does an athlete have to take in more protein than specified in the RDA, or is the normal diet adequate? The answer, confusing as it may seem, appears to be yes.

Protein Requirement During Exercise

Adequacy of protein intake has been based primarily on nitrogen (N) balance studies. Protein is about 16% N by weight, and when N intake (dietary protein) equals N excretion, the person is in N balance. Excretion of less N than one consumes is called positive N balance, and the excretion of more N than one consumes is called negative N balance. This latter condition, if maintained, is inconsistent with good health due to the potential loss of muscle. Based on these N balance studies it was generally believed that the 0.8 gm $\cdot$ kg^{-1} $\cdot$ d^{-1} RDA standard was adequate for those engaged in prolonged exercise (76). In these studies, urinary N excretion was usually used as an index of N excretion, since about 85% of N is excreted this way (53). However, recent experiments suggest this method of measurement may have underestimated amino acid utilization in exercise. Lemon and Mullin (54) found that while there was no difference in urinary N excretion compared to rest, the loss of N in sweat increased 60–150-fold during exercise, suggesting that as much as 10% of the energy requirement of the exercise was met by the oxidation of amino acids.

Other studies, using different techniques, supported these observations. Muscle has been shown to release the amino acid alanine in proportion to exercise intensity (35), and the alanine is used in gluconeogenesis in the liver to generate new plasma glucose. White and Brooks (68), using a radioactive isotope of the amino acid leucine, showed that it was metabolized faster during exercise, compared to rest. These results were later confirmed in humans (22). Taken as a group, these studies suggest that amino acids are used as a fuel during exercise to a greater extent than previously believed. They also suggest that the protein requirement for those involved in prolonged exercise is higher than the RDA (53). However, there is more to the story.

Oxidation of Amino Acids

Part of the justification for a greater protein requirement in those who exercise is based on work using isotopes of amino acids whose metabolism could be traced during exercise. That is, if an amino acid is metabolized, the "labeled" CO_2 is exhaled and can be used as a marker of its rate of use. The essential amino acid leucine has been used as being representative of the amino acid pool. The previously mentioned work by White and Brooks (68) and Davies et al. (22) showed that leucine oxidation is increased with exercise. This implies that the catabolism of protein is higher during exercise compared to rest. Wolfe et al. (75) confirmed this greater rate of leucine oxidation during exercise but failed to show an increase in urea production, a primary index of protein catabolism. It was concluded that the N contained in leucine does not find its way to plasma urea N as a result of exercise (74), instead the N in leucine is transferred to intermediates (pyruvate) to form alanine, which is later used in the liver in gluconengenesis.

These results raised additional questions, so another experiment was conducted to see if leucine was, in fact, representative of the amino acid pool. The investigators used the amino acid lysine and found different results for the same experimental procedures. On the basis of their experiments, Wolfe et al. (74) concluded that leucine cannot be used as a model of whole-body protein metabolism during exercise, that changes (or lack of) in urea production during exercise may not reflect an accurate picture of protein breakdown, and finally, that *the data provide no rationale for increasing protein intake when exercising* (73).

Whole Body Nitrogen Balance Studies

The ability to maintain N balance during exercise appears to be dependent on the training state, total calories consumed, carbohydrate stores, and the amount of exercise done (11, 53). If measurements of protein utilization are made during the first few days of an exercise program, formally sedentary subjects show a negative N balance (figure 23.3). However, after about twelve to fourteen days of training, this condition disappears and the person can maintain N balance (41). So, depending on the point into the training program

Figure 23.3 **Effect of exercise on nitrogen balance.**

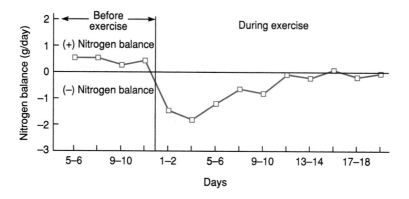

where the measurements are made, one could conclude that either more protein is needed (during the adaptation to exercise) or that protein needs can be met by the RDA (after the adaptation is complete) (10).

Another factor influencing the conclusion one would reach about protein needs during exercise is whether the person is in caloric balance, that is, taking in enough kcal to cover the cost of the added exercise. For example, it has been shown that by increasing the energy intake *15% more* than that needed to maintain weight, an increase in N retention occurred during exercise when these subjects consumed only $0.57 \text{ g} \cdot \text{kg}^{-1} \cdot \text{d}^{-1}$ of egg white protein (11). In a parallel study by the same group (66), a *15% deficit* in energy intake was created while subjects consumed either 0.57 or 0.8 g $\cdot \text{ kg}^{-1} \cdot \text{d}^{-1}$ egg white protein. When taking in 15% fewer calories than needed, the 0.8 g $\cdot$ kg$^{-1} \cdot$ d^{-1} protein intake was associated with a negative N balance of 1 g $\cdot$ d^{-1}. However, when the subjects did one or two hours of exercise the negative N balance improved to a loss of only 0.51, or 0.27 g $\cdot$ d^{-1}, respectively. During the treatment in which the subjects were in caloric balance, the RDA of 0.8 g $\cdot$ kg$^{-1} \cdot$ d^{-1} was sufficient to achieve a positive N balance for both durations of exercise. It is clear, then, that in order to make proper judgements about the adequacy of the protein intake, the person must be in energy balance.

A final nutritional factor that can influence the rate of amino-acid metabolism during exercise is the availability of carbohydrate. Lemon and Mullin (54) showed that the quantity of urea found in sweat was cut in half when subjects were carbohydrate loaded as opposed to carbohydrate depleted (see figure 23.4). Further, as figure 23.5 shows, the ingestion of glucose during the latter half of a three-hour exercise test at 50% $\dot{V}O_2$ max reduces the rate of oxidation of the amino acid leucine (22). So, not only is caloric balance important in protein metabolism, but the ability of the diet to provide adequate carbohydrate must also be considered.

Dietary Goals for Athletes

So, how much protein does an athlete need? One way to approach this question is to consider the protein requirement of a human from childhood to adulthood. The RDA for protein is 2.2 gm $\cdot$ kg$^{-1} \cdot$ d^{-1} during the first year of life, decreases to 1.2 gm $\cdot$ kg$^{-1} \cdot$ d^{-1} by ages seven to ten, and reaches the adult value of .8 gm $\cdot$ kg$^{-1} \cdot$ d^{-1} by ages nineteen to twenty-two (see appendix E). During this period of growth in which an individual increases body weight by a factor of 10 (15 to 150 lb), the highest RDA is 2.2 g $\cdot$ kg$^{-1} \cdot$ d^{-1}. Once growth has been achieved the value decreases to a stable 0.8 g $\cdot$ kg$^{-1} \cdot$ d^{-1}. This is not unlike, but to a much smaller degree, what was previously mentioned about the adaptation to exercise. During the initial days

Figure 23.4 Effect of initial muscle glycogen levels on sweat urea nitrogen excretion during exercise. A high muscle glycogen level decreases the excretion of urea nitrogen in sweat during exercise.

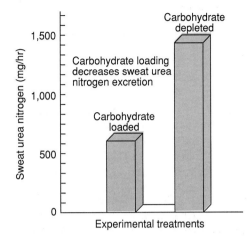

Figure 23.5 Effect of glucose ingestion on the rate of metabolism of the amino acid leucine. Glucose ingestion decreases the rate of amino acid oxidation.

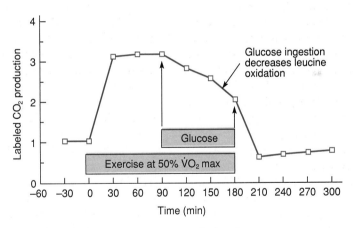

of an exercise training program, while the body is adapting to the new exercise, the protein requirement might be higher than 0.8 gm · kg⁻¹ · d⁻¹, and data of Goutzea (40) support this proposition. However, once the person has adapted to the exercise, the requirement would revert to the RDA, and research studies involving both endurance training (11) and weight training (65) support this idea. In fact, when individuals take in more protein than required (3 × RDA), the proportion of N retained by the body is considerably less than when protein intake equals the RDA, *as long as energy intake is adequate* (10). In summary, if energy intake is adequate, a protein intake of 0.8 g · kg⁻¹ · d⁻¹ is sufficient to meet the body's needs for protein during training. However, when energy balance is negative, the protein requirement may have to be higher than when it is maintained (10).

At the beginning of this section on protein requirements for athletes a question was raised: Does an athlete have to take in more protein than the RDA, or is the normal diet adequate? During a transition state from one level of activity to another, there may be a temporary need for a protein intake that is higher than normal. So the answer is "yes" to that part of the question. It is also "yes" to the second part, in that the average person typically takes in 50% more than the RDA for protein. While the dietary goal for the protein is 12% of total kcal, Brotherhood (9) reports that an average athlete's diet is about 16% protein, exceeding $1.5 \text{ g} \cdot \text{kg}^{-1} \cdot \text{d}^{-1}$. (*88% more than RDA!*). These values exceed the RDA of young children who are in a chronic state of positive nitrogen balance. It would appear that while scientists deal with the questions of the effect of exercise on the oxidation of amino acids, and whether or not the RDA for athletes is greater than $0.8 \text{ g} \cdot \text{kg}^{-1} \cdot \text{d}^{-1}$, the person following a normal dietary pattern will consume more than enough protein to meet the needs associated with exercise.

Some concern has been raised about too much dietary protein, especially with regard to amenorrheic athletes (10). Ca^{++} is excreted at a higher rate with high protein diets (46), and given that amenorrheic athletes have a lower bone density than those with a normal menstrual cycle (30), a high-protein diet may exacerbate the problem.

Water and Electrolytes

Chapter 12 described in some detail the need to dissipate heat during exercise in order to minimize the increase in core temperature. The primary mechanism for heat loss at high work rates in a comfortable environment, and at all work rates in a hot environment, is the evaporation of sweat. Sweat rates increase linearly with exercise intensity, and in hot weather sweat rates can reach 2.8 liters per hour (16). In spite of attempts to replace water during marathon races, some runners lose 8% of their body weight (16). Given that

water losses in excess of 3% are regarded as potentially harmful (70), there is a clear need to maintain water balance. Of course, more than water is lost in sweat. An increased sweat rate means that a wide variety of electrolytes, such as Na^+, K^+, Cl^-, and Mg^{++} are lost as well (16). These electrolytes are needed for normal functioning of excitable tissues, enzymes, and hormones. It should be no surprise then, that investigators have been concerned about the optimal way to replace water and electrolytes to reduce the chance of health-related problems and increase the chance of optimal performance.

Water Replacement – Before Exercise
Knowing that one is going to lose water weight during exercise, some investigators have tried to anticipate this by providing a volume of water or electrolyte beverage prior to the start of exercise. In these studies the subjects drank 1–3 liters of water and/or dilute saline prior to exercise. Williams (70) and Herbert (47) report that subjects generally have lower heart rate and body temperature responses to exercise in the hyperhydrated state than in the control condition. In practical terms, while an athlete would not consume such large volumes prior to an event, smaller fluid volumes (0.5 liters) might be consumed fifteen to thirty minutes prior to exercise.

Water Replacement – During Exercise
If an athlete can't "replace" water before it is lost, then water replacement during an activity is the next step. Fortunately, for some sports where play is intermittent (football, tennis, golf), water replacement during the activity is possible. However, in other sports like marathon running, there are no formal breaks in the activity to allow for replacement. It is in these latter sports, where the rate of heat production is high, coupled with the potential problems of environmental heat and humidity, that the athlete is at great risk. Figure 23.6, taken from the classic study by Pitts et al. (58), shows the advantage of replacing water as one exercises. A soldier marched for five hours under high heat (100° F), but with a moderate relative humidity (35%–40%). When water was replaced as fast as it was lost

Figure 23.6 Effect of water consumption on marching in the heat. Six experiments on subject J.S. at a temperature of 100° F, relative humidity of 35%–45%.

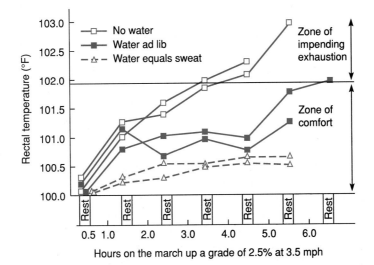

Hours on the march up a grade of 2.5% at 3.5 mph

during the rest periods (water balance), body temperature achieved a plateau. When water was taken to simply quench his thirst (ad lib), the subject's body temperature was slightly higher, but without water replacement the body temperature rose steadily.

These results have been supported by those of Dill et al. (27), who used a very dilute saline solution (1 gm · l⁻¹) during long walks in the desert heat, and by Herbert (47), who used a 16-km running test in an environmental chamber set at 35° C and RH = 50%. In this latter experiment, the heart rate and core temperature were lower during the treatment in which the subject was force-fed 400-ml volumes of a cold dilute glucose-electrolyte solution. Given that fluid replacement during exercise is clearly beneficial, how much fluid should be taken at one time? Should it be warm or cold? Should it contain glucose?

Costill and colleagues (15, 19) provided some of the original answers to these questions. One study examined the effects of fluid volume, temperature, glucose concentration, and the intensity of exercise on the rate at which fluid leaves the stomach to the small intestine. They determined this by giving the subject the fluid in question and fifteen minutes later,

aspirating the contents of the stomach. Figure 23.7 summarizes the results of that study. A glucose concentration above 139 mM (2.5%) slowed gastric emptying (figure 23.7 a). Colder drinks appeared to be emptied faster, and the optimal volume to ingest was 600 ml (figure 23.7 b and c). Finally, exercise had no effect until the intensity exceeded 65%–70% $\dot{V}O_2$ max (figure 23.7 d). A second study, which compared three glucose-electrolyte fluids to water, supported the findings that drinks high in glucose slowed the exit of water from the stomach to the small intestine, where it is absorbed into the blood (19). Recently, however, these results have been questioned.

In the previously discussed studies, the effectiveness of a drink was evaluated fifteen minutes after ingestion by aspirating the contents of the stomach. Davis and colleagues (25, 26) questioned the use of the aspiration technique since it simply measures how much fluid leaves the stomach, not how much is actually absorbed into the blood from the small intestine. They used heavy water (D_2O) as a tracer of fluid absorption from the gastrointestinal tract to the blood and found that a 6% glucose-electrolyte solution was absorbed as fast or faster than water at rest (25) or during

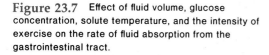

Figure 23.7 Effect of fluid volume, glucose concentration, solute temperature, and the intensity of exercise on the rate of fluid absorption from the gastrointestinal tract.

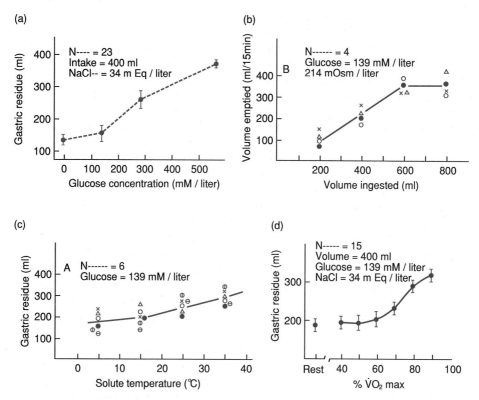

exercise (26). Two additional studies that used the aspiration technique (55, 56) found that when either a 10% glucose solution or glucose polymer solutions containing 5%–10% carbohydrate were ingested at fifteen to twenty-minute intervals during prolonged exercise at 65%–70% $\dot{V}O_2$ max, there was no difference in the gastric emptying rate of these solutions compared to water. The improved performance of the carbohydrate drinks in the most recent studies may be related to the experimental procedures which included the ingestion of small volumes (~200 ml) at regular intervals (fifteen to twenty minutes) during prolonged exercise with the aspiration occurring at the end of the entire exercise session (not fifteen minutes after ingestion). An additional benefit of these glucose solutions is that the extra carbohydrate helps to maintain the blood glucose during exercise. It must be added, however, that drinks containing 12% glucose remain in the stomach longer, with subjects complaining of gastrointestinal distress (26).

Salt (NaCl)

One of the United States Dietary Guidelines presented in chapter 18 was to decrease the intake of sodium. While the point was made that Americans consume two to three times the amount needed for optimal health, is the dietary intake sufficient for an athlete who participates in regular vigorous physical activity? The mass of sodium in the body determines the water content, given the way water is reabsorbed at the kidney. If a person becomes sodium depleted, body water will be decreased, and the risk of heat injury is increased. An untrained and unacclimatized individual (see chapter 24) loses more Na^+ in sweat than a trained and acclimatized person. If the unacclimatized person has 1.9 gm Na^+ per liter of sweat and loses 5 liters of sweat (11 pounds), the person would lose 9.5 grams of Na^+ per day. As the person becomes acclimatized, the sodium content in sweat decreases to about half that and Na^+ loss is about 5 gm/day. Given that Na is 40% of NaCl by weight, a person would have to consume 12.5 gm of salt per day to meet that demand. Interestingly, that is about what an average American, eating an average diet, now consumes. It is generally believed that an individual with a high Na^+ loss can stay in sodium/water balance by simply adding salt to food at mealtime, rather than consume salt tablets (70). *The best single test of the success of the salt/water replacement procedures is to have an athlete weigh in each day.* The general dietary routine followed by athletes must be successful since early morning body weight remains relatively constant despite large daily sweat losses (9).

Minerals

Iron

As mentioned in chapter 18, iron deficiency is the most common nutritional deficiency. The stages of iron deficiency are spelled out in table 23.1, as well as the tests used to detect deficiencies (43). An analysis of the literature suggested that both male and female athletes have higher rates of depleted iron stores and/or iron deficiency anemia (9, 12, 43). Given that hemoglobin is a necessary part of the oxygen-transport process, it is not surprising that in individuals with very low hemoglobin values ($<11 g \cdot dl^{-1}$), endurance and work performance are decreased (38, 39). Interestingly, when the low hemoglobin condition is corrected in iron-deficient animals by transfusion, $\dot{V}O_2$ max is brought back to normal but not endurance time. This suggests (1) that iron deficiency affects the iron-containing cytochromes (electron transport chain) that are involved in oxidative phosphorylation and (2) while hemoglobin levels may be high enough to achieve a normal $\dot{V}O_2$ max, endurance performance may still be affected (23). In a similar study (24), iron supplementation brought the $\dot{V}O_2$ max back to normal values faster than that of endurance performance (see figure 23.8).

What causes iron deficiency in athletes? Inadequate intake of dietary iron, as in the general population, has been cited as a primary cause of iron deficiency in women athletes (13). In addition, exercise has been associated with increased hemoglobin loss in feces (63) and sweat (57). When this is coupled with evidence showing a greater hemolysis of red blood cells due to simple "pounding" of the foot on the pavement during running (21), one can understand why some athletes are at risk of iron deficiency anemia. Consistent with this, Diehl et al. (28) have shown decreases in serum ferritin over the course of a field hockey season, and from one hockey season to the next in female athletes. The average value at the end of the season on third-year players was 10.5 $\mu g \cdot l^{-1}$, or below the 12 $\mu g \cdot l^{-1}$ standard, indicating iron depletion (43).

Generally, when a person has a deficiency in iron stores there is an increased uptake of dietary iron. Unfortunately, athletes do not appear to follow that pattern; studies show that athletes absorb less than half the dietary iron that a comparable group of sedentary anemic individuals absorb (32). This absorption problem increases the difficulty of returning to normal iron status: athletes may have a higher need and yet, when deficient, do not absorb the iron as well as sedentary individuals. Given that the total kcal intake of some athletes (especially small athletes) will be inadequate in terms of iron intake (6 mg iron per 1,000 kcal in the average American diet), supplementation may be needed (13). Prior to supplementation, a complete physical exam with blood work describing the extent of the problem is recommended. In this way the success of the treatment can be monitored (12). Oral supplements of 36–74 mg of a ferrous salt taken three times a day is recommended. As mentioned in chapter 18, when taken with vitamin C, iron absorption is enhanced (12). Haynes (43) makes a special note that the studies reporting beneficial results from such supplementation had a high proportion of iron-deficient subjects.

Table 23.1 Stages of iron deficiency

Stages	Description	Test
Iron depletion	Lack of iron stores in the bone and liver due to long-term dietary iron deficiency	Bone marrow biopsy; serum ferritin $<12 \, \mu g \cdot l^{-1}$
Iron-deficient erythropoiesis	Red blood cell production decreases due to inadequate hemoglobin formation	Unbound protoporphyrin (used in the formation of hemoglobin) increases due to low iron stores
Iron deficiency anemia	Hemoglobin fall to low levels	Men: $<13 \, g \cdot dl^{-1}$ Women: $12 \, g \cdot dl^{-1}$; *with* evidence that first two stages exist

From: Haymes (43).

Figure 23.8 Recovery of various physiological capacities with iron repletion. Note that recovery of endurance lagged behind $\dot{V}O_2$ max.

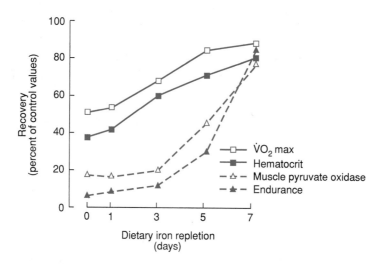

Vitamins

Chapter 18 provided the detail about the RDA for each vitamin. Many of these vitamins are directly involved in energy production, acting as coenzymes in mitochondrial reactions associated with aerobic metabolism. Unfortunately, the old adage that "if a little is good, more will be better," has been applied to the question of whether or not the RDA for athletes is higher than for normal people, rather than a factual research base. In general, the major reviews of this issue over the past *thirty years* have systematically concluded that:

1. vitamin supplementation is unnecessary for the athlete on a well-balanced diet,
2. people who are **clearly deficient** in certain vitamins have improved performance when values return to normal, and

3. individuals taking large doses of fat soluble vitamins or vitamin C should be concerned about toxicity (5, 67, 70).

The central concern issued by these reviewers is for the small athlete on a low-energy diet who may not make wise food selections. In those situations a single RDA multi-vitamin/mineral pill might be appropriate (5).

Pregame Meal

The two most important nutritional practices associated with optimal performance are (1) to eat a high (about 70%) carbohydrate diet in the *days preceding* competition when the intensity and duration of workouts are reduced and (2) to drink water at regular intervals *during* the competition. The purposes of the pregame meal are (42, 70):

1. to provide adequate hydration;
2. provide carbohydrate to "top off" already high carbohydrate stores in the liver, without interfering with the mobilization of fuel (i.e., effect of glucose intake prior to work);
3. to avoid the sensation of hunger on a relatively empty stomach; and
4. minimize G.I. tract problems (gas, diarrhea).

Unfortunately, the type of pregame meal served at various universities throughout this country may rely more on tradition than nutrition. The standard rare steak before a boxing match or football game to bring out the animal instinct or careful planning to make sure that the color of the Jello® is the same as that when the team won last year's championship are less than rational, but may be useful in pulling the team together to get ready for competition. The problem arises when the pregame meal can actually be responsible for poor performance because of its own characteristics (high fat and protein) or the ability of the athlete to tolerate the meal without vomiting or experiencing diarrhea due to the emotion associated with competition. These latter conditions would cause a dehydration inconsistent with optimal performance. It is

Jello® is a registered trademark of General Foods, Inc.

clear that beyond what is recommended in the nutrient make-up of a pregame meal, the ability of the athlete to tolerate it must be considered (70).

Nutrients in Pregame Meal

The number of kcal in a pregame meal should be about 500–1,000, and the primary nutrient should be complex carbohydrates, because they are easily digested and would provide glucose to increase liver glycogen. It is generally recommended that large amounts of simple sugars should not be consumed immediately prior to competition (70). The reasons for this were presented earlier. The fat content of the pregame meal should be kept to a minimum since fat is more slowly digested and is not needed as a fuel for exercise since body stores are more than adequate. The protein content of the pregame meal should be small. The digestion and metabolism of protein increases the quantity of acids in the blood that must be buffered and finally excreted by the kidneys (42, 70). Table 23.2 presents two pregame meals that meet these considerations (70). These meals should be eaten about three hours prior to competition.

Some coaches and athletes prefer one of the commercially available liquid meals (Exceed®, Sustagen®, Ensure®, SustaCal®, Ensure-Plus®) as the pregame meal because of convenience, and also because they are consistent with the recommendations previously mentioned. The following are examples (69).

	Sustagen®	Exceed®
Calories	390	360
Carbohydrate (g/%)	66.5/68%	47/53%
Fat (g/%)	3.5/8%	12/30%
Protein (g/%)	23.5/24%	15/17%

These liquid meals can also be used throughout the day (along with additional water) when events or games are scheduled over long periods of time. Given that some people may not react favorably to any new "food," these liquid meals should be tried on practice days rather than on game day to make sure they are suitable.

Table 23.2 Suggested pre-game meals

Breakfast	Calories	Lunch	Calories
4 ounces orange juice	60	4 ounces tomato juice	25
8 ounces skim milk	80	2 ounces turkey	100
2 slices toast	140	2 slices bread	140
2 tablespoons preserves	110	8 ounces skim milk	80
1 poached egg	80	1 orange	60
		2 plain cookies	120
Total calories	470		545

From M. H. Williams, *Nutritional Aspects of Human Physical and Athletic Performance*, 2d ed., 1985. Courtesy of Charles C. Thomas, Publisher, Springfield, Ill.

Body Composition and Performance

A simple observation of the track and field events at the Olympic Games suggests that the physical characteristics of those successful in the shot put are different from those successful in the marathon. The purpose of this section is to reinforce that observation by providing a brief review of **somatotype** and body fatness related to performance.

Somatotype

In 1940 Sheldon (60) published **The Varieties of Human Physique,** in which he introduced the concept of the somatotype. In his scheme each person could be characterized as possessing a certain amount of the following three components of body form:

Endomorphy—relative predominance of soft roundness and large digestive visera. He used the prefix *endo* as it relates to the *endo*dermal embryonic layers from which the digestive track is derived.

Mesomorphy—relative predominance of muscle, bone and connective tissue ultimately derived from the *meso*dermal embryonic layer.

Ectomorphy—relative predominance of linearity and fragility with a great surface area to mass ratio giving great sensory exposure to the environment. The nervous system is derived from the *ecto*dermal embryonic layer.

Sheldon photographed 4,000 *college men* and ranked each of these three components on a scale of 1 to 7, with 1 representing the least amount of a component and 7 representing the greatest amount. A somatotype is a three-number sequence (e.g., 171 is one-seven-one) characterizing the endomorphic, mesomorphic, and ectomorphic components, respectively. Figure 23.9 shows the extremes of each somatotype. It must be remembered that somatotype considers only body form or shape and does not consider size. Tanner (64) used a two-dimensional plot of the original somatotypes of Sheldon's 4,000 college students on whom the 1-to-7 scale was based. This distribution of somatotypes is shown in figure 23.10 where a contrasting distribution is also presented, showing the somatotypes of 137 Olympic track-and-field athletes. Not surprisingly, the body form or type associated with world-class performance is different from that of the average population and differs by sport and event.

The values used in these figures were based on the Sheldon photographs (61), but according to the somatotyping method of Heath-Carter (44), Sheldon's 1-to-7 scale was too confining in that there are components in certain body types that exceed that given the value of 7. Using their method of somatotyping,

Figure 23.9 Extremes of somatotypes.

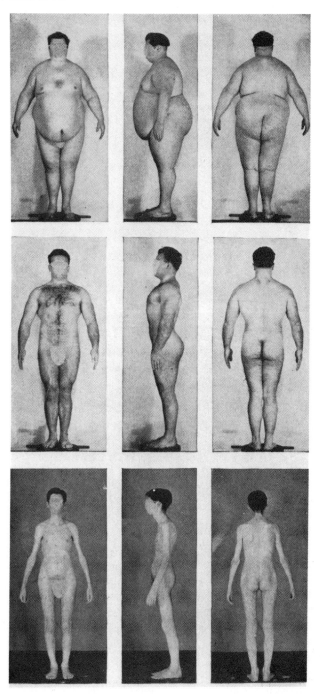

Figure 23.10 Contrast of the somatotypes of American college students with Olympic track-and-field athletes.

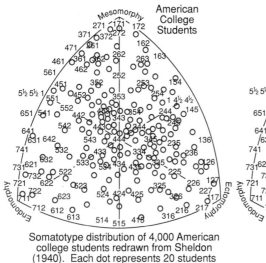

Somatotype distribution of 4,000 American college students redrawn from Sheldon (1940). Each dot represents 20 students

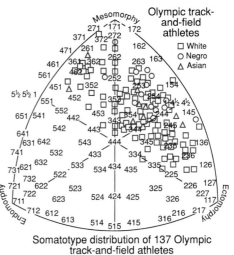

Somatotype distribution of 137 Olympic track-and-field athletes

Heath-Carter (44) cite the following examples of extremes in somatotypes: (1) extremely obese individuals having endomorphy values as high as 12, (2) members of the Manu tribe of the Admirality Islands with values of 9.5 for mesomorphy, and (3) members of the Nilote tribe in Africa having ectomorphic values of 8 and 9. When Olympic athletes were rated with this Heath-Carter scale weight lifters and throwers were outside the normal distribution of Sheldon's mesomorphy scale. As one moved from these weight lifters and throwers to the distance runners and basketball players the somatotype becomes progressively more ectomorphic. The distribution of somatotypes for the women athletes was shifted down and to the left, indicating smaller mesomorphic and larger endomorphic components (27).

Further, Heath-Carter view the somatotype, especially the endomorphic and mesomorphic components, to be dynamic with the potential to change over time. Sheldon had viewed the somatotype as more of a permanent form for a given individual. The Heath-Carter method sees the endomorphic component as being equivalent to relative fatness or leanness and is closely tied to the sum of skinfolds. The mesomorphic component is viewed as being an estimate of the relative musculoskeletal development and similar to lean body mass. This latter translation of somatotype values into body composition values is a good lead into our next section.

Body Fatness and Performance

The somatotype of the athletes involved in the Olympic Games represented low relative fatness (low endomorphy) and high relative fat-free mass (high mesomorphy). This two-component system of body composition was described in detail in chapter 18, where optimal body fatness goals were presented for health and fitness:

Males: 10%–20% fat
Females: 15%–25% fat

The question is, are these values optimal for athletic performance?

Table 23.3 lists a summary of body fatness values by sport (72). These are average values and do not represent the range that might be observed in a study. For example, a study might find an average value of

Table 23.3 Percent body fat values for male and female athletes

Athletic Group or Sport	Male	Female
Baseball	11.8–14.2	—
Basketball	7.1–10.6	20.8–26.9
Canoeing	12.4	—
Football		
Backs	9.4–12.4	
Linebackers	13.7	
Linemen	15.5–19.1	
Quarterbacks, kickers	14.1	
Gymnastics	4.6	9.6–23.8
Ice hockey	13–15.1	—
Jockeys	14.1	—
Orienteering	16.3	18.7
Pentathalon	—	11.0
Racketball	8.3	14.0
Skiing		
Alpine	7.4–14.1	20.6
Cross-country	7.9–12.5	15.7–21.8
Nordic combined	8.9–11.2	—
Ski jumping	14.3	—
Soccer	9.6	—
Speed skating	11.4	—
Swimming	5.0–8.5	20.3
Tennis	15.2–16.3	20.3
Track and field		
Distance runners	3.7–18.0	15.2–19.2
Middle distance runners	12.4	—
Sprinters	16.5	19.3
Discus	16.3	25.0
Jumpers/hurdlers	—	20.7
Shot put	16.5–19.6	28.0
Volleyball	—	21.3–25.3
Wrestling	4.0–14.4	

From J. H. Wilmore, "Body Composition in Sport Medicine: Directions for Future Research," in *Medicine and Science in Sports Medicine* 15:21-31, 1983. Copyright © 1983 American College of Sports Medicine, Madison, Wis.

12% body fat for a group of football players, but the range might be 5%–19%. In a sport or activity where body weight must be carried along (e.g., running or jumping), there is a negative correlation between body fatness and performance (72).

There is little question that regular measurements of body composition are useful for athletes in order to monitor changes during the season as well as over the off-season. In this way the athlete will know whether changes in body weight represent gains or losses of body fatness. What is more difficult is providing a fixed absolute recommendation about what body fatness should be for optimal performance for each individual.

One of the main reasons one must be careful in making absolute recommendations, such as "This athlete should reduce her percent body fat from 15.6% to 14.0%," is that the athlete may already be 14% body fat. Each *individual estimate* of body fatness, even done by the underwater weighing technique, has an error in measurement that cannot be ignored. The conversion of a body density value to a percent body fat value has an error of $\pm 2.5\%$ for underwater weighing and $\pm 3.7\%$ for skinfold techniques (see discussion in chapter 18). So when an athlete is measured as 15.6% body fat the true value may actually be 13.1% or 18.1%.

Another reason caution must be used in making absolute recommendations for each individual athlete is that it ignores the normal variation in body fatness found in elite athletes in any particular sport. An elite group of volleyball players may have an average value of 12%, but the range among the team members might be 6%–16%. No one would think of telling the athlete with 6% body fat to increase body fatness to reach the team average, and the same advice holds true for the one at 16% body fatness who is playing with world-class skill. A recommendation to alter body composition to achieve better performance must be made against the background of present performance, and general health status as seen in sleeping patterns, adequate diet, mental outlook, etc. The implementation of longer workouts or a reduction in caloric intake might change the % body fat in the appropriate direction, but either one could adversely affect the athlete's ability to hold a workout or to study for exams. Wilmore's (72) observation of one of the best female distance runners who held most of the American middle distance records should be remembered when making such recommendations: the champion was 17% body fat when most of the elite female runners were <12%.

Monitoring body fatness in athletes by skinfold or underwater weighing is a reasonable procedure to follow because it allows a coach or trainer to observe **changes** in body fatness over the course of a season and from one year to the next. The information is also useful to the athletes who, when they finish their competitive careers, must attend to what is a reasonable body weight in order to be within the optimal body fatness range for health and fitness.

Summary

1. Performance in endurance events is improved by a diet high in carbohydrates due primarily to the increase in muscle glycogen. The recommended dietary goal for Americans to have 58% of their caloric intake as carbohydrate would provide for a high muscle glycogen content. However, procedures have been developed to cause a "supercompensation" of the glycogen store.
2. Glucose ingestion prior to performance can induce an insulin response that accelerates glycogen depletion and is inconsistent with optimal performance.
3. The ingestion of glucose polymer solutions can extend performance limitations, especially in those who experience hypoglycemia during exercise.
4. Protein utilization during exercise may be higher than at rest based on measurements of nitrogen lost in sweat and the release of the amino acid alanine from muscle. However, studies using radioactively labeled amino acids fail to support the need for additional protein.
5. It is clear that the protein requirement for an athlete is dependent on both an adequate carbohydrate and caloric intake. While an athlete may need more protein, the average diet of an athlete contains 16% protein, more than enough to cover this need given the higher caloric intake.
6. Fluid replacement during exercise reduces the heart rate and body temperature responses to exercise, in contrast to not drinking water. Drinking water to quench thirst is not as effective as taking in water to balance sweat loss.
7. Cold drinks are absorbed faster than warm drinks, with the optimal volume being 600 ml. If exercise intensity exceeds 65%–70% $\dot{V}O_2$ max, gastric emptying decreases.
8. Salt needs are easily met at mealtime and salt tablets are not needed. In fact, most Americans take in more salt than is required.
9. Iron deficiency in American athletes may be related to an inadequate intake of dietary iron as well as a potentially greater loss in sweat and feces. Strangely, in spite of this deficiency athletes may absorb less than half of what a sedentary group of anemic individuals absorb. Iron supplementation, following a clinical assessment of the condition, is recommended.
10. Vitamin supplementation is unnecessary for an athlete on a well-balanced diet, however, for those with a clear deficiency, supplementation is warranted.
11. The pregame meal should provide for hydration and adequate carbohydrate to "top off" stores while minimizing hunger symptoms, gas, and diarrhea. A variety of commercially available liquid meals are consistent with these goals.
12. A somatotype is a numerical (1–to–7 scale) representation of the degree to which a person possesses a high level endomorphy, mesomorphy, and ectomorphy. Athletes are clearly different from the ordinary population, indicating a natural predisposition needed for success.
13. The body fat percentage consistent with excellence in performance is different for men and women and varies within gender and from sport to sport. Average values for a team should not be applied to any single individual without regard to overall health status as seen in diet, sleep, and mental outlook. Further, it is "natural" for some athletes to have a higher body fatness than others in order to perform optimally.

Study Questions

1. What procedures would you follow to cause a supercompensation of muscle glycogen?
2. How much of a change in carbohydrate intake would be required for an individual who already achieves the dietary goal for carbohydrate?
3. How could glucose ingestion prior to exercise actually increase the rate of glycogen depletion?
4. What type of person would benefit from carbohydrate intake during exercise? Why?
5. Is the protein requirement of an athlete higher than that of a sedentary person? Should protein intake be increased?
6. How would you recommend that a person replace water loss due to exercise?
7. Are glucose/electrolyte drinks better than water in replacing fluid loss? Explain.
8. How would you recommend that a potential iron deficiency anemia condition be dealt with?
9. Does an athlete need additional vitamins for optimal performance? Why?
10. What are the primary considerations in a pregame meal?
11. What is a somatotype and how is it different for athletes compared to the average college population?
12. Given a female distance runner with a 17% body fat, what should you consider before making a recommendation for change?

Suggested Reading

Williams, M. H. 1985. *Nutritional Aspects of Human Physical and Athletic Performance*. Springfield, Ill.: Charles C. Thomas.

References

1. Ahlborg, B. et al. 1967. Muscle glycogen and muscle electrolytes during prolonged physical exercise. *Acta Physiologica Scandinavica* 70:129–42.
2. Ahlborg, G., and P. Felig. 1976. Influence of glucose ingestion on fuel-hormone response during prolonged exercise. *Journal of Applied Physiology* 41:683–88.
3. ———. 1982. Lactate and glucose exchange across the forearm, legs, and splanchnic bed during and after prolonged exercise. *Journal of Clinical Investigation* 69:45–54.
4. ———. 1977. Substrate utilization during prolonged exercise preceded by ingestion of glucose. *American Journal of Physiology* 233:E188–E194.
5. Belko, A. Z. 1987. Vitamins and exercise—an update. *Medicine and Science in Sports and Exercise* 19:S191–S196.
6. Bergstrom, J., and E. Hultman. 1966. Muscle glycogen synthesis after exercise: An enhancing factor localized to the muscle cells in man. *Nature* 210:309.
7. Bergstrom, J. et al. 1967. Diet, muscle glycogen and physical performance. *Acta Physiologica Scandinavica* 71:140–50.
8. Blom, Per C. S. et al. 1987. Effect of different post-exercise sugar diets on the rate of muscle glycogen synthesis. *Medicine and Science in Sports and Exercise* 19:491–96.
9. Brotherhood, J. R. 1984. Nutrition and sports performance. *Sports Medicine* 1:350–89.
10. Butterfield, G. E. 1987. Whole-body protein utilization in humans. *Medicine and Science in Sports and Exercise* 19:S157–S165.
11. Butterfield, G. E., and D. H. Calloway. 1984. Physical activity improves protein utilization in young men. *British Journal of Nutrition* 51:171–84.
12. Clement, D. B., and L. L. Sawchuk. 1984. Iron status and sports performance. *Sports Medicine* 1:65–74.
13. Clement, D. B., and R. C. Asmundson. 1982. Nutritional intake and hematological parameters in endurance runners. *Physician and Sportsmedicine* 10:37–43.
14. Costill, D. L. 1977. Sweating: Its composition and effects on body fluids. *Annals of the New York Academy of Sciences* 301:160–74.

15. Costill, D. L., and B. Saltin. 1974. Factors limiting gastric emptying during rest and exercise. *Journal of Applied Physiology* 37:679–83.

16. Costill, D. L. et al. 1977. Effects of elevated plasma FFA and insulin on muscle glycogen usage during exercise. *Journal of Applied Physiology* 43:695–99.

17. Costill, D. L. et al. 1981. The role of dietary carbohydrates in muscle glycogen resynthesis after strenuous running. *American Journal of Clinical Nutrition* 34:1831–36.

18. Coyle, E. F., and A. R. Coggan. 1984. Effectiveness of carbohydrate feeding in delaying fatigue during prolonged exercise. *Sports Medicine* 1:446–58.

19. Coyle, E. F. et al. 1978. Gastric-emptying rates of selected athletic drinks. *Research Quarterly* 49:119–24.

20. Coyle, E. F. et al. 1983. Carbohydrate feeding during prolonged strenuous exercise can delay fatigue. *Journal of Applied Physiology* 55:230–35.

21. Davidson, R. J. L. 1969. March or exertioneal haemoglobinuria. *Seminars in Hematology* 6:150–61.

22. Davies, C. T. M. et al. 1982. Glucose inhibits CO_2 production from leucine during whole body exercise in man. *Journal of Physiology* 332:40–41.

23. Davies, K. J. A. et al. 1984. Distinguishing effects of anemic and muscle iron deficiency on exercise bioenergetics in the rat. *American Journal of Physiology* 246:E535–E543.

24. Davies, K. J. A. et al. 1982. Muscle mitochondrial bioenergetics, oxygen supply, and work capacity during dietary iron deficiency and repletion. *American Journal of Physiology* 242:E418–E427.

25. Davis, J. M. et al. 1987. Accumulation of deuterium oxide in body fluids after ingestion of D_2O-labeled beverages. *Journal of Applied Physiology* 63:2060–66.

26. Davis, J. M. et al. 1988. Effects of ingesting 6% and 12% glucose/electrolyte beverages during prolonged intermittent cycling in the heat. *European Journal of Applied Physiology* 57:563–69.

27. de Garay, A., L. Levine, and J. Carter. 1974. *Genetic and Anthropological Studies of Olympic Athletes.* New York: Academic Press, Inc.

28. Diehl, D. M. et al. 1986. Effects of physical training and competition on the iron status of female hockey players. *International Journal of Sports Medicine* 264–70.

29. Dill, D. B., M. K. Yousef, and J. D. Nelson. 1973. Responses of men and women to two-hour walks in the desert heat. *Journal of Applied Physiology* 35:231–35.

30. Drinkwater, B. L. et al. 1984. Bone mineral content of amenorrheic and eumenorrheic athletes. *New England Journal of Medicine* 311:277–81.

31. Edgerton, V. R. et al. 1979. Iron-deficiency anaemia and its effect on worker productivity and activity patterns. *British Medical Journal* 2:1546–49.

32. Ehn, L., B. Carlwark, and S. Hoglund. 1980. Iron status in athletes involved in intense physical activity. *Medicine and Science in Sports and Exercise* 12:61–64.

33. Essen, B. 1977. Intramuscular substrate utilization during prolonged exercise. *Annals of the New York Academy of Science* 301:30–44.

34. Felig, P. et al. 1982. Hypoglycemia during prolonged exercise in normal men. *New England Journal of Medicine* 306:895–900.

35. Felig, P., and J. Wahren. 1971. Amino acid metabolism in exercising man. *Journal of Clinical Investigation* 50:2703–14.

36. Foster, C., D. L. Costill, and W. J. Fink. 1979. Effects of preexercise feedings on endurance performance. *Medicine and Science in Sports* 11:1–5.

37. ———. 1980. Gastric emptying characteristics of glucose and glucose ploymer solutions. *Research Quarterly for Exercise and Sport* 51:299–305.

38. Gardner, G. W. et al. 1977. Physical work capacity and metabolic stress in subjects with iron deficiency anemia. *American Journal of Clinical Nutrition* 30:910–17.

39. Gledhill, N. 1985. The influence of altered blood volume and oxygen transport capacity on aerobic performance. In (R. L. Terjung, ed.) *Exercise and Sport Sciences Reviews,* vol. 13, 75–93.

40. ———. 1974. The influence of muscular activity on nitrogen balance, and on the need of man for protein. *Nutrition Reports International* 10:35–43.

41. Gontzea, I., P. Sutzescu, and S. Dumitrache. 1975. The influence of adaptation of physical effort on nitrogen balance in man. *Nutrition Reports International* 11:231–36.

42. Guild, W. R. 1960. Pre-event nutrition, with some implications for endurance athletes. In *Exercise and Fitness.* Chicago: The Athletic Institute.

43. Haymes, E. M. 1987. Nutritional concerns: need for iron. *Medicine and Science in Sports and Exercise* 19:S197–S200.

44. Heath, B. H., and J. E. L. Carter. 1967. A modified somatotype method. *American Journal of Physical Anthropology* 27:57–74.

45. Hecker, A. L. 1983. Digestive, absorptive, and metabolic characteristics of glucose polymers. In *Nutrient Utilization During Exercise,* 35–43. Columbus, Oh.: Ross Laboratories.

46. Hegsted, M. et al. 1981. Urinary calcium and calcium balance in young men affected by level of protein and inorganic phosphate intake. *Journal of Nutrition* 111:553–62.

47. Herbert, W. 1983. Water and electrolytes. In (M. A. Williams, ed.) *Ergogenic Aids in Sports.* Champaign, Ill.: Human Kinetics Publishers.

48. Hermansen, L., E. Hultman, and B. Saltin. 1967. Muscle glycogen during prolonged severe exercise. *Acta Physiologica Scandinavica* 71:129–39.

49. Ivy, J. L. et al. 1979. Influence of caffeine and carbohydrate feedings on endurance performance. *Medicine and Science in Sports* 11:6–11.

50. Ivy, J. L. et al. 1983. Endurance improved by the ingestion of a glucose polymer supplement. *Medicine and Science in Sports and Exercise* 15:466–71.

51. Karlsson, J., and B. Saltin. 1971. Diet, muscle glycogen, and endurance performance. *Journal of Applied Physiology* 31:203–6.

52. Lamb, D. R., and G. R. Brodowicz. 1986. Optimal use of fluids of varying formulations to minimise exercise-induced disturbances in homeostasis. *Sports Medicine* 3:247–74.

53. Lemon, P. W. R. 1987. Protein and exercise: update 1987. *Medicine and Science in Sports and Exercise* 19:S179–S190.

54. Lemon, P. W. R., and J. P. Mullin. 1980. Effect of initial muscle glycogen levels on protein catabolism during exercise. *Journal of Applied Physiology* 48:624–29.

55. Levine, L. et al. 1983. Fructose and glucose ingestion and muscle glycogen use during submaximal exercise. *Journal of Applied Physiology* 55:1767–71.

56. Mitchell, J. B. et al. 1988. Effects of carbohydrate ingestion on gastric emptying and exercise. *Medicine and Science in Sports and Exercise* 20:110–15.

57. Owen, M. D. et al. 1986. Effects of ingesting carbohydrate beverages during exercise in the heat. *Medicine and Sciences in Sports and Exercise* 18:568–75.

58. Paulev, P. E., R. Jordal, and N. S. Pedersen. 1983. Dermal excretion of iron in intensely trained athletes. *Clinical Chimica Acta* 127:19–27.

59. Pitts, G., R. Johnson, and F. Consolazio. 1944. Work in the heat as affected by intake of water, salt and glucose. *American Journal of Physiology* 142:353–59.

60. Seiple, R. S. et al. 1983. Gastric-emptying characteristics of two glucose polymer-electrolyte solutions. *Medicine and Science in Sports and Exercise* 15:366–69.

61. Sheldon, W. H. 1940. *The Varieties of Human Physique.* New York: Harper & Brothers Publishers.

62. Sheldon, W. H., C. W. Dupertuis, and E. McDermott. 1954. *Atlas of Men.* New York: Harper & Brothers.

63. Sherman, W. M. 1983. Carbohydrates, muscle glycogen, and muscle glycogen super compensation. In (M. H. Williams, ed.) *Ergogenic Aids in Sports,* Chapter 1, 3–26.

64. Stewart, J. G. et al. 1984. Gastrointestinal blood loss and anemia in runners. *Annals of Internal Medicine* 100:843–45.

65. Tanner, J. M., S. S. Stevens, and W. B. Tucker. 1964. *The Physique of the Olympic Athlete.* London: George Allen and Unwin, Ltd.

66. Tarnopolsky, M. D. et al. 1986. Dietary protein requirements for body builders versus sedentary controls (abstract). *Medicine and Science in Sports and Exercise* 18:S64.

67. Todd, K. S., G. Butterfield, and D. H. Calloway. 1984. Nitrogen balance in men with adequate and deficit energy intake at 3 levels of work. *Journal of Nutrition* 114:2107–18.

68. Van der Beek, E. J. 1985. Vitamins and endurance training: Food for running or faddish claims? *Sports Medicine* 2:175–97.

69. White, T. P., and G. A. Brooks. 1981. [U-^{14}C] glucose, -alanine, and -leucine oxidation in rats at rest and two intensities of running. *American Journal of Physiology* 241:E155–E165.

70. Williams, M. H. 1985. *The Nutrition for Fitness Answer Book.* Dubuque, Ia.: Wm. C. Brown Publishers.

71. ———. 1985. *Nutritional Aspects of Human Physical and Athletic Performance.* Springfield, Ill.: Charles C. Thomas.

72. Wilmore, J. H. 1984. Body composition and sports medicine: Research considerations. In *Report of the Sixth Ross Conference on Medical Research* 78–82. Columbus, Ohio: Ross Laboratories.

73. ———. 1983. Body composition in sport and exercise: Directions for future research. *Medicine and Science in Sports and Exercise* 15:21–31.

74. Wolfe, R. R. 1987. Does exercise stimulate protein breakdown in humans?: Isotopic approaches to the problem. *Medicine and Science in Sports and Exercise* 19:S172–S178.

75. Wolfe, R. R. et al. (1984). Isotopic determination of amino acid-urea interactions in exercise in humans. *Journal of Applied Physiology* 56:221–29.

76. Wolfe, R. R. et al. 1982. Isotopic analysis of leucine and urea metabolism in exercising humans. *Journal of Applied Physiology: Respiration, Environmental, and Exercise Physiology* 52:458–66.

77. Young, D. R., R. Pelligra, and R. R. Adachi. 1960. Serum glucose and free fatty acids in man during prolonged exercise. *Journal of Applied Physiology* 21:1047–52.

24 Exercise and the Environment

Objectives

*B*y studying this chapter, you should be able to do the following:
1. Describe the changes in atmospheric pressure (PO_2), air temperature, and air density with increasing altitude.
2. Describe how altitude affects sprint performances and explain why that is the case.
3. Explain why distance running performance decreases at altitude.
4. Draw a graph to show the effect of altitude on $\dot{V}O_2$ max and list the reasons for this response.
5. Graphically describe the effect of altitude on the heart rate and ventilation responses to submaximal work, and offer an explanation of why these changes are appropriate.
6. Describe the process of adaptation to altitude, and the degree to which this adaptation can be complete.
7. Explain why such variability existed among athletes in the decrease in $\dot{V}O_2$ max upon exposure to altitude, the degree of improvement in $\dot{V}O_2$ max at altitude, and the gains made upon return to sea level.
8. Describe the potential problems associated with training at high altitude and how one might get around them.
9. Explain the circumstances that caused physiologists to reevaluate their conclusions that humans could not climb Mount Everest without oxygen.
10. Explain the role that hyperventilation plays in helping to maintain a high oxygen-hemoglobin saturation at extreme altitudes.
11. List and describe the factors influencing the risk of heat injury.
12. Provide suggestions for the fitness participant to follow to minimize the likelihood of heat injury.
13. Describe in general terms the guidelines suggested for running road races in the heat.
14. Describe the three elements in the heat stress index, and explain why one is more important that the other two.
15. List the factors influencing hypothermia.
16. Explain what the Windchill Index is relative to convective heat loss.
17. Explain why exposure to cold water is more dangerous than exposure to air of the same temperature.
18. Describe what the clo unit is and how recommendations for insulation change when one does exercise.
19. Describe the role of subcutaneous fat and energy production in the development of hypothermia.
20. List the steps to follow to deal with hypothermia.
21. Explain how carbon monoxide can influence performance, and list the steps that should be taken to reduce the impact of pollution on performance.

Outline

Key Terms

clo
hypoxia
hyperoxia
normoxia

By now it should be clear that performance is dependent on more than simply having a high $\dot{V}O_2$ max. We have just seen the role of diet and body composition on performance, and in the next chapter we will formally consider "ergogenic" or work-inducing aids and performance. Sandwiched between these chapters will be a discussion of how the environmental factors of altitude, heat, cold, and pollution can influence performance.

Altitude

In the late 1960s, when the Olympic Games were scheduled to be held in Mexico City, our attention was directed at the question of how altitude (2,300 meters [7,400 feet] at Mexico City) would affect performance. Previous experience at altitude suggested that many performances would not equal former Olympic standards or, for that matter, the athlete's own personal record (PR) at sea level. On the other hand, some performances were actually expected to be better because they were conducted at altitude. Why? What happens to $\dot{V}O_2$ max with altitude? Can a sea-level resident ever completely adapt to altitude? We will address these and other questions after a brief review of the environmental factors that change with increasing altitude.

Atmospheric Pressure

The atmospheric pressure at any spot on earth is a measure of the weight of a column of air directly over that spot. At sea level the weight (and height) of that column of air is greatest, but as one climbs to higher and higher altitudes the height, and of course, the weight of the column is reduced. Consequently, atmospheric pressure decreases with increasing altitude, the air is less dense, and each liter of air contains fewer molecules of gas. Since the *percentages* of O_2, CO_2, and N_2 are the same at altitude as at sea level, any change in the *partial pressure* of each gas is due solely to the change in the atmospheric or barometric pressure (see chapter 10). The decrease in the partial pressure of O_2 (PO_2) with increasing altitude has a direct effect on the saturation of hemoglobin and, consequently, oxygen transport. This lower PO_2 is called **hypoxia,** with **normoxia** being the term to describe the PO_2 under sea-level conditions. The term, **hyperoxia,** describes a condition in which the inspired PO_2 is greater than that at sea level (see chapter 25). In addition to the hypoxic condition at altitude, the air temperature and humidity are lower, adding potential temperature regulation problems to the hypoxic stress of altitude. How do these changes affect performance? In order to answer that question we will divide performances into short-term anaerobic performances and long-term aerobic performances.

Short-Term Anaerobic Performance

In chapters 3 and 19 we described the importance of the anaerobic sources of ATP in maximal performances lasting two minutes or less. If this information is correct, and we think it is, then the short-term anaerobic races shouldn't be affected by the low PO_2 at altitude since O_2 transport to the muscles is not limiting performance. Table 24.1 shows this to be the case when the sprint performances of the 1968 Mexico City Olympic Games were compared to those in the 1964 Tokyo Olympic Games. The performances improved

Table 24.1 *Comparison of performances in short races in the 1964 and 1968 Olympic Games*

Olympic Games	Short Races: Men				Short Races: Women			
	100 m	200 m	400 m	800 m	100 m	200 m	400 m	800 m
1964 (Tokyo)	10.0 s	20.3 s	45.1 s	1 m 45.1 s	11.4 s	23.0 s	52.0 s	2 m 1.1 s
1968 (Mexico City)	9.9 s	19.8 s	43.8 s	1 m 44.3 s	11.0 s	22.5 s	52.0 s	2 m 0.9 s
% change*	+1.0	+2.5	+2.9	+0.8	+3.5	+2.2	0	+0.2

* + sign indicates improvement over 1964 performance.
From E. T. Howley, "Effect of Altitude on Physical Performance," in G. A. Stull and T. K. Cureton, *Encyclopedia of Physical Education, Fitness, and Sports: Training, Environment, Nutrition, and Fitness.* Copyright © 1980 Brighton Publishing Company, Salt Lake City, Utah.

Box 24.1

In the 1968 Olympic Games in Mexico City, Bob Beamon shattered the world record in the long jump with a leap of 29 feet, 2.5 inches. Due to the fact that the record was achieved at altitude where air density is less than at sea level, some questions were raised about the true magnitude of the achievement. Recent progress in biomechanics has made it possible to determine just how much would have been gained by doing the long jump at altitude (71). The calculations had to consider the mass of the jumper, a drag coefficient based on the frontal area exposed to the air while jumping, and the difference in the air density between sea level and Mexico City. The result indicated that approximately 2.4 cm, less than an inch, would have been gained by doing the jump at altitude where the air density is less. Beamon's record stands out as one of the greatest performances in recorded history.

---

in all but one case, in which the time for the 400-meter run for the women was the same. The reasons for the improvements in performance include the "normal" gains made over time from one Olympic Games to the next and the fact that the *less dense air* at altitude offers less resistance to movements at high speeds. This latter reason sparked controversy over Bob Beamon's fantastic performance in the long jump in the Mexico City Games (see box 24.1).

Long-Term Aerobic Performance
Maximal performances in excess of two minutes are primarily dependent on oxygen delivery, and, in contrast to the short-term performances, are clearly affected by the lower PO_2 at altitude. Table 24.2 shows the results of the distance running events from 1,500 meters up through the marathon and the 50,000-meter walk, and as you can see, performance was diminished at all distances but the 1,500-meter run. This performance is worthy of special note given that it was expected to be affected as were the others. It is more

Table 24.2 Comparison of performances in long races in the 1964 and 1968 Olympic Games

Olympic Games	Long Races: Men					
	1,500 m	3,000 m	5,000 m	10,000 m	Marathon	50,000 m Walk
1964 (Tokyo)	3 m 38.1 s	8 m 30.8 s	13 m 48.8 s	28 m 24.4 s	2 h 12 m 11.2 s	4 h 11 m 11.2 s
1968 (Mexico City)	3 m 34.9 s	8 m 51.0 s	14 m 05.0 s	29 m 27.4 s	2 h 20 m 26.4 s	4 h 20 m 13.6 s
% change*	+1.5	−3.9	−1.9	−3.7	−6.2	−3.6

* + sign indicates improvement over 1964 performance.
From E. T. Howley, "Effect of Altitude on Physical Performance," in G. A. Stull and T. K. Cureton, *Encyclopedia of Physical Education, Fitness, and Sports: Training, Environment, Nutrition, and Fitness.* Copyright © 1980 Brighton Publishing Company, Salt Lake City, Utah.

than just a passing interest that the record setter was Kipchoge Keino, who was born and raised in Kenya at an altitude similar to that of Mexico City. Did he possess a special adaptation due to his birth place? We will come back to this question in a later section. We would like to continue our discussion of the effect of altitude on performance by asking why did the performance fall off by as much as 6.2% in the long distance races?

Maximal Aerobic Power and Altitude

The decrease in distance running performance at altitude is similar to what occurs when a trained runner becomes untrained—it would clearly take longer to run a marathon! The similarity in the effect is related to a decrease in maximal aerobic power that occurs with detraining and with increasing altitude. Figure 24.1 shows that $\dot{V}O_2$ max decreases in a linear fashion, being about 12% lower at 2,400 meters (7,400 feet), 20% lower at 3,100 meters (10,200 feet), and 27% lower at about 4,000 meters (13,100 feet) (8, 14, 16, 20). While it should be no surprise that endurance performance decreases with such changes in $\dot{V}O_2$ max, why does $\dot{V}O_2$ max decrease?

Cardiovascular Function at Altitude

Maximal oxygen uptake is equal to the product of the maximal cardiac output and the maximal arteriovenous oxygen difference, $\dot{V}O_2 = CO \times (CaO_2 - C\bar{v}O_2)$. Given this relationship, the decrease in $\dot{V}O_2$ max with increasing altitude could be due to a decrease in cardiac output and/or a decrease in oxygen extraction.

Maximal cardiac output is equal to the product of maximal heart rate and maximal stroke volume. In several studies the maximal heart rate was unchanged at altitudes of 2,300 meters (20, 54), 3,100 meters (26), and 4,000 meters (8), while changes in maximal stroke volume were somewhat inconsistent (41). If these two variables, maximal stroke volume and maximal heart rate, do not change with increasing altitude then the decrease in $\dot{V}O_2$ max must be due to a difference in oxygen extraction.

While oxygen extraction ($CaO_2 - C\bar{v}O_2$) could decrease due to a decrease in the arterial oxygen content (CaO_2) or an increase in the mixed venous oxygen content ($C\bar{v}O_2$), the primary cause is the desaturation of the arterial blood due to the low PO_2 at altitude. As you recall from chapter 10, as the arterial PO_2 falls there is a reduction in the volume of oxygen bound to

Figure 24.1 Changes in maximal aerobic power with increasing altitude. The sea-level value for maximal aerobic power is set to 100%.

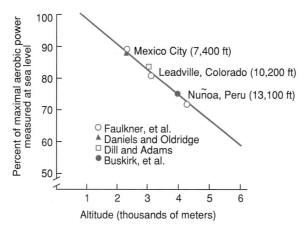

hemoglobin. At sea level, hemoglobin is about 96%–98% saturated with oxygen. However, at 2,300 meters and 4,000 meters, saturation falls to 88% and 71%, respectively. These decreases in the oxygen saturation of hemoglobin are similar to the reductions in $\dot{V}O_2$ max described earlier at these altitudes. Since maximal oxygen transport is the product of the maximal cardiac output and the arterial oxygen content, the capacity to transport oxygen to the working muscles at altitude is reduced due to desaturation, even though maximal cardiac output may be unchanged up to altitudes of 4,000 meters (41). However, it must be added that there are a variety of studies that have shown a decrease in maximal heart rate at altitude. While some of these decreases have been observed at altitudes of 3,100 meters (16) and 4,300 meters (20), it is more common to find lower maximal heart rates above altitudes of 4,300 meters. For example, compared to sea level, maximal HR was observed to be 24–33 beats/minute lower at 4,650 meters (15,300 feet) and 47 beats/minute lower at about 6,100 meters (20,000 feet) (31, 56). This depression in maximal heart rate is reversed by acute restoration of normoxia, or atropine (32). This altitude-induced bradycardia suggests that myocardial hypoxia may trigger the slower heart rate to decrease the work and, therefore, the oxygen demand

of the heart muscle. Given this lower maximal HR, it means that $\dot{V}O_2$ max may decrease at a faster rate at the higher altitudes due to the combined effects of the desaturation of hemoglobin and the decrease in maximal cardiac output.

This desaturation of arterial blood at altitude affects more than $\dot{V}O_2$ max. The cardiovascular responses to submaximal work are also influenced. Due to the fact that each liter of blood is carrying less oxygen, more liters of blood must be pumped per minute in order to compensate. This is accomplished through an increase in the HR response, since the stroke volume response is at its highest point already, or it is actually lower at altitude due to the hypoxia (3). This elevated HR response is shown in figure 24.2 (26). This has implications for more than the performance-based athlete. The average person who participates in an exercise program will have to decrease the intensity of exercise at altitude in order to stay in the target heart zone. Remember, the exercise prescription needed for a cardiovascular training effect includes a proper duration of exercise to achieve a total caloric expenditure of about 200–300 kcal, and if the intensity is too high the person will not be able to complete the workout.

Figure 24.2 The effect of altitude on the heart-rate response to submaximal exercise.

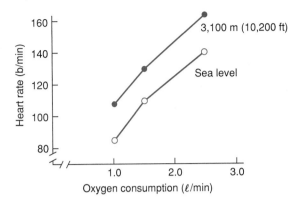

Figure 24.3 The effect of altitude on the ventilation response to submaximal exercise.

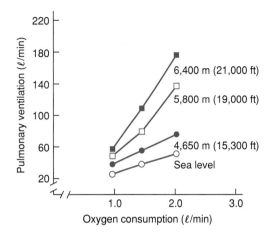

Respiratory Function at Altitude

In the introduction to this section we mentioned that the air is less dense at altitude. This means that there are fewer O_2 molecules per liter of air, and if a person wished to consume the same number of liters of O_2, pulmonary ventilation would have to increase. At 5,600 meters (18,400 feet) the atmospheric pressure is one-half that of sea level and the number of molecules of O_2 per liter of air is reduced by one-half; therefore, a person would have to breathe twice as much air to take in the same amount of O_2. The consequences of this are shown in figure 24.3, which shows a subject who exercised at work rates demanding about a $\dot{V}O_2$ of 1–2 l · min^{-1} at sea level and at three altitudes exceeding 4,000 meters. The pulmonary ventilation is elevated at all altitudes, reaching values of almost 180 l · min^{-1} at 6,400 meters (21,000 feet) (57). This extreme ventilatory response requires the respiratory muscles, primarily the diaphragm, to work so hard that fatigue may occur. We will see more on this in a later section dealing with the assault on Mount Everest.

Adaptation to High Altitude

The body's response to the low PO_2 at altitude is to produce additional red blood cells to compensate for the desaturation of hemoglobin. In the mining community of Morococha, Peru, where people reside at altitudes above 4,540 meters, hemoglobin levels of 211 g · l^{-1} have been measured, in contrast to the normal

156 g · l^{-1} of the sea-level residents in Lima. This higher hemoglobin compensates rather completely for the low PO_2 at those altitudes (40):

Sea Level: 156 g · l^{-1} times 1.34 ml O_2 · g^{-1}
                  at 98% saturation = 206 ml · l^{-1}
4,540 m: 211 g · l^{-1} times 1.34 ml O_2 · g^{-1}
                  at 81% saturation = 224 ml · l^{-1}.

Probably the best test of the degree to which these altitude residents have adapted is found in the $\dot{V}O_2$ max values measured at altitude. Average values of 46–50 ml · kg^{-1} · min^{-1} were obtained on the altitude natives (42, 47), which compares favorably with sea level natives in that country and in ours.

There is no question that any sea-level resident who makes a journey to altitude and stays a while will experience an increase in red blood cell number. However, the adaptation will probably never be complete. This conclusion is drawn from a study that compared $\dot{V}O_2$ max values of Peruvian lowlanders and Peace Corps volunteers who came to altitude as adults, to those of lowlanders who came to altitude as children and spent their growing years at altitude, and finally, to those of permanent altitude residents (21). The $\dot{V}O_2$ max values were 46 ml · kg^{-1} · min^{-1} for the altitude residents and those who arrived there as children. In contrast, the lowlanders who arrived as adults and spent only one to four years at altitude had values of 38 ml · kg^{-1} · min^{-1}. This indicates that in order to have complete adaptation one must spend the developmental years at high altitude. This may help explain the surprisingly good performance of Kipchoge Keino's performance in the 1,500-meter run at the Mexico City Olympic Games mentioned earlier, since he spent his childhood at an altitude similar to that of Mexico City.

Training for Competition at Altitude

It was clear to many of the middle- and long-distance runners who competed in the Olympic Trials or Games in 1968 that the altitude was going to have a detrimental effect on performance. Using $\dot{V}O_2$ max as an indicator of the impact on performance, scientists studied the effect of immediate exposure to altitude, the rate of recovery in $\dot{V}O_2$ max as the individual stayed at altitude, and whether or not $\dot{V}O_2$ max was higher than the pre-altitude value upon return to sea level. The results were interesting, not due to the general trends that were expected, but to the extreme variability in response among the athletes. For example, the decrease in $\dot{V}O_2$ max upon ascent to a 2,300-meter altitude ranged from 8.8%–22.3% (56), at 3,090 meters it ranged from 13.9%–24.4% (16), and at 4,000 meters the decrease ranged from 24.8%–34.3% (8). One of the major conclusions that could be drawn from these data is that the best runner at sea level might not be the best at altitude if that person had the largest drop in $\dot{V}O_2$ max. Why such variability? A recent study of this phenomenon suggests that the variability in the decrease in $\dot{V}O_2$ max across individuals relates to the degree that athletes experience desaturation of arterial blood during maximal work (43). Chapter 10 described the effect that arterial desaturation has on $\dot{V}O_2$ max of superior athletes *at sea level*. If such desaturation can occur under sea-level conditions, then the altitude condition will have an additional impact, with the magnitude of the impact being greater on those who suffer some desaturation at sea level. Exposure to a simulated altitude of 3,000 meters resulted in 20.8% decrease in $\dot{V}O_2$ max for trained subjects and only a 9.8% decrease for untrained subjects (43).

The decrease in the $\dot{V}O_2$ max upon exposure to altitude was not the only physiological response that varied among the athletes. There was also a variable response in the size of the increase in $\dot{V}O_2$ max as the subjects stayed at altitude and continued to train. One study lasting twenty-eight days at 2,300 meters found the $\dot{V}O_2$ max to increase from 1%–8% over that time (56). Some found the $\dot{V}O_2$ max to gradually improve over a period of ten to twenty-eight days (5, 14, 16, 56), while others (20, 26) did not. In addition, when the subjects returned to sea level and were retested, some found the $\dot{V}O_2$ max to be higher than before they left (5, 14, 16), while others found no improvements (8, 20, 26). Why was there such variability in response?

There are several possibilities. If an athlete is not in peak condition before ascending to altitude, then the stress of the exercise and altitude could increase the $\dot{V}O_2$ max over time while at altitude and show a gain when returned to sea level. There is evidence to both support (62) and not support (2) the idea that the combination of altitude and exercise stress leads to greater changes in $\dot{V}O_2$ max than exercise stress alone. Another reason for the variability is related to the altitude at which the training was conducted. When runners trained at high (4,000 meters) altitude the intensity of the runs (relative to sustained sea-level speeds) had to be reduced in order to complete a workout, due to the reduction in $\dot{V}O_2$ max that occurs at altitude. As a result, the runner might actually "detrain" while at altitude and subsequent performance at sea level might not be as good as it was before going to altitude (8). Daniels and Oldridge (14) provided a way around this problem by having runners alternate training at altitude (seven to fourteen days) and sea level (five to eleven days). Using an altitude of only 2,300 meters, the runners were still able to train at "race pace" and detraining did not occur. In fact, thirteen personal records were achieved by the athletes when they raced at sea level.

Figure 24.4 The highest altitudes attained by climbers in this century. In 1924 the climbers ascended within 300 meters of the summit without oxygen. It took another fifty-four years to climb those last 300 meters.

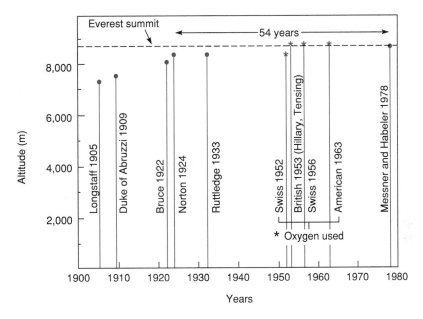

The Quest for Everest

The most obvious tie between exercise and altitude is mountain climbing. The climber faces the stress of altitude, cold, radiation, and, of course, the work of climbing up steep slopes or sheer rock walls. A goal of some mountaineers has been to climb Mt. Everest, at 8,848 meters, the highest mountain on Earth. Figure 24.4 shows the various attempts to climb Everest during this century (73). Special note should be made of Hillary and Tensing, who were the first to do it, and Messner and Habeler, who, to the amazement of all, did it without supplementary oxygen in 1978. This achievement brought scientists back to Everest in 1981 asking how this was possible. This section provides some background to this fascinating story.

In 1924, Norton's climbing team attempted to scale Everest without O_2, and almost succeeded—they stopped only 300 meters from the summit (52). This 1924 expedition was noteworthy because data were collected on the climbers and porters by physicians and scientists associated with the attempt. The story of this assault is good reading for those interested in mountain climbing and provides evidence of the keen powers of observation of the scientists. Major Hingston noted the respiratory distress associated with climbing to such heights, stating that at 5,800 meters (19,000 feet) "the very slightest exertion, such as the tying of a bootlace, the opening of a rationbox, the getting into a sleeping bag, was associated with marked respiratory distress." At 8,200 meters (27,000 feet) one climber "had to take seven, eight, or ten complete respirations for every single step forward. And even at that slow rate of progress he had to rest for a minute or two every twenty or thirty yards" (52). Pugh, who made observations during a 1960–61 expedition to Everest, believed that fatigue of the respiratory muscles may be the primary factor limiting such endeavors at extreme altitudes (54). Further, Pugh's observations of the decreases in $\dot{V}O_2$ max at the extreme altitudes suggested that $\dot{V}O_2$ max would be just above basal metabolism at the

Figure 24.5 Plot of maximal oxygen uptake measured at a variety of altitudes, expressed as inspired PO_2 values. The 1964 data of Pugh et al. predicted the $\dot{V}O_2$ max to be equal to basal metabolic rate. The estimation based on the finding that the barometric pressure (and PO_2) was higher than expected as the summit shifts the estimate to about 15 ml · kg^{-1} · min^{-1}.

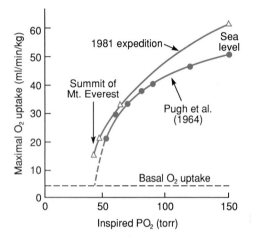

summit, making the task an unlikely one at best. How then did Messner and Habeler climb Everest without O_2?

This was one of the primary questions addressed by the 1981 expedition to Everest. As mentioned earlier, $\dot{V}O_2$ max decreases with altitude due to the lower barometric pressure which causes a lower PO_2 and a desaturation of hemoglobin. In effect, the $\dot{V}O_2$ max at the summit of Everest was predicated on the observed rate of decrease in $\dot{V}O_2$ max at lower altitudes and then extrapolated to the barometric pressure at the top of the mountain. One of the first major findings of the 1981 expedition was that the barometric pressure at the summit was 17 mm Hg higher than previously believed (75, 76). This higher barometric pressure increased the estimated inspired PO_2 and made a big difference in the predicted $\dot{V}O_2$ max. Figure 24.5 shows that the $\dot{V}O_2$ max predicted from the 1960–61 expedition was near the basal metabolic rate while the value predicted from the 1981 expedition was closer to 15 ml · kg^{-1} · min^{-1} (75, 76). The small difference in

the predicted $\dot{V}O_2$ max helps to explain how the climbers reached the summit without the aid of supplementary oxygen. However, it was not the only reason.

The arterial saturation of hemoglobin is dependent upon the arterial PO_2, PCO_2, and pH (chapter 10). A low PCO_2 and a high pH causes the oxygen hemoglobin curve to shift to the left, so that hemoglobin is more saturated under these conditions than under normal conditions. A person who can ventilate great volumes in response to hypoxia can exhale more CO_2 and cause the pH to become elevated. It has been shown that those who successfully deal with altitude have strong hypoxic ventilatory drives, allowing them to have a higher arterial PO_2 and oxygen saturation (66). In fact, when alveolar PCO_2 values were obtained at the top of Mt. Everest in the 1981 expedition, the climbers had values much lower than expected (74). This ability to hyperventilate, coupled with the barometric pressure being higher than expected, resulted in higher arterial PO_2, and of course, $\dot{V}O_2$ max values.

One final note in this regard: It is clear from figure 24.5 that the climbers in the 1981 expedition had $\dot{V}O_2$ max values at sea level that were higher than those of the 1960–61 expedition. In fact, several of the climbers had been competitive marathon runners (75), and, given the need to transport oxygen at these high altitudes in order to do work, having such a high $\dot{V}O_2$ max would appear to be a prerequisite to success in climbing without oxygen. Subsequent measurements on other mountaineers who had scaled 8,500 meters or more without oxygen confirmed this by showing them to possess primarily type I muscle fibers and have an average $\dot{V}O_2$ max of 60 ± 6 ml · kg^{-1} · min^{-1} (53). However, there was one notable exception. One of the subjects in this study was Messner, who had climbed Everest without oxygen; his $\dot{V}O_2$ max was 48.8 ml · kg^{-1} · min^{-1} (53). West et al. (77) provide food for thought in this regard, "It remains for someone to elucidate the evolutionary processes responsible for man being just able to reach the highest point on Earth while breathing ambient air."

Table 24.3 Heat-related problems

Heat Illness	Signs and Symptoms	Immediate Care
Heat Syncope	Headache Nausea	Normal intake of fluids
Heat Cramps	Muscle cramping (calf is very common) Multiple cramping (very serious)	Isolated cramps: Direct pressure to cramp and release, stretch muscle slowly and gently, gentle massage, ice Multiple cramps: Danger of heat stroke, *treat as heat exhaustion*
Heat Exhaustion	Profuse sweating Cold, clammy skin Normal temperature or slightly elevated Pale Dizzy Weak, rapid pulse Shallow breathing Nausea Headache Loss of consciousness	Move individual out of sun to a well-ventilated area Place in shock position (feet elevated 12–18 in); prevent heat loss or gain Gentle massage of extremities Gentle range of motion of the extremities Force fluids Reassure Monitor body temperature and other vital signs Refer to physician
Heat Stroke	Generally, no perspiration Dry skin Very hot Temperature as high as 106° F Skin color bright red or flushed (blacks—ashen) Rapid and strong pulse Labored breathing—semi-reclining position	This is an *extreme medical emergency* Transport to hospital quickly Remove as much clothing as possible without exposing the individual Cool quickly starting at the head and continuing down the body; use any means possible (fan, hose down, pack in ice) Wrap in cold, wet sheets for transport Treat for shock; if breathing is labored, place in a semi-reclining position

From Sue Carver, "Injury Prevention and Treatment," In E. T. Howley and B. D. Franks, *Health/Fitness Instructor's Handbook*, 211-32, 1986. Copyright © 1986 Human Kinetics Press, Inc., Champaign, Ill.

Heat

Chapter 12 described the changes in body temperature with exercise, how heat loss mechanisms are activated, and the benefits of acclimatization. This section will extend that discussion by considering the prevention of thermal injuries during exercise.

Hyperthermia

Our core temperature stays within a few degrees of a value that could lead to death due to thermal injury. Given that, and the fact that distance running races, triathalons, fitness programs, and football games occur during the warmer part of the year, the potential for heat injury is increased (9, 28, 39). Heat injury is not an all-or-none affair, but includes a series of stages that need to be recognized and attended to in order to prevent a progression from the least to the most serious. Table 24.3 summarizes each stage, identifying signs, symptoms, and the immediate care that should be provided (11). While it is important to recognize and deal with these problems, it is better to prevent them from happening.

Figure 24.6 Factors affecting heat injury.

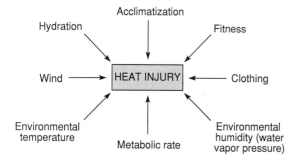

Figure 24.7 The effect of different types of uniforms on the body temperature response to treadmill running.

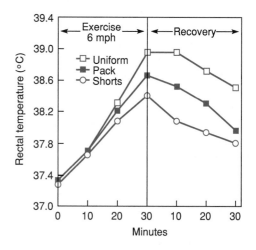

Figure 24.6 shows the major factors related to heat injury. Each one independently influences susceptibility to heat injury:

Fitness—A high level of fitness is related to a lower risk of heat injury (24). Fit subjects can tolerate more work in the heat (17) and will acclimatize faster (9).

Acclimatization—Exercise in the heat increases the capacity to sweat and reduce salt loss. This leads to lower body temperature and HR responses during exercise and a reduced chance of salt depletion (9).

Hydration—Inadequate hydration reduces sweat rate and increases the chance of heat injury (9, 63, 64, 65). Chapter 23 discussed the procedures for fluid replacement. Generally, there is no difference between water and electrolyte drinks in replacing water following dehydration (13).

Environmental Temperature—Convection and radiation heat loss mechanisms are dependent on a temperature gradient from skin to environment. Exercising in temperatures greater than skin temperatures result in a heat *gain*. Evaporation of sweat must then compensate if body temperature is to remain at a safe value.

Clothing—Expose as much skin surface as possible to encourage evaporation. Choose materials, such as cotton, that will "wick" sweat to the surface for evaporation. Materials impermeable to water will increase the risk of heat injury. Figure 24.7 shows the influence of different uniforms on the body temperature response to treadmill running (46).

Humidity (water vapor pressure)—Evaporation of sweat is dependent on the water vapor pressure gradient between skin and environment. In warm/hot environments the relative humidity is a good index of the water vapor pressure, with a lower relative humidity facilitating evaporation.

Metabolic rate—Given that core temperature is proportional to work rate, metabolic heat production plays an important role in the overall heat load experienced by the body during exercise. Decreasing the work rate decreases this heat load, as well as the strain on the physiological systems that must deal with it.

Wind—Wind places more air molecules into contact with the skin and can influence heat loss in two ways. If a temperature gradient for heat loss exists between the skin and the air, wind will increase the rate of heat loss by convection. In a similar manner, wind increases the rate of evaporation assuming the air can accept moisture.

Implications for Fitness

The person exercising for fitness needs to be educated about all of the previously listed factors. Suggestions might include:

• providing information on heat illness symptoms: cramps, lightheadedness, etc.

- exercising in the cooler part of the day to avoid heat gain from the sun or structures heated by the sun
- gradually increasing exposure to high heat/humidity to safely acclimatize
- drinking water before, during, and after exercise and weighing in each day to monitor hydration
- wearing only shorts and a tank top to expose as much skin as possible
- taking heart rate measurements several times during the activity and reducing exercise intensity to stay in the THR zone

The latter recommendation is most important. The heart rate is a sensitive indicator of dehydration, environmental heat load, and acclimatization. Variation in any of these factors will modify the heart rate response to any fixed submaximal exercise. It is therefore important for fitness participants to monitor heart rate on a regular basis and to slow down to stay within the THR zone.

Implications for Performance

Heat injury has been a concern in athletics for decades. Initially, the vast majority of attention was focused on football because of the large number of heat-related deaths associated with that sport (10). This problem has diminished over the last twenty years due to an emphasis on replacing water **during** practice and games, the use of a pre-season conditioning program to increase fitness and initiate acclimatization, weighing in each day to monitor hydration, the development of new materials for jerseys, and the improved recognition of the potential for heat-related injury. While the risk of heat injuries was decreasing for football players, it was increasing in another athletic activity—long distance road races (28, 39). In response to this problem, and on the basis of sound research, the American College of Sports Medicine developed a Position Stand on The Prevention of Thermal Injuries During Distance Running (4). The elements recommended in this position statement are consistent with what we previously presented:

Medical Director	• Work with race director to prevent heat injury and coordinate first-aid measures.
Race Organization	• Minimize environmental heat load by planning races for the cooler months, and at a time of day (before 8:00 A.M. or after 6:00 P.M.) to reduce solar heat gain. • Use an environmental heat stress index (see next section) to help make decisions about whether or not to run a race. • Have a water station every 2–3 km; encourage runners to drink 100–200 milliters of water per station. • Clearly identify the race monitors and have them look for those who might be in trouble due to heat injury. • Have traffic control for safety. • Use radio communication throughout the race course.
Medical Support	• Medical director coordinates ambulance service with local hospitals and has the authority to evaluate or stop runners who appear to be in trouble. • Coordinates medical facilities at race site to provide first aid.
Competitor Education	• Provide information about factors related to heat illness that were previously discussed. • Encourage the "buddy system" (see chapter 17).

The primary focus in these recommendations, be they for the fitness participant involved in a "fun run" or the marathon runner, is safety.

Environmental Heat Stress

The previous discussion mentioned high temperature and relative humidity as factors increasing the risk of heat injuries. In order to quantify the overall heat stress associated with any environment, a Wet Bulb Globe Temperature (WBGT) guide has been developed (4).

This overall heat stress index is composed of the following measurements:

Dry Bulb Temperature (T_{db}) —ordinary measure of air temperature taken in the shade

Black Globe Temperature (T_g) —measure of the radiant heat load measured in direct sunlight

Wet Bulb Temperature (T_{wb}) —measurement of air temperature with a thermometer whose mercury bulb is covered with a wet cotton wick. This measure is sensitive to the relative humidity (water vapor pressure) and provides an index of the ability to evaporate sweat

The formula used to calculate the WBTG temperature shows the importance of this latter wet bulb temperature in determining heat stress (4):

$$WBGT = 0.7\ T_{wb} + 0.2\ T_g + 0.1\ T_{db}$$

The risk of heat stress is given by the following color-coded flags on the race course:

- Red Flag $WBGT = 23–28°\ C$ $(73–82°\ F)$ High risk
- Amber Flag $WBGT = 18–23°\ C$ $(65–73°\ F)$ Moderate risk
- Green Flag $WBGT < 18°\ C$ $(<65°\ F)$ Low risk of heat injury
- White Flag $WBTG < 10°\ C$ $(<50°\ F)$ Low risk of hyperthermia, but possibility of hypothermia

Cold

Altitude and heat stress are not the only environmental factors having an impact on performance. As mentioned in the "White Flag" category of heat stress, a WBGT of 10° C or less is associated with hypothermia. Hypothermia is the result of a higher rate of heat loss from the body compared to heat production.

Cold air facilitates this process in more ways than are readily apparent. First, and most obvious, when air temperature is less than skin temperature a gradient for heat loss exists for convection, and physiological mechanisms involving peripheral vasoconstriction and shivering come into play to counter this gradient. Second, and less obvious, cold air has a low water vapor pressure, which encourages the evaporation of moisture from the skin to further cool the body. The combined effects can be deadly, as witnessed in Pugh's report of three deaths during a "walking" competition over a forty-five-mile distance (57).

Figure 24.8 shows the factors related to hypothermia. These include environmental factors such as temperature, water vapor pressure, wind, and whether air or water are involved; insulating factors such as clothing and subcutaneous fat; and the capacity for sustained energy production. We will now comment on each of these relative to hypothermia.

Environmental Factors

Heat loss mechanisms introduced in chapter 12 included conduction, convection, radiation, and evaporation. Given that hypothermia is the result of a higher rate of heat loss compared to heat production, understanding how these mechanisms are involved will facilitate a discussion of how to deal with this problem.

Conduction, convection, and radiation are dependent on a temperature gradient between skin and environment; the larger the gradient the greater the rate of heat loss. What is surprising is that the environmental temperature does not have to be below freezing in order to help hypothermia along. In effect, there are other environmental factors that interact with temperature to create the dangerous condition by facilitating heat loss, namely, wind and water.

Windchill Index

The rate of heat loss at any given temperature is directly influenced by the wind speed. Wind increases the number of cold air molecules coming into contact with the skin so that heat loss is accelerated. The windchill index indicates what the "effective" temperature is for any combination of temperature and wind speed. Siple and Passel (68) developed a formula

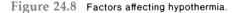

Figure 24.8 Factors affecting hypothermia.

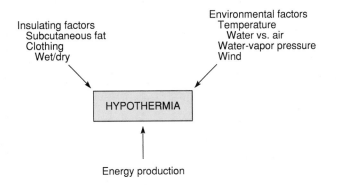

for predicting how fast heat would be lost at different wind speeds and temperatures:

$$\text{Windchill (kcal} \cdot m^{-2} \cdot h^{-1})$$
$$= [\sqrt{WV \times 100} + 10.45 - WV]$$
$$\times (33 - T_A)$$

Where: WV = wind velocity (m · sec^{-1}); 10.45 is a constant; 33 is 33° C, which is taken as the skin temperature; and T_A = ambient dry bulb temperature in °C.

If the windchill value equals 800, the conditions are classified as "cold," at 1,200, "bitterly cold," while at 2,000, exposed flesh would freeze in one minute, and at 2,300, exposed flesh would freeze in thirty seconds (23). This information has been translated into a familiar windchill chart shown in Table 24.4, which allows you to properly gauge the conditions at a variety of wind velocities and temperatures. The term "danger" refers to the 2,000 windchill value and "great danger" refers to the 2,300 value. Please keep in mind that if you are running, riding, or cross country skiing into the wind you must add your speed to the wind speed to evaluate the full impact of the windchill. For example, cycling at 20 mph into calm air at 0° F is equivalent to −35° F! However, wind is not the only factor that can increase the rate of heat loss at any given temperature.

Water
The thermal conductivity of water is about twenty-five times greater than that of air so you can lose heat twenty-five times faster in water compared to air of the same temperature (36). Figure 24.9 shows how few hours it takes to cause death when a person is shipwrecked in cold water. Unlike air, water offers little or no insulation at the skin-water interface, so heat is rapidly lost from the body. Given that movement in such cold water would increase heat loss from the arms and legs, the recommendation is to stay as still as possible in long-term immersions (36).

Insulating Factors
The rate at which heat is lost from the body is inversely related to the insulation between the body and the environment. The insulating quality is related to the thickness of subcutaneous fat, the ability of clothing to trap air, and whether or not the clothing is wet or dry.

Subcutaneous Fat
An excellent indicator of total body insulation per unit surface area (through which heat is lost) is the average subcutaneous fat thickness (33). Pugh and Edholm's (55) observation that a "fat" man was able to swim for seven hours in 16° C water with no change in body temperature while a "thin" man had to leave the water in thirty minutes with a core temperature

Table 24.4 Windchill index

Wind Speed in MPH	50	40	30	20	10	0	−10	−20	−30	−40	−50	−60
					Equivalent Temperature (°F)							
Calm	50	40	30	20	10	0	−10	−20	−30	−40	−50	−60
5	48	37	27	16	6	−5	−15	−26	−36	−47	−57	−68
10	40	28	16	4	−9	−21	−33	−46	−58	−70	−83	−95
15	36	22	9	−5	−18	−36	−45	−58	−72	−85	−99	−112
20	32	18	4	−10	−25	−39	−53	−67	−82	−96	−110	−124
25	30	16	0	−15	−29	−44	−59	−74	−88	−104	−118	−133
30	28	13	−2	−18	−33	−48	−63	−79	−94	−109	−125	−140
35	27	11	−4	−20	−35	−49	−67	−82	−98	−113	−129	−145
40	26	10	−6	−21	−37	−53	−69	−85	−100	−116	−132	−148

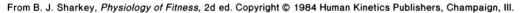

(Wind speeds greater than 40 MPH have little additional effect)

Little Danger (for properly clothed person)

Increasing Danger

Great Danger

Danger from freezing of exposed flesh

Figure 24.9 The effect of different water temperatures on the survival time of shipwrecked individuals.

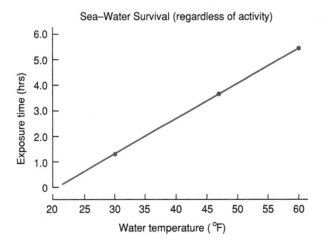

Figure 24.10 Changes in the insulation requirement of clothing (plus air) with increasing rates of energy expenditure over environmental temperatures of −50 to +30° C.

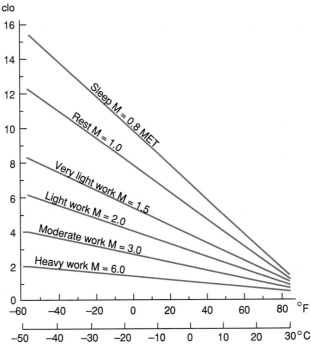

of 34.5° C, supports this statement. Long-distance swimmers tend to be fatter than short-course swimmers, and the higher body fatness does more than help maintain body temperature; fatter swimmers are more buoyant, requiring less energy to swim at any set speed (35).

Clothing

Clothing can extend our natural subcutaneous fat insulation to allow us to sustain very cold environments. The insulation quality of clothing is given in **clo** units, where one clo is the insulation needed at rest (1 MET) to maintain core temperature when the environment is 21° C, the RH = 50%, and the air movement is 6 m · min^{-1} (7). Still air next to the body has a clo rating of 0.8. As the air temperature falls, clothing with a higher clo value must be worn to maintain core temperature since the gradient between skin and environment is increasing. Figure 24.10 shows the insulation needed at different energy expenditures across a broad range of temperatures from −60 to +80° F (7). It is clear that as energy production increases, insulation must decrease to maintain core temperature. By wearing clothing in layers, insulation can be removed piece by piece, since less insulation is needed to maintain core temperature. By following these steps, sweating, which can rob the clothing of its insulating value, will be minimized. A practical example of how clothing helps maintain body temperature (and comfort) can be seen in the following study. Heat loss from the head increases linearly from +32° C to −21° C, with about *half* of the entire heat production being lost through the head when the temperature is −4° C.

Wearing a simple "helmet" with a clo rating of 3.5 allows an individual to stay out indefinitely at 0° C (22).

Clothing offers insulation by trapping air, a poor conductor of heat. If the clothing becomes wet, the insulating quality decreases since the water can now conduct heat away from the body at a faster rate (36). A primary goal, then, is to avoid wetness, due either to sweat or to weather. This problem is exacerbated by the cold environment's very low water vapor pressure. Recall from chapter 12 that the water vapor pressure in the environment is the primary factor influencing evaporation and that at low environmental temperatures the water vapor pressure is low even when the relative humidity is high. Think of the time when you have finished playing a game indoors and stepped outside into cold damp weather to cool off. You notice "steam" coming off your body; how is this possible when the RH is near 100%? The water vapor pressure is high at the skin surface since the skin temperature is elevated and, thus, a gradient for water vapor pressure exists; you will cool off very fast under these circumstances. This is why *cold, wet, windy* environments carry an extra risk of hypothermia. The wind not only provides for greater convective heat loss as described in the windchill, but it also accelerates evaporation (29).

Energy Production

Figure 24.10 showed that the amount of insulation needed to maintain core temperature decreased as energy expenditure increased. This is also true for our "natural" insulation, subcutaneous fat. McArdle et al. (44) showed that when fat men (27.6% fat) were immersed for one hour in 20° C, 24° C, and 28° C water, the resting $\dot{V}O_2$ and core temperature did not change compared to values measured in air. In thinner men (<16.8% fat) the $\dot{V}O_2$ increased to counter the rapid loss of heat, however, the core temperature still decreased. When these same subjects did exercise in the cold water, requiring a $\dot{V}O_2$ of 1.7 l · min^{-1}, the fall in body temperature was either prevented or retarded (45), showing the importance of high rates of energy production in preventing hypothermia.

Dealing with Hypothermia

As body temperature falls the person's ability to carry out coordinated movements is reduced, speech is slurred, and judgement is impaired (67). People can die from hypothermia, and the condition must be dealt with when it occurs. The following steps on how to do this are taken from Sharkey (67):

- Get person out of the cold, wind, and rain.
- Remove all wet clothing.
- Provide warm drinks, dry clothing, and a warm, dry sleeping bag for a mildly impaired person.
- If semiconscious, keep the person awake, remove clothing, and put into a sleeping bag with another person.
- Find a source of heat (e.g., camp fire).

Air Pollution

Air pollution includes a variety of gases and particulates that are products of the combustion of fossil fuels. The "smog" that results when these pollutants are in high concentration can have detrimental effects on health and performance. The gases can affect performance by decreasing the capacity to transport oxygen, increasing airway resistance, and altering the perception of effort required when the eyes "burn" and the chest "hurts." This section will focus on carbon monoxide, the most common and widely distributed pollutant (58).

Carbon Monoxide

Carbon monoxide (CO) is derived from the burning of fossil fuel, coal, oil, gasoline, and wood, as well as from cigarette smoke. Carbon monoxide can bind to hemoglobin (HbCO) and decrease the capacity for oxygen transport. This has the potential to affect the physiological responses to submaximal exercise (34) as well as $\dot{V}O_2$ max, as does altitude. The carbon monoxide concentration [HbCO] in blood is generally less than 1% in nonsmokers, but may be as high as 10% in smokers (58). Horvath et al. (37) found that the critical concentration of HbCO needed to decrease $\dot{V}O_2$ max was 4.3%. Figure 24.11 shows the relationship between the blood HbCO concentration and the decrease in $\dot{V}O_2$ max (59).

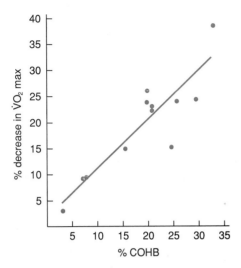

Figure 24.11 The effect of the concentration of carbon monoxide in the blood on the change in $\dot{V}O_2$ max.

In contrast, when one performs light work, at about 40% $\dot{V}O_2$ max, the [HbCO] can be as high as 15% before endurance is affected. There is simply a greater capacity of the cardiovascular system to respond with a larger cardiac output when the HbO_2 concentration is reduced during submaximal work. Unfortunately, it is difficult to predict what the actual [HbCO] will be in any given environment. One must consider the previous exposure to the pollutant, as well as the length of time and rate of ventilation associated with the current exposure. As a result, Raven (58) provides the following guidelines for exercising in an area with air pollution:

- Reduce exposure to the pollutant prior to exercise since the physiological effects are time- and dose-dependent
- Stay away from areas where you might receive a "bolus" dose of CO: smoking areas, high traffic areas, urban environment
- Schedule activities around the times when pollutants are at their highest levels: 7–10 A.M., and 4–7 P.M., due to traffic

Summary

1. The atmospheric pressure, PO_2, air temperature, and air density decrease with altitude.
2. The lower air density at altitude offers less resistance to high-speed movement, and sprint performances are either not affected or are improved.
3. Distance-running performances are adversely affected by altitude due to the reduction in the PO_2, which causes a decrease in hemoglobin saturation and $\dot{V}O_2$ max.
4. Submaximal performances conducted at altitude require higher heart rate and ventilation responses due to the lower oxygen content of arterial blood and the reduction in the number of oxygen molecules per liter of air, respectively.
5. Persons adapt to altitude by producing more red blood cells to counter the desaturation caused by the lower PO_2. Altitude residents who spent their growing years at altitude show a rather complete adaptation as seen in their arterial oxygen content and $\dot{V}O_2$ max values. Lowlanders who arrive as adults show only a modest adaptation.
6. When athletes go to altitude some experience a greater decline in $\dot{V}O_2$ max than others. This may be due to differences in the degree to which each athlete experiences a desaturation of hemoglobin. Remember, some athletes experience desaturation during maximal work at sea level.
7. Some athletes show an increase in $\dot{V}O_2$ max while training at altitude while others do not. This may be due to the degree to which the athlete was trained before going to altitude. In addition, some athletes show an improved $\dot{V}O_2$ max upon return to sea level, while others do not. Part of the reason may be the altitude at which they train. Those who train at high altitudes may actually "detrain" due to the fact that the quality of their workouts suffer at

the high altitudes. To get around this problem one can alternate low-altitude and sea-level exposures.

8. Mount Everest was climbed without oxygen in 1978. This surprised scientists who thought $\dot{V}O_2$ max would be just above resting $\dot{V}O_2$ at that altitude. They later found that the barometric pressure was actually higher than they previously had thought and that the estimated $\dot{V}O_2$ max was about 15 ml $\cdot$ kg^{-1} $\cdot$ min^{-1} at this altitude. In addition, those who are successful at these high altitudes have a great capacity to hyperventilate, driving down the PCO_2 and the [H$^+$] in blood, allowing more oxygen to bind with hemoglobin at the same arterial PO_2.

9. Heat injury is influenced by environmental factors such as temperature, water vapor pressure, acclimatization, hydration, clothing, and metabolic rate. The fitness participant should be educated about the signs and symptoms of heat injury, the importance of drinking water before, during, and after the activity, gradually becoming acclimated to the heat, exercising in the cooler part of the day, dressing appropriately, and checking the HR on a regular basis.

10. Road races conducted in the heat and humidity need to reflect the coordinated wisdom of the race director and medical director to minimize heat and other injuries. Concerns include running the race at the correct time of the day and season of the year, frequent water stops, traffic control, race monitors to identify and stop those in trouble, and communication between race monitors, medical director, ambulance services, and hospitals.

11. The heat stress index includes dry bulb, wet bulb, and globe temperatures. The wet bulb temperature, which is a good indicator of the vapor pressure, is more important than the other two in determining the overall heat stress.

12. Hypothermia is influenced by natural and added insulation, environmental temperature, vapor pressure, wind, water immersion, and energy production. The Windchill Index describes how wind lowers the effective temperature at the skin such that convective heat loss is greater than what it would be in calm air at that same temperature. Water causes heat to be lost by convection twenty-five times faster than it would be by exposure to air of the same temperature.

13. Subcutaneous fat is the primary "natural" insulation and is very effective in preventing rapid heat loss when a person is exposed to cold water. Clothing extends this insulation, and the insulation value of clothing is described in clo units, where a value of 1 describes what is needed to maintain core temperature while sitting in a room set at 21° C and 50% RH. The amount of insulation needed to maintain core temperature is less when one exercises because the metabolic heat production helps maintain the core temperature. Clothing should be worn in layers when exercising in order to shed one insulating layer at a time as body temperature increases.

14. If a person becomes hypothermic, get the person out of the wind, rain, and cold; remove wet clothing and put on dry clothing; use a sleeping bag for warmth; and if it is a severe case, remove clothing from the person and have another person climb into the sleeping bag to provide warmth; finally, provide some source of heat.

15. Carbon monoxide binds to hemoglobin and reduces oxygen transport in much the same way that altitude does. To prevent problems associated with pollution of any type, reduce exposure time; stay away from "bolus" amounts of the pollutant; and schedule activity at the least polluted part of the day.

Study Questions

1. Describe the changes in barometric pressure, PO_2, and air density with increasing altitude.
2. Why is sprint performance not affected by altitude?
3. Explain why maximal aerobic power decreases at altitude and what effect this has on performance in long-distance races.
4. Graphically describe the effect of altitude on the HR and ventilation responses to submaximal work and provide recommendations for fitness participants who occasionally exercises at altitude.
5. Describe the process by which an individual adapts to altitude, and contrast the adaptation of the permanent residents of high altitude with that of the lowlander who arrives there as an adult.
6. While training at altitude can be beneficial, how could someone "detrain"? How can you work around this problem?
7. It was formally believed that a person could not climb Mt. Everest without oxygen because the estimated $\dot{V}O_2$ max at altitude was close to basal metabolic rate. When two climbers accomplished the feat in 1978 scientists had to determine how this was possible. What were the primary reasons allowing the climb to take place without oxygen?
8. List and describe the factors related to heat injury.
9. What is the heat stress index and why is the wet bulb temperature weighed so heavily in the formula?
10. List the factors related to hypothermia.
11. Explain what the Windchill Index is relative to convective heat loss.
12. What is a clo unit, and why is the insulation requirement less when you exercise?
13. What would you do if a person has hypothermia?
14. Explain how carbon monoxide can influence $\dot{V}O_2$ max and endurance performance.
15. What steps would you follow to minimize the effect of pollution on performance?

Suggested Readings

Pandolf, K. B., M. N. Sawka, and R. R. Gonzalez. 1988. *Human Performance Physiology and Environmental Medicine at Terrestrial Extremes.* Indianapolis, Id.: Benchmark Press, Inc.

West, J. B., and S. Lahiri, eds. 1984. *High Altitude and Man.* Baltimore, Md.: The Williams & Wilkins Co.

References

1. Abbrecht, P. H., and J. K. Littell. 1972. Plasma erythropoietin in men and mice during acclimatization to different altitudes. *Journal of Applied Physiology* 32:54–58.
2. Adams, W. C. et al. 1975. Effects of equivalent sea-level and altitude training on $\dot{V}O_2$ max and running performance. *Journal of Applied Physiology* 39:262–66.
3. Alexander, J. K. et al. 1967. Reduction of stroke volume during exercise in man following ascent to 3,100 m altitude. *Journal of Applied Physiology* 23:849–58.
4. American College of Sports Medicine 1985. The prevention of thermal injuries during distance running. *Medicine and Science in Sports and Exercise* 19:529–33, 1985.
5. Balke, B., F. J. Nagle, and J. Daniels. 1965 (Nov.) Altitude and maximum performance in work and sports activity. *Journal of the American Medical Association* 194:646–49.
6. Billings, C. E. et al. 1971. Cost of submaximal and maximal work during chronic exposure at 3,800 m. *Journal of Applied Physiology* 30:406–8.
7. Burton, A. C., and O. G. Edholm. 1955. *Man in a Cold Environment,* 273. London: Edward Arnold Publishers Ltd.
8. Buskirk, E. R. et al. 1967. Maximal performance at altitude and on return from altitude in conditioned runners. *Journal of Applied Physiology* 23:259–66.
9. Buskirk, E. R., and D. E. Bass. 1974. Climate and Exercise. In (W. R. Johnson and E. R. Buskirk, eds.) *Science and Medicine of Exercise and Sport,* 190–205. New York: Harper & Row.
10. Buskirk, E. R., and W. C. Grasley. 1974. Heat injury and conduct of athletics. In (W. R. Johnson and E. R. Buskirk, eds.) *Science and Medicine of Exercise and Sport,* 206–10. New York: Harper & Row, Publishers.

11. Carver, Sue. 1986. Injury Prevention and Treatment. In (E. T. Howley and B. Don Franks) *Health/Fitness Instructor's Handbook,* 211–32. Champaign, Ill.: Human Kinetics Publishers.

12. Cerretelli, P. 1976. Limiting factors to oxygen transport on Mount Everest. 1976. *Journal of Applied Physiology* 40:658–67.

13. Costill, D. L. et al. 1975. Water and electrolyte replacement during repeated days of work in the heat. *Aviation, Space and Environmental Medicine* 46 (6) 795–800, 1975.

14. Daniels, J., and N. Oldridge. 1970. The effects of alternate exposure to altitude and sea level on world-class middle-distance runner. *Medicine and Science in Sports* 2:107–12.

15. DeJours, P., R. H. Kellogg, and N. Pace. 1963. Regulation of respiration and heart rate response in exercise during altitude acclimatization. *Journal of Applied Physiology* 18:10–18.

16. Dill, D. B., and W. C. Adams. 1971. Maximal oxygen uptake at sea level and at 3,090-m altitude in high school champion runners. *Journal of Applied Physiology* 30:854–59.

17. Drinkwater, B. L. et al. 1976. Aerobic power as a factor in women's response to work with in hot environments. *Journal of Applied Physiology* 41:815–21.

18. Drinkwater, B. L. et al. 1979. Response of women mountaineers to maximal exercise during hypoxia. *Aviation, Space, and Environmental Medicine* 50:657–62.

19. Eaton, J. W., G. J. Brewer, and R. F. Grover. 1969 (April). Role of red cell 2, 3-diphosphglycerate in the adaptation of man to altitude. *Journal of Laboratory and Clinical Medicine* 73:603–9.

20. Faulkner, J. A. et al. 1968. Maximum aerobic capacity and running performance at altitude. *Journal of Applied Physiology* 24:685–91.

21. Frisancho, A. R. et al. 1973. Influence of developmental adaptation on aerobic capacity at high altitude. *Journal of Applied Physiology* 34:176–80.

22. Froese, G. and A. C. Burton. 1957. Heat loss from the human head. *Journal of Applied Physiology* 10:235–41.

23. Gates, D. M. 1972. *Man and His Environment: Climate.* New York: Harper and Row.

24. Gisolfi, G. V., and J. Cohen. 1979. Relationships among training, heat acclimation, and heat tolerance in men and women: The controversy revisited. *Medicine and Science in Sports* 11:56–59.

25. Gold, A. J., T. F. Johnson, and L. C. Costello. 1973. Effects of altitude stress on mitochondrial function. *American Journal of Physiology* 224:946–49.

26. Grover, R. et al. 1967. Muscular exercise in young men native to 3,100 m altitude. *Journal of Applied Physiology* 22:555–64.

27. Hannon, J. P., J. L. Shields, and C. W. Harris. 1969. Effects of altitude acclimatization on blood composition of women. *Journal of Applied Physiology* 26:540–47.

28. Hanson, P. G., and S. W. Zimmerman. 1979. Exertional heatstroke in novice runners. *Journal of the American Medical Association* 242:154–57.

29. Hardy, J. D., and P. Bard. 1974. Body temperature regulation. In (V. B. Mountcastle, ed.) *Medical Physiology,* 13th ed., vol. 2, 1305–42. St. Louis: The C.V. Mosby Company.

30. Harris, C. W., and J. E. Hansen. 1966. Electrocardiographic changes during exposure to high altitude. *American Journal of Cardiology* 18:183–90.

31. Hartley, L. H., J. A. Vogel, and J. C. Cruz. 1974. Reduction of maximal exercise heart rate at altitude and its reversal with atropine. *Journal of Applied Physiology* 36:362–65.

32. Hartley, L. H. et al. 1967. Subnormal cardiac output at rest and during exercise in residents at 3,100 m altitude. *Journal of Applied Physiology* 23:839–48.

33. Hayward, M. G., and W. R. Keatinge. 1981. Roles of subcutaneous fat and thermoregulatory reflexes in determining ability to stabilize body temperature in water. *Journal of Physiology* (London) 320:229–51.

34. Hirsch, G. L. et al. 1985. *Journal of Applied Physiology* 58:1975–81.

35. Holmer, I. 1979. Physiology of swimming man. In (R. S. Hutton and D. I. Miller, eds.), *Exercise and Sport Sciences Reviews* 7.

36. Horvath, S. M. 1981. Exercise in a cold environment. In (D.I. Miller, ed.) *Exercise and Sport Sciences Reviews* 9 (1981):221–63.

37. Horvath, S. M. et al. 1975. Maximal aerobic capacity of different levels of carboxyhemoglobin. *Journal of Applied Physiology* 38:300–3.

38. Howley, E. T. 1980. Effect of altitude on physical performance. In (G. A. Stull and T. K. Cureton, eds.) *Encyclopedia of Physical Education, Fitness, and Sports: Training, Environment, Nutrition, and Fitness,* 177–87. Salt Lake City: Brighton Publishing Company.

39. Hughson, R. L. et al. 1980. Heat Injuries in Canadian mass participation runs. *Canadian Medicine Medical Association Journal* 122:1141–44.

40. Hurtado, A. 1964. Animals in high altitudes: resident man. In (D. B. Dill, ed.) *Handbook of Physiology: Section 4—Adaptation to the Environment,* Washington, D.C.: American Physiological Society.

41. Kollias, J., and E. Buskirk. 1974. Exercise and Altitude. In (W. R. Johnson and E. R. Buskirk, eds.) *Science and Medicine of Exercise and Sport,* 2d ed. New York: Harper & Row.

42. Kollias, J. et al. 1968. Work capacity of long-time residents and newcomers to altitude. *Journal of Applied Physiology* 24:792–99.

43. Lawler, J., S. K. Powers, and D. Thompson. 1988. Linear relationship between $\dot{V}O_2$ max and $\dot{V}O_2$ max decrement during exposure to acute hypoxia. *Journal of Applied Physiology* 64:1486–92.

44. McArdle, W. D. et al. 1984. Thermal adjustment to cold-water exposure in resting men and women. *Journal of Physiology: Respiratory, Environmental, and Exercise Physiology* 56:1565–71.

45. McArdle, W. D. et al. 1984. Thermal adjustment to cold-water exposure in exercising men and women. *Journal of Applied Physiology: Respiratory, Environmental, and Exercise Physiology* 56:1572–77.

46. Mathews, D. K., E. L. Fox, and D. Tanzi. 1969. Physiological responses during exercise and recovery in a football uniform. *Journal of Applied Physiology* 26:611–15.

47. Mazess, R. B. 1969. Exercise performance at high altitude in Peru. *Federation Proceedings* 28:1301–6.

48. ———. 1969. Exercise performance of Indian and white high-altitude residents. *Human Biology* 41:494–518.

49. ———. 1970. Cardiorespiratory characteristics and adaptations to high altitudes. *American Journal of Physical Anthropology* 32:267–78.

50. Milledge, J. S. et al. 1983. Cardiorespiratory response to exercise in men repeatedly exposed to extreme altitude. *Journal of Applied Physiology: Respiratory, Environmental, and Exercise Physiology* 55:1379–85.

51. Moore, L. G. et al. 1986. Low acute hypoxic ventilatory response and hypoxic depression in acute altitude sickness. *Journal of Applied Physiology* 60:1407–12.

52. Norton, E. F. 1925. *The Fight for Everest* 1924. New York: Longmans, Green.

53. Oelz, O. et al. 1986. Physiological profile of world-class high-altitude climbers. *Journal of Applied Physiology* 60:1734–42.

54. Pugh, L. G. C. 1964. Deaths from exposure in Four Inns Walking Competition, *Lancet* 1(March 14–15):1210–12.

55. Pugh, L. G. C., and O. G. Edholm. 1955. The physiology of Channel swimmers. *Lancet* 2:761–68.

56. Pugh, L. G. C. E. 1967. Athletes at altitude. *Journal of Physiology* (London) 192:619–46.

57. Pugh, L. G. C. E. et al. 1964. Muscular exercise at great altitudes. *Journal of Applied Physiology* 19:431–40.

58. Raven, P. B. 1980. Effects of air pollution on physical performance. In *Encyclopedia of Physical Education, Fitness, and Sports: Training, Environment, Nutrition, and Fitness,* Vol. 2, 201–16. Salt Lake City: Brighton Publishing Company.

59. Raven, P. B. et al. 1974. Effect of carbon monoxide and peroxyacetyl nitrate on man's maximal aerobic capacity. *Journal of Applied Physiology* 36:288–93.

60. Rennie, D. W. et al. 1962. Physical insulation of Korean diving women. *Journal of Applied Physiology* 17:961–66.

61. Reynafarje, B. 1962. Myoglobin content and enzymatic activity of muscle and altitude adaptation. *Journal of Applied Physiology* 17:301–5.

62. Roskamm, H. et al. 1969. Effects of a standardized ergometer training program at three different altitudes. *Journal of Applied Physiology* 27:840–47.

63. Saltin, B. 1964. Circulatory response to submaximal and maximal exercise after thermal dehydration. *Journal of Applied Physiology* 19:1125–32, 1984.

64. Sawka, M. N. et al. 1985. Thermoregulatory and blood responses during exercise at graded hypohydration levels. *Journal of Applied Physiology* 59:1394–1401.

65. Sawka, M. N. et al. 1984. Influence of hydration level and body fluids on exercise performance in the heat. *Journal of the American Medical Association* 252(9) 1165–69.

66. Schoene, R. B. et al. 1984. Relationship of hypoxic ventilatory response to exercise performance on Mount Everest. *Journal of Applied Physiology: Respiratory, Environmental, and Exercise Physiology* 56:1478–83.

67. Sharkey, B. J. 1984. *Physiology of Fitness.* 2d ed. Champaign, Ill.: Human Kinetics Publishers.

68. Siple, P. A., and C. F. Passel. 1945. Measurements of dry atmospheric cooling in subfreezing temperatures. *Proceedings of the American Philosophical Society* 89:177–99.

69. Sutton, J. R. et al. 1976. Pulmonary gas exchange in acute mountain sickness. *Aviation, Space, and Environmental Medicine* 47:1032–37.

70. Sutton, J. R. et al. 1983. Exercise at altitude. *Annual Review of Physiology* 45:427–37.

71. Ward-Smith, A. J. 1983. The influence of aerodynamic and biomechanic factors on long jump performance. *Journal of Biomechanics* 16:655–58.

72. West, J. B. Man at extreme altitude. 1982. *Journal of Applied Physiology: Respiratory, Environmental, and Exercise Physiology* 52:1393–99.

73. West, J. B., and P. D. Wagner. 1980. Predicted gas exchange on the summit of Mt. Everest. *Respiration Physiology* 42:1–16.

74. West, J. B. et al. 1983. Pulmonary gas exchange on the summit of Mount Everest. *Journal of Applied Physiology: Respiratory, Environmental, and Exercise Physiology* 55:678–87.

75. West, J. B. et al. 1983. Barometric pressures at extreme altitudes on Mt. Everest: physiological significance. *Journal of Applied Physiology* 54:1188–94.

76. West, J. B. et al. 1983. Maximal exercise at extreme altitudes on Mt. Everest. *Journal of Applied Physiology* 55:688–98.

77. West, J. B. et al. 1962. Arterial oxygen saturation during exercise at high altitude. *Journal of Applied Physiology* 17:617–21.

25 *Ergogenic Aids*

Objectives

*B*y studying this chapter, you should be able to do the following:
1. Define ergogenic aid.
2. Explain why a "placebo" treatment in a "double-blind design" is used in research studies involving ergogenic aids.
3. Describe the effect of additional oxygen on performance; distinguish between hyperbaric oxygenation and that accomplished by breathing oxygen-enriched gas mixtures.
4. Describe blood doping and its potential for improving endurance performance.
5. Explain the mechanism by which ingested buffers might improve anaerobic performances.
6. Explain how amphetamines might improve exercise performance.
7. Describe the various mechanisms by which caffeine might improve performance.
8. Identify the risks associated with using chewing tobacco to obtain a nicotine "high".
9. Describe the risks of cocaine use and how it can cause death.
10. Describe the physiological and psychological effects of different types of warm-up.

Outline

Key Terms

autologous transfusion
blood boosting
blood doping
dental caries
double-blind design
ergogenic aid
erythrocythemia
hyperbaric chamber
hyperoxia
homologous transfusion
induced erythrocythemia
normocythemia
placebo
sham reinfusion
sham withdrawal
sympathomimetic

*T*he preceding chapters have described exercise and dietary plans related to performance. However, no presentation of factors affecting performance would be complete without a discussion of **ergogenic aids.** Ergogenic aids are defined as work-producing substances or phenomena believed to increase performance (37).

Ergogenic aids include nutrients, drugs, warm-up exercises, hypnosis, stress management, blood doping, oxygen breathing, music, and extrinsic biomechanical aids. The reader is referred to the texts by Williams (58) and Morgan (37) which cover these and more ergogenic aids. We decided to discuss nutrients in chapter 24 (Nutrition and Performance) because we view them more as being an extension of optimal nutrition, rather than ergogenic aids per se. In this chapter we will discuss ergogenic aids related to aerobic performance (oxygen inhalation and blood doping) and anaerobic performance (blood buffers), as well as various drugs (amphetamines, caffeine, cocaine, and nicotine) and physical warm-up. Please note that anabolic steroids and growth hormone were discussed in chapter 5.

While the attention of the reader will be focused on athletic performance, where an improvement of less than 1% would alter world records, it must be noted that industrial physiologists have long been concerned about the relationship of lighting, environmental temperature, and background noise (music) to performance in the workplace (37). Research work in this area must be carefully done, with special attention to the research design due to the number of factors that can influence the outcome of the study.

Research Design Concerns

It is sometimes difficult to compare the results of one research study with another. The reason for this is that the effect of an ergogenic aid is dependent on a number of variables (37):

1. Amount —too little or too much may show no effect
2. Subject —the ergogenic aid may be effective in "untrained" subjects but not "trained" subjects, or vice versa
   —"value" of an ergogenic aid is determined by the subject
3. Task —may work in short-term power-related tasks, but not in endurance tasks, or vice versa
   —may work for gross-motor, large-muscle activities and not with fine-motor activities, or vice versa
4. Use —an ergogenic aid used on an acute (short-term) basis may show a positive effect, but in the long run may compromise performance, or vice versa.

Given these variables, scientists must be careful in designing experiments in order not to be "fooled" by the result. For example, an *athlete* may improve performance because he or she believes the substance improves performance, so the "belief" is more important than the substance in determining the outcome. Further, an *investigator* may "believe" in the ergogenic aid and inadvertently offer different levels of encouragement during the testing of athletes under the influence of the ergogenic aid. These problems are

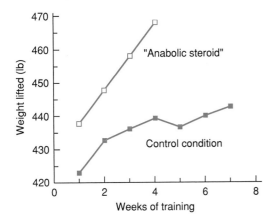

Figure 25.1 Changes in performance when subjects were told they were taking an anabolic steroid, but were really taking a placebo.

controlled for by using a **placebo** as a treatment condition, and using a **double-blind research design,** respectively.

A placebo is a "look-alike" substance relative to the ergogenic aid under consideration, but contains nothing that will influence performance. The need for such a control is seen in figure 25.1, which describes the gain in strength by a group that was taking a placebo, but *told* it was an anabolic steroid. It is contrasted with their performance prior to taking the placebo. The rate of strength gain was higher with the placebo, indicating the need for such a control if one is to isolate the true effect of a substance (2).

A double-blind research design is one in which neither the subject nor the investigator knows who is receiving the placebo or the substance under investigation. The subjects are randomly assigned to receive pill "x" or pill "y". After all data are collected the "code" is broken to find out which pill (x or y) was the placebo and which was the substance under investigation. These designs are very complex and difficult to carry out but reduce the chance of subject or investigator bias (37).

The scientist must also be careful in the selection of subjects. If a substance is tested as a potential aid to sprinters, it would be reasonable to select subjects from that population so the results can be generalized

to that group. Further, the tests used by the investigator should be as close as, or actually be, the performance task (e.g., 100-meter dash). In short, results obtained on a proper subject population, but under controlled laboratory conditions using conventional physiological tests, may not be useful when taken to the "field" (37).

Aerobic Performance

Chapter 20 detailed the various tests used to evaluate the physiological factors related to endurance performance. Clearly, an increased ability to transport O_2 to the muscles and a delay in the onset of lactate production are related to improved performance. Two ergogenic aids have been used to try to influence O_2 delivery: the breathing of O_2-enriched mixtures and blood doping.

Oxygen

Given the importance of aerobic metabolism in the production of ATP for muscular work, it is not surprising that scientists have been interested in the effect of additional oxygen (hyperoxia) on performance. But in order to discuss this issue we must ask the following question: How and when was the O_2 administered to achieve a higher PO_2 in the blood? In his recent and insightful review of this topic, Welch (54) stressed the difficulty of comparing results from studies in which hyperoxia is achieved by increasing the percent of O_2 in the inspired air with those that use a **hyperbaric** (high-pressure) chamber with 21% or higher O_2 mixtures. Figure 25.2 shows that performance improves throughout the range of inspired oxygen pressures when O_2-enriched mixtures are used at a normal pressure of 1 atmosphere ("constant pressure"), compared to the use of a hyperbaric chamber ("increasing pressure"). The second part of the question is related to the time of administration of the supplemental O_2. Results vary depending on whether the O_2 is administered prior to, during, or following exercise. For that latter reason this section on oxygen will be organized by those conditions.

Figure 25.2 The effect of PO₂ on performance. Constant pressure experiments used oxygen-enriched gas mixtures at sea-level pressure, while the increasing pressure experiments used a hyperbaric chamber to increase the PO₂.

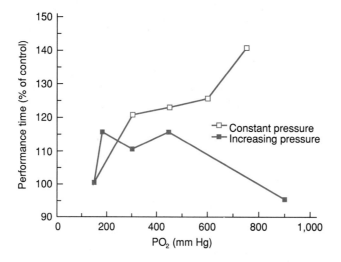

Prior to Exercise

The rationale for the use of supplemental oxygen prior to exercise is to try to "store" additional oxygen in the blood so that more would be available at the onset of the exercise. It has been estimated that the hemoglobin in arterial blood is about 97% saturated with O_2 at rest (200 ml O_2/l blood). Breathing 100% O_2 would increase this value by only 3%, or 6 milliliters. However, the amount of oxygen physically dissolved in solution is proportional to the arterial PO_2, and when the PO_2 increases from about 100 mm Hg (breathing 21% O_2 at sea level) to about 700 mm Hg (breathing 100% O_2) the dissolved oxygen increases from 3 ml/l to 21 ml/l. If a person has a total blood volume of 5 liters, approximately 100 milliliters of additional O_2 can be "stored" prior to exercise. However, if the person breathes several times between the time the O_2 breathing stops and the event begins, the O_2 store will return to that associated with air breathing (60).

The focus of attention on the use of oxygen prior to exercise has been on short-term exercise. In general, in runs of 880 yards or less, weight lifting, stair climbing, and swims of 200 yards or less the O_2 seemed to be beneficial (38, 60). In addition, evidence suggested that the O_2 breathing needed to take place within two minutes prior to the task (60). Some concern has been expressed about these findings due to the fact that in some cases the subjects knew they were breathing O_2, a factor that could have affected the results (60). Overall, considering the fact that O_2 cannot be breathed up to the start of a sprint event in swimming or track, any effect would be lost before the starter's gun is fired. Therefore, unless one participates in a breath holding event, oxygen breathing prior to exercise will have little effect on performance.

During Exercise

The rationale for the use of oxygen during exercise to improve performance is based on the proposition that muscle is hypoxic during exercise and additional O_2 delivery will alleviate the problem (54). If this is the case then the additional O_2 in the blood during O_2 breathing should increase the delivery of O_2 to the muscle and improve performance. However, Welch et al. (55) showed that when breathing hyperoxic gas mixtures, the increase in the O_2 content of arterial blood (CaO_2) is balanced by a *decrease* in blood flow to the working muscles such that O_2 delivery ($CaO_2 \times$ flow) was not different from normoxic (21% O_2) conditions. $\dot{V}O_2$ max is increased by only 2%–5% with hyperoxia, which is about what would be expected since maximal cardiac output doesn't change and the a-$\bar{v}$ O_2 difference does not increase more than 5%–6% (54) [$\dot{V}O_2$ max = $\dot{Q}_{max}$ × (Ca O_2^- C$\bar{v}$ O_2) max].

In spite of similarities in O_2 delivery during hyperoxia and normoxia, *performance* has been shown to increase dramatically as a result of an increase in inspired O_2. Figure 25.2, presented in the introduction to this section, showed a performance increase of 40% while breathing 100% O_2. How could this be if O_2 delivery to muscles is not substantially different? The increased availability of O_2 has been shown to decrease pulmonary ventilation and reduce the work of breathing, a change that should lead to an increase in performance (54, 62). In addition, those athletes who experience "desaturation" of hemoglobin during maximal work (see chapters 9 and 24) while breathing 21% O_2 could benefit by breathing oxygen-enriched gas mixtures (44). Finally, the additional O_2 slows glycolysis (Pasteur effect) during heavy exercise, resulting in a slower accumulation of lactate and H^+ in the plasma and extending the time to exhaustion (24, 54). Given the impracticality of trying to provide O_2 mixtures to athletes *during* performance, this research on hyperoxia is more useful as a tool to answer questions related to the age-old question of what factor, O_2 delivery or the muscle's capacity to consume O_2, limits aerobic performance (54).

After Exercise

The rationale associated with the use of supplemental oxygen after exercise is that the subject might recover more quickly following exercise and be ready to go again. Some of the early work showed just that, but because the subjects knew what gas they were breathing, the results have to be interpreted with caution (38, 60). Wilmore (60) summarized the effects of several studies and concluded that there was no benefit of O_2 breathing during recovery on heart rate, ventilation and post-exercise oxygen uptake. This conclusion was supported by a study showing no effect of O_2 breathing on subsequent performance in all-out exercise (56). In summary, oxygen breathing before or after exercise seems to have little or no effect on performance, while oxygen breathing during exercise improves endurance performance.

Blood Doping

In chapter 13 we described how $\dot{V}O_2$ max is limited by maximal cardiac output, given the constraint that blood pressure had to be maintained by vasoconstriction of the active muscle mass. Since maximal O_2 transport is equal to the product of maximal cardiac output (Q_{max}) and the O_2 content of arterial blood (CaO_2), one way to improve O_2 delivery to tissue when Q_{max} cannot change is to increase the quantity of hemoglobin in each liter of blood. **Blood doping** refers to the infusion of red blood cells (RBC) in an attempt to increase the hemoglobin concentration ([Hb]) and, consequently, O_2 transport (CaO_2 is equal to the [Hb] × 1.34 ml O_2/gmHb). Other terms to describe this are **blood boosting** and **blood packing**, with **induced erythrocythemia** being the proper medical term.

In blood doping, a subject receives a transfusion of blood, which may be his or her own (**autologous transfusion**) or blood from a matched donor (**homologous transfusion**). The latter procedure is acceptable in times of medical emergencies, but carries the risk of infection and blood-type incompatibility (19); it is therefore not recommended in blood-doping procedures. The constraint to use your own blood in order to achieve the goal of a higher [Hb] creates some interesting problems that led to confusion in the early days of research in this area. The primary problem was related to the mismatch between the maximum time blood could be refrigerated and the time period needed for the subject to produce new RBC and bring the [Hb] back to normal before the reinfusion. Maximum storage time with refrigeration is three weeks, during which time about 1% of the RBC are lost per day. In addition, some RBCs adhere to the storage containers or become so fragile that they will not function upon reinfusion. Due to these problems only about 60% of the removed RBCs could be reinfused (19). The normal time period for replacement of the RBCs following a 400-milliliter donation is three to four weeks, and following a 900-milliliter donation, five to six weeks or more are required. If the blood were reinfused at the end of the three-week maximal storage time, the investigator might not have been able to achieve the condition of an increased [Hb] due to RBC loss (decreased 40%) and the below normal (anemic) [Hb]

Figure 25.3 Changes in hemoglobin levels in blood following removal (phlebotomy) and reinfusion.

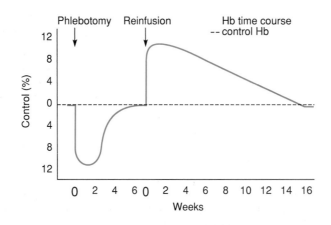

values in the subjects. Gledhill (19) makes a strong case for this as a primary reason why studies prior to 1978 showed inconsistent changes in $\dot{V}O_2$ max and performance with blood doping. Another major problem encountered in these early studies was the lack of an adequate research design. There was a need to have a group undergoing a **"sham" withdrawal** (needle placed in the arm but no blood is removed) and a **"sham" reinfusion** (needle placed in the arm but blood is not returned) to act as "placebo" controls.

The central factor allowing a more careful study of blood doping was the introduction of the freezer-preservation technique that allows the blood to be stored frozen for years with only a 15% RBC loss. This allows plenty of time for the subject to become **normocythemic** (achieve normal [Hb]), so that any effect of the reinfusion can be correctly evaluated (19).

The general findings were that reinfusions of single units (~450 milliliter) of blood showed small but insignificant increases in [Hb], $\dot{V}O_2$ max, and performance, while the infusion of two units (~900 milliliter) significantly increased the [Hb] (8%–9%), $\dot{V}O_2$ max (4%–5%), and performance (<3%–34%). The infusion of three units (1,350 milliliters) of blood caused slightly greater increases in [Hb] (10.8%) and $\dot{V}O_2$ max (6.6%). This large reinfusion caused borderline **erythrocythemia** to be approached, so 1,350-milliliter

infusion probably represents the upper limit that can be used. Figure 25.3 shows a gradual reduction in [Hb] toward the normal value following reinfusion, indicating that increased O_2 transport is maintained for ten to twelve weeks. This is an important point as far as performance gains are concerned (17).

The improvements in performance (3%–34%) were much more variable than the changes in [Hb] or $\dot{V}O_2$ max. Part of the reason for this variation was the type of performance test used. The greatest change was observed in a running test to exhaustion that lasted less than ten minutes while the smallest change was observed in a 5-mile time trial, with the improvement being fifty-one seconds compared to a preinfusion run time of 30:17 (59). Given that the laboratory results show consistent gains, the question raised by Eichner, "Does it work in the field?," still needs to be answered (10). Until that time blood doping will continue to be a useful laboratory tool to study the factors limiting $\dot{V}O_2$ max.

While the blood doping issue will always raise a question of ethics, Gledhill presents what amounts to a moral dilemma in the use of blood doping in getting athletes ready for performance at altitude. In chapter 24 we have already discussed the changes in $\dot{V}O_2$ max and performance at altitude. Those athletes who stay at altitude experience a natural increase in RBC production to deal with the hypoxia. As Gledhill (19) points out, those athletes who can afford to train at altitude accomplish what blood doping does in a manner that is acceptable to the International Olympic Committee.

Anaerobic Performance

Improvements in endurance performance focus on the supply of carbohydrate and oxygen to muscle (see previous sections on oxygen and blood doping in this chapter and on carbohydrate in chapter 24). However, in short-term, all-out performances in which anaerobic energy sources provide the vast majority of energy for muscle contraction, the focus of attention shifts to the buffering of the H^+ released from muscle. This section will consider a means by which investigators have tried to buffer the H^+ and improve performance.

Blood Buffers

Elevations in the $[H^+]$ in muscle can decrease the activity of PFK (51), which may slow glycolysis, as well as interfere with excitation-contraction coupling events by reducing Ca^{++} efflux from the terminal cisternae of the sarcoplasmic reticulum (16) and the binding of Ca^{++} to troponin (39). Decreases in muscle force development have been shown to be linked to increases in muscle lactate in both frog muscle (13) and human muscle (50). Finally, when Adams and Welch (1) showed that performance times in heavy exercise (90% $\dot{V}O_2$ max) could be altered by breathing 60% O_2 compared to 21% or 17% O_2, the point of exhaustion was associated with the same arterial $[H^+]$. The mechanisms involved in the regulation of the plasma $[H^+]$ were described in detail in chapter 11. Briefly, the primary means by which H^+ are buffered *during* exercise is through its reaction with the plasma bicarbonate reserve to form carbonic acid, which subsequently yields CO_2 that is exhaled (respiratory compensation). As the bicarbonate buffer store decreases, the ability to buffer H^+ is reduced and the plasma $[H^+]$ will increase. Knowing this, scientists have explored ways of increasing the plasma buffer store to slow down the rate of H^+ increase during strenuous exercise.

Dill (8) induced alkalosis in a subject (means unknown) and showed that run time to exhaustion could be extended (5:22 to 6:04). Jones et al. (27) used 0.3 gm/kg body weight sodium bicarbonate and contrasted it with 0.3 g/kg calcium carbonate, used as the control condition, and 0.3 gm/kg ammonium chloride, which caused a plasma acidosis. Subjects worked at 33% and 66% $\dot{V}O_2$ max for twenty minutes each, followed by work to exhaustion at 95% $\dot{V}O_2$ max. The ammonium chloride condition decreased the duration of the ride to exhaustion (160 seconds) while the sodium bicarbonate treatment increased the ride time (438 seconds) over control (270 seconds). Wilkes et al. (57) supported these findings in a study in which they used sodium bicarbonate to induce alkalosis and compared it with a calcium carbonate placebo condition, as well as a control trial with no placebo. The subjects were six varsity track athletes and the test was an 800-meter run. The sodium bicarbonate resulted in a significantly faster time (2:02.9) compared to either the control (2:05.8) or placebo (2:05.1) runs. Work by Robertson et al. (45) supported these studies by showing a lower RPE during work at 80% $\dot{V}O_2$ max with sodium bicarbonate.

The usefulness of the procedure may depend on the length of the anaerobic exercise bout. In studies in which the duration of the work task was thirty seconds (40), sixty seconds (29) or one-hundred seconds (28) the induced alkalosis did not result in a significant improvement over the control condition. This is surprising given the expectation that glycolysis is more important in these activities. It may be that some short-term anaerobic activities are more dependent on the plasma $[H^+]$ as a primary cause of fatigue than others. Welch (54) indicates that while subjects may stop at the same $[H^+]$ within any exercise protocol, the differences that exist among studies in the "terminal" $[H^+]$ suggest the other factors are more limiting as far as performance is concerned. The use of these agents to cause an alkalosis is not without risks. Large doses of sodium bicarbonate can cause diarrhea and vomiting, both of which are sure to affect performance (18).

Drugs

A variety of drugs have been used to aid performance. Some drugs are as common and "legal" as caffeine and nicotine, while others, like amphetamines and cocaine, are banned from use. We will briefly examine each of these drugs, exploring how they might work to improve performance, as well as the evidence about whether or not they do.

Amphetamines

Amphetamine is a stimulant that has been used primarily to recover from fatigue and improve endurance. In 1972 Golding (21) indicated that it was the most abused group of drugs at that time. Amphetamines are readily absorbed in the small intestine and while the effects reach a peak two to three hours after ingestion, they persist for twelve to twenty-four hours (25, 31). Amphetamines are both a **sympathomimetic** drug (simulates catecholamine effects), and a central nervous system stimulant. The drug produces its effects by altering the metabolism and synthesis of catecholamines, or receptor affinity for catecholamines (25, 31).

The most consistent effect of amphetamines is to increase one's arousal or wakefulness, leading to a perception of increased energy and self-confidence (25). The drug affects the redistribution of blood flow, driving it away from the skin and splanchnic areas and delivering more to muscle or brain. This could lead to problems related to a decrease in lactic acid removal (see chapter 3) and an increase in body temperature (see chapter 12). Animal studies show that amphetamines can increase endurance-type performances. However, the dose of the drug was shown to be important, in that smaller doses (1–2 mg/kg) were not different from control and large doses (16 mg/kg) appeared to reduce the ability of the rat to swim. Data collected using run tests on rats indicate the same detrimental effect of high doses (7.5–10 mg/kg) of amphetamines (25).

Ivy (25) concluded from an analysis of studies on human subjects that amphetamines extend endurance and hasten recovery from fatigue. Time to exhaustion was increased in spite of no effect on submaximal or maximal $\dot{V}O_2$ (6, 25). Two explanations have been offered. Ivy (25) feels that the endurance aspect of performance can be improved due to amphetamines' catecholamine-like effect in mobilizing FFA and sparing muscle glycogen, similar to that of caffeine (see the caffeine section, this chapter). Chandler and Blair (6) believe that the amphetamines may simply mask fatigue and interfere with the perception of the normal biological signals that fatigue has occurred. It is this latter conclusion that has raised the most concern about the safety of the athlete, in that during prolonged submaximal work, especially in a hot and/or humid environment, the decreased blood flow to the skin could cause hyperthermia, leading to death (24, 31).

As mentioned at the beginning of this section, amphetamines' major effect is in increasing wakefulness and producing a state of arousal. However, while amphetamines have restored reaction time in fatigued subjects, the drug does not have this effect on alert, motivated, and nonfatigued subjects. Given that athletes are usually alert and motivated prior to competition, Golding (21) suggests that amphetamines would be counterproductive, making users hyperirritable and interfering with their sleep. Finally, it is risky to extrapolate from data collected under tightly controlled laboratory conditions using discrete measures related to performance ($\dot{V}O_2$ max, endurance time, reaction time) to the actual performance in a skilled sport in front of a hostile audience for a national championship.

Caffeine

Caffeine is a stimulant that is found in a wide variety of common foods, drinks, and over-the-counter drugs (see table 25.1). Caffeine has been viewed as an on-again, off-again ergogenic aid. Caffeine was banned by the International Olympic Committee (IOC) in 1962, removed from the list of banned drugs in 1972 and in 1984, the IOC again banned "high levels" (15 μg/ml) in the urine that might have been the result of caffeine injections or suppositories (52). Caffeine is absorbed rapidly from the GI tract, significantly elevated in the blood at fifteen minutes, and peaking at sixty minutes (52). Caffeine is diluted by body water and the physiological response is proportional to the

Table 25.1 Caffeine content of popular foods, beverages, soft drinks, and drug preparations

Caffeine Content of Popular Beverages and Food

Item	Caffeine (mg)*
Coffee (5-oz Cup)	
Drip method	110–150
Percolated	64–124
Instant	40–108
Decaffeinated	2–5
Instant decaffeinated	2
Tea (Loose or Bags) (5-oz Cup)	
One-minute brew	9–33
Three-minute brew	20–46
Five-minute brew	20–50
Tea Products	
Instant tea (5-oz cup)	12–28
Iced tea (12-oz cup)	22–36
Cocoa	
Made from mix	6
Milk chocolate (1 oz)	6
Baking Chocolate (1 oz)	35

Caffeine Content of Various Soft Drinks

Soft Drinks	Caffeine (mg per 12-oz Serving)
Sugar-Free Mr. PIBB	58
Mountain Dew	54
Mello Yello	52
TAB	46
Coca-Cola	46
Diet Coke	46
Shasta Cola	44
Shasta Diet Cola	44
Mr. PIBB	40
Dr Pepper	40
Sugar-Free Dr Pepper	40
Pepsi Cola	38.4
Diet Pepsi	36
Pepsi Light	36
RC Cola	36
Diet Rite	0
Canada Dry Diet Cola	0

Caffeine in Drug Preparations*

Classification	Caffeine (mg per Tablet or Capsule)
Over-the-Counter Stimulants	
No Doz Tablets	100
Vivarin Tablets	200
Pain Relievers	
Anacin	32
Excedrin	65
Midol	32
Plain aspirin, any brand	0
Vanquish	33

Caffeine in Drug Preparations*

Classification	Caffeine (mg per Tablet or Capsule)
Diuretics	
Aqua Ban	100
Cold Remedies	
Coryban-D	30
Dristan	0
Triaminicin	30
Weight-Control Aids	
Dexatrim	200
Prolamine	140
Prescription Pain Relievers	
Cafergot	100
Darvon Compound	32.4
Fiorinal	40
Migralam	100

From J. L. Slavin, and D. J. Joensen, "Caffeine and Sport Performance," in *The Physician and Sportsmedicine* 13:191, 193. May 1985. Copyright © 1985. McGraw-Hill Healthcare Group, Minneapolis, Minn.

concentration in the body water. There is a natural variability in how people respond to caffeine and chronic users are less responsive than abstainers (52).

While caffeine can affect a wide variety of tissues, figure 25.4 shows its role as an ergogenic aid is based on its effects on skeletal muscle, the central nervous system, and in the mobilization of fuels for muscular work. The evidence for the enhanced function of skeletal muscle is based primarily on *in vitro* and *in situ* muscle preparations and shows that caffeine can increase tension production (42, 52). This was shown most clearly in fatigued muscle and was believed to be due to enhanced Ca^{++} availability (34). In one human study caffeine had no effect on maximum voluntary contraction or the maximal tension elicited by electrical stimulation. However, there was greater tension development at lower levels of electrical stimulation in both rested and fatigued muscles. The change in endurance time measured by time at 50% MVC was variable and nonsignificant (33).

Caffeine has long been recognized as a stimulator of the CNS. Caffeine can pass the blood-brain barrier and affect a variety of brain centers that usually leads to an increased alertness and decreased drowsiness (42, 52). The best evidence supporting caffeine as a CNS stimulant is in the decreased perception of fatigue during prolonged exercise in subjects who took caffeine (7).

The role of caffeine in the mobilization of fuel has received considerable attention as the primary means by which it exerts its ergogenic effect. Caffeine has been shown to cause an elevation of both glucose and an increase in fatty acid utilization. The elevated glucose could be due to the stimulation of the sympathetic nervous system and the resulting increase in catecholamines, which would increase the mobilization of glucose from the liver. On the other hand, the glucose concentration could be elevated due to a decreased rate of removal related to the suppression of insulin release by catecholamines (see chapter 5) (52).

Lipid mobilization has been shown to be increased as a result of caffeine ingestion. Figure 25.5 shows that the mechanism of action could be related to either the elevated catecholamines increasing the level of cyclic AMP in the adipose cell or to the caffeine's blocking of phosphodiesterase activity, which is responsible for breaking down the cyclic AMP. Van Handle (52) feels that the latter mechanism is less likely given the dose of caffeine needed. Plasma free fatty acids increase quickly *at rest* after ingestion of caffeine (15 minutes) and continue to increase over the next several hours (52). *During exercise* plasma FFA have been shown not to be significantly elevated as a result of caffeine ingestion. However, the respiratory exchange ratio was lower, indicating a greater use of fat as fuel (7, 11, 26). The caffeine effect seemed to be mediated by increasing the utilization of intramuscular triglycerides (11). Independent of the mechanism, the bottom line in these studies is that caffeine was effective in increasing total work time, making it an "ergogenic aid."

This ergogenic effect is dose dependent and may vary with the type of subject. While some studies show physiological change with doses as low as 5–7 mg/kg (7,11) others find a 10 mg/kg dose to be inadequate (35). In fact, in another study from this same research group (36), a dose of 15 mg/kg was needed to see an increase in fat metabolism (35,36). Finally, there is evidence that habitual caffeine users who abstain from caffeine for four days are more responsive to caffeine during exercise than in their normal mode of daily caffeine use (12). Van Handel (52) makes the point that what an investigator might observe in a controlled laboratory setting may be masked by a normal sympathetic nervous system response to competition. Given the potential side effects such as diuresis, insomnia, diarrhea, anxiety, tremulousness, and irritability (52) and the variability among subjects in how they respond to caffeine, one should not expect much of an improvement in performance (9).

Cocaine

Cocaine is presented in this section on ergogenic aids because of the recent publicity surrounding its use by professional athletes. It is meant to provide information about the drug rather than to describe cocaine's role in athletic performance. Cocaine acts as a local anaesthetic and a powerful stimulator of the cardiovascular and central nervous systems. Peruvian natives used it as an ergogenic aid in the sixth century

Figure 25.4 Factors influenced by caffeine that might cause an improvement in performance.

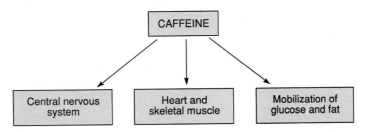

Figure 25.5 Mechanisms by which caffeine might increase free-fatty-acid mobilization.

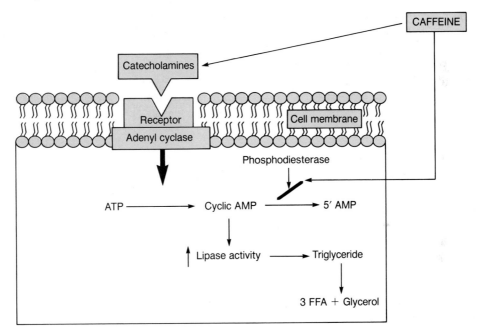

to improve work performance at altitude (32). Cocaine can be taken in a variety of ways:

1. Sniffing—inhaled through nose to be absorbed through the nasal mucosa. The "high" is rapid and peaks in about twenty minutes

2. Smoking—coca paste: rapid onset, short-acting

—free-basing: onset is rapid, intense "rush," short-acting

3. Intravenous injection—rapid onset, peaks in three to five minutes

4. "Crack"—almost pure cocaine smoked in pipe or cigarette. Similar to intravenous injection method (32)

Figure 25.6 Mechanisms by which cocaine can kill.

From John D. Cantwell, "Cocaine and cardiovascular events," in *The Physician and Sportsmedicine* 14(11):77–82, 1986. Copyright © 1986 McGraw-Hill Healthcare Group, Minneapolis, Minn.

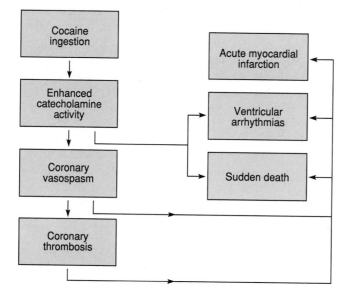

Figure 25.7 Schematic representation of how nicotine can have both a relaxing and stimulating effect.

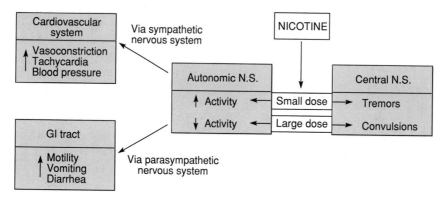

Cocaine gives a person a sense of euphoria and feelings of increased mental and physical power. However, the drug is psychologically addictive, becoming the focal point in a user's life. The dark side of this drug's effects is when euphoria leads to paranoia, anxiety, insomnia, hallucinations, and delusions (32). An overdose of cocaine can lead to arrhythmias, coma, seizures, hyperthermia, and death (32). Figure 25.6 presents an outline of the mechanism by which cocaine may have caused the death of two professional athletes (4).

Nicotine

Nicotine is a drug with no therapeutic application. However, the fact that it is a part of cigarette and chewing tobacco makes it one of the most abused substances. Nicotine has unpredictable effects due to the fact that it can simultaneously increase sympathetic, parasympathetic, and central nervous system activities (see figure 25.7). Small doses of nicotine increase autonomic activity, while large doses lead to a blocking of the response. The cardiovascular system responds with increases in heart rate and blood pressure due to increased sympathetic nerve activity and the GI tract responds with an increase in activity via parasympathetic nerve stimulation. Nicotine is easily absorbed through the lungs, mucous membranes, and the skin, and the half-life of nicotine is about thirty to sixty minutes (49).

Nicotine is primarily taken in by either smoking or chewing tobacco, and independent of whether it has a calming or a stimulating effect on an individual, the smoking and chewing of tobacco are associated with major health problems. We already know from the precursors identified in the health risk appraisal (chapter 14) that cigarette smoking is linked directly to a variety of cancers and heart and lung diseases. That alone is motivation enough to not encourage smoking, independent of the fact that it increases the work of breathing (46) and decreases $\dot{V}O_2$ max (30). The point is, of course, that cigarette smoke contains more than nicotine, specifically, carbon monoxide and various carcinogens. But what if the nicotine could be obtained without the cigarette smoke?

Smokeless tobacco has become a part of the American sport scene. Athletes can be observed using it on the field and selling it in one of the many commercials on TV. Smokeless tobacco includes (1) loose leaf tobacco that is placed between the cheek and lower gum and is "chewed," (2) snuff, moist or dry powdered tobacco, that is "dipped" and placed between the cheek or lip and lower gum, and (3) compressed tobacco, a "plug," that is used as loose leaf tobacco (20).

In addition to athletes, there has been a tremendous increase in the use of smokeless tobacco in the general population. In 1986 Glover et al. (20) reported data from the American Cancer Society and the National Institutes of Health suggesting that seven to twelve million Americans use smokeless tobacco. The greatest potential problem is related to the high rate at which this practice has been adopted by public school students, with evidence that some begin using this product before the age of ten.

While one might be worried about a young person becoming addicted to nicotine through the use of smokeless tobacco, the greatest concern is with regard to damage to teeth (**dental caries**) and gums (peridontal disease), including oral cancer (20). The increase in dental caries (2.4 times more than nonusers) is related, in part, to the sugar content in the pouch (35%) and plug (24%) tobacco (20). However, it is more important to focus attention on peridontal disease and cancer. The withdrawal of the gum from a tooth's surface exposes the tooth to greater damage that can lead to the loss of the tooth and potentially, to bone loss. The loss of the gum is in the area where the tobacco is held in the mouth, indicating a clear link. Further, lesions of the mucosa can develop which can ultimately lead to cancer. While it is known that regular smoking can cause oral cancer, smokeless tobacco users are actually at a greater risk. Independent of any potential beneficial effect of nicotine on performance, the use of smokeless tobacco should be discouraged. Once "hooked," the habit is more difficult to break than that associated with cigarette smoking (20).

Physical Warm-Up

"Warming-up" prior to moderate or strenuous activity is a general recommendation made for those involved in fitness programs or athletes involved in various types of performance. While most of us accept this as a reasonable recommendation, is there good scientific support for it? In Franks' original 1972 review (14) he found that 53% of the studies supported the proposition that warm-up was better than no warm-up, 7% the opposite, and 40% found no difference between the two. Concerns were raised about the wide variety of tasks and the methods used to evaluate the effectiveness of warm-up. In his 1983 review, Franks (15) analyzed the role of the participant (trained or untrained), the duration and intensity of the warm-up, and the type of performance as the variables involved in a determination of the effectiveness of warm-up. Before we summarize these findings a few definitions must be presented.

Warm-up refers to exercise conducted prior to a performance, whether or not muscle or body temperature is elevated. Warm-up activities can be *identical to the performance* (baseball pitcher throwing with normal form and high speed to a catcher prior to the batter stepping up), *directly related to the performance* (shot putter practicing at 75% of normal effort prior to a competition), or *indirectly related to a performance* (general activities to increase body temperature or arousal) (15). Generally all three are used in a typical warm-up prior to performance, in the reverse order of the above descriptions.

The theoretical benefits of warm-up are separated into physiological, psychological, and safety-related. Physiological benefits would include less muscle resistance and faster enzymatic reactions at high body temperatures. This might lower the oxygen deficit at the onset of work or decrease the RER during the subsequent activity (23). Increases in body temperature as a result of warm-up have been linked to improved performance (15). Skilled performances benefit from identical and direct warm-up, with indirect warm-up sometimes acting in a facilitatory manner. The warm-up procedures can increase arousal, which is good up to a point, and provide the optimal "mental set" for improved performance (15).

Most students of exercise physiology are familiar with the role of warm-up in the prevention of injuries and in improving the transition from rest to strenuous exercise. However, Franks (15) indicates that little evidence exists showing that warm-up prevents injury. On the other hand, there is some evidence that warm-up reduces the "stress" experienced when doing strenuous work. In Barnard et al.'s (3) classic study, six of ten fire fighters who did not warm-up experienced an ischemic response (reduced myocardial blood flow) as shown by a depressed ST segment on the ECG during strenuous exercise. All had normal ECG responses when a gradual warm-up preceded the strenuous exercise.

With this information as background, table 25.2 provides a summary of the factors influencing an optimal warm-up (15). Identical and direct warm-up focuses the participant's attention on the task at hand and provides the correct mental set for the performance. Indirect warm-up with large muscle groups increases core temperature and increases arousal. The indirect warm-up activities should be at least ten minutes in duration at an intensity of 60%–80% of $\dot{V}O_2$ max. This will cause the appropriate changes to occur quickly, without fatigue or use of the limited carbohydrate store. Given the fact that these physiological and psychological changes are reversible, it is recommended that performance take place less than sixty seconds after the warm-up. Conditioned and skilled participants can sustain the warm-up without fatigue compared to their less well-conditioned counterparts. It should be noted that the recommended warm-up intensity is also the training stimulus for cardiovascular *fitness* (chapter 16). It is clear that these warm-up recommendations are for those interested in *performance*. Finally, performance of gross motor tasks seems to benefit more than with fine motor tasks (15). In fine-motor tasks a lower arousal level may be more appropriate.

Table 25.2 Summary of research on optimal warm-up

Warm-Up Components	Physiological Aspects	Psychological Aspects
Type of Warm-Up		
Direct warm-up	↑ Muscle temperature	Focus on task
Indirect warm-up with large muscle groups	↑ Core temperature without local fatigue	↑ Arousal
Similar activities	—	Optimal mental set
Characteristics of Warm-Up		
Moderate intensity (60%–80% $\dot{V}O_2$ max)	↑ Core temperature in short period of time	↑ Arousal
Moderate duration (<ten min)	Minimize carbohydrate utilization	—
Short rest interval (<sixty sec)	Retain effect of the warm-up	Retain effect of the warm-up
Type of Participant		
Skilled players	—	Can increase arousal and focus on task without fatigue
Conditioned participants	↑ Body temperature without fatigue	Can increase arousal without fatigue
Type of Task		
Short-explosive, uninhibited	Benefits most from physiological changes	High levels of arousal is consistent with good performance

From B. D. Franks, "Physical Warm-Up," in M. H. Williams, *Ergogenic Aids in Sport*. Copyright © 1983 Human Kinetics Publishers, Inc., Champaign, Ill.

Summary

1. Ergogenic aids are defined as substances or phenomena that are work-producing and are believed to increase performance.
2. Due to the fact that an athlete's *belief* in a substance may influence performance, scientists use a placebo or look-alike substance to control for this effect. In addition, scientists use a double-blind research design in which the investigator and subject are both unaware of the treatment.
3. Additional oxygen provided by oxygen-enriched gas mixtures improves endurance performance; hyperbaric oxygenation results in poorer performances at high air pressures.
4. Oxygen breathing within two minutes of performance *may* improve performance in short-term events. However, in practical terms, it is difficult to implement.
5. Oxygen breathing during endurance exercise improves performance even though oxygen delivery to muscle may be unaffected.

6. Oxygen breathing does not enhance recovery from exercise.
7. Blood doping refers to the reinfusion of red blood cells in order to increase the hemoglobin concentration and oxygen-carrying capacity of the blood.
8. Due to improvement in blood storage techniques, blood doping has been shown to be effective in improving $\dot{V}O_2$ max and endurance performance.
9. In an attempt to improve short-term anaerobic performances that generate large amounts of lactate, athletes have ingested buffers. There is evidence showing both improvement in performance as well as no effect on performance.
10. Amphetamines have a catecholamine-like effect that leads to an increased arousal and a perception of increased energy and self-confidence.
11. While amphetamines improve performance of fatigued subjects, the drug does not have this effect on alert, motivated, and nonfatigued subjects.
12. Caffeine could potentially improve performance at the muscle, central nervous system, or in the delivery of fuel for muscular work. Caffeine can elevate blood glucose and simultaneously increase the utilization of fat.
13. Caffeine's positive effect on performance is dose-related and is less in subjects who are daily users of caffeine.
14. Cocaine is a powerful stimulator of the cardiovascular and central nervous systems. It provides a sense of euphoria and feelings of increased mental and physical power, however, it is psychologically addictive and potentially deadly.
15. Nicotine has varied effects depending on whether the parasympathetic or sympathetic nervous systems is stimulated. The use of smokeless tobacco can cause dental caries, gum disease, and oral cancer.
16. Warm-up activities can be identical to performance, directly related to performance, or indirectly related to performance (general warm-up). Warm-up causes both physiological and psychological changes that are beneficial to performance.

Study Questions

1. What is an ergogenic aid?
2. Why must an investigator use a "placebo" treatment to evaluate the affect of an ergogenic aid?
3. What is a double-blind research design?
4. Does breathing 100% O_2 improve performance? Recovery?
5. Breathing hyperoxic gas mixtures improves performance without changing O_2 delivery to tissue. How is this possible?
6. What is blood doping and why does it appear to improve performance now when it did not in the earliest investigations?
7. How might ingested buffers improve short-term performances?
8. While amphetamines improve performance in fatigued individuals they might not have this effect on motivated subjects. Why?
9. How might caffeine improve long-term performances? Can the results be extrapolated to "real" performances in the field?
10. Chewing tobacco may provide a nicotine "high," but not without risks. What are they?
11. Describe the different types of warm-up activities and the mechanisms by which they may improve performance.

Suggested Reading

Williams, M. H. 1983. *Ergogenic Aids in Sports.* Champaign, Ill.: Human Kinetics Publishers.

References

1. Adams, R. P., and H. G. Welch. 1980. Oxygen uptake, acid-base status, and performance with varied inspired oxygen fractions. *Journal of Applied Physiology: Respiratory, Environmental, and Exercise Physiology* 49:863–68.

2. Ariel, G., and W. Saville. 1972. Anabolic steroids: the physiological effects of placebos. *Medicine and Science in Sports* 4:124–26.

3. Barnard, R. J. et al. 1973. Cardiovascular responses to sudden strenuous exercise—heart rate, blood pressure and ECG. *Journal of Applied Physiology* 34:833–37.

4. Cantwell, John D. 1986. Cocaine and cardiovascular events. *The Physician and Sportsmedicine* 14(11):77–82.

5. Casal, S. C., and A. S. Leon. 1985. Failure of caffeine to affect substrate utilization during prolonged running. *Medicine and Science in Sports and Exercise* 17:174–79.

6. Chandler, J. V., and S. N. Blair. 1980. The effect of amphetamines on selected physiological components related to athletic success. *Medicine and Science in Sports and Exercise* 12:65–69.

7. Costill, D. L., G. Dalsky, and W. Fink. 1978. Effects of caffeine ingestion on metabolism and exercise performance. *Medicine and Science in Sports* 10:155–58.

8. Dill, D. B., H. T. Edwards, and J. H. Talbot. 1932. Alkalosis and the capacity for work. *Journal of Biological Chemistry* 97:LVII–LIX.

9. Eichner, E. R. 1986. The caffeine controversy: effects on endurance and cholesterol. *The Physician and Sportsmedicine* 14:124–32.

10. Eichner, E. R. 1987. Blood doping results and consequences from the laboratory and the field. *The Physician and Sportsmedicine* 15(1):121–29.

11. Essig, D., D. L. Costill, and P. J. Van Handel. 1980. Effect of caffeine ingestion on utilization of muscle glycogen and lipid during leg ergometer cycling. *International Journal of Sport Medicine* 1:86–90.

12. Fisher, S. M. et al. 1986. Influence of caffeine on exercise performance in habitual caffeine users. *International Journal of Sports Medicine* 7:276–80.

13. Fitts, R. H., and J. O. Holloszy. 1976. Lactate and contractile force in frog muscle during development of fatigue and recovery. *American Journal of Physiology* 231:430–33.

14. Franks, B. D. 1972. Physical warm-up. In (W. P. Morgan, ed.), *Ergogenic Aids and Muscular Performance,* Chapter 6, 160–91. New York: Academic Press.

15. Franks, B. D. 1983. Physical warm-up. In (M. H. Williams, ed.), *Ergogenic Aids in Sport,* Chapter 13, 340–75. Champaign, Ill.: Human Kinetics Publishers.

16. Fuchs, F., V. Reddy, and F. N. Briggs. 1970. The interaction of cations with the calcium-binding site of troponin. *Biochemistry Biophysics Acta* 221:407–9.

17. Gledhill, N. 1982. Blood doping and related issues: A brief review. *Medicine and Science in Sports and Exercise* 14:183–89.

18. Gledhill, N. 1984. Bicarbonate ingestion and anaerobic performance. *Sports Medicine* 1:177–80.

19. Gledhill, N. 1985. The influence of altered blood volume and oxygen transport capacity on aerobic performance. In (R. L. Terjung, ed.), *Exercise and Sport Sciences Reviews,* Vol. 13, 75–94. New York: Macmillan Publishing Company.

20. Glover, E. D. et al. 1986. Implications of smokeless tobacco use among athletes. *The Physician and Sportsmedicine* 14(Dec.): 95–105.

21. Golding, L. A. 1972. Drugs and hormones. In (W. P. Morgan, ed.), *Ergogenic Aids and Muscular Performance.* New York: Academic Press.

22. Goodman, L. S., and A. Gilman., eds. 1985. *The Pharmacological Basis of Therapeutics,* 7th ed. London: The MacMillian Company.

23. Hetzler, R. K. et al. 1986. Effect of warm-up on plasma free fatty acid responses and substrate utilization during submaximal exercise. *Research Quarterly for Exercise and Sport* 57:223–28.

24. Hogan, M. C., R. H. Cox, and H. G. Welch. 1983. Lactate accumulation during incremental exercise with varied inspired oxygen fractions. *Journal of Applied Physiology* 55:1134–40.

25. Ivy, John L. 1983. Amphetamines. In *Ergogenic Aids in Sport.* Champaign, Ill.: Human Kinetics Publishers.

26. Ivy, J. L. et al. 1979. Influence of caffeine and carbohydrate feedings on endurance performance. *Medicine and Science in Sports and Exercise* 11:6–11.

27. Jones, N. L. et al. 1977. Effect of pH on cardiorespiratory and metabolic responses to exercise. *Journal of Applied Physiology* 43:959–64.

28. Katz, A. et al. 1984. Maximal exercise tolerance after induced alkalosis. *International Journal of Sports Medicine* 5:107–10.

29. Kinderman, W., J. Keul, and G. Huber. 1977. Physical exercise after induced alkalosis (bicarbonate or Tris-buffer). *European Journal of Applied Physiology* 37:197–204.

30. Klausen, K., S. Andersen, and S. Nandrup. 1983. Acute effects of cigarette smoking and inhalation of carbon monoxide during maximal exercise. *European Journal of Applied Physiology* 51:371–79.

31. Lombardo, J. A. 1986. Stimulants and athletic performance (part 1 of 2): amphetamines and caffeine. *The Physician and Sportsmedicine* 14 (11):128–42.

32. Lombardo, J. A. 1986. Stimulants and athletic performance (part 2): Cocaine and nicotine. *The Physician and Sportsmedicine* 14 (12):85–89.

33. Lopes, J. M. et al. 1983. Effect of caffeine on skeletal muscle function before and after fatigue. *Journal of Applied Physiology: Respiratory, Environmental, and Exercise Physiology* 54:1303–5.

34. MacIntosh, B. R., R. W. Barbee, and W. N. Stainsby. 1981. Contractile response to caffeine of rested and fatigued skeletal muscle. *Medicine and Science in Sports and Exercise* 13:95.

35. McNaughton, L. R. 1986. The influence of caffeine ingestion on incremental treadmill running. *British Journal of Sports Medicine* 20:109–12.

36. McNaughton, L. 1987. Two levels of caffeine ingestion on blood lactate and free fatty acid responses during incremental exercise. *Research Quarterly for Exercise and Sport* 58:255–59.

37. Morgan, W. P. 1972. Basic considerations. In (W. P. Morgan, ed.) *Ergogenic Aids and Muscular Performance*. New York: Academic Press.

38. Morris, A. F. 1983. Oxygen. In *Ergogenic Aids in Sport*. Champaign, Ill.: Human Kinetics Publishers.

39. Nakamura, Y., and S. Schwartz. 1972. The influence of hydrogen ion concentration on calcium binding and release by skeletal muscle sarcoplasmic reticulum. *Journal of General Physiology* 59:22–32.

40. Parry-Billings, M., and D. M. MacLaren. 1986. The effect of sodium bicarbonate and sodium citrate ingestion on anaerobic power during intermittent exercise. *European Journal of Applied Physiology* 55:524–29.

41. Perkins, R., and M. H. Williams. 1975. Effect of caffeine upon maximal muscular endurance of females. *Medicine of Science and Sports* 7:221–24.

42. Powers, S. K., and S. Dodd. 1985. Caffeine and endurance performance. *Sports Medicine.* 2:165–74.

43. Powers, S. K. et al. 1983. Effect of caffeine ingestion on metabolism and performance during graded exercise. *European Journal of Applied Physiology* 50:301–7.

44. Powers, S. K. et al. 1989. Effects of incomplete pulmonary gas exchange on $\dot{V}O_2$ max. *Journal of Applied Physiology* 66:2491–95.

45. Robertson, R. et al. (1982). Effect of induced alkalosis on differentiated perceptions of exertion during arm and leg ergometry. *Medicine and Science in Sports and Exercise* 14:158.

46. Rode, A., and R. J. Shepard. 1971. The influence of cigarette smoking on the oxygen cost of breathing in near maximal exercise. *Medicine and Science in Sports* 3:51–55.

47. Rupp, J. C. et al. 1983. Effect of sodium bicarbonate ingestion on blood and muscle pH and exercise performance. *Medicine and Science in Sports and Exercise* 15:115.

48. Slavin, J. L., and D. J. Joensen. 1985. Caffeine and sport performance. *The Physician and Sportsmedicine* 13:191–93.

49. Taylor, P. 1980. Ganglionic stimulating and blocking agents. In (A. G. Gilman, L. S. Goodman, and A. Gilman, eds.), *Goodman and Gilman's The Pharmocological Basis of Therapeutics,* 6th ed. New York: MacMillan Publishing Co.

50. Tesch, P. et al. 1978. Muscle fatigue and its relation to lactate accumulation and LDH activity in man. *Acta Physiologica Scandinavia* 103:413–20.

51. Trevedi, B., and W. H. Danforth. 1966. Effect of pH on the kinetics of frog muscle phosphofructokinase. *Journal of Biological Chemistry* 241:4110–12.

52. Van Handel, P. 1983. Caffeine. In (M. H. Williams, ed.) *Ergogenic Aids in Sports*. Champaign, Ill.: Human Kinetics Publishers.

53. Weir, J. et al. 1987. A high carbohydrate diet negates the metabolic effects of caffeine during exercise. *Medicine and Science in Sports and Exercise* 19:100–5.

54. Welch, H. G. 1987. Effects of hypoxia and hyperoxia on human performance. In (K. B. Pandolf, ed.) *Exercise and Sports Sciences Reviews,* Vol. 15, 191–222. New York: Macmillan Publishing Company.

55. Welch, H. G. et al. (1977). Effects of hyperoxia on leg blood flow and metabolism during exercise. *Journal of Applied Physiology* 42:385–90.

56. Weltman, A. L. et al. 1977. Exercise recovery, lactate removal, and subsequent high intensity exercise performance. *Research Quarterly* 48:786–96.

57. Wilkes, D., N. Gledhill, and R. Smyth. 1983. Effect of acute induced metabolic alkalosis on 800-m racing time. *Medicine and Science in Sports and Exercise* 15:277–80.

58. Williams, M. H. 1983. *Ergogenic Aids in Sports.* Champaign, Ill.: Human Kinetics Publishers.

59. Williams, M. H. et al. 1981. *Medicine and Science in Sports and Exercise* 13:169–75.

60. Wilmore, J. H. 1972. Oxygen. In (W. P. Morgan, ed.) *Ergogenic Aids and Muscular Performance,* 321–42. New York: Academic Press.

61. Wilson, G. D., and H. G. Welch. 1975. Effects of hyperoxic gas mixtures on exercise tolerance in man. *Medicine and Science in Sports* 7:48–52.

62. Wilson, G. D., and H. G. Welch. 1980. Effects of varying concentrations of N_2/O_2 and He/O_2 on exercise tolerance in man. *Medicine and Science in Sports and Exercise* 12:380–84.

Appendix A

Calculation of Oxygen Uptake and Carbon Dioxide Production

Calculation of Oxygen Consumption

Calculation of oxygen consumption is a relatively simple process that involves subtracting the amount of oxygen exhaled from the amount of oxygen inhaled:

(1) Oxygen consumption ($\dot{V}O_2$) =
[volume of O_2 inspired] − [volume of O_2 expired]

The volume of O_2 inspired (I) is computed by multiplying the volume of air inhaled per minute ($\dot{V}_I$) times the fraction (F) of air that is made up of oxygen. Room air is 20.93% O_2. Expressed as a fraction, 20.93% becomes .2093 and is symbolized as F_IO_2. When we exhale, the fraction of O_2 is lowered (i.e., O_2 diffuses from the lung to the blood) and the fraction of O_2 in the expired (E) gas is represented by F_EO_2. The volume of expired O_2 is calculated by the product of the volume of expired gas ($\dot{V}_E$) and F_EO_2. Equation (1) can now be symbolized as:

(2) $\dot{V}O_2 = (F_IO_2 \cdot \dot{V}_I) - (F_EO_2 \cdot \dot{V}_E)$

The exercise values for F_IO_2, F_EO_2, $\dot{V}_I$, and $\dot{V}_E$ for a subject are easily measured in most exercise physiology laboratories. In practice, F_IO_2 is not generally measured but is assumed to be a constant value of .2093 if the subject is breathing room air. F_EO_2 will be determined by a gas analyzer, and $\dot{V}_I$ and $\dot{V}_E$ can be measured by a number of different laboratory devices capable of measuring airflow. Note that it is not necessary to measure both $\dot{V}_I$ and $\dot{V}_E$. This is true because if $\dot{V}_I$ is measured, $\dot{V}_E$ can be calculated (and vice versa). The formula used to calculate $\dot{V}_E$ from the measurement of $\dot{V}_I$ is called the "Haldane transformation" and is based on the fact that nitrogen (N_2) is neither used nor produced in the body. Therefore, the volume of N_2 inhaled must equal the volume of N_2 exhaled:

(3) $[\dot{V}_I \cdot F_IN_2] = [\dot{V}_E \cdot F_EN_2]$

Therefore, $\dot{V}_I$ can be computed if $\dot{V}_E$, F_IO_2, and F_EO_2 are known. For example, to solve for $\dot{V}_I$:

(4) $\dot{V}_I = \dfrac{(\dot{V}_E \cdot F_EN_2)}{F_IN_2}$

Likewise, if $\dot{V}_I$ was measured, $\dot{V}_E$ can be computed as:

(5) $\dot{V}_E = \dfrac{(\dot{V}_I \cdot F_IN_2)}{F_EN_2}$

The values for F_IN_2 and F_EN_2 are obtained in the following manner. If the subject is breathing room air, F_IN_2 is considered to be a constant .7904. The final remaining piece to the puzzle is F_EN_2. Recall that the three principal gases in air are N_2, O_2, and CO_2 and the sum of their fractions must add up to 1.0 (i.e., $F_ECO_2 + F_EO_2 + F_EN_2 = 1.0$). Therefore, F_EN_2 can be computed by subtracting the sum of F_ECO_2 and F_EO_2 from 1(i.e., $F_EN_2 = 1 - (F_ECO_2 + F_EO_2)$). Since the expired fractions of O_2 and CO_2 will be determined by gas analyzers, F_EN_2 can then be calculated.

Calculation of Carbon Dioxide Production

The volume of carbon dioxide produced ($\dot{V}CO_2$) can be calculated in a manner similar to $\dot{V}O_2$. That is, the volume of CO_2 produced is equal to:

(6) $\dot{V}CO_2$ = [Volume of CO_2 expired] − [Volume of CO_2 inspired]

or

$$(7) \quad \dot{V}CO_2 = (\dot{V}_E \cdot F_ECO_2) - (\dot{V}_I \cdot F_ICO_2)$$

The steps in performing this calculation are the same as in the computation of $\dot{V}O_2$. That is, $\dot{V}_E$ and $\dot{V}_I$ must be measured (or calculated) and the fraction of expired carbon dioxide (F_ECO_2) must be determined by a gas analyzer. Similar to F_IO_2, the fraction of inspired carbon dioxide (F_ICO_2) is considered to be a constant value of .0003.

Standardization of Gas Volumes

By convention, $\dot{V}O_2$ or $\dot{V}CO_2$ are expressed in liters $\cdot$ min^{-1} and standardized to a reference condition called "STPD." STPD is an acronym for "standard temperature pressure dry." In a similar manner, pulmonary ventilation is expressed in liters $\cdot$ min^{-1} and standardized to a reference standard called BTPS (an acronym for "body temperature pressure saturated"). The purpose of these reference standards is to allow comparison of gas volumes measured in laboratories throughout the world, which may vary in ambient temperature and barometric pressures. Standardization of gas volumes to a specified temperature and pressure is necessary because gas volume is dependent upon both temperature and pressure. For instance, a given number of gas molecules will occupy a greater volume at a higher temperature and lower pressure when compared to a lower temperature and higher pressure. This means that a fixed number of gas molecules would change volume as a function of the ambient temperature and barometric pressure. This poses a serious problem to researchers trying to make comparsions of respiratory gas exchange since temperature and pressures vary day-by-day and vary from one laboratory to another. By standardizing temperature and pressure conditions for gases, the scientist or technician knows that two equal volumes of gas contain the same number of molecules. It is for these reasons that respiratory gases must be corrected to a reference temperature and volume.

Correction of Gas Volumes to Reference Conditions

Before we begin a discussion of "how to" calculate gas volume corrections, it is necessary to introduce two important gas laws. The first, called "Charles's Law," states that the relationship between temperature and gas volume is directly proportional. That is, the gas volume is directly related to temperature, so that increasing or decreasing the temperature of a gas (at a constant pressure) causes a proportional volume increase or decrease, respectively. This relationship is expressed mathematically in the following way:

$$(8) \quad \frac{T_1}{T_2} = \frac{V_1}{V_2}$$

The units for temperature in equation (8) are the Kelvin (K) or Absolute (A) scale, where $0°$ C $=$ $273°$ K [i.e. $20°$ C $= (273° + 20°) = 293°$ K]. In using Charles's Law for gas temperature corrections, we rearrange equation (8) to solve for V_2:

$$(9) \quad V_2 = \frac{V_1 \cdot T_2}{T_1}$$

Let's leave Charles's Law for the moment and introduce a second gas law known as Boyle's Law. Boyle's Law states that at a constant temperature, the number of gas molecules in a given volume varies inversely with the pressure and is represented mathematically in the following equation:

$$(10) \quad P_1V_1 = P_2V_2$$

Again, rearranging equation (10) to solve for V_2:

$$(11) \quad V_2 = \frac{P_1 \cdot V_1}{P_2}$$

Pressure in equations (10) and (11) is expressed in mm Hg or Torr. Note that when respiratory gases are corrected for pressure differences that a correction is often made for water vapor, even though water vapor pressure is dependent only upon temperature (since respiratory gas is saturated with water vapor). When the gas volume is to be corrected to "0" water vapor pressure or "dried" as in STPD, the vapor pressure of water (PH_2O) at the ambient temperature is subtracted from the ambient or initial pressure (P_1) in Boyle's Law as follows:

$$(12) \quad V_2 = \frac{V_1(P_1 - PH_2O)}{P_2}$$

Combined Correction Factors

We can now combine Charles's Law and Boyle's Law (complete with water vapor correction) into one equation for STPD and BTPS conditions. Let's consider the STPD correction first.

STPD Correction

Gas volumes measured in the laboratory under room conditions of temperature and pressure are expressed as "ambient temperature pressure and saturated" (ATPS). This means that the gas volume is not a standardized volume but rather a volume that is subject to the ambient conditions of temperature and pressure. As previously stated, since ATPS conditions may vary from laboratory to laboratory, there is a need to correct VO_2 and VCO_2 volumes to the reference volume, STPD. Correcting a volume to STPD requires the standardization of temperature to 0° C (273° K), pressure to 760 mm Hg (sea level), and a correction for vapor pressure. For simplicity we will divide the gas correction procedure into two parts: (1) temperature and (2) pressure correction.

Step 1: Temperature Correction

Let's consider the temperature correction first. For this correction, we use equation (9) (Charles' Law):

$$V_2 = \frac{V_1 \cdot T_2}{T_1}$$

where:

V_2 = volume corrected to standard temperature (V_{ST})
V_1 = ATPS volume (V_{ATPS})

T_1 = absolute temperature in ambient surroundings (273° K + T_a° C)
where: T_a = ambient temperature
T_2 = absolute standard temperature (273° K)

Therefore, correcting an ATPS gas volume to V_{ST} is performed using the following equation:

$$(13) \quad V_{ST} = V_{ATPS} \left[\frac{273°}{(273° + T_a)} \right]$$

Step 2: Barometric pressure and water vapor pressure correction

To correct for barometric pressure and vapor pressure, we use equation (12), where:

V_1 = volume ATPS
V_2 = volume corrected to standard pressure and dry (V_{SPD})
P_1 = ambient barometric pressure in mm Hg
P_2 = standard barometric pressure (760 mm Hg)
PH_2O = partial pressure of water vapor at ambient temperature (see table A.1 for a list of vapor pressures at various ambient temperatures)

Therefore, when correcting V_{SPD} from ATPS volumes, the following equation is used:

$$(14) \quad V_{SPD} = V_{ATPS} \left[\frac{P_1 - PH_2O}{P_2} \right]$$

At this point we are ready to combine both the temperature correction factor (equation 13) and the pressure and vapor pressure correction factor (equation 14) into one equation and compute one single STPD correction factor. Combining equations (13) and (14) we arrive at:

$$(15) \quad V_{STPD} = V_{ATPS} \left[\frac{273°}{(273° + T_a)} \right] \left[\frac{(P_1 - PH_2O)}{P_2} \right]$$

Let's consider a sample problem to illustrate correction of ATPS volumes to STPD volumes.
Given:

V_{ATPS} = 90.0 liters
Laboratory temperature = 21° C

Table A.1 Water vapor pressure as a function of ambient temperature

Temperature (° C)	Saturation Water Vapor Pressure (mm Hg)
18	15.5
19	16.5
20	17.5
21	18.7
22	19.8
23	21.1
24	22.4
25	23.8
26	25.2
27	26.7

Ambient barometric pressure = 742 mm Hg
H_2O vapor pressure at 21° C (from table A.1)
= 18.7 mm Hg

Using the above sample conditions and equation (15), the STPD correction would be as follows:

$$V_{STPD} = 90 \left[\frac{273°}{(273° + 21°)} \right] \left[\frac{742 - 18.7}{760} \right]$$
$$= 79.53 \text{ liters STPD}$$

It is important to point out that if inspired gas volumes are measured and the relative humidity of the inspired gas is not 100%, then equation (15) must be modified by multiplying the relative humidity (RH) of the inspired gas (expressed as a fraction) by the partial pressure of water vapor at ambient temperature (e.g., if RH = 80%, then use $.8 \times PH_2O$).

BTPS Correction

As previously mentioned, all ventilatory volumes are corrected to BTPS conditions. This correction procedure is similar to the STPD correction procedure with two exceptions: 1. Standard temperature is 310° K instead of 273° K (e.g., 310° = 273° K + 37° C

[normal core temperature]). This correction is necessary because body temperature value is usually greater than ambient temperature and results in an increase in gas volume. 2. The partial pressure of vapor pressure at body temperature is subtracted from P_2 in equation (13). This correction is necessary because the partial pressure of water vapor at body temperature is generally greater than PH_2O at ambient conditions (i.e., at 37° the PH_2O = 47 mm Hg).

Therefore, correcting from ATPS to BTPS would involve the following equation:

$$(16) \quad V_{BTPS} = V_{ATPS} \left[\frac{310°}{273° + T_a} \right] \left[\frac{P_1 - PH_2O}{P_2 - 47} \right]$$

Let's consider a sample calculation of converting V_{ATPS} to V_{BTPS} using the following conditions:

Laboratory temperature = 20° C
Ambient barometric pressure = 752 mm Hg
PH_2O at 20° C = 17.5 mm Hg
V_{ATPS} = 60 liters

Therefore:

$$V_{BTPS} = 60 \left[\frac{310°}{273° + 20°} \right] \left[\frac{752 - 17.5}{752 - 47} \right]$$
$$= 65.39 \text{ liters BTPS}$$

Problems

1. Calculate $\dot{V}O_2$ and $\dot{V}CO_2$ given:
   $\dot{V}_E$ (ATPS) = 100 liters · min^{-1}
   F_EO_2 = .1768
   F_ECO_2 = .0399
   Assume F_IO_2 = .2093 and F_ICO_2 = .0003.
   Ambient Temperature = 21° C
   Barometric pressure = 749 mm Hg
2. Calculate the respiratory exchange ratio (R) from $\dot{V}O_2$ and $\dot{V}CO_2$ values computed in question number 1.
3. Calculate V_{BTPS} and V_{STPD} given:
   V_{ATPS} = 45.3 liters
   Laboratory temperature = 19° C
   Ambient barometric temperature = 746 mm Hg
   Body temperature = 37° C

Appendix B

Estimated Energy Expenditure during Selected Activities

It is often desireable to estimate energy expenditure during various types of physical activities. The following table provides a means of computing an estimated energy expenditure (per minute) based on the body weight of the subject. For example, to compute the caloric expenditure per minute for a 70-kg person during archery, multiply the calorie expenditure coefficent times body weight (i.e., $70 \times 0.065 = 4.55$ kcal $\cdot$ min^{-1}). This means that for every minute that this individual engages in archery 4.55 kcal are expended.

Activity	Calorie Expenditure Coefficent (kcal $\cdot$ min^{-1} $\cdot$ kg^{-1})
Archery	0.065
Badminton	0.097
Basketball	0.138
Billiards	0.042
Circuit weight training	
Hydra-Fitness	0.132
Universal Gym	0.116
Nautilus	0.092
Free weights	0.086
Dancing	
Aerobic (medium intensity)	0.103
Aerobic (high intensity)	0.135
Ballroom	0.051
Field hockey	0.134
Football (American)	0.132
Golf	0.085
Gymnastics	0.066
Judo	0.195
Jumping rope	
70/min	0.162
80/min	0.164
125/min	0.177
Racquetball	0.178
Running (horizontal)	
140 meters $\cdot$ min^{-1}	0.135
180 meters $\cdot$ min^{-1}	0.193
200 meters $\cdot$ min^{-1}	0.208
240 meters $\cdot$ min^{-1}	0.228
281 meters $\cdot$ min^{-1}	0.252
307 meters $\cdot$ min^{-1}	0.289
Swimming	
Back stroke	0.169
Breast stroke	0.162
Crawl (fast)	0.156
Crawl (slow)	0.128
Side stroke	0.122
Tennis	0.109
Volleyball	0.050

*Adapted from: McArdle, W., F. Katch, and V. Katch. 1986. *Exercise Physiology: Energy, Nutrition, and Human Performance*. Philadelphia: Lea & Febiger.

Appendix C

THE
CARTER CENTER
OF EMORY UNIVERSITY

Healthier People
Health Risk Appraisal

No. _____

Detach this coupon and put it in a safe place.
You will need it to claim your appraisal results.

✄ _

Healthier People
Health Risk Appraisal
The Carter Center of Emory University

No. _____

_____

Health Risk Appraisal is an educational tool. It shows you choices you can make to keep good health and avoid the most common causes of death for a person your age and sex. This Health Risk Appraisal is not a substitute for a check-up or physical exam that you get from a doctor or nurse. It only gives you some ideas for lowering your risk of getting sick or injured in the future. It is NOT designed for people who already have HEART DISEASE, CANCER, KIDNEY DISEASE, OR OTHER SERIOUS CONDITIONS. If you have any of these problems and you want a Health Risk Appraisal anyway, ask your doctor or nurse to read the report with you.
DIRECTIONS: To keep your answers confidential DO NOT write your name or any identification on this form. Please keep the coupon with your participant number on it. You will need it to claim your computer report. To get the most accurate results answer as many questions as you can and as best you can. If you do not know the answer leave it blank. Questions with a ★ (star symbol) are important to your health, but are not used by the computer to calculate your risks. However, your answers may be helpful in planning your health and fitness program.

Please put your answers in the empty boxes. (Examples: ☒ or ⌐125⌐)

1. SEX	1 ☐ Male 2 ☐ Female
2. AGE	☐ Years
3. HEIGHT (Without shoes) (No fractions)	☐ Feet ☐ Inches
4. WEIGHT (Without shoes) (No fractions)	☐ Pounds
5. Body frame size	1 ☐ Small 2 ☐ Medium 3 ☐ Large
6. Have you ever been told that you have diabetes (or sugar diabetes)?	1 ☐ Yes 2 ☐ No
7. Are you now taking medicine for high blood pressure?	1 ☐ Yes 2 ☐ No
8. What is your blood pressure now?	☐ / ☐ Systolic (High number) / Diastolic (Low number)
9. If you *do not* know the numbers, check the box that describes your blood pressure.	1 ☐ High 2 ☐ Normal or Low 3 ☐ Don't Know
10. What is your TOTAL cholesterol level (based on a blood test)?	☐ mg/dl
11. What is your HDL cholesterol (based on a blood test)?	☐ mg/dl
12. How many cigars do you usually smoke per day?	☐ cigars per day
13. How many pipes of tobacco do you usually smoke per day?	☐ pipes per day
14. How many times per day do you usually use smokeless tobacco? (Chewing tobacco, snuff, pouches, etc.)	☐ times per day

A–6

Health Risk Appraisal is an educational tool. It shows you choices you can make to keep good health and avoid the most common causes of death for a person your age and sex. This Health Risk Appraisal is not a substitute for a check-up or physical exam that you get from a doctor or nurse. It only gives you some ideas for lowering your risk of getting sick or injured in the future. It is NOT designed for people who already have HEART DISEASE, CANCER, KIDNEY DISEASE, OR OTHER SERIOUS CONDITIONS. If you have any of these problems and you want a Health Risk Appraisal anyway, ask your doctor or nurse to read the report with you.

Your report may be picked up at _____ on _____.

---

15. CIGARETTE SMOKING
How would you describe your cigarette smoking habits?

1 ☐ Never smoked   ☛ Go to 18
2 ☐ Used to smoke   ☛ Go to 17
3 ☐ Still smoke   ☛ Go to 16

16. STILL SMOKE
How many cigarettes a day do you smoke?
    ☛ GO TO QUESTION 18

[ ] cigarettes per day ☛ Go to 18

17. USED TO SMOKE
a. How many years has it been since you smoked cigarettes fairly regularly?

[ ] years

b. What was the average number of cigarettes per day that you smoked in the 2 years before you quit?

[ ] cigarettes per day

---

18. In the next 12 months how many thousands of miles will you probably travel by each of the following? (NOTE: U.S. average = 10,000 miles)
    a. Car, truck, or van:
    b. Motorcycle:

[ ] ,000 miles
[ ] ,000 miles

---

19. On a typical day how do you USUALLY travel?

(Check one only)

1 ☐ Walk
2 ☐ Bicycle
3 ☐ Motorcycle
4 ☐ Sub-compact or compact car
5 ☐ Mid-size or full-size car
6 ☐ Truck or van
7 ☐ Bus, subway, or train
8 ☐ Mostly stay home

---

20. What percent of the time do you usually buckle your safety belt when driving or riding?

[ ] %

---

21. On the average, how close to the speed limit do you usually drive?

1 ☐ Within 5 mph of limit
2 ☐ 6-10 mph over limit
3 ☐ 11-15 mph over limit
4 ☐ More than 15 mph over limit

---

22. How many times in the last month did you drive or ride when the driver had perhaps too much alcohol to drink?

[ ] times last month

---

23. How many drinks of alcoholic beverages do you have in a typical week?

☛ (MEN GO TO QUESTION 33)

(Write the number of each type of drink)
[ ] Bottles or cans of beer
[ ] Glasses of wine
[ ] Wine coolers
[ ] Mixed drinks or shots of liquor

WOMEN
24. At what age did you have your first menstrual period?

[ ] years old

---

25. How old were you when your first child was born?

[ ] years old
(If no children write 0)

26. How long has it been since your last breast x-ray (mammogram)?	1 ☐ Less than 1 year ago 2 ☐ 1 year ago 3 ☐ 2 years ago 4 ☐ 3 or more years ago 5 ☐ Never
27. How many women in your natural family (mother and sisters only) have had breast cancer?	☐ women
28. Have you had a hysterectomy operation?	1 ☐ Yes 2 ☐ No 3 ☐ Not sure
29. How long has it been since you had a pap smear test?	1 ☐ Less than 1 year ago 2 ☐ 1 year ago 3 ☐ 2 years ago 4 ☐ 3 or more years ago 5 ☐ Never
★ 30. How often do you examine your breasts for lumps?	1 ☐ Monthly 2 ☐ Once every few months 3 ☐ Rarely or never
★ 31. About how long has it been since you had your breasts examined by a physician or nurse?	1 ☐ Less than 1 year ago 2 ☐ 1 year ago 3 ☐ 2 years ago 4 ☐ 3 or more years ago 5 ☐ Never
★ 32. About how long has it been since you had a rectal exam?	1 ☐ Less than 1 year ago 2 ☐ 1 year ago 3 ☐ 2 years ago 4 ☐ 3 or more years ago 5 ☐ Never
☞ (WOMEN GO TO QUESTION 34)	
MEN ★ 33. About how long has it been since you had a rectal or prostate exam?	1 ☐ Less than 1 year ago 2 ☐ 1 year ago 3 ☐ 2 years ago 4 ☐ 3 or more years ago 5 ☐ Never
★ 34. How many times in the last year did you witness or become involved in a violent fight or attack where there was a good chance of a serious injury to someone?	1 ☐ 4 or more times 2 ☐ 2 or 3 times 3 ☐ 1 time or never 4 ☐ Not sure
★ 35. Considering your age, how would you describe your overall physical health?	1 ☐ Excellent 2 ☐ Good 3 ☐ Fair 4 ☐ Poor
★ 36. In an average week, how many times do you engage in physical activity (exercise or work which lasts at least 20 minutes without stopping and which is hard enough to make you breathe heavier and your heart beat faster)?	1 ☐ Less than 1 time per week 2 ☐ 1 or 2 times per week 3 ☐ At least 3 times per week
★ 37. If you ride a motorcycle or all-terrain vehicle (ATV) what percent of the time do you wear a helmet?	1 ☐ 75% to 100% 2 ☐ 25% to 74% 3 ☐ Less than 25% 4 ☐ Does not apply to me

★ 38. Do you eat some food every day that is high in fiber, such as whole grain bread, cereal, fresh fruits or vegetables? 1 ☐ Yes   2 ☐ No

★ 39. Do you eat foods every day that are high in cholesterol or fat, such as fatty meat, cheese, fried foods, or eggs? 1 ☐ Yes   2 ☐ No

★ 40. In general, how satisfied are you with your life?
1 ☐ Mostly satisfied
2 ☐ Partly satisfied
3 ☐ Not satisfied

★ 41. Have you suffered a personal loss or misfortune in the past year that had a serious impact on your life? (For example, a job loss, disability, separation, jail term, or the death of someone close to you.)
1 ☐ Yes, 1 serious loss or misfortune
2 ☐ Yes, 2 or more
3 ☐ No

★ 42a. Race
1 ☐ Aleutian, Alaska native, Eskimo or American Indian
2 ☐ Asian
3 ☐ Black
4 ☐ Pacific Islander
5 ☐ White
6 ☐ Other
7 ☐ Don't know

★ 42b. Are you of Hispanic origin such as Mexican-American, Puerto Rican, or Cuban? 1 ☐ Yes   2 ☐ No

★ 43. What is the highest grade you completed in school?
1 ☐ Grade school or less
2 ☐ Some high school
3 ☐ High school graduate
4 ☐ Some college
5 ☐ College graduate
6 ☐ Post graduate or professional degree

★ 44. What is your job or occupation?   (Check only one)
1 ☐ Health professional
2 ☐ Manager, educator, professional
3 ☐ Technical, sales or administrative support
4 ☐ Operator, fabricator, laborer
5 ☐ Student
6 ☐ Retired
7 ☐ Homemaker
8 ☐ Service
9 ☐ Skilled crafts
10 ☐ Unemployed
11 ☐ Other

★ 45. In what industry do you work (or did you last work)?   (Check only one)
1 ☐ Electric, gas, sanitation
2 ☐ Transportation, communication
3 ☐ Agriculture, forestry, fishing
4 ☐ Wholesale or retail trade
5 ☐ Financial and service industries
6 ☐ Mining
7 ☐ Government
8 ☐ Manufacturing
9 ☐ Construction
10 ☐ Other

V.3.0

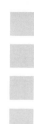

Appendix D

**Physical Activity
Prescriptions**

PARx

PHYSICAL ACTIVITY PRESCRIPTIONS*

PARx is a checklist of medical conditions requiring that a degree of precaution and/or special advice be considered for adults undertaking physical activities. Three categories are provided, and conditions are grouped by system or otherwise as appropriate. Comments under Special Prescriptive Conditions/Advice are general, since details and alternatives require clinical judgment in each individual instance.

ABSOLUTE CONTRAINDICATIONS	RELATIVE CONTRAINDICATIONS	SPECIAL PRESCRIPTIVE CONDITIONS/ ADVICE		System
• Permanent restriction, or temporary restriction until condition is treated, stable, and/or past acute phase.	• Highly variable. Value of exercise testing and/or program may exceed risk. Activity may be restricted. • Desirable to maximize control of condition. • Direct or indirect medical supervision of exercise program may be desirable.	• Individualized prescriptive advice generally appropriate: • limitations imposed and/or • special exercises prescribed • May require medical following and/or initial medical supervision in exercise program.		Comments
☐ aortic aneurysm (dissecting) ☐ aortic stenosis (severe) ☐ congestive heart failure ☐ crescendo angina ☐ myocardial infarction (acute) ☐ myocarditis (active or recent) ☐ pulmonary or systemic embolism – acute ☐ thrombophlebitis ☐ ventricular tachycardia and other dangerous dysrhythmias (e.g. multi-focal ventricular activity)	☐ aortic stenosis (moderate) ☐ subaortic stenosis (severe) ☐ marked cardiac enlargement ☐ supraventricular dysrhythmias (uncontrolled or high rate) ☐ ventricular ectopic activity (repetitive or frequent) ☐ ventricular aneurysm ☐ hypertension – untreated or uncontrolled severe (systemic or pulmonary)	☐ aortic (or pulmonic) stenosis – mild angina pectoris and other manifestations of coronary insufficiency (e.g. post-acute infarct) ☐ cyanotic heart disease ☐ shunts (intermittent or fixed) ☐ conduction disturbances • complete AV block • left BBB • Wolff-Parkinson-White syndrome ☐ dysrhythmias – controlled ☐ fixed rate pacemakers	• clinical exercise test may be warranted in selected cases, for specific determination of functional capacity and limitations and precautions (if any). • slow progression of exercise to levels based on test performance and individual tolerance. • consider individual need for initial conditioning program under medical supervision (indirect or direct)	Cardio-vascular
		☐ intermittent claudication	progressive exercise to tolerance	
		☐ hypertension: systolic 160 · 180; diastolic 105+	progressive exercise; care with medications (serum electrolytes; post-exercise syncope; etc.)	
☐ acute infectious disease (regardless of etiology)	☐ subacute/chronic/recurrent infectious diseases (e.g. malaria, others)	☐ chronic infections	variable as to condition	Infections
PHYSICAL ACTIVITY RECOMMENDATIONS	☐ uncontrolled metabolic disorders (diabetes, thyrotoxicosis, myxedema)	☐ renal, hepatic & other metabolic insufficiency ☐ obesity (25-50+ pounds overweight)	variable as to status dietary moderation, and initial light exercises with slow progression (walking, swimming, cycling)	Metabolic
Provided as a physician checklist or patient handout	☐ complicated pregnancy (e.g. toxemia, hemorrhage, incompetent cervix, etc.)	☐ advanced pregnancy (late 3rd trimester)	taper off intensity near term	Pregnancy
		☐ chronic pulmonary disorders ☐ obstructive lung disease ☐ asthma ☐ "exercise-induced asthma"	special relaxation and breathing exercises; breath control during endurance exercises to tolerance; avoid polluted air; avoid hyperventilation during exercise	Lung
		☐ anemia – severe (< 10 Gm/dl) ☐ electrolyte disturbances	control preferred; exercise as tolerated	Blood
		☐ hernia	minimize straining and isometrics; strengthen abdominal muscles	Hernia
		☐ convulsive disorder not completely controlled by medication	minimize exercise in hazardous environments and/or exercising alone (e.g. swimming, mountain climbing, etc.)	CNS
		☐ low back conditions (pathological, functional) ☐ arthritis—acute (infective, rheumatoid, gout) ☐ arthritis – subacute ☐ arthritis – chronic (osteoarthritis and above conditions) ☐ orthopedic	avoid forced extreme flexion, extension, and violent twisting, correct posture, proper back exercises treatment, plus judicious blend of rest, splinting and gentle movement progressive increase of active exercise therapy maintenance of mobility and strength; endurance exercises to minimize joint trauma (e.g. cycling, swimming, etc.) highly variable and individualized	Musculo-skeletal
		☐ antianginal ☐ antiarrhythmic ☐ antihypertensive ☐ anticonvulsant ☐ beta-blockers ☐ digitalis preparations ☐ diuretics ☐ ganglionic blockers ☐ others	NOTE: consider underlying condition. Potential for: exertional syncope, electrolyte imbalance, bradycardia, dysrhythmias, impaired coordination and reaction time, heat intolerance. May alter resting and exercise ECG's and exercise test performance.	Medications
		☐ post-exercise syncope ☐ heat intolerance ☐ temporary minor illness	moderate program; prolong cool-down with light activities postpone until recovered	Other

* REFER TO SPECIAL PUBLICATIONS FOR ELABORATION AS REQUIRED.

PHYSICAL ACTIVITY RECOMMENDATIONS

If you have been cleared by your physician for unrestricted activity and/or a progressive exercise program, these key points may be of assistance to you.

☐ Components of a balanced exercise program (the 3S's)
- Strength – arms, shoulders, back, abdomen and legs
- Suppleness – stretch and relaxation of body and limbs
- Stamina – endurance fitness through aerobic activities (large muscle action that increases the heart rate)

☐ Progression – slow and easy, gradually increase the volume and vigor of your activities over several weeks.

☐ Warm-up and cool-down – quiet entry and exit of a few minutes each, such as with calisthenics and light activities.

☐ FITT is a guide to your Stamina (endurance) activities.

FREQUENCY	INTENSITY	TIME	TYPE
3 to 5 times per week	Work up to and sustain a target heart rate (for your age) during exercise	Once your body is accustomed to exercise, attempt to keep moving for at least 15 minutes (even if it means slowing down a little)	Any endurance exercise – walking, jogging, swimming, cycling, skipping, vigorous ball games, ski touring, etc.

☐ Pulse count is a good method to assess your response to aerobic exercises. Count for 10 seconds *immediately* after stopping your activity. Have your physician or exercise professional show you how to count your pulse. The chart below is age-adjusted. Be content to work at the lower FIT START heart rate initially until your condition improves, then slowly increase the intensity of your activity until your heart rate is reaching the KEEP FIT level. Remember, enter and exit your activity gently.

FIT START

AGE	HEART RATE
20 · 29	118
30 · 39	112
40 · 49	106
50 · 59	100
60 · 69	94

Progress Slowly

KEEP FIT

AGE	HEART RATE
20 · 29	146 · 164
30 · 39	138 · 156
40 · 49	130 · 148
50 · 59	122 · 140
60 · 69	116 · 132

Derived from the "Half-As-Much" approach, B.C. Department of Health

MAJOR REFERENCES FOR PARx CHART:

1. Fox, S.M. III, Naughton, J.P., and Haskell, W.C. Physical Activity and the Prevention of Coronary Heart Disease. Ann. Clin. Res. 3: 404-432, 1971.
2. American College of Sports Medicine. Guidelines for Graded Exercise Testing and Exercise Prescription. Lea and Febiger, 1975.
3. Committee on Exercise and Physical Fitness. Evaluation for Exercise Participation – The Apparently Healthy Individual. JAMA 219: 900-01, 1972.
4. Cooper, K.H. Guidelines in the Management of the Exercising Patient. JAMA 211: 1663-67, 1970.
5. Licht, S. Therapeutic Exercise Volume III. Waverly Press, 1965.
6. Recommendations and Guidelines of the Canadian Heart Foundation for Exercise Testing and Exercise Programmes for Improving Cardiopulmonary and General Physical Fitness. 1975.

From *British Columbia Medical Journal* 17(11), November 1975.
Copyright © 1975 British Columbia Medical Association, Vancouver, British Columbia, Canada.

1980 Recommended Dietary Allowances

Food and Nutrition Board, National Academy of Sciences-National Research Council Recommended Daily Dietary Allowance[a]
Revised 1980

	Age (years)	Weight		Height		Protein (g)	Fat-soluble vitamins				
		(kg)	(lbs)	(cm)	(in)		Vitamin A (μg R.E.)[b]	Vitamin D (μg)[c]	Vitamin E (mg α T.E.)[d]	Vitamin C (mg)	Thiamin (mg)
Infants	0.0-0.5	6	13	60	24	kg×2.2	420	10	3	35	0.3
	0.5-1.0	9	20	71	28	kg×2.0	400	10	4	35	0.5
Children	1-3	13	29	90	35	23	400	10	5	45	0.7
	4-6	20	44	112	44	30	500	10	6	45	0.9
	7-10	28	62	132	52	34	700	10	7	45	1.2
Males	11-14	45	99	157	62	45	1,000	10	8	50	1.4
	15-18	66	145	176	69	56	1,000	10	10	60	1.4
	19-22	70	154	177	70	56	1,000	7.5	10	60	1.5
	23-50	70	154	178	70	56	1,000	5	10	60	1.4
	51+	70	154	178	70	56	1,000	5	10	60	1.2
Females	11-14	46	101	157	62	46	800	10	8	50	1.1
	15-18	55	120	163	64	46	800	10	8	60	1.1
	19-22	55	120	163	64	44	800	7.5	8	60	1.1
	23-50	55	120	163	64	44	800	5	8	60	1.0
	51+	55	120	163	64	44	800	5	8	60	1.0
Pregnant						+30	+200	+5	+2	+20	+0.4
Lactating						+20	+400	+5	+3	+40	+0.5

[a]The allowances are intended to provide for individual variations among most normal persons as they live in the United States under usual environmental stresses. Diets should be based on a variety of common foods in order to provide other nutrients for which human requirements have been less well defined.

[b]Retinol equivalents. 1 Retinol equivalent = 1 μg retinol or 6 μg carotene.

[c]As cholecaliciferol. 10 μg cholecaliciferol = 400 I.U. vitamin D.

[d]α tocopheral equivalents. 1 mg d-α-tocopheral = 1αT.E.

Water-soluble vitamins							Minerals			
Riboflavin (mg)	Niacin (mg N.E.)[e]	Vitamin B_6 (mg)	Folacin[f] (μg)	Vitamin B_{12} (μg)	Calcium (mg)	Phosphorus (mg)	Magnesium (mg)	Iron (mg)	Zinc (mg)	Iodine (μg)
0.4	6	0.3	30	0.5[g]	360	240	50	10	3	40
0.6	8	0.6	45	1.5	540	360	70	15	5	50
0.8	9	0.9	100	2.0	800	800	150	15	10	70
1.0	11	1.3	200	2.5	800	800	200	10	10	90
1.4	16	1.6	300	3.0	800	800	250	10	10	120
1.6	18	1.8	400	3.0	1,200	1,200	350	18	15	150
1.7	18	2.0	400	3.0	1,200	1,200	400	18	15	150
1.7	19	2.2	400	3.0	800	800	350	10	15	150
1.6	18	2.2	400	3.0	800	800	350	10	15	150
1.4	16	2.2	400	3.0	800	800	350	10	15	150
1.3	15	1.8	400	3.0	1,200	1,200	300	18	15	150
1.3	14	2.0	400	3.0	1,200	1,200	300	18	15	150
1.3	14	2.0	400	3.0	800	800	300	18	15	150
1.2	13	2.0	400	3.0	800	800	300	18	15	150
1.2	13	2.0	400	3.0	800	800	300	10	15	150
+0.3	+2	+0.6	+400	+1.0	+400	+400	+150	[h]	+ 5	+25
+0.5	+5	+0.5	+100	+1.0	+400	+400	+150	[h]	+10	+50

[e]1 NE (niacin equivalent) is equal to 1 mg of niacin or 60 mg of dietary tryptophan.

[f]The folacin allowances refer to dietary sources as determined by *Lactobacillus casei* assay after treatment with enzymes ("conjugases") to make polyglutamyl forms of the vitamin available to the test organism.

[g]The RDA for vitamin B_{12} in infants is based on average concentration of the vitamin in human milk. The allowances after weaning are based on energy intake (as recommended by the American Academy of Pediatrics) and consideration of other factors such as intestinal absorption.

[h]The increased requirement during pregnancy cannot be met by the iron content of habitual American diets nor by the existing iron stores of many women; therefore the use of 30–60 mg of supplement iron is recommended. Iron needs during lactation are not substantially different from those of non-pregnant women, but continued supplementation of the mother for 2–3 months after parturition is advisable in order to replenish stores depleted by pregnancy.

Source: Food and Nutrition Board, National Academy of Sciences—National Research Council Recommended Daily Dietary Allowances, Revised 1980, Washington, D.C.

Appendix F

1979 RDAs—Estimated safe and adequate daily dietary intakes of additional selected vitamins and minerals[a]

Subjects	Vitamins			Trace elements[b]						Electrolytes		
Age (years)	Vitamin K (µg)	Biotin (µg)	Pantothenic acid (mg)	Copper (mg)	Manganese (mg)	Fluoride (mg)	Chromium (mg)	Selenium (mg)	Molybdenum (mg)	Sodium (mg)	Potassium (mg)	Chloride (mg)
Infants												
0–0.5	12	35	2	0.5–0.7	0.5–0.7	0.1–0.5	0.01–0.04	0.01–0.04	0.03–0.06	115–350	350–925	275–700
0.5–1	10–20	50	3	0.7–1.0	0.7–1.0	0.2–1.0	0.02–0.06	0.02–0.06	0.04–0.08	250–750	425–1,275	400–1,200
Children and adolescents												
1–3	15–30	65	3	1.0–1.5	1.0–1.5	0.5–1.5	0.02–0.08	0.02–0.08	0.05–0.1	325–975	550–1,650	500–1,500
4–6	20–40	85	3–4	1.5–2.0	1.5–2.0	1.0–2.5	0.03–0.12	0.03–0.12	0.06–0.15	450–1,350	775–2,325	700–2,100
7–10	30–60	120	4–5	2.0–2.5	2.0–3.0	1.5–2.5	0.05–0.2	0.05–0.2	0.10–0.3	600–1,800	1,000–3,000	925–2,775
11	50–100	100–200	4–7	2.0–3.0	2.5–5.0	1.5–2.5	0.05–0.2	0.05–0.2	0.15–0.5	900–2,700	1,525–4,575	1,400–4,200
Adults	70–140	100–200	4–7	2.0–3.0	2.5–5.0	1.5–4.0	0.05–0.2	0.05–0.2	0.15–0.5	1,100–3,300	1,875–5,625	1,700–5,100

[a]Because there is less information on which to base allowances, these figures are not given in the main table of the RDA and are provided here in the form of ranges of recommended intakes

[b]Since the toxic levels for many trace elements may be only several times usual intakes, the upper levels for the trace elements given in this table should not be habitually exceeded

From: Recommended Dietary Allowances, Revised 1980. Food and Nutrition Board National Academy of Sciences-National Research Council. Washington, D.C.

1980 RDAs—Mean heights and weights and recommended energy intake

Category	Age (years)	Weight (kg)	(lb)	Height (cm)	(in)	Energy Needs (with range) (Calories)	(MJ)
Infants	0.0–0.5	6	13	60	24	kg × 115 (95–145)	kg × .48
	0.5–1.0	9	20	71	28	kg × 105 (80–135)	kg × .44
Children	1–3	13	29	90	35	1,300 (900–1,800)	5.5
	4–6	20	44	112	44	1,700 (1,300–2,300)	7.1
	7–10	28	62	132	52	2,400 (1,650–3,300)	10.1
Males	11–14	45	99	157	62	2,700 (2,000–3,700)	11.3
	15–18	66	145	176	69	2,800 (2,100–3,900)	11.8
	19–22	70	154	177	70	2,900 (2,500–3,300)	12.2
	23–50	70	154	178	70	2,700 (2,300–3,100)	11.3
	51–75	70	154	178	70	2,400 (2,000–2,800)	10.1
	76 +	70	154	178	70	2,050 (1,650–2,450)	8.6
Females	11–14	46	101	157	62	2,200 (1,500–3,000)	9.2
	15–18	55	120	163	64	2,100 (1,200–3,000)	8.8
	19–22	55	120	163	64	2,100 (1,700–2,500)	8.8
	23–50	55	120	163	64	2,000 (1,600–2,400)	8.4
	51–75	55	120	163	64	1,800 (1,400–2,200)	7.6
	76+	55	120	163	64	1,600 (1,200–2,000)	6.7
Pregnancy						+300	
Lactation						+500	

Source: Food and Nutrition Board, National Academy of Sciences—National Research Council Recommended Daily Dietary Allowances, Revised 1980, Washington, D.C.

Diet Analysis Using Food Composition Data

This diet analysis of a food intake record was done by a twenty-year-old woman.

Item	Amount	Protein (g)	Fat (g)	Carbo-hydrate (g)	Calcium (mg)	Irom (mg)	Vitamin A (IU)	Thiamin (mg)	Vitamin C (mg)
Egg bagel	1	6	2	28			30	.14	0
Jelly	1 T.	0	0	13	9	1.2	0	0	1
7-Up	12 oz.	0	0	36	4	0.3	0	0	0
McDonald's Cheeseburgers	2	32	26	62	0	0	744	.48	3
Potato chips	2 oz.	3	24	30	316	5.8	0	.12	9
McDonald's Cookies	small box	4	11	45	24	1.2	47	.28	1
Cola drink	12 oz.	0	0	37	10	1.4	0	0	0
Pork chop	3 oz	21	28	0	0	0	0	.83	0
Baked potato	1 avg.	4	0	33	11	3.0	0	.15	31
Frozen peas	½ c.	4	0	10	14	1.1	480	.22	11
Butter	2 t	0	8	0	15	1.5	288	0	0
Iceberg lettuce	2 c.	0	0	4	2	0	360	.06	6
French dressing	2 T.	0	12	6	22	0.6	0	0	0
2% milk	½ c.	4	3	6	4	0.2	250	.05	1
Graham crackers	2 pq.	1	1	10	147	0	0	.02	0
Totals		79	115	320	584	16.8	2,199	2.35	63
Your RDA		44			800	180	4,000	1.1	60
% of your RDA		180			73	93	55	214	105

Appendix I

Percent Fat Estimate for Men: Sum of Triceps, Chest, and Subscapula Skinfolds

Sum of Skinfolds (mm)	Age to Last Year								
	Under 22	23–27	28–32	33–37	38–42	43–47	48–52	53–57	Over 57
8–10	1.5	2.0	2.5	3.1	3.6	4.1	4.6	5.1	5.6
11–13	3.0	3.5	4.0	4.5	5.1	5.6	6.1	6.6	7.1
14–16	4.5	5.0	5.5	6.0	6.5	7.0	7.6	8.1	8.6
17–19	5.9	6.4	6.9	7.4	8.0	8.5	9.0	9.5	10.0
20–22	7.3	7.8	8.3	8.8	9.4	9.9	10.4	10.9	11.4
23–25	8.6	9.2	9.7	10.2	10.7	11.2	11.8	12.3	12.8
26–28	10.0	10.5	11.0	11.5	12.1	12.6	13.1	13.6	14.2
29–31	11.2	11.8	12.3	12.8	13.4	13.9	14.4	14.9	15.5
32–34	12.5	13.0	13.5	14.1	14.6	15.1	15.7	16.2	16.7
35–37	13.7	14.2	14.8	15.3	15.8	16.4	16.9	17.4	18.0
38–40	14.9	15.4	15.9	16.5	17.0	17.6	18.1	18.6	19.2
41–43	16.0	16.6	17.1	17.6	18.2	18.7	19.3	19.8	20.3
44–46	17.1	17.7	18.2	18.7	19.3	19.8	20.4	20.9	21.5
47–49	18.2	18.7	19.3	19.8	20.4	20.9	21.4	22.0	22.5
50–52	19.2	19.7	20.3	20.8	21.4	21.9	22.5	23.0	23.6
53–55	20.2	20.7	21.3	21.8	22.4	22.9	23.5	24.0	24.6
56–58	21.1	21.7	22.2	22.8	23.3	23.9	24.4	25.0	25.5
59–61	22.0	22.6	23.1	23.7	24.2	24.8	25.3	25.9	26.5
62–64	22.9	23.4	24.0	24.5	25.1	25.7	26.2	26.8	27.3
65–67	23.7	24.3	24.8	25.4	25.9	26.5	27.1	27.6	28.2
68–70	24.5	25.0	25.6	26.2	26.7	27.3	27.8	28.4	29.0
71–73	25.2	25.8	26.3	26.9	27.5	28.0	28.6	29.1	29.7
74–76	25.9	26.5	27.0	27.6	28.2	28.7	29.3	29.9	30.4
77–79	26.6	27.1	27.7	28.2	28.8	29.4	29.9	30.5	31.1
80–82	27.2	27.7	28.3	28.9	29.4	30.0	30.6	31.1	31.7
83–85	27.7	28.3	28.8	29.4	30.0	30.5	31.1	31.7	32.3
86–88	28.2	28.8	29.4	29.9	30.5	31.1	31.6	32.2	32.8
89–91	28.7	29.3	29.8	30.4	31.0	31.5	32.1	32.7	33.3
92–94	29.1	29.7	30.3	30.8	31.4	32.0	32.6	33.1	33.4
95–97	29.5	30.1	30.6	31.2	31.8	32.4	32.9	33.5	34.1
98–100	29.8	30.4	31.0	31.6	32.1	32.7	33.3	33.9	34.4
101–103	30.1	30.7	31.3	31.8	32.4	33.0	33.6	34.1	34.7
104–106	30.4	30.9	31.5	32.1	32.7	33.2	33.8	34.4	35.0
107–109	30.6	31.1	31.7	32.3	32.9	33.4	34.0	34.6	35.2
110–112	30.7	31.3	31.9	32.4	33.0	33.6	34.2	34.7	35.3
113–115	30.8	31.4	32.0	32.5	33.1	33.7	34.3	34.9	35.4
116–118	30.9	31.5	32.0	32.6	33.2	33.8	34.3	34.9	35.5

Percent Fat Estimate for Women: Sum of Triceps, Abdomen, and Suprailium Skinfolds

Sum of Skinfolds (mm)	Age to Last Year								Over 57
	18–22	23–27	28–32	33–37	38–42	43–47	48–52	53–57	
8–12	8.8	9.0	9.2	9.4	9.5	9.7	9.9	10.1	10.3
13–17	10.8	10.9	11.1	11.3	11.5	11.7	11.8	12.0	12.2
18–22	12.6	12.8	13.0	13.2	13.4	13.5	13.7	13.9	14.1
23–27	14.5	14.6	14.8	15.0	15.2	15.4	15.6	15.7	15.9
28–32	16.2	16.4	16.6	16.8	17.0	17.1	17.3	17.5	17.7
33–37	17.9	18.1	18.3	18.5	18.7	18.9	19.0	19.2	19.4
38–42	19.6	19.8	20.0	20.2	20.3	20.5	20.7	20.9	21.1
43–47	21.2	21.4	21.6	21.8	21.9	22.1	22.3	22.5	22.7
48–52	22.8	22.9	23.1	23.3	23.5	23.7	23.8	24.0	24.2
53–57	24.2	24.4	24.6	24.8	25.0	25.2	25.3	25.5	25.7
58–62	25.7	25.9	26.0	26.2	26.4	26.6	26.8	27.0	27.1
63–67	27.1	27.2	27.4	27.6	27.8	28.0	28.2	28.3	28.5
68–72	28.4	28.6	28.7	28.9	29.1	29.3	29.5	29.7	29.8
73–77	29.6	29.8	30.0	30.2	30.4	30.6	30.7	30.9	31.1
78–82	30.9	31.0	31.2	31.4	31.6	31.8	31.9	32.1	32.3
83–87	32.0	32.2	32.4	32.6	32.7	32.9	33.1	33.3	33.5
88–92	33.1	33.3	33.5	33.7	33.8	34.0	34.2	34.4	34.6
93–97	34.1	34.3	34.5	34.7	34.9	35.1	35.2	35.4	35.6
98–102	35.1	35.3	35.5	35.7	35.9	36.0	36.2	36.4	36.6
103–107	36.1	36.2	36.4	36.6	36.8	37.0	37.2	37.3	37.5
108–112	36.9	37.1	37.3	37.5	37.7	37.9	38.0	38.2	38.4
113–117	37.8	37.9	38.1	38.3	39.2	39.4	39.6	39.8	39.2
118–122	38.5	38.7	38.9	39.1	39.4	39.6	39.8	40.0	40.0
123–127	39.2	39.4	39.6	39.8	40.0	40.1	40.3	40.5	40.7
128–132	39.9	40.1	40.2	40.4	40.6	40.8	41.0	41.2	41.3
133–137	40.5	40.7	40.8	41.0	41.2	41.4	41.6	41.7	41.9
138–142	41.0	41.2	41.4	41.6	41.7	41.9	42.1	42.3	42.5
143–147	41.5	41.7	41.9	42.0	42.2	42.4	42.6	42.8	43.0
148–152	41.9	42.1	42.3	42.4	42.6	42.8	43.0	43.2	43.4
153–157	42.3	42.5	42.6	42.8	43.0	43.2	43.4	43.6	43.7
158–162	42.6	42.8	43.0	43.1	43.3	43.5	43.7	43.9	44.1
163–167	42.9	43.0	43.2	43.4	43.6	43.8	44.0	44.1	44.3
168–172	43.1	43.2	43.4	43.6	43.8	44.0	44.2	44.3	44.5
173–177	43.2	43.4	43.6	43.8	43.9	44.1	44.3	44.5	44.7
178–182	43.3	43.5	43.7	43.8	44.0	44.2	44.4	44.6	44.8

Glossary

absolute $\dot{V}O_2$ the amount of oxygen consumed over a given time period; expressed as liters $\cdot$ min^{-1}.

acidosis an abnormal increase in blood hydrogen ion concentration (i.e., arterial pH below 7.35).

acids a compound capable of giving up hydrogen ions into solution.

acromegaly a condition caused by hypersecretion of growth hormone from the pituitary gland; characterized by enlargement of the extremities, such as the jaw, nose, and fingers.

actin a structural protein of muscle that works with myosin in permitting muscular contraction.

action potential the all-or-none electrical event in the neuron or muscle cell in which the polarity of the cell membrane is rapidly reversed and then reestablished.

adenosine diphosphate (ADP) a molecule that combines with inorganic phosphate to form ATP.

adenosine triphosphate (ATP) the high-energy phosphate compound synthesized and used by cells to release energy for cellular work.

adenyl cyclase enzyme found in cell membranes that at catalyzes the conversion of ATP to cyclic AMP.

adrenal cortex the outer portion of the adrenal gland. Synthesizes and secretes corticosteroid hormones, such as cortisol, aldosterone, and androgens.

adrenocorticotrophic hormone (ACTH) a hormone secreted by the anterior pituitary gland that stimulates the adrenal cortex.

aerobic in the presence of oxygen.

afferent neuron sensory neuron carrying information toward the central nervous system.

aldosterone a corticosteroid hormone involved in the regulation of electrolyte balance.

alkalosis an abnormal increase in blood concentration of OH$^-$ ions, resulting in a rise in arterial pH above 7.45.

alpha receptors a subtype of adrenergic receptors located on cell membranes of selected tissues.

alveoli microscopic air sacs located in the lung where gas exchange occurs between respiratory gases and the blood.

amenorrhea the absence of menses.

anabolic steroid a prescription drug that has anabolic, or growth-stimulating, characteristics similar to that of the male androgen, testosterone.

anaerobic without oxygen.

anaerobic threshold a commonly used term meant to describe the level of oxygen consumption at which there is a rapid and systematic increase in blood lactate concentration. Also termed the lactate threshold.

anatomical dead space the total volume of the lung (i.e., conducting airways) that does not participate in gas exchange.

androgenic a compound that has the qualities of an androgen; associated with masculine characteristics.

androgens male sex hormones. Synthesized in the testes and in limited amounts in the adrenal cortex. Steroids that have masculinizing effects.

angina a sharp pain. Used almost exclusively to describe angina pectoris (*see* angina pectoris).

angina pectoris chest pain due to a lack of blood flow (ischemia) to the myocardium.

angioplasty an invasive medical procedure used to open partially blocked coronary arteries.

angiotensin I and II these compounds are polypeptides formed from the cleavage of a protein (angiotensinogen) by the action of the enzyme renin produced by the kidneys, and converting enzyme in the lung, respectively.

anorexia nervosa an eating disorder characterized by rapid weight loss due to failure to consume adequate amounts of nutrients.

anterior hypothalamus the anterior portion of the hypothalamus. The hypothalamus is an area of the brain below the thalamus that regulates the autonomic nervous system and the pituitary gland.

anterior pituitary the anterior portion of the pituitary gland that secretes follicle-stimulating hormone, luteinizing hormone, adrenocorticotropic hormone, thyroid stimulating hormone, growth hormone, and prolactin.

antidiuretic hormone (ADH) hormone secreted by the posterior pituitary gland which promotes water retention by the kidney.

aortic bodies receptors located in the arch of the aorta that are capable of detecting changes in arterial PO_2.

apophyses sites of muscle-tendon insertion in bones.

arrhythmia abnormal electrical activity in the heart (i.e., a premature ventricular contraction).

arteries large vessels that carry arterialized blood away from the heart.

arterioles a small branch of an artery that communicates with a capillary network.

articular cartilage cartilage that covers the ends of bones in a synovial joint.

atherosclerosis a pathological condition in which fatty substances collect inside the lumen of arteries.

ATPase enzyme capable of breaking down ATP to ADP + Pi + energy.

ATP-CP system term used to describe the metabolic pathway involving muscle stores of ATP and the use of creatine phosphate to rephosphorylate ADP. This pathway is used at the onset of exercise and during short-term, high-intensity work.

atrioventricular node a specialized mass of muscle tissue located in the interventricular septum of the heart; functions in the transmission of cardiac impulses from the atria to the ventricles.

autologous transfusion blood transfusion where the individual receives his or her own blood.

autonomic nervous sytem portion of the nervous system that functions to control the actions of visceral organs.

autoregulation mechanism by which an organ regulates blood flow to match the metabolic rate.

axon a nerve fiber that conducts a nerve impulse away from the neuron cell body.

ballistic stretching a rapid stretching movement (e.g., bobbing to touch your toes).

bases a compound that ionizes in water to release hydroxyl ions (OH⁻) or other ions that are capable of combining with hydrogen ions.

beta receptor agonist a molecule that is capable of binding to and activating a beta receptor.

beta receptors an adrenergic receptor located on cell membranes. Combines mainly with epinephrine and, to some degree, with norepinephrine.

bioenergetics the chemical processes involved with production of cellular ATP.

biological control systems a control system capable of maintaining homeostasis within a cell or organ system in a living creature.

blood boosting a term that applies to the increase of the blood's hemoglobin concentration by infusion of additional red blood cells. Medically termed as "induced erythrocythemia."

blood doping blood boosting.

Bohr effect the right shift of oxyhemoglobin curve due to a decrease of blood pH. Results in a decreased affinity for oxygen.

bradycardia a resting heart rate to less than sixty beats per minute.

brainstem portion of the brain that includes midbrain, pons, and medulla.

buffers substances capable of accepting hydrogen ions or hydroxyl ions and, therefore, resist a change in pH.

bulimia an eating disorder characterized by eating and forced regurgitation.

bulk flow movement of molecules from an area of high pressure to an area of lower pressure.

capillaries microscopic blood vessels that connect arterioles and venules. Portion of vascular system where blood/tissue gas exchange occurs.

cardiac accelerator nerves part of the sympathetic nervous system that stimulates the SA node to increase heart rate.

cardiac output the amount of blood pumped by the heart per unit of time; equal to product of heart rate and stroke volume.

cardiovascular control center the area of the medulla that regulates the cardiovascular system.

carotid bodies chemoreceptors located in the internal carotid artery; respond to changes in arterial PO_2, PCO_2, and pH.

catecholamines organic compounds that includes epinephrine, norepinephrine, and dopamine.

cell body the soma, or major portion of the body of a nerve cell. Contains the nucleus.

cell membrane the bilayer-lipid envelope that encloses cells. Called the sarcolemma in muscle cells.

central command the control of the cardiovascular or pulmonary system by cortical impulses.

central nervous system portion of the nervous system that consists of the brain and spinal cord.

cerebellum portion of the brain that is concerned with fine coordination of skeletal muscle during movement.

cerebrum superior aspect of the brain that occupies the upper cranial cavity. Contains the motor cortex.

cholesterol a twenty-seven-carbon lipid that can be synthesized in cells or consumed in the diet. Cholesterol serves as a precursor of steroid hormones and plays a role in the development of atherosclerosis.

clo units that describe the insulation quality of clothing.

conduction process of body heat movement into the molecules of cooler objects in contact with the body. This term may also be used in association with the conveyance of neural impulses.

conductivity capacity for conduction.

convection the transmission of heat from one object to another through the circulation of heated molecules.

coronary artery bypass graft surgery (CABGS) the replacement of a blocked coronary artery with another vessel to permit blood flow to the myocardium.

cortisol a glucocorticoid secreted by the adrenal cortex upon stimulation by ACTH.

coupled reactions the linking of energy-liberating chemical reactions to "drive" energy-requiring reactions.

creatine phosphate (CP) a compound found in skeletal muscle used to resynthesize ATP from ADP.

cromolyn sodium a drug used to stabilize the membranes of mast cells and prevent an asthma attack.

crude fiber an estimate of fiber percentage in foods based on harsh chemical analysis.

cycle ergometer a stationary exercise cycle that allows accurate measurement of work output.

cyclic AMP a substance produced from ATP through the action of adrenyl cyclase that alters several chemical processes in the cell.

cytoplasm the contents of the cell surrounding the nucleus. Called sarcoplasm in muscle cells.

deficiency a shortcoming of some essential nutrient.

degenerative diseases diseases not due to infection, which result in a progressive decline in some bodily function.

delayed onset muscle soreness (DOMS) muscle soreness that occurs twelve to twenty-four hours after the exercise bout.

dendrites portion of the nerve fiber that transmits action potentials toward the nerve cell body.

dental caries tooth decay; related to sugar content in foods.

deoxyhemoglobin hemoglobin not in combination with oxygen.

diabetes mellitus a condition characterized by high blood glucose levels due to inadequate insulin. Type I diabetics are insulin dependent, whereas Type II are not.

diabetic coma unconscious state induced by a lack of insulin.

diaphragm the major respiratory muscle responsible for inspiration. Dome shaped—separates the thoracic cavity from the abdominal cavity.

diastole period of filling of the heart between contractions (i.e., resting phase of the heart).

diastolic blood pressure arterial blood pressure during diastole.

dietary (edible) fiber an accurate estimate of fiber percentage in foods.

direct calorimetry assessment of the body's metabolic rate by direct measurement of the amount of heat produced.

double-blind design an experimental design in which the subjects and the principal investigator are not aware of the experimental treatment order.

double product the product of heart rate and systolic blood pressure.

dynamic refers to an isotonic muscle contraction.

dysmenorrhea painful menstruation.

dyspnea shortness of breath or labored breathing. May be due to various types of lung or heart diseases.

ectomorphy category of somatotype that is rated for linearity of body form.

effector organ or body part that responds to stimulation by a efferent neuron (e.g., skeletal muscle in a withdrawal reflex).

efferent neuron conducts impulses from the CNS to the effector organ (e.g., motorneuron).

ejection fraction the proportion of end-diastolic volume that is ejected during a ventricular contraction.

electrocardiogram a recording of the electrical activity of the heart. Used clinically to diagnose various types of cardiac pathology.

electron transport chain a series of cytochromes in the mitochrondia that are responsible for oxidative phosphorylation.

elements a single chemical substance composed of only one type of atom (e.g., calcium or potassium).

endergonic reactions energy-requiring reactions.

endocrine gland a gland that produces and secretes its products directly into the blood or interstitial fluid (ductless glands).

endomorphy the somatotype category that is rated for roundness (fatness).

endomysium the inner layer of connective tissue surrounding a muscle fiber.

endorphin a neuropeptide produced by the pituitary gland having pain-suppressing activity.

end plate potential depolarization of a membrane region by a sodium influx.

energy of activation energy required to initate a chemical reaction.

enzymes proteins that lower the energy of activation and, therefore, catalyze chemical reactions. Enzymes regulate the rate of most metabolic pathways.

epilepsy a neurological disorder manifested by muscular seizures.

epimysium the outer layer of connective tissue surrounding muscle.

epinephrine a hormone synthesized by the adrenal medulla; also called adrenaline.

epiphyseal plate or growth plate cartilagious layer between the head and shaft of a long bone where growth takes place.

EPOC an acronym for "excess post-exercise oxygen consumption"; often referred to as the oxygen debt.

EPSP excitatory post synaptic potential. A graded depolarization of a post synaptic membrane by a neurotransmitter.

ergogenic aid a substance or aid that improves performance.

ergometer instrument for measuring work.

erythrocythemia an increase in the number of erthrocytes in the blood.

estrogens female sex hormones, including estradiol and estrone. Produced primarily in the ovary and also produced in adrenal cortex.

evaporation the change of water from a liquid form to a vapor form. Results in the removal of heat.

exercise a subclass of physical activity.

exergonic reactions chemical reactions that release energy.

extensors muscles that function to extend a limb, that is, increases the angle at a joint.

external respiration movement of gas in and out of the lungs (pulmonary ventilation).

FAD flavin adenine dinucleotide. Serves as an electron carrier in bioenergetics.

fasciculi a small bundle of muscle fibers.

fast twitch fibers one of several types of muscle fibers found in skeletal muscle; also called Type II fibers; characterized as having low oxidative capacity but high glycolytic capacity.

ferritin the iron-carrying molecule used as an index of whole-body iron status.

field test a test of physical performance performed in the field (outside the laboratory).

flexors muscle groups that cause flexion of limbs, that is, decreasing the angle at a joint.

follicle stimulating hormone (FSH) a hormone secreted by the anterior pituitary gland that stimulates the development of an ovarian follicle in the female and the production of sperm in the male.

food records the practice of keeping dietary food records for determining nutrient intake.

free fatty acid a type of fat that combines with glycerol to form triglycerides. Can be used as an energy source.

gain refers to the amount of correction that a control system is capable of achieving.

General Adaptation Syndrome (GAS) a term defined by Selye in 1936 that describes the organism's response to chronic stress. In response to stress the organism reacts in a three-stage response: (1) alarm reaction; (2) stage of resistance; and (3) readjustment to the stress or exhaustion.

glucagon a hormone produced by the pancreas that acts to increase blood glucose and free fatty acid levels.

glucocorticoids any one of a group of hormones produced by the adrenal cortex that influences carbohydrate, fat, and protein metabolism.

gluconeogenesis the synthesis of glucose from non-carbohydrate sources.

glucose a simple sugar that is transported via the blood and metabolized by tissues.

glucose polymer a complex sugar molecule that contains multiple simple sugar molecules linked together.

glycogen a glucose polymer synthesized in cells as a means of storing carbohydrate.

glycogenolysis the breakdown of glycogen into glucose.

glycolysis a metabolic pathway in the cytoplasm of the cell that results in the degradation of glucose into pyruvate or lactate.

Golgi tendon organ a tension receptor located in series with skeletal muscle.

gross efficiency a simple measure of exercise efficiency defined as: work performed/energy expended $\times$ 100%.

growth hormone hormone synthesized and secreted by the anterior pituitary that stimulates growth of the skeleton and soft tissues during the growing years.

HDL cholesterol (high density lipoprotein cholesterol) cholesterol that is transported in the blood via high-density proteins; related to low risk of heart disease.

hemoglobin a heme containing protein in red blood cells that is responsible for transporting oxygen to tissues. Hemoglobin also serves as a weak buffer within red blood cells.

hemosiderin an insoluble form of iron stored in tissues.

high density lipoproteins proteins used to transport cholesterol in blood; high levels appear to offer some protection from atherosclerosis.

homeostasis the maintenance of a constant internal environment.

homeotherms animals that maintain a fairly constant internal temperature.

homologous transfusion a blood transfusion of matching blood from another donor.

hormone a chemical substance that is synthesized and released by an endocrine gland and transported to a target organ via the blood.

hydrogen ion (H^+) a free hydrogen ion in solution that results in a decrease in pH of the solution.

hyperbaric chamber chamber where the absolute pressure is increased above atmospheric pressure.

hyperoxia oxygen concentration in an inspired gas that exceeds 21%.

hyperplasia an increase in the number of cells present in a tissue.

hyperthermia an above-normal increase in body temperature.

hypertrophy an increase in cell size.

hypothalamic somatostatin hypothalamic hormone that inhibits growth hormone secretion; also secreted from the delta cells of the islets of Langerhans.

hypothalamus brain structure that integrates many physiological functions to maintain homeostasis; site of secretion of hormones released by the posterior pituitary; also releases hormones that control anterior pituitary secretions.

hypothermia a condition in which heat is lost from the body faster than it is produced.

hypoxia a relative lack of oxygen (e.g., at altitude).

immunotherapy procedure in which the body is exposed to specific substances to elicit an immune response in order to offer better protection upon subsequent exposure.

indirect calorimetry estimation of heat or energy production on the basis of oxygen consumption, carbon dioxide production, and nitrogen excretion.

induced erythrocythemia causing an elevation of the red blood cell (hemoglobin) concentration by infusing blood; also called blood doping or blood boosting.

infectious diseases diseases due to the presence of pathogenic microorganisms in the body (e.g., viruses, bacteria, fungi, and protozoa).

inorganic relating to substances that do not contain carbon (C).

inorganic phosphate (Pi) a stimulator of cellular metabolism; split off, along with ADP, from ATP when energy is released; used with ADP to form ATP in the electron transport chain.

insulin hormone released from the beta cells of the islets of Langerhans in response to elevated blood glucose and amino acid concentrations; increases tissue uptake of both.

insulin shock condition brought on by too much insulin, which causes an immediate hypoglycemia; symptoms include tremors, dizziness, and possibly convulsions.

integrating center the portion of a biological control system that processes the information from the receptors and issues an appropriate response relative to its set point.

intercalated discs portion of cardiac muscle cell where one cell connects to the next.

intermediate fibers muscle fiber type that generates high force at a moderate speed of contraction, but has a relatively large number of mitochondria (type IIa).

internal respiration refers to the utilization of oxygen at the mitochondria where ATP is produced; distinguished from external respiration in which atmospheric air is brought into the lungs (*see* external respiration).

ion a single atom or small molecule containing a net positive or negative charge due to an excess of either protons or electrons, respectively (e.g., Na^+, Cl^-).

IPSP inhibitory post-synaptic potential that moves the post synaptic membrane further from threshold.

irritability a trait of certain tissues that enables them to respond to stimuli (e.g., nerve and muscle).

isocitrate dehydrogenase rate-limiting enzyme in the Krebs Cycle that is inhibited by ATP and stimulated by ADP and Pi.

isokinetic action in which the rate of movement is constantly maintained through a specific range of motion even though maximal force is exerted.

isometric contraction in which the muscle develops tension, but does not shorten; also called a static contraction. No movement occurs.

isotonic contraction in which a muscle shortens against a constant load or tension, resulting in movement.

ketosis acidosis of the blood caused by the production of ketone bodies (e.g., acetoacetic acid) when fatty acid mobilization is increased, as in uncontrolled diabetes.

kilocalorie a measure of energy expenditure equal to the heat needed to raise the temperature of one kg of water 1 degree Celsius; also equal to 1,000 calories and sometimes written as Calorie rather than kilocalorie.

kilogram-meter a unit of work in which 1 kg of force (1 kg mass accelerated at 1 G) is moved through a vertical distance of 1 meter; abbreviated as kg-m, kg · m, or kgm.

kinesthesia a perception of movement obtained from information about the position and rate of movement of the joints.

Krebs cycle metabolic pathway in the mitochondria in which energy is transferred from carbohydrates, fats, and amino acids to NAD for subsequent production of ATP in the electron transport chain.

lactate threshold a point during a graded exercise test when the blood lactate concentration increases abruptly.

lactic acid an end product of glucose metabolism in the glycolytic pathway; formed in conditions of inadequate oxygen and in muscle fibers with few mitochondria.

LDL cholesterol form of low-density lipoprotein responsible for the transport of plasma cholesterol; high levels are indicative of a high risk of coronary heart disease.

lipase an enzyme responsible for the breakdown of triglycerides to free fatty acids and glycerol.

lipolysis the breakdown of triglycerides in adipose tissue to free fatty acids and glycerol for subsequent transport to tissues for metabolism.

lipoprotein protein involved in the transport of cholesterol and triglycerides in the plasma.

low density lipoproteins form of lipoprotein that transports a majority of the plasma cholesterol; see LDL cholesterol.

luteinizing hormone (LH) also called Interstitial Cell Stimulating Hormone; a surge of LH stimulates ovulation in middle of menstrual cycle; LH stimulates testosterone production in men.

Maragaria power test test of anaerobic power, primarily related to high energy phosphates, in which a subject runs up stairs with time monitored to the nearest hundredth of a second.

mast cell connective tissue cell that releases histimine and other chemicals in response to certain stimuli (e.g., injury).

maximal oxygen uptake greatest rate of oxygen uptake by the body measured during severe dynamic exercise, usually on a cycle ergometer or a treadmill; dependent on maximal cardiac output and the maximal arteriovenous oxygen difference.

membrane potential a voltage difference between the inside and outside of a cell membrane; due to membrane permeability and the charge separation across the membrane that causes a flux of ions across the membrane.

mesomorphy one component of a somatotype that characterizes the muscular form or lean body mass aspect of the human body.

MET an expression of the rate of energy expenditure at rest; equal to approximately $3.5 \text{ ml} \cdot \text{kg}^{-1} \cdot \text{min}^{-1}$, or $1 \text{ kcal} \cdot \text{kg}^{-1} \cdot \text{hr}^{-1}$.

mineralocorticoids steroid hormones released from the adrenal cortex that are responsible for Na^+ and K^+ regulation (e.g., aldosterone).

minerals ions or substances that do not contain carbon (*see* inorganic) (e.g., calcium, iron, sulfur, sodium, chloride, magnesium, and potassium). Important aspects of a balanced diet.

mitochondrion the subcellular organelle responsible for the production of ATP with oxygen; contains the enzymes for the Krebs Cycle, Electron Transport Chain, and the Fatty Acid Cycle.

motor cortex portion of the cerebral cortex containing large motor neurons whose axons descend to lower brain centers and spinal cord; associated with the voluntary control of movement.

motor neurons efferent neurons that conduct action potentials from the central nervous system to the muscles.

motor unit a motor neuron and all the muscle fibers innervated by that single motor neuron; responds in an "all-or-none" manner to a stimulus.

muscle spindle a muscle stretch receptor oriented parallel to skeletal muscle fibers; the capsule portion is surrounded by afferent fibers, and intrafusal muscle fibers can alter the length of the capsule during muscle contraction and relaxation.

myocardial infarction death of a portion of heart tissue that no longer conducts electrical activity nor provides force to move blood.

myocardial ischemia a condition in which the myocardium experiences an inadequate blood flow; sometimes accompanied by irregularities in the electrocardiogram (arrhythmias and ST-segment depression) and chest pain (angina pectoris).

myocardium cardiac muscle; provides the force of contraction to eject blood; muscle type with many mitochondria that is dependent on a constant supply of oxygen.

myofibrils the portion of the muscle containing the thick and thin contractile filaments; a series of sarcomeres where the repeating pattern of the contractile proteins gives the striated appearance to skeletal muscle.

myoglobin protein in muscle that can bind oxygen and release it at low PO_2 values; aids in diffusion of oxygen from capillary to mitochondria.

myosin contractile protein in the thick filament of a myofibril that contains the cross-bridge that can bind actin and split ATP to cause tension development.

NAD coenzyme that transfers hydrogen and the energy associated with those hydrogens; in the Krebs Cycle NAD transfers energy from substrates to the electron transport chain.

negative feedback describes the response from a control system that reduces the size of the stimulus, e.g., an elevated blood glucose concentration causes the secretion of insulin which, in turn, lowers the blood glucose concentration.

neuroendocrinology study of the role of the nervous and endocrine systems in the automatic regulation of the internal environment.

neuromuscular junction synapse between axon terminal of a motor neuron and the motor end plate of a muscle's plasma membrane.

neuron nerve cell; composed of a cell body with dendrites (projections) that bring information to the cell body and axons that take information away from the cell body to influence neurons, glands, or muscles.

norepinephrine a hormone and neurotransmitter; released from postganglionic nerve ending and the adrenal medulla.

normocythemia a normal red blood cell concentration.

normoxia a normal PO_2.

nucleus membrane-bound organelle containing most of the cell's DNA.

nutrient density the degree to which foods contain selected nutrients, e.g., protein.

open-circuit spirometry indirect calorimetry procedure in which either inspired or expired ventilation is measured and oxygen consumption and carbon dioxide production is calculated.

organic describes substances that contain carbon.

osteoporosis a decrease in bone density due to a loss of cortical bone; common in older women and implicated in fractures; estrogen and Ca^{++} therapy used to correct the condition.

overload a principle of training describing the need to increase the load (intensity) of exercise to cause a further adaptation of a system.

oxidative phosphorylation mitochondrial process in which inorganic phosphate (Pi) is coupled to ADP as energy is transferred along the electron transport chain in which oxygen is the final electron acceptor.

oxygen debt the elevated post-exercise oxygen consumption; related to replacement of creatine phosphate, lactic acid resynthesis to glucose, and elevated body temperature, catecholamines, heart rate, breathing, etc.

oxygen deficit a measure of the energy production not provided by oxidative phosphorylation in the transition from rest to exercise; ATP provided by high energy phosphates and anaerobic glycolysis.

oxyhemoglobin hemoglobin combined with oxygen; 1.34 ml of oxygen can combine with 1 g Hb.

pancreas gland containing both exocrine and endocrine portions; exocrine secretions include enzymes and bicarbonate to digest food in the small intestine; endocrine secretions include insulin, glucagon, and somatostatin, which are released into the blood.

parasympathetic nervous system portion of the autonomic nervous system that primarily releases acetylcholine from its postganglionic nerve endings.

partial pressure the fractional part of the barometric pressure due to the presence of a single gas, e.g., PO_2, PCO_2, and PN_2.

percent grade a measure of the elevation of the treadmill; calculated as the sine of the angle.

percutaneous transluminal coronary angioplasty a balloon-tipped catheter is inserted into a blocked coronary artery and plaque is pushed back to artery wall to open the blood vessel.

perimysium the connective tissue surrounding the fasiculus of skeletal muscle fibers.

peripheral nervous system portion of the nervous system located outside the spinal cord and brain.

pH a measure of the acidity of a solution; calculated as the negative $\log_{10}$ of the $[H^+]$ in which 7 is neutral, values that are >7 are basic and <7 are acidic.

phosphodiesterase an enzyme that catalyzes the breakdown of cyclic AMP, moderating the effect of the hormonal stimulation of adenyl cyclase.

phosphofructokinase rate-limiting enzyme in glycolysis that is responsive to ADP, Pi, and ATP levels in the cytoplasm of the cell.

physical activity characterizes all types of human movement; associated with living, work, play, and exercise.

physical fitness a broad term describing healthful levels of cardiovascular function, strength, and flexibility; fitness is specific to the activities performed.

pituitary gland a gland at the base of the hypothalamus of the brain having an anterior portion that produces and secretes numerous hormones that regulate other endocrine glands and a posterior portion that secretes hormones that are produced in the hypothalamus.

placebo an inert substance that is used in experimental studies, e.g., drug studies, to control for any subjective reaction to the substance being tested.

pleura a thin lining of cells that is attached to the inside of the chest wall and to the lung; the cells secrete a fluid that facilitates the movements of the lungs in the thoracic cavity.

posterior pituitary gland portion of the pituitary gland secreting oxytocin and antidiuretic hormone (vasopressin) that are produced in the hypothalamus.

power a rate of work; work per unit time; $P = W/t$.

power test a test measuring the quantity of work accomplished in a time period; anaerobic power tests include the Margaria stair climb test and the Wingate test; aerobic power tests include the 1.5-mile run and cycle ergometer and treadmill tests in which power output and oxygen consumption are measured.

precursor a warning sign associated with and preceding specific diseases or death; a risk factor; an inactive substance that precedes the active form.

primary risk factor a sign (e.g., high blood pressure) or a behavior (e.g., cigarette smoking) that is directly related to the appearance of certain diseases independent of other risk factors.

progressive resistance exercise (PRE) a training program in which the muscles must work against a gradually increasing resistance; an implementation of the overload principle.

proprioceptors receptors that provide information about the position and movement of the body; includes muscle and joint receptors as well as the receptors in the semicircular canals of the inner ear.

protein kinase an enzyme involved in the transfer of a phosphate group to protein.

provitamin a precursor of a vitamin.

pulmonary circuit the portion of the cardiovascular system involved in the circulation of blood from the right ventricle to the lungs and back to the left atrium.

radiation process of energy exchange from the surface of one object to the surface of another that is dependent on a temperature gradient but does not require contact between the objects; an example is the transfer of heat from the sun to the earth.

RDA Recommended Dietary Allowances; standards of nutrition associated with good health for the majority of people. Standards exist for protein, vitamins, and minerals for children and adults.

receptor in the nervous system, a receptor is a specialized portion of an afferent neuron (or a special cell attached to an afferent neuron) that is sensitive to a form of energy in the environment; receptor is also a term that applies to unique proteins on the surface of cells that can bind specific hormones or neurotransmitters.

reciprocal inhibition when extensor muscles (agonists) are contracted there is a reflex inhibition of the motor neurons to the flexor muscles (antagonists), and vice versa.

relative $\dot{V}O_2$ oxygen uptake (consumption) expressed per unit body weight (e.g., $ml \cdot kg^{-1} \cdot min^{-1}$).

releasing hormone hypothalamic hormones released from neurons into the anterior pituitary that control the release of hormones from that gland.

renin enzyme secreted by special cells in the kidney that converts angiotensinogen to angiotensin I.

repetition the number of times an exercise is repeated within a single exercise "set."

residual volume volume of air in the lungs following a maximal expiration.

respiration external respiration is the exchange of oxygen and carbon dioxide between the lungs and the environment; internal respiration describes the use of oxygen by the cell (mitochondria).

respiratory compensation the buffering of excess H^+ in the blood by plasma bicarbonate (HCO_3^-), and the associated elevation in ventilation to exhale the resulting CO_2.

respiratory exchange ratio (R) the ratio of CO_2 production to O_2 consumption; indicative of substrate utilization during steady state exercise in which a value of 1.0 represents 100% carbohydrate metabolism and 0.7 represents 100% fat metabolism.

resting membrane potential the voltage difference measured across a membrane that is related to the concentration of ions on each side of the membrane and the permeability of the membrane to those ions.

rest interval the time period between bouts in an interval training program.

reversibility a principle of training that describes the temporary nature of a training effect; adaptations to training are lost when the training stops.

sarcolemma the cell (plasma) membrane surrounding a muscle fiber.

sarcomeres the repeating contractile unit in a myofibril bounded by Z-lines.

sarcoplasmic reticulum a membranous structure that surrounds the myofibrils of muscle cells; location of the terminal cisternae or lateral sacs that store the Ca^{++} needed for muscle contraction.

Sargent's jump and reach test a test of anaerobic power dependent on the high-energy phosphates; a vertical jump test in which the subject jumps as high as possible.

Schwann cell the cell that surrounds peripheral nerve fibers forming the myelin sheath.

second messenger a molecule (cyclic AMP) or ion (Ca^{++}) that increases in a cell as a result of an interaction between a "first messenger" (e.g., hormone or neurotransmitter) and a receptor that alters cellular activity.

secondary risk factor a characteristic (age, gender, race, body fatness) or behavior (inactivity) that increases the risk of coronary heart disease when primary risk factors are present.

set a basic unit of a workout containing the number of times (repetitions) a specific exercise is done (e.g., do three sets of five repetitions with 100 pounds).

sex steroids a group of hormones, androgens and estrogens, secreted from the adrenal cortex and the gonads.

sham reinfusion an experimental treatment at the end of a blood doping experiment in which a needle is placed in a vein, but the subject does not receive a reinfusion of blood.

sham withdrawal an experimental treatment at the beginning of a blood doping experiment in which a needle is placed in a vein and blood is not withdrawn.

sliding filament theory a theory of muscle contraction describing the sliding of the thin filaments (actin) past the thick filaments (myosin).

slow twitch fibers muscle fiber type that contracts slowly and develops relatively low tension but displays great endurance to repeated stimulation; contains many mitochondria, capillaries, and myoglobin.

somatomedins groups of growth-stimulating peptides released primarily from the liver in response to growth hormone.

somatostatin hormone produced in the hypothalamus that inhibits growth hormone release from the anterior pituitary gland; secreted from cells in the islet of Langerhans and causes a decrease in intestinal activity.

somatotype body-type (form) classification method used to characterize the degree to which an individual's frame is linear (ectomorphic), muscular (mesomorphic), and round (endomorphic); Sheldon's scale rates each component on 1–7 scale.

specificity a principle of training indicating that the adaptation of a tissue is dependent on the type of training undertaken, e.g., muscles hypertrophy with heavy resistance training but show an increase in mitochondria number with endurance training.

spirometry measurement of various lung volumes.

static stationary; describes a muscle contraction in which tension is developed but the muscle does not shorten (isometric contraction).

static stretching stretching procedure in which a muscle is stretched and held in the stretched position for ten to thirty seconds; in contrast to dynamic stretching which involves motion.

steady-state describes the tendency of a control system to achieve a balance between an environmental demand and the response of a physiological system to meet that demand to allow the tissue (body) to function over a period of time.

steroids a class of lipids, derived from cholesterol, that includes the hormones testosterone, estrogen, cortisol, and aldosterone.

strong acids an acid that completely ionizes when dissolved in water to generate H^+ and its anion.

strong bases a base (alkaline substance) that completely ionizes when dissolved in water to generate OH^- and its cation.

ST segment depression an electrocardiographic change reflecting an ischemia (inadequate blood flow) in the heart muscle; indicative of coronary heart disease.

summation repeated stimulation of a muscle that leads to an increase in tension compared to a single twitch.

supercompensation an increase in the muscle glycogen content above normal levels following an exercise-induced muscle glycogen depletion and an increase in carbohydrate intake.

sympathetic nervous system portion of the autonomic nervous system that releases norepinephrine from its postganglionic nerve endings; epinephrine is released from the adrenal medulla.

sympathomimetic substance that mimics the effects of epinephrine or norepinephrine, which are secreted from the sympathetic nervous systems.

synapses junctions between nerve cells (neurons) where the electrical activity of one neuron influences the electrical activity of the other neuron.

systole portion of the cardiac cycle in which the ventricles are contracting.

systolic blood pressure the highest arterial pressure measured during a cardiac cycle.

target heart rate (THR) range the range of heart rates describing the optimum intensity of exercise consistent with making gains in maximal aerobic power; equal to 70%–85% HR max.

terminal cisternae portion of the sarcoplasmic reticulum near the transverse tubule containing the Ca^{++} that is released upon depolarization of the muscle; also called lateral sac.

testis the sex gland, gonad, of the male; (pl.: testes).

testosterone the steroid hormone produced in the testes; involved in growth and development of reproductive tissues, sperm, and secondary sex characteristics.

tetanus highest tension developed by a muscle in response to a high frequency of stimulation.

theophylline a drug used as a smooth muscle relaxant in the treatment of asthma.

thermogenesis the generation of heat as a result of metabolic reactions.

thyroid gland endocrine gland located in the neck that secretes triiodothyronine (T_3) and thyroxine (T_4), which increase the metabolic rate.

tidal volume volume of air inhaled or exhaled in a single breath.

tonus low level of muscle activity at rest.

total lung capacity the total volume of air the lung can contain; equal to the sum of the vital capacity and the residual volume.

toxicity a condition resulting from an chronic ingestion of vitamins, especially fat soluble vitamins, in quantities well above that needed for health.

transferrin plasma protein that binds iron and is representative of the whole body iron store.

transverse tubules an extension, invagination, of the muscle membrane that conducts the action potential into the muscle to depolarize the terminal cisternae which contains the Ca^{++} needed for muscle contraction.

tropomyosin protein covering the actin binding sites that prevents the myosin cross bridge from touching actin.

troponin protein, associated with actin and tropomyosin, that binds Ca^{++} and initiates the movement of tropomyosin on actin to allow the myosin cross bridge to touch actin and initiate contraction.

twenty-four-hour recall a technique of recording the type and amount of food (nutrients) consumed during a twenty-four-hour period.

twitch the tension-generating response following the application of a single stimulus to muscle.

underwater weighing procedure to estimate body volume by the loss of weight in water; result is used to calculate body density and, from that, body fatness.

U.S. Dietary Goals a series of nutritional goals to achieve better health for the American population: 58% carbohydrate; 30% fat (no more than 10% saturated fat), and 12% protein.

U.S. RDA nutritional information on foods that expresses the degree to which the food meets the adult RDA value for various nutrients.

vagus nerve a major parasympathetic nerve.

variable resistance exercise strength training equipment in which the resistance varies throughout the range of motion.

veins the blood vessel that accepts blood from the venules and brings it back to the heart.

ventilation the movement of air into or out of the lungs (e.g., pulmonary or alveolar ventilation); external respiration.

venules small blood vessels carrying capillary blood to veins.

vestibular apparatus sensory organ consisting of three semicircular canals that provides needed information about body position to maintain balance.

vital capacity the volume of air that can be moved into or out of the lungs in one breath; equal to the sum of the inspiratory and expiratory reserve volumes and the tidal volume.

whole body density a measure of the weight to volume ratio of the entire body; high values are associated with low body fatness.

Windgate test anaerobic power test to evaluate maximal rate at which glycolysis can deliver ATP.

work the product of a force and the distance through which that force moves ($W = F \times D$).

work interval in interval training, the duration of the work phase of each work-to-rest interval.

Credits

Chapter 3

Figure 3.1: From Ross M. Durham, *Human Physiology: Functions of the Human Body.* Copyright © 1989 Wm. C. Brown Publishers, Dubuque, Iowa. All Rights Reserved. Reprinted by permission; **Figures 3.2, 3.3, 3.4, 3.6, 3.7, 3.9, 3.11, and 3.14:** From Stuart Ira Fox, *Human Physiology,* 2d ed. Copyright © 1987 Wm. C. Brown Publishers, Dubuque, Iowa. All Rights Reserved. Reprinted by permission; **Figures 3.8, 3.10, 3.12, and 3.13:** From Leland G. Johnson, *Biology,* 2d ed. Copyright © 1987 Wm. C. Brown Publishers, Dubuque, Iowa. All Rights Reserved. Reprinted by permission.

Chapter 4

Figure 4.8: Reprinted by permission of the American Alliance for Health, Physical Education, Recreation and Dance, 1900 Association Drive, Reston, VA 22091; **Figure 4.11:** Figure constructed from data from S. Dodd, "Blood Lactate Disappearance at Various Intensities of Recovery Exercise" in *Journal of Applied Physiology,* 57:1462–65, 1984. Copyright © The 1984 American Physiological Society, Bethesda, MD. Used by permission.

Chapter 5

Figure 5.1 and 5.6: From A. J. Vander, et al., *Human Physiology: The Mechanisms of Body Function,* 4th ed. Copyright © 1985 McGraw-Hill Book Company, New York, NY. Reprinted by permission; **Figures 5.2 and 5.3:** From Stuart Ira Fox, *Human Physiology,* 2d ed. Copyright © 1987 Wm. C. Brown Publishers, Dubuque, Iowa. All Rights Reserved. Reprinted by permission; **Figure 5.5:** From John W. Hole, Jr., *Human Anatomy and Physiology,* 3d ed. Copyright © 1984 Wm. C. Brown Publishers, Dubuque, Iowa. All Rights Reserved. Reprinted by permission; **Figure 5.7:** Figure constructed from data from V. A. Convertino, et al., "Plasma Volume, Renin and Vasopression Responses to Graded Exercise After Training" in *Journal of Applied Physiology: Respiration Environment Exercise Physiology,* 54:508–14, 1983. Copyright © 1983 The American Physiological Society, Bethesda, MD; **Figure 5.9:** Figure constructed from data from J. T. Maher, et al., "Aldosterone Dynamics during Graded Exercise at Sea Level and High Altitude" in *Journal of Applied Physiology,* 39:18–22, 1975. Copyright © 1975 The American Physiological Society, Bethesda, MD; **Figure 5.13:** From Leland G. Johnson, *Biology,* 2d ed. Copyright © 1987 Wm. C. Brown Publishers, Dubuque, Iowa. All Rights Reserved. Reprinted by permission; **Figure 5.14:** Figure constructed from data from J. E. Jurkowski, et al., "Ovarian Hormonal Responses to Exercise" in *Journal of Applied Physiology: Respiration Environment Exercise Physiology,* 44:109–14, 1978. Copyright © 1978 The American Physiological Society, Bethesda, MD; **Figure 5.15:** From B. Saltin and J. Karlsson, "Muscle Glycogen Utilization during Work of Different Intensities" in *Muscle Metabolism During Exercise,* 289–99, 1971, edited by B. Pernow and B. Saltin. Copyright © 1971 Plenum Press, New York, NY; **Figure 5.16:** Figure constructed from data from P. C. Painter, et al., "Changes in Plasma CAMP and Catecholamines in Men Subjected to the Same Relative Amount of Physical Work Stress" in *Aviation, Space, and Environmental Medicine,* 56:683–86, 1982; **Figure 5.20:** Figure constructed from data from C. T. M. Davies and J. D. Few, "Effects of Exercise on Adrenocortical Function" in *Journal of Applied Physiology,* 35:887–91, 1973. Copyright © 1973 The American Physiological Society, Bethesda, MD; **Figure 5.22a:** Figure constructed from data from J. Sutton and L. Lazarus, "Growth Hormone in Exercise: Comparison of Physiological and Pharmacological Stimuli" in *Journal of Applied Physiology,* 41:523–27, 1976. Copyright © 1976 The American Physiological Society, Bethesda, MD; **Figure 5.22b:** Figure constructed from data from J. C. Bunt et al., "Sex and Training Differences in Human Growth Hormone Levels during Prolonged Exercise" in *Journal of Applied Physiology,* 61:1796–1801.5, 1986. Copyright © 1986 The American Physiological Society, Bethesda, MD; **Figure 5.24:** Figure constructed from data from Scott Powers et al., "A Different Cathecholamine Response during Prolonged Exercise and Passive Heating" in *Medicine and Science in Sports and Exercise,* 14:435–39, 1982. Copyright © 1982 American College of Sports Medicine; **Figure 5.25:** Figure constructed from data from W. W. Winder et al., "Time Course of Sumpathadrenal Adaptation to Endurance Exercise Training in Man" in *Journal of Applied Physiology: Respiration Environment Exercise Physiology* 45:370–74, 1978. Copyright © 1978 The American Physiological Society, Bethesda, MD; **Figure 5.27a:** Figure constructed from data from L. H. Hartley et al., "Multiple Hormonal Responses to Graded Exercise in Relation to Physical Training" in *Journal of Applied Physiology* 33:602–6, 1972. Copyright © 1972 The American Physiological Society, Bethesda, MD; **Figures 5.27b and 5.28:** Figure constructed from data from F. Gyntelberg et al., "Effect of Training on the Response of Plasma Glucagon to Exercise" in *Journal of Applied Physiology: Respiration Environment Exercise Physiology* 43:302–5, 1977. Copyright © 1977 The Physiological Association, Bethesda, MD.

Model for Pulmonary Rehabilitation" in *Journal of Cardiopulmonary Rehabilitation* 6:368–71, 1986. Copyright © 1986 J. B. Lippincott, Philadelphia, PA.

Chapter 18

Figure 18.3: From T. G. Lohman, "The Use of Skinfold to Estimate Body Fatness in Children and Youth" in *Journal of Health, Physical Education, Recreation and Dance* 98:102, November-December 1987. Copyright © 1987 American Alliance for Health, Physical Recreation and Dance, Reston, VA; **Figure 18.4:** Figure constructed from data from L. Sjostrom and P. Bjorntorp, "Body Composition and Adipose Tissue Cellularity in Human Obesity" in *Acta Medica Scandinavica* 195:201–11, 1974. Copyright © 1974 Almqvist & Wiksell International, Stockholm, Sweden; **Figure 18.5:** From M. Krotkiewski, et al., "Adipose Tissue Cellularity in Relation to Prognosis for Weight Reduction" in *International Journal of Obesity* 1:395–416, 1977. Copyright © 1977 John Libbey & Co., London, England; **Figure 18.6:** From S. Garn and D. C. Clark, "Trends in Fatness and the Origins of Obesity" in *Pediatrics* 57:443–56, 1976. Copyright © 1976 American Academy of Pediatrics, Evanston, IL; **Figure 18.7:** Reprinted with permission from *The New England Journal of Medicine* 314:193–98, 1986; **Figures 18.8 and 18.9:** From D. A. Booth, "Acquired Behavior Controlling Energy Intake and Output" in *Obesity*, 101–43, 1980, edited by A. J. Stunkard. Copyright © 1980 Saunders College-Harcourt Brace Jovanovich, Orlando, FL; **Figure 18.10:** From A. Keys et al., *The Biology of Human Starvation,* Vol. 1. Copyright © 1950 University of Minnesota Press, Minneapolis, MN; **Figure 18.11:** Figure constructed from data from W. P. T. James and P. Trayhurn, "Thermogenesis and Obesity" in *British Medical Bulletin* 37:43–48, 1981. Copyright © 1981 British Council, Edinburgh, Scotland; **Figure 18.12:** From J. Mayer et al., "Exercise, Food Intake, and Body Weight in Normal Rats and Genetically Obese Mice" in *American Journal of Physiology* 177:544–48, 1954. Copyright © 1954 American Physiological Society, Bethesda, MD. Used by permission; **Figure 18.13:** From J. Mayer et al., "Relation between Caloric Intake, Body Weight and Physical Work: Studies in an Industrial Male Population in West Bengal" in *American Journal of Clinical Nutrition* 4:169–75, 1956. Copyright © 1956 American Society for Clinical Nutrition, Inc., Bethesda, MD.

Chapter 19

Figure 19.1: From P. Astrand and K. Rodahl, *Textbook of Work Physiology,* 2d ed. Copyright © 1977 McGraw-Hill Book Company, New York, NY. Reprinted by permission; **Figure 19.2:** From H. Gibson and R. H. T. Edwards, "Muscular Exercise and Fatigue" in *Sports Medicine,* 2:120–32, 1985. Copyright © 1985 Adis Press, Langhorn, PA; **Figure 19.3:** From D. G. Sale, "Influence of Exercise and Training on Motor Unit Activation" in K. B. Pandolf, *Exercise and Sport Sciences Reviews* 15:95–151, 1987. Copyright © Macmillan Publishing Company, New York, NY.

Chapter 20

Figure 20.7: Figure constructed from data from P. Astrand and K. Rodahl, *Textbook of Work Physiology.* Copyright © 1986 McGraw-Hill Book Company, New York, NY. Reprinted by permission.

Chapter 21

Figure 21.1: Figure constructed from data from M. Ikai and T. Fukunaga, "Calculation of Muscle Strength per Unit of Cross Sectional Area of a Human Muscle by Means of Ultrasonic Measurements" in *Internationale Zeitschrift fuer Angewandte Physiologie* 26: 26–31, 1968. Copyright © 1968 Springer-Verlag, Heidelberg, West Germany; **Figure 21.2:** Figure constructed from data from J. Wilmore, "Alterations in Strength, Body Composition, and Anthrometric Measurements Consequent to a 10-Week Weight Training Program," in *Medicine and Science in Sports,* 6:133–139, 1974. Copyright © 1974 by American College of Sports Medicine; **Figure 21.3:** From R. Armstrong, "Mechanisms of Exercise-induced Delayed Onset of Muscular Soreness: A Brief Review" in *Medicine and Science in Sports and Exercise* 16:529–38, 1984. Copyright © 1984 American College of Sports Medicine.

Chapter 22

Figure 22.2: Figure constructed from data from C. Feicht et al., "Secondary Amenorrhea in Athletes" in *Lancet* 2:1145–46, 1978. Copyright © 1978 Lancet, Ltd., London, England. Reprinted by permission of the publisher.

Chapter 23

Figure 23.1: From J. Bergstrom et al., "Diet, Muscle Glycogen and Physical Performance" in *Acta Physiologica Scandinavica,* 71:140–150, 1967. Copyright © 1967 Scandinavian Physiological Society, Stockholm, Sweden. Used with permission; **Figure 23.2:** From W. M. Sherman, "Carbohydrates, Muscle Glycogen, and Muscle Glycogen Super Compensation" in *Erogenic Aids in Sports,* 3–26, 1983, edited by M. H. Williams. Copyright © 1983 Human Kinetics Publishers, Inc., Champaign, IL. Used with permission; **Figure 23.3:** Figure constructed from data from I. Gontzia et al., "The Influence of Adaptation of Physical Effort on Nitrogen Balance in Man" in *Nutrition Reports International* 11:231–36, 1975. Copyright © 1975 Geron-x Inc., Publishers, Los Altos, CA; **Figure 23.4:** From P. W. R. Lemon and J. P. Mullin, "Effect of Initial Muscle Glycogen Levels on Protein Catabolism during Exercise" in *Journal of Applied Physiology,* 48:624–29, 1980. Copyright © 1980 The American Physiological Society, Bethesda, MD; **Figure 23.5:** Figure constructed from data from C. T. M. Davis, et al., "Glucose Inhibits CO_2 Production from Leucine during Whole Body Exercise in Man" in *Journal of Physiology* 332:40–41, 1982. Copyright © 1982 Cambridge University Press, Cambridge, England; **Figure 23.6:** From G. Pitts et al., "Work in the Heat as Affected by Intake of Water, Salt and Glucose" in *American Journal of Physiology,* 142:353–59, 1944. Copyright © 1944 American Physiological Society, Bethesda, MD. Used by permission; **Figure 23.7:** From D. L. Costill and B. Saltin, "Factors Limiting Gastric Emptying during Rest and Exercise" in *Journal of Applied Physiology* 37:679–83, 1974. Copyright © 1974 American Physiological Society, Bethesda, MD; **Figure 23.8:** From K. Davies et al., "Muscle Mitochondrial Bioenergetics, Oxygen Supply, and Work Capacity during Dietary Iron Deficiency and Repletion" in *American Journal of Physiology* 242:E418-E427, 1982. Copyright © 1982 The American Physiological Society, Bethesda, MD; **Figure 23,10:** From J. M. Tanner et al., *The*

Physique of the Olympic Athlete. Copyright © 1964 George Allen & Unwin Publishers, Ltd., London, England.

Chapter 24

Figure 24.1: From E. T. Howley, "Effects of Altitude on Physical Performance" in G. A. Stull and T. K. Cureton, *Encyclopedia of Physical Education, Fitness, and Sports: Training, Environment, Nutrition, and Fitness.* Copyright © 1980, American Alliance for Health, Physical Education, Recreation and Dance, Reston, VA; **Figure 24.2:** From R. Grover et al., "Muscular Exercise in Young Men Native to 3,100 m Altitude" in *Journal of Applied Physiology* 22:555–64, 1967. Copyright © 1967 American Physiological Society, Bethesda, MD; **Figure 24.3:** From L. G. C. E. Pugh, "Muscular Exercise at Great Altitudes" in *Journal of Applied Physiology* 19:431–440, 1964. Copyright © 1964 American Physiological Society, Bethesda, MD; **Figure 24.4:** From J. B. West and P. D. Wagner, "Predicted Gas Exchange on the Summit of Mt. Everest" in *Respiration Physiology* 42:1–16, 1980. Copyright © 1980 Elsevier Biomedical Press, Amsterdam, The Netherlands; **Figure 24.5:** From J. B. West et al., "Barometric Pressures at Extreme Altitudes on Mt. Everest: Physiological Significance" in *Journal of Applied Physiology* 54:1188–94, 1983. Copyright © American Physiological Society, Bethesda, MD; **Figure 24.7:** From D. K. Mathews et al., "Physiological Responses during Exercise and Recovery in a Football Uniform" in *Journal of Applied Physiology* 26:611–15, 1969. Copyright © 1969 American Physiological Society, Bethesda, MD; **Figure 24.10:** From A. C. Burton and O. G. Edholm, *Man in a Cold Environment.*

Copyright © 1955 Edward Arnold Publishers, Ltd, London, England; **Figure 24.11:** From P. B. Raven et al., "Effect of Carbon Monoxide and Peroxacetyle Nitrate on Man's Maximal Aerobic Capacity" in *Journal of Applied Physiology* 36:288–93, 1974. Copyright © 1974 American Physiological Society, Bethesda, MD.

Chapter 25

Figure 25.1: Figure constructed from data from G. Ariel and W. Saville, "Anabolic Steroids: The Physiological Effects of Placebos" in *Medicine and Science in Sports* 4:124–26, 1972. Copyright © 1972 American College of Sports Medicine, Madison, WI; **Figure 25.2:** From H. W. Welch, "Effects of Hypoxia and Hyperoxia on Human Performance" in *Exercise and Sports Sciences Reviews,* Vol. 15. Copyright © 1987 Macmillan Publishing Company, New York, NY; **Figure 25.3:** From N. Gledhill, "Blood Doping and Related Issues: A Brief Review" in *Medicine and Science in Sports and Exercise,* 14:183–89, 1982. Copyright © 1982 American College of Sports Medicine, Madison, WI; **Figure 25.6:** From John D. Cantwell, "Cocaine and Cardiovascular Events" in *The Physician and Sports Medicine* 14(11):77–82, 1986. Copyright © 1986 McGraw-Hill Book Company, New York, NY.

Index

blood glucose and homeostasis, 20
control of secretion, 72
control of substrate mobilization during exercise, 91
fast-acting, 100, 102–5, 107
hypothalamus and pituitary gland, 76
mechanism of action, 73
metabolism and excretion, 72
neuroendocrinology, 71–72
pancreas, 84–86
parathyroid gland, 80
permissive and slow-acting, 97, 99–100
plasma volume, 72–73
posterior pituitary gland, 78–79
sex, 33
substrate interaction, 107, 109
thyroid gland, 79–80
Humidity, evaporation and heat loss, 255–56, 508
Hydration, heat injury, 508
Hydrogen
anaerobic ATP production, 35, 37
ions
acids, bases, and pH, 242
production during exercise, 243–44
Hyperoxia, 499
Hyperplasia, 453
Hyperpolarization, neurons, 138
Hypertension, 180
Hyperthermia, 261, 507
Hypertrophy, 453
Hypoglycemia
carbohydrates and performance, 477–78
diabetes and exercise, 346, 348
homeostasis and exercise, 71
Hypothalamic somatostatin, 77
Hypothalamus
hormone regulation and action, 76
temperature regulation, 253, 256–58
Hypothermia, 263, 510, 514
Hypothyroid, 79
Hypoxemia, 229–30
Hypoxia, 499, 502

I bands, 152, 154
Illinois Research Laboratory, 9
Immunotherapy, 349
Indirect calorimetry, 122–23
Induced erythrocythemia, 525–27
Industrial engineering, 121
Inhibitory postsynaptic potential (IPSP), 138
Inorganic compounds, 26
Inorganic phosphate (Pi), 33
Inspiration, 212
Insulation, cold and hypothermia, 511, 513–14

Insulin
blood glucose concentration, 20
control of secretion, 72
diabetes and exercise, 345–46, 464
fast-acting hormones, 103–6, 107
pancreas, 84–85
regulation
carbohydrate metabolism, 60
fat metabolism, 60–61
Integrating center, control system, 18
Intercalated discs, 176–77
Intermediate fibers, 160, 161
Interval training, 450–51
Iron, dietary, 372, 485
Irritability, neurons, 134
Isocitrate dehydrogenase, 46
Isotope dilution, 382

Jogging, 336–38, 339
Journals, exercise physiology, 10
Journal of Applied Physiology, 10
Jumping, determination of anaerobic power, 435–36

Keino, Kipchoge, 501, 504
Kennedy, John F., 7
Ketosis
insulin and acidosis, 345
low-carbohydrate diets, 396
Kidneys
acid-base balance, 246–47
metabolism and excretion of hormones, 72
renin, 81
Kilocalorie (kcal), 121
Kinases, 30–31
Kinesthetic receptors, 138–39
Krebs cycle
aerobic ATP production, 37–38, 40, 42
control, 46
Krebs, Hans, 38
Krogh, August, 4

Lactate dehydrogenase (LDH)
lactate threshold, 55–56
naming system, 31
Lactate threshold
high-intensity, continuous exercise, 451–52
metabolic response to exercise, 54–57
performance evaluation, 431–32
regulation of fat metabolism, 61
Lactic acid
acid-base balance regulation, 248
acidosis, 244
anaerobic ATP production, 37
exercise intensity, 54

slow-twitch fibers, 159, 160, 161, 162, 164, 165
spindles, 166, 168
strength
 evaluation, 438–39
 soreness, 455–56
 training, 452–55
structure, 150–52
Muscle pump, 185
Myelin, 134
Myocardial ischemia
 fitness programs and rehabilitation, 353, 354
 fitness testing and diagnosis, 312
Myocardium, 176–77
Myofibrils, 151, 152
Myoglobin
 oxygen transport in muscle, 225–26
 slow-twitch fibers, 159
Myosin
 muscular contraction, 154
 myofibril structure, 151, 152

Negative feedback
 ATP-CP system, 45
 baroreceptor system, 19–20
 control system, 18
 gain, 19
Neuroendocrinology, 71
Neuromuscular junction
 fatigue, 419
 skeletal muscle function, 152–53
Neurons
 electrical activity, 134
 peripheral nervous system, 132
 structure, 132, 134
Neurotransmitters, 137–38
Nicotinamide adenine dinucleotide (NAD)
 electron transport chain, 42, 44
 hydrogen transportation, 35, 37
 Krebs cycle, 38
Nicotine, 533, 535
Nitrogen, balance studies and protein intake, 479–80
Nobel Prize, 4
Nodes of Ranvier, 134
Noll Laboratory, 10
Norepinephrine (NE)
 adrenal medulla, 81
 endurance training, 102–3
 fast-acting hormones, 100, 102–3
 insulin and glucagon, 105
 intense exercise and concentration, 63
Normoxia, 499, 502
Nuclear Magnetic Resonance (NMR), 384
Nucleus, cell structure, 26

Nutrition
 Basic Four Food Group Plan, 378–80
 carbohydrates, 373, 376–78
 Exchange System, 380
 health objectives, 299
 menstrual cycle, 88, 91
 minerals, 368, 372–73
 osteoporosis, 355
 pregame meal, 487
 proteins, 378
 standards, 366–67
 vitamins, 368
 water, 367–68
 See also Diet; Weight control

Obesity
 body composition, 381–82, 384–88
 health and weight control, 390–91, 393–95
Olympic Games, Mexico City, 499–501
Open-circuit spirometry, 123
Organic compounds, 26
Osmolality, plasma and ADH, 78–79
Osteoporosis
 athletic amenorrhea, 91
 fitness programs and the elderly, 355
 nutrition and calcium, 372
Ovaries, 86, 87–88, 91
Overload
 principles of training, 269
 strength training, 453
Oxaloacetic acid, 61
Oxidative phosphorylation
 aerobic ATP production, 38
 efficiency, 44
Oxygen
 blood and altitude, 501–2
 enriched mixtures and aerobic performance, 523–25
 estimation of energy expenditure, 123–24
 function of lung, 207
 heat production, 122–23
 transport
  blood, 221–25
  hemoglobin, 221–22
  muscle, 225–26
 treadmill walking and running, 125
Oxygen debt, 62
Oxygen deficit
 biochemical adaptations, 277–78
 definition, 52–53
Oxyhemoglobin
 dissociation curve, 222–25
 oxygen transport and chemical bond, 221
Oxytocin, 78